34.99

369 0289662

KU-407-119

FIRST AID FOR THE ®

Medicine Clerkship

Third Edition

Alistair Mackenzie Library
Wishaw General Hospital
50 Netherton Street
Wishaw
ML2 0DP

MATTHEW S. KAUFMAN, MD

Assistant Professor
Albert Einstein College of Medicine
Department of Hematology
North Shore–Long Island Jewish Medical Center
New Hyde Park, New York

LATHA G. STEAD, MD, MS, FACEP

Chief, Division of Clinical Research
Professor of Emergency Medicine
University of Florida College of Medicine at Gainesville
Adjunct Professor of Emergency Medicine
Mayo Clinic, College of Medicine
Rochester, Minnesota
Editor-in-Chief, *International Journal of Emergency Medicine*

ARTHUR RUSOVICI, MD

Cardiology Fellow
Division of Cardiology
University of Medicine and Dentistry of New Jersey
Newark, New Jersey
Formerly Chief Medical Resident
Department of Internal Medicine
North Shore–Long Island Jewish Medical Center
New Hyde Park, New York

 Medical

New York / Chicago / San Francisco / Lisbon / London / Madrid / Mexico City
Milan / New Delhi / San Juan / Seoul / Singapore / Sydney / Toronto

ALISTAIR MACKENZIE LIBRARY
Barcode: 369028966 2
Class no: W 49 KAU

The McGraw-Hill Companies

First Aid for the® Medicine Clerkship, Third Edition

Copyright © 2010 by The McGraw-Hill Companies, Inc. All rights reserved. Printed in the United States of America. Except as permitted under the United States Copyright Act of 1976, no part of this publication may be reproduced or distributed in any form or by any means, or stored in a data base or retrieval system, without the prior written permission of the publisher.

First Aid for the® is a registered trademark of The McGraw-Hill Companies, Inc.

1 2 3 4 5 6 7 8 9 0   WDQ/WDQ   14 13 12 11 10

ISBN 978-0-07-163382-6
MHID 0-07-163382-0

NOTICE

Medicine is an ever-changing science. As new research and clinical experience broaden our knowledge, changes in treatment and drug therapy are required. The authors and the publisher of this work have checked with sources believed to be reliable in their efforts to provide information that is complete and generally in accord with the standards accepted at the time of publication. However, in view of the possibility of human error or changes in medical sciences, neither the authors nor the publisher nor any other party who has been involved in the preparation or publication of this work warrants that the information contained herein is in every respect accurate or complete, and they disclaim all responsibility for any errors or omissions or for the results obtained from use of the information contained in this work. Readers are encouraged to confirm the information contained herein with other sources. For example and in particular, readers are advised to check the product information sheet included in the package of each drug they plan to administer to be certain that the information contained in this work is accurate and that changes have not been made in the recommended dose or in the contraindications for administration. This recommendation is of particular importance in connection with new or infrequently used drugs.

This book was set in Electra LH by Rainbow Graphics.
The editors were Catherine A. Johnson and Cindy Yoo.
The production supervisor was Catherine Saggese.
Production management was provided by Rainbow Graphics.
World Color Dubuque was printer and binder.

This book is printed on acid-free paper.

Library of Congress Cataloging-in-Publication Data

Kaufman, Matthew S.
   First aid for the medicine clerkship / Matthew S. Kaufman, Latha G.
Stead, Arthur Rusovici. -- 3rd ed.
      p. ; cm.
   Other title: Medicine clerkship
   Rev. ed. of: First aid for the medicine clerkship / series editors,
Latha G. Stead, S. Matthew Stead, Matthew S. Kaufman ; supervising
editor and contributing author, Samy I. McFarlane. 2nd ed. 2005.
   Includes index.
   ISBN-13: 978-0-07-163382-6 (pbk. : alk. paper)
   ISBN-10: 0-07-163382-0 (pbk. : alk. paper) 1. Clinical clerkship.
I. Stead, Latha G. II. Rusovici, Arthur . III. Title. IV. Title:
Medicine clerkship.
   [DNLM: 1. Clinical Clerkship--Handbooks. 2. Career
Choice--Handbooks. 3. Fellowships and Scholarships--Handbooks. 4.
First Aid--Handbooks. W 49 K21f 2010]
   R839.F57 2010
   610.71'1--dc22
                                    2010011625

McGraw-Hill books are available at special quantity discounts to use as premiums and sales promotions, or for use in corporate training programs. To contact a representative please e-mail us at bulksales@mcgraw-hill.com

DEDICATION

To my mother, Madeleine, and stepfather, Costas, for their love and support. — MK

To my parents, Ganti and Prabha Rao, for giving me the peace and encouragement to excel, always. — LS

I would like to dedicate this book to my family. Mom, Dad, Tommy, and Grandma, I love you dearly and I thank you for the lessons, the care, and the support you have all given me. — AR

CONTENTS

Alistair Mackenzie Library
Wishaw General Hospital
50 Netherton Street
Wishaw
ML2 0DP

M12 0DE

PREFACE

In the 2010 edition of *First Aid for the® Medicine Clerkship*, a complete and thorough revision has been done to make the book an even more effective tool to ace both the clerkship and the shelf exam. These changes have been made carefully according to valuable feedback from extensive student and faculty reviews.

In addition to stylistic updates, the following changes have been made:

- An overhaul of topic organization with additions to some and reductions of others to emphasize the most relevant information.
- Update of information according to newer guidelines and data.
- The addition of minicases which provide classic exam scenarios.
- Additional exam tips to point out the favorite tested facts.

We are grateful to all of the student and faculty contributors who made this edition the best yet and we welcome additional feedback for the continued improvement of *First Aid for the® Medicine Clerkship*. (See How to Contribute, p. ix.)

New Hyde Park, New York	Matthew Kaufman
Rochester, New York	Latha Stead

HOW TO CONTRIBUTE

We are grateful for and welcome any updates, corrections, and study hints. Contributors will receive compensation and credit at the discretion of the authors. Also let us know about material in this edition that you feel is low yield and should be deleted.

The preferred way to submit entries, suggestions, or corrections is via e-mail:

Mattkaufman1@gmail.com; Latha.Stead@gmail.com;
firstaidclerkships@gmail.com; Catherine_Johnson@mcgraw-hill.com.

NOTE TO CONTRIBUTORS

All contributions become property of the authors and are subject to editing and reviewing. Please verify all data and spellings carefully. In the event that similar or duplicate entries are received, only the first entry received will be used. Include a reference to a standard textbook to facilitate verification of the fact. Please follow the style, punctuation, and format of this edition if possible.

CONTRIBUTORS

Jian Li Campian, MD, PhD

Resident
North Shore–LIJ Health System
Long Island Jewish Medical Center
New Hyde Park, New York
Endocrinology

Bella Fradlis, MD

Medical Student
Department of Medicine
Columbia University Medical Center
New York–Presbyterian Hospital
New York, New York
Dermatology

Abhishek Jaiswal, MBBS

Resident, Department of Internal Medicine
Long Island Jewish Medical Center
New Hyde Park, New York
Gastroenterology
Health Maintenance and Evidence Based Medicine

Tim Johnson, MD

Internal Medicine
Emergency Medicine
Critical Care
Long Island Jewish Medical Center
New Hyde Park, New York
Neurology

Pralay K. Sarkar, MD, MRCP(UK)

Attending Physician
Hospitalist Division, Department of Internal Medicine
Long Island Jewish Medical
New Hyde Park, New York
Pulmonary Diseases

Peter Bryan Schrier, MD

Resident
Internal Medicine
Long Island Jewish Medical Center
New Hyde Park, New York
Nephrology and Acid-Base Disorders

Bilal K. Siddiqui, MD

Resident
Long Island Jewish Medical Center
New Hyde Park, New York
Hematology-Oncology

Avneet Singh, MD, MRCP(UK)

Resident
Internal Medicine Residency Program
Long Island Jewish Medical Center
New Hyde Park, New York
Cardiology
Rheumatology

Joshua N. Vernatter, MD

Resident
Long Island Jewish Medical Center
New Hyde Park, New York
Infectious Disease

FACULTY EDITOR

Samy I. McFarlane, MD, MPH, MBA, FACP

Professor of Medicine
Division of Endocrinology
Medical Director of Clinical Research
College of Medicine
State University of New York–Dowstate Medical Center
Kings County Hospital
Brooklyn, New York

STUDENT REVIEWERS

Jean C. Ancelet

Medical Student
LSUHSC New Orleans School of Medicine

Mary M. Bonar

Medical Student
Ohio University College of Osteopathic Medicine

Kenneth Marc Fomberstein

Class of 2010
Albert Einstein College of Medicine

Dmitriy Kedrin

Medical Student
Albert Einstein College of Medicine

Eileen Kisilis

Medical Student
Albert Einstein College of Medicine

Vibhuti Kowluru

Medical Student
Albert Einstein College of Medicine

Christy Nolan

Medical Student
Lake Erie College of Medicine

Brian Park

Medical Student
Albert Einstein College of Medicine

Sharon Rose

Medical Student
Albert Einstein College of Medicine

Matthew Saybolt

Medical Student
UMDNJ Robert Wood Johnson Medical School

David Scoville

Medical Student
Kansas University Medical Center

How to Succeed in the Medicine Clerkship

Be on Time

Most medical ward teams begin rounding between 7 and 8 AM. If you are expected to "pre-round," you should give yourself at least 10 minutes per patient that you are following to see the patient and learn about the events that occurred overnight. Like all working professionals, you will face occasional obstacles to punctuality, but make sure this is occasional. When you first start a rotation, try to show up at least 15 minutes early until you get the routine figured out. If the morning vitals are not yet recorded, take them yourself. Also, look at the chart to update yourself on any developments.

Dress in a Professional Manner

Even if the resident wears scrubs and the attending wears stiletto heels, you must dress in a professional, conservative manner. Wear a *short* white coat over your clothes unless discouraged (as in pediatrics).

- **Men** should wear long pants, with cuffs covering the ankle, a long collared shirt, and a tie. No jeans, no sneakers, no short-sleeved shirts.
- **Women** should wear long pants or knee-length skirt and a blouse or dressy sweater. No jeans, no sneakers, no heels greater than 1½ inches, no open-toed shoes.
- **Both men and women** may wear scrubs occasionally, during overnight call or in the operating room. Do not make this your uniform.

Act in a Pleasant Manner

The medical rotation is often difficult, stressful, and tiring. Smooth out your experience by being nice to be around. Smile a lot and learn everyone's name. Don't be afraid to ask how your resident's weekend was. If you do not understand or disagree with a treatment plan or diagnosis, do not "challenge." Instead, say, "I'm sorry, I don't quite understand, could you please explain. . ." Show kindness and compassion toward your patients. Never participate in callous talk about patients.

Be Aware of the Hierarchy

The way in which this will affect you will vary from hospital to hospital and team to team, but it is always present to some degree. In general, address your questions regarding ward functioning to interns or residents. Address your medical questions to attendings; make an effort to be somewhat informed on your subject prior to asking attendings medical questions. It's always good to make your residents look good on rounds (. . . "Dr. Smith was nice enough to teach me about . . ."). Make sure the resident knows new patient developments ASAP.

Address Patients and Staff in a Respectful Way

Address patients as Sir, Ma'am, or Mr., Mrs., or Miss. Try not to address patients as "honey," "sweetie," and the like. Although you may feel these names are friendly, patients will think you have forgotten their name, that you are being inappropriately familiar, or both. Address all physicians as "doctor," unless told otherwise.

Show Initiative

Often, residents are busy with work and neglect their teaching responsibilities. Read up on your patient's condition, find an article, and offer to summarize in a few minutes what you learned. Give a copy of the article to your resident. This kind of initiative goes a long way in evaluations.

Take Responsibility for Your Patients

Know everything there is to know about your patients: their history, test results, details about their medical problem, and prognosis. Keep your intern or resident informed of new developments that they might not be aware of, and ask them for any updates you might not be aware of. Assist the team in developing a plan; speak to radiology, consultants, and family. Never give bad news to patients or family members without the assistance of your supervising resident or attending.

Respect Patients' Rights

1. All patients have the right to have their personal medical information kept private. This means do not discuss the patient's information with family members without that patient's consent, and do not discuss any patient in hallways, elevators, or cafeterias.
2. All patients have the right to refuse treatment. This means they can refuse treatment by a specific individual (you, the medical student) or of a specific type (no nasogastric tube). Patients can even refuse lifesaving treatment. The only exceptions to this rule are if the patient is deemed to not have the capacity to make decisions or understand situations, in which case a health care proxy should be sought, or if the patient is suicidal or homicidal.
3. All patients should be informed of the right to seek advance directives on admission. Often, this is done by the admissions staff, in a booklet. If your patient is chronically ill or has a life-threatening illness, address the subject of advance directives with the assistance of your attending.

Volunteer

Be self-propelled, self-motivated. Volunteer to help with a procedure or a difficult task. Volunteer to give a 20-minute talk on a topic of your choice. Volunteer to take additional patients. Volunteer to stay late. If the answer is "You don't have to," do it anyway.

Be a Team Player

Help other medical students with their tasks; teach them information you have learned. Support your supervising intern or resident whenever possible. Never steal the spotlight, steal a procedure, or make a fellow medical student look bad. Making other people look good always helps you, too.

Be Honest

If you don't understand, don't know, or didn't do it, make sure you always say that. Never say or document information that is false (a common example: "bowel sounds normal" when you did not listen). This can get you into serious trouble.

Keep Patient Information Handy

Use a clipboard, notebook, or index cards to keep patient information, including a miniature history and physical, and lab and test results, at hand. The first day of the rotation, learn the computer system so that you can get lab and test results on your own. Know all of these results *before* your resident does; don't ask him or her what a test showed, tell them!

Present Patient Information in an Organized Manner

Here is a template for the "bullet" presentation:

> "This is a [age]-year-old [gender] with a history of [major history such as HTN, DM, coronary artery disease, CA, etc.] who presented on [date] with [major symptoms, such as cough, fever, and chills] and was found to have [working diagnosis]. [Tests done] showed [results]. Yesterday, the patient [state important changes, new plan, new tests, new medications]. This morning the patient feels [state the patient's words], and the physical exam is significant for [state major findings]. Plan is [state plan].

The newly admitted patient generally deserves a longer presentation following the complete history and physical format.

Some patients have extensive histories. The whole history should be present in the admission note, but in ward presentation, it is often too much to absorb. In these cases, it will be very much appreciated by your team if you can generate a **good summary** that maintains an accurate picture of the patient. This usually takes some thought, but it's worth it.

Document Information in an Organized Manner

A complete medical student initial History and Physical is neat, legible, organized, and usually two to three pages long. Major topics should include: chief complaint, history of present illness, medical history, surgical history, medications, allergies, sexual history, smoking and alcohol history, occupation, travel, review of systems, vital signs, physical exam, lab results, test results, assessment or problem list, and plan.

HOW TO ORGANIZE YOUR LEARNING

The main advantage to doing the medical clerkship is that you get to see patients. The patient is the key to learning medicine, and the source of most satisfaction and frustration on the wards. Plan your learning before the rotation starts as follows.

Make a List of Core Material to Learn

This list should reflect common symptoms, illnesses, and areas in which you have particular interest, or in which you feel particularly weak. Do not try to learn every possible topic. The Committee of Directors in Internal Medicine (*www.im.org/cdim/*) publishes a list of core content, on which this book is based. The CDIM emphasizes:

Symptoms and Lab Tests
- Abdominal pain
- Altered mental status
- Anemia
- Back pain
- Chest pain
- Cough
- Dysuria
- Fluid, electrolyte, and acid-base disorders

Common Illnesses
- Chronic obstructive pulmonary disease (COPD)
- Congestive heart failure
- Depression
- Diabetes mellitus
- Dyslipidemia
- Human immunodeficiency virus (HIV) infection
- Hypertension
- Smoking cessation
- Substance abuse
- Common cancers

We Also Recommend
- Adult vaccinations
- Domestic violence
- Dysrhythmias
- Nutritional disorders

Select Your Study Material

We recommend:

- This review book, *First Aid for the Clinical Clerkship in Medicine*
- A major medicine textbook such as *Harrison's Principles of Internal Medicine* (costs about $135)
- A full-text online journal database, such as www.mdconsult.com (subscription is $99/year for students)
- A small pocket reference book to look up lab values, clinical pathways, and the like, such as *Maxwell Quick Medical Reference* (costs $7)
- A small book to look up drugs, such as *Pocket Pharmacopoeia* (Tarascon Publishers, $9.95)

Make a Schedule to Learn the Illness-Based Topics

This schedule should reflect the rotation you are doing. For example, for the time you are going to be rotating in a clinic or office, make a schedule to study smoking cessation, dyslipidemia, depression, and diabetes. First, read this review book on each topic, then read the major textbook, taking notes. Make sure to include all chosen topics in your schedule, but leave room at least 2 weeks before the clerkship exam for review.

As You See Patients, Note Their Major Symptoms and Diagnosis for Review

Your reading on the symptom-based topics above should be done with a specific patient in mind. For example, if a patient comes to the office with cough, fever, and night sweats and is thought to have tuberculosis, read about chronic and acute cough, postnasal drip, asthma, gastroesophageal reflux disease (GERD), pneumonia, and tuberculosis in this review book that night.

Prepare a Talk on a Topic

You may be asked to give a small talk once or twice during your rotation. If not, you should volunteer! Feel free to choose a topic that is on your list; however, realize that this may be considered dull by the people who hear the lecture. The ideal topic is slightly uncommon but not rare, for example, cardiomyopathy. To prepare a talk on a topic, read about it in a major textbook and a review article not more than 2 years old, and then search online or in the library for recent developments or changes in treatment.

HOW TO PREPARE FOR THE CLINICAL CLERKSHIP EXAM

If you have read about your core illnesses and core symptoms, you will know a great deal about medicine. To study for the clerkship exam, we recommend:

2–3 weeks before exam: Read this entire review book, taking notes.
10 days before exam: Read the notes you took during the rotation on your core content list and the corresponding review book sections.
5 days before exam: Read this entire review book, concentrating on lists and mnemonics.
2 days before exam: Exercise, eat well, skim the book, and go to bed early.
1 day before exam: Exercise, eat well, review your notes and the mnemonics, and go to bed on time. Do not have any caffeine after 2 PM.

Other helpful studying strategies include:

Study with Friends

Group studying can be very helpful. Other people may point out areas that you have not studied enough and may help you focus on the goal. If you tend to get distracted by other people in the room, limit this to less than half of your study time.

Study in a Bright Room

Find the room in your house or in your library that has the best, brightest light. This will help prevent you from falling asleep. If you don't have a bright light, get a halogen desk lamp or a light that simulates sunlight (not a tanning lamp).

Eat Light, Balanced Meals

Make sure your meals are balanced, with lean protein, fruits and vegetables, and fiber. A high-sugar, high-carbohydrate meal will give you an initial burst of energy for 1–2 hours, but then you'll drop.

Take Practice Exams

The point of practice exams is not so much the content that is contained in the questions, but the training of sitting still for 3 hours and trying to pick the best answer for each and every question.

Tips for Answering Questions

All questions are intended to have one best answer. When answering questions, follow these guidelines:

Read the answers first. For all questions longer than two sentences, reading the answers first can help you sift through the question for the key information.

Look for the words "EXCEPT, MOST, LEAST, NOT, BEST, WORST, TRUE, FALSE, CORRECT, INCORRECT, ALWAYS, and NEVER." If you find one of these words, circle or underline it for later comparison with the answer.

Evaluate each answer as being either true or false. Example:

Which of the following is *least* likely to be associated with pulmonary embolism?
   A.   Tachycardia **T**
   B.   Tachypnea **T**
   C.   Chest pain? **F not always**
   D.   Deep venous thrombosis? **T not always**
   E.   Back pain? **F aortic dissection**

By comparing the question, noting LEAST, to the answers, "E" is the best answer.

As the Boy Scouts say, "BE PREPARED."

POCKET CARDS FOR THE WARDS

The "cards" on the following page contain information that is often helpful in family practice. We advise that you make a copy of these cards, cut them out, and carry them in your coat pocket.

History

CC: complaint (pt's words)
HPI: - age, race, sex
       - chronological description of illness, include relevant PMH
       - include dates, times, sx, prior occurrences & treatment
       - sx description: location, duration, frequency, timing, quality, radiation, aggravating or relieving factors, & associated sx

PMH: illnesses not mentioned in HPI
PSH: surgeries not mentioned in HPI
OBH: ob/gyn Hx in women (if not in HPI)
Psy: psychiatric Hx, if present
All: drugs (foods, insects, pollen, etc.), transfusion rxns, describe rxn
Med: current medications, home remedies, vitamins
FH: ages, health, causes of death, HTN, HD, DM, CA, arthritis, hereditary diseases, Sx similar to pt's
SH: occupations (past & present), home situation, lifestyle, sexual practices, religion
Trv: country of origin, travel history
Tox: - toxic habits (tobacco, alcohol, illicit drugs)
       - CAGE: Cut down/Annoyed/Guilty/Eye-opener
ROS: Gen: fever, weight change, appetite, sleep, night sweats
       Skin: rash, itch, growths, color change, hair loss/growth
       Head: headaches, trauma
       Eyes: acuity, spots, flashes, diplopia, pain
       Ears: acuity, tinnitus, vertigo, infection, discharge
       Nose: bleed, sinusitis, congestion, rhinorrhea, acuity
       Mouth: lesions, sore throat, teeth/gums, bruxism, TMJ
       Neck: pain, stiffness, swollen glands
       Lung: cough, wheeze, sputum (color), SOB, pleuritic pain, emphysema, bronchitis, TB, last CXR
       Heart: CP, palpitations, HTN, edema, orthopnea, murmurs
       GI: pain, N/V, diarrhea/constipation, bleeding, abd girth
       GU: pain, dysuria/frequency/urgency, nocturia, discharge, masses, STDs, sexual dysfunction/libido
       Gyn: menarche/menopause, hot flashes, contraception LMP, meno/metrorrhagia, dyspareunia
       Breast: pain, lumps, discharge, self-exam
       Musc: cramps, bone pain, joint pain/swelling, arthritis, gout
       Vasc: varicose, DVTs, claudication/rest pain, Raynaud's
       Endo: heat/cold intolerance, polydipsia/uria, polyphagia
       Heme: anemia, excess bleeding, easy bruising
       Neuro: seizures, syncope, weakness/paralysis, paresthesias, tics, tremors, memory deficits, blackouts
       Psych: anxiety/tension, depression/suicide, insomnia, concentration, mood swings, paranoia, voices

Physical

VS: T, HR, RR, BP (upright vs recumbent, R arm vs leg), O_2 sat pain
Gen: appearance, distress/anxiety, obese/wasted, apparent age
Skin: texture, color, turgor, temp, lesions, rashes, scars, hair texture/distribution, cyanosis, edema
Hands: deformities, arthritic nodes, nail pitting/stippling, capillary refill, clubbing
LN: axillary, cervical, postauricular, supraclavicular, inguinal (mobility, size, texture)
H/N: size, symmetry, trauma (palpate), neck ROM, thyroid, carotid pulses/bruits, JVD
Eyes: pupils, EOMs, alignment, acuity, visual fields, conjunctiva/sclera, fundi, nystagmus, strabismus
Ears: location/symmetry, auditory acuity, TMs, discharge
Nose: discharge, congestion, frontal/maxillary sinus tenderness
Mouth: pharynx (erythema, exudate), uvula, tonsils, palate, gums, lips, tongue
Back: alignment, spinal/CV tenderness, ROM
Chest: symmetry, retractions, air entry, breath sounds, percussion
CVS: PMI, thrills, heart sounds, murmurs, rhythm, peripheral pulses
Murm: grade (I - VI), timing (midsystolic, diastolic, etc), quality (rumbling, click, vibratory, etc.) location (e.g. lower left sternal border), radiation (axilla, neck, back, etc.), accentuating maneuvers (squatting, Valsalva, etc.)
Breast: symmetry, dimples, masses, pain, nipple shape/discharge
Abd: bowel sounds/bruits, distention, tenderness, rebound, guarding, rigidity, liver borders (palpation, percussion, scratch test), hepatojugular reflux, Murphy's, spleen, masses, aorta (AAA), percussion (tympany), shifting dullness/fluid wave
Rectal: sphincter tone, prostate, mass, hemorrhoid/fissure/abscess, guaiac
♂ GU: lesions, meatal discharge, pain, scrotal veins/mass/swelling, (transilluminate) inguinal/femoral masses (reducible)
♀ GU: lesions, discharges, odors, swelling, pelvic if indicated
Neuro: strength (0-5), tone, DTRs (0-4+, 2+ N), Babinski, FTN/HTS, rapidly alternating movements, gait, sensory (light touch, pin prick, vibration, joint position), Romberg, mini MS if indicated
CN: I - smell, II/III/IV/VI - EOMs/visual fields/pupils/acuity, V - bite (masseter, temporalis)/facial sensation, VII - facial expression, VIII - hearing, IX/X - gag/swallow/uvula midline, XI - turn head/shrug shoulders, XII - stick out tongue

Laboratory Values

	♂ 13.5-18.0 Hb ♀ 12.5-16.0	
WBC 4.0-10.5	♂ 42-52 Hct ♀ 37-47	Plt 150-450

57-67N / 23-33L / 3-7M / 1-3E / 0-1B
neutrophils: 54-62 segs, ≤5 bands
absolute 1.5-6.6

Na^+ 135-145	Cl^- 98-106	BUN 7-18	Glu 70-115
K^+ 3.5-5.1	HCO_3^- 22-29	Cr 0.6-1.2	

Ca^{2+} total 8.4-10.2, ionized 4.6-5.3
Mg^{2+} 1.3-2.1
PO_4^{2-} ♂ 2.3-3.7, ♀ 2.8-4.1, >60y 2.7-4.5

Fe	♂ 65-175, ♀ 50-170
TIBC	250-450
Fe sat	♂ 20-50, ♀ 15-50
Ferritin	♂ 20-250, ♀ 10-120

ABG:
pH	$PaCO_2$	PaO_2	HCO_3^-	O_2 Sat	B.E.
7.35-7.45	35-45	80-100	20-28	>95	±2

VBG:
pH	$PvCO_2$	PvO_2	HCO_3^-	O_2 Sat	B.E.
7.32-7.42	45-50	37-43	22-30	60-80	±2

Urinalysis:
Color	yellow
Clarity	clear
Spec. grav.	1.001-1.035
pH	4.6-8.0

Negative: Bilirubin, Ketones, Blood, Glucose, Protein, Nitrites, Leukocyte esterase

CSF:
Opening pressure:	70-180
WBC	5-10
RBC	0
Protein	15-45
Glucose	45-80

Cardiac enzymes:
CK	♂ 38-174, ♀ 26-140
CK-MB	<5
Troponin I	I <0.6, T <0.1
Myoglobin	serum <90, urine <2

RBC	♂ 4.7-6.0, ♀ 4.2-5.4
Retic	0.5-1.5
MCV	78-100
MCH	27-31
MCHC	31-37
RDW	11.5-14.0

Haptoglobin	40-270
Bilirubin	total <1.0, direct <0.6
AST (SGOT)	♂ 15-45, ♀ 5-30
ALT (SGPT)	♂ 10-40, ♀ 5-35
LD	50-150

PT	11-15
aPTT	20-35
Bleeding Time	2-7
Thrombin Time	6.3-11.1
FDP	<10
D-dimers	<200

GGT	♂ 9-50, ♀ 8-40
CPK	♂ 38-174, ♀ 26-140
ESR	♂ <15, ♀ <20
CRP	<0.8

Alk Phos	♂ 38-126, ♀ 70-230
Protein	total 6.0-8.0
	albumin 3.5-5.5

Amylase	25-125
Lipase	10-140, >60y 18-180
C peptide	0.7-1.9
HbA_{1c}	4.0-6.7

Tot Chol	<200
LDL	<130
HDL	♂ >29, ♀ >35
Trig	♂ 40-160, ♀ 35-135

TFTs:
T4	5.0-12.0
FreeT4	0.8-2.3
T3	100-200
TBG	15-34
TSH	<10

Serum drug levels:
	peak	trough
Gentamicin	5-10	<2
Tobramycin	5-10	<2
Amikacin	15-25	<5
Vancomycin	30-40	5-10

	therapeutic	toxic
Lidocaine	1.5-5.0	>7
Theophylline	10-20	>20
Digoxin	0.1-2.0	>2.4
Phenobarbital	15-40	>50
Phenytoin	10-20	>20
Carbamazepine	8-12	>15
Valproic acid	50-100	>200

Formulae

Anion Gap:
$$(Na^+) - (HCO_3^- + Cl^-)$$

Osmolality:
$$(2 \times Na^+) + (Glu / 18) + (BUN / 2.8)$$

Creatinine Clearance:
$$\frac{(\text{urine Cr}) \times (\text{urine volume [mL]})}{(\text{serum Cr}) \times (\text{time [min]})}$$
$$\frac{(140 - \text{age}) \times (\text{weight [Kg]}) \times (0.85 \text{ for } ♀)}{72 \times (\text{serum Cr})}$$

Fractional Excretion of Sodium:
$$\frac{(\text{urine Na}^+) \times (\text{serum Cr})}{(\text{serum Na}^+) \times (\text{urine Cr})}$$
$$\frac{\left(\frac{\text{urine Na}^+}{\text{serum Na}^+}\right)}{\left(\frac{\text{urine Cr}}{\text{serum Cr}}\right)}$$

Maintenance Fluids:
100 mL/d/kg for 1st 10 kg plus
50 mL/d/kg for 2nd 10 kg plus
20 mL/d/kg for remaining weight

4 mL/hr/kg for 1st 10 kg plus
2 mL/hr/kg for 2nd 10 kg plus
1 mL/hr/kg for remaining weight

Body Water Deficit [Liters]:
$$\frac{0.6 \times (\text{weight [kg]}) \times (Na^+ - 140)}{140}$$

Unit Conversions:
1 in = 2.54 cm	1 cm = 0.394 in
1 ft = 0.305 m	1 m = 3.28 ft
1 mi = 1.61 km	1 km = 0.621 mi
1 ft ≈ 30 cm	

1 fl oz = 29.6 mL	1 mL = 0.0338 fl oz
1 qt = 0.946 L	1 L = 1.06 qt
1 gal = 3.79 L	1 L = 0.264 gal
1 tsp = 5 mL	1 tbs = 15 mL
	1 cc = 1 mL

1 oz = 28.4 g	1 g = 0.0353 oz
1 lb = 0.454 kg	1 kg = 2.20 lb
70 kg = 154 lb	

$$°F = (1.8 \times °C) + 32 \qquad °C = \frac{(°F - 32)}{1.8}$$

Aa Gradient:
$$\frac{(713 \times FIO_2) - PaCO_2}{0.8} - PaO_2$$

ABG Rule:
$$\Delta 10\ PaCO_2 = \Delta 0.08\ pH$$

Corrected Total Ca^{2+}:
$$Ca^{2+} + 3.6 - (0.8 \times \text{albumin})$$

Corrected Na^+:
$$Na^+ + \left(\frac{Glu}{62.5}\right) - 1.6$$

Regular Insulin Sliding Scale (RISS):
$$\left(\frac{Glu}{25}\right) - 6\ \text{units, for } 200 \le Glu \le 450$$

Mean Arterial Pressure (MAP):
$$\frac{\text{systolic} + 2(\text{diastolic})}{3}$$

Body Surface Area:
$$\frac{\sqrt{\text{height [cm]} \times \text{weight [kg]}}}{60}$$

Body Mass Index:
$$\frac{\text{weight [kg]}}{(\text{height [m]})^2}$$

Normal Weights (lbs) for ♂ and ♀:
Height	Age 19-34	Age ≤ 35
5'0"	97-128	108-138
5'1"	101-132	111-143
5'2"	104-137	115-148
5'3"	107-141	119-152
5'4"	111-146	122-157
5'5"	114-150	126-162
5'6"	118-156	130-167
5'7"	121-160	134-172
5'8"	125-164	138-178
5'9"	129-169	142-183
5'10"	132-174	146-188
5'11"	136-179	151-194
6'0"	140-184	155-199
6'1"	144-189	159-205
6'2"	148-195	164-210

First Aid for the® Medicine Clerkship, 3/E; copyright © 2010 McGraw-Hill. All rights reserved.

SECTION II

High-Yield Facts in Internal Medicine

Cardiology

- **Myocardial infarction (MI)/angina:** Chest heaviness, pressure, or pain, typically radiating to left arm, shoulder, or jaw. *Diaphoresis is a key symptom also*. Shortness of breath is another. Often described as "An elephant sitting on my chest."
- **Pericarditis:** Chest pain radiating to shoulder, neck, or back, worse with deep breathing or cough (pleuritic), relieved by sitting up and leaning forward.
- **Aortic dissection:** Severe chest pain radiating to the back, can be associated with unequal pulses or unequal blood pressure in right and left arms.
- **Thoracic abscess or mass:** Often sharp, localized pain, can be pleuritic.
- **Pulmonary embolism:** Often pleuritic. Frequently associated with tachypnea and tachycardia.
- **Pneumonia:** Pleuritic, frequently associated with cough, sputum, and hypoxia if severe.
- **GERD/esophageal spasm/tear:** Burning pain, midline, substernal, may be associated with dysphagia. Pain made worse with lying flat, certain foods, also bitter taste in mouth known as "water brash." May be similar to pain of MI.
- **Costochondritis/musculoskeletal:** Sharp, localized pain with *reproducible tenderness* (touch chest wall and feel the pain); often exacerbated by exercise (second or third costochondral junction inflammation, aka Tietze's syndrome).
- **Other causes:** Peptic ulcer disease, biliary disease, herpes zoster, anxiety, pneumothorax, pleuritis (infection, systemic lupus erythematosus [SLE]), pulmonary embolus.

Myocardial infarction can be *silent*, with no symptoms or atypical symptoms in diabetics (due to neuropathy) or heart transplant (denervated heart).

Criteria for **family history** of coronary artery disease:
MI before age 40 in men
MI before age 55 in women

Modifiable
- Smoking
- Hypercholesterolemia
- Hypertension
- Obesity (central)
- Diabetes mellitus
- Physical inactivity
- Metabolic syndrome

Nonmodifiable
- Age
- Male sex/ postmenopausal female
- Family history

A 55 year-old male with HTN complains of claudication. Further questioning reveals increasing shortness of breath with exertion. Coronary artery disease should be suspected and stress testing should be performed.

Stress Tests

A stress test is a noninvasive test to assess for possible coronary artery disease (CAD) or risk of MI. There are different types.

- Indications for stress test:
  - Symptoms consistent with angina (to rule out, or in CAD).
  - Post MI (to evaluate risk of having another; poor exercise tolerance correlates with higher mortality).

The *normal* maximum heart rate is estimated as: [220 – patient's age].

- **Exercise stress test:** Patients are asked to walk on a treadmill at ↑ levels of difficulty to reach a heart rate that is 85% of predicted maximum for age. Patients should not be taking meds that prevent heart rate from rising (beta blockers or digoxin).
- **Pharmacologic stress test: Agents** such as dobutamine may be administered IV to stimulate myocardial function (and cause cardiac exertion) in a patient who cannot exercise.
- Electrocardiographic (ECG) monitoring during the procedure detects changes.
- A test is considered positive for CAD if the patient develops:
  - ECG changes (ST elevation or depression).
  - ↓ blood pressure.
  - Failure to exercise more than 2 minutes due to cardiac symptoms.

Stress Myocardial Perfusion Imaging

This is similar to other stress tests except imaging allows the visualization of the amount of blood perfusion in the myocardium. "Defects" indicate that the blood is not getting to a part of the myocardial tissue (fixed defects = infarct, reversible = inducible ischemia). Thallium or technetium is typically used.

Echocardiography

- Echocardiography, or ultrasound of the heart, provides a picture of the heart and can evaluate its function. It is used to evaluate many different types of heart disease, from valvular defects to the strength of the heart muscle (described as ejection fraction). It can demonstrate a myocardial infarction (either acute or old) by showing a defect in movement of one of the walls (called "wall motion abnormality").
- In transthoracic echocardiography (TTE) the probe is placed on the chest wall. Transesophageal echo requires the probe to be placed into the esophagus (TEE); it is used for more precise imaging of valves and aorta.
- For specific uses of echocardiography, see Table 2.1-1.

Cardiac Catheterization

- Cardiac catheterization is used for diagnosis and treatment of many different types of heart disease. In left heart catheterization, a wire is inserted through a vessel (usually the radial or femoral artery) and threaded up to the coronary vessels. Dye is injected into the coronary vessels (angiogram), and stenosis (narrowing) or blockage can be visualized. The dye also allows visualization of heart function. These are *diagnostic*. Cardiac catheterizations can include therapeutic *intervention*, such as angioplasty or stenting (see below). A right heart catheterization is the same as above but through a vein.
- For other uses of cardiac catheterization, see Table 2.1-2.

TABLE 2.1-1.   Uses of Echocardiography

DISORDER	USE OF ECHO
Myocardial infarction	Assess wall motion abnormalities, or new valve abnormalities induced by the MI.
Heart failure	Assess ventricular function, ejection fraction.
Heart murmur	Identify and evaluate valvular disease.
Pericardial effusion	Assess volume of effusion and tamponade.
Aortic dissection	Identify presence of tear (especially TEE).
Pulmonary embolism	Identify saddle emboli or evidence of ↑ right-sided heart pressure caused by the PE.
Patent foramen ovale	Assess bubbles traversing PFO (air administered through peripheral IV).
Endocarditis	Identify vegetation, abscess (sensitivity TEE > TTE).
Congenital heart disease	Identify coarctation of the aorta, pulmonary stenosis, tetralogy of Fallot, ventricular septal defect (VSD), atrial septal defect (ASD).

TABLE 2.1-2.   Uses of Cardiac Catheterization

DISORDER	THERAPY
Myocardial infarction and unstable angina	Coronary artery angiography (visualize the blockage); also can intervene with balloon dilatation of stenoses, stent placement (percutaneous transluminal coronary angioplasty [PTCA]), or laser techniques.
Valvular heart disease	"Balloon valvuloplasty": Dilatation of valves with a balloon. This can be used for mitral stenosis, pulmonary stenosis, aortic stenosis.
Dysrhythmias	When a patient has an arrhythmia, the cause can be located and removed. This is called "electrophysiologic mapping" and radiofrequency ablation.
Myocardial disease	Biopsy of myocardium for cardiomyopathies.
Congenital heart disease	Can diagnose valvular disorder and correct in some cases (ASDs, VSDs, PFOs).
Pericardial disease	Simultaneous left and right heart catheterization will measure heart pressures and diagnose a pericardial abnormality such as restriction.

CARDIOLOGY

Typically left-sided chest pain caused by temporary myocardial ischemia.

- **Stable angina:** A chronic, episodic, predictable, pain syndrome due to temporary myocardial ischemia. Pattern of pain is similar to that of acute MI, but resolves with rest or medication. Doesn't change (ie, it's stable). **Treatment:** Beta blocker (reduces myocardial oxygen demand); aspirin; nitroglycerin.
- **Unstable angina** (further discussed in next section; a type of acute coronary syndrome). Defined as (1) new onset of anginal pain, (2) anginal pain that accelerates or changes in pattern location or severity, (3) anginal pain at rest. **Treatment:** See Acute Coronary Syndromes section.
- **Prinzmetal's angina (variant angina):** Angina due to coronary vasospasm, not linked to exertion. Distinguished from unstable angina by chronic, intermittent nature. Pain usually occurs at a specific hour in the early morning. Coronary vessels are normal (no stenosis or plaques). ECG may show transient ST elevations. **Treatment:** Calcium channel blockers and nitrates to reduce vasospasm.

 A 62-year-old smoker presents complaining of three episodes of severe chest heaviness this morning. Each episode lasted 3–5 minutes, but he has no pain now. He has never had this type of pain before. *Think: Unstable angina.*

A middle-aged woman comes to the ER with severe chest pain and ST elevations on ECG. She is rushed for a cardiac catherization, which shows no obstruction in her coronary arteries. What is it? *Variant angina (aka Prinzmetal's angina/vasospasm).*

A 62-year-old man presents with frequent episodes of dull chest pain on and off for 8 months. He says the pain wakes him from sleep. *Think: Prinzmetal's angina.*

ACUTE CORONARY SYNDROMES (ACS)

- Acute coronary syndromes (ACS) refers to unstable angina (chest pain in which an MI can happen at any second) or an actual MI. On a physiologic level, this is due to an imbalance of myocardial oxygen supply and demand. The most common cause of ↓ oxygen supply is narrowing of coronary artery by thrombus or plaque that has become unstable.
- **Ischemia** is reversible insult to the tissue by oxygen deprivation.

- **Infarction** is when the damage is permanent (as in MI). When there is tissue damage (infarction), there is enzyme leakage (eg, creatinine phosphokinase [CPK] and troponin see below).
- **ACS events are classified according to the changes on ECG:** (1) **non-ST-elevation** (includes non-ST elevation myocardial infarction or unstable angina) or (2) **ST-elevation** (includes ST-elevation MI [STIMI]).

Serum Markers for MI

- Myoglobin: Elevated within 1 hour of MI; peak 6 hours; nonspecific.
- Creatinine phosphokinase (CPK): Elevated within 4–8 hours; peak 18–24 hours of MI; total is nonspecific but CK MB is specific. CK MB isoenzyme is the subgroup of CPK specific for myocardial tissue damage. The extent of elevation correlates with the amount of cardiac damage.
- Troponin T or I: Very sensitive and specific markers for cardiac muscle injury. Elevated within 3 hours and can stay elevated for more than a week. Renal insufficiency can → high levels that can be mistaken for cardiac damage. Troponin may also be slightly chronically elevated in CHF.
- "Serial enzymes": Consists of cardiac biomarkers followed every 6–8 hours for a 24-hour period. This is standard practice for patients presenting to the hospital for chest pain and when you want to rule out or in an MI.

ENZYME	ONSET (HRS)	PEAK (HRS)	DURATION
Myoglobin	1–4	6–8	24 hrs
Troponin T/I	3–12	18–24	7–10 days
Creatinine kinase (total and CK MB)	3–12	18–24	3–4 days
Lactate dehydrogenase	6–12	24–48	6–8 days

A 47-year-old man presents to the ER with left-sided chest pain at rest. He is a chronic smoker with family history of diabetes and hypertension. On examination, he is found to have stable vitals. ECG showed new ST flattening in II, III, and AVF. ASA, Plavix and nitrate were administered and patient still complained of pain. **Next step:** Start heparin drip and send patient for cardiac catheterization.

What Do You Do With a Patient Suspected of ACS?

- Detailed history and physical:
  - **Typical symptoms for any anginal/MI:** Left-sided/substernal chest pressure with radiation to the left shoulder, arm, or jaw. Patient may characterize this by putting a closed fist over the chest (Levine's sign), shortness of breath, diaphoresis, nausea or vomiting.

Patients presenting with ACS should be given MONA + beta blocker (unless contraindicated):
   Oxygen
   Nitrate
   Aspirin
   Morphine
Note: Morphine should be the last medication given. It may mask angina and should only be given when a diagnosis of ACS is certain and the patient still has severe pain.

- Specific situations:
  - **Syncope or cardiac arrest** (arrhythmia can result from the ischemic insult).
  - **Unstable angina** is associated with ↑ frequency and/or severity of symptoms, symptoms at rest or new onset of symptoms
  - **Atypical presentation:** No symptoms or just one. Presentation may be atypical in diabetics (they may have a neuropathy that blunts the sensation of pain; many diabetics have "silent MIs" where the MI has no symptoms). Women may also have atypical symptoms.
- **Initial tests:** (1) ECG, and (2) cardiac enzymes.

Initial Treatment for All ACS

- Patients should also be placed on a cardiac monitor (telemetry) because during ischemia they are at high risk for arrhythmias.
- Beta blockers ↓ cardiac oxygen demand and have been shown to ↓ mortality.
- Antiplatelet and anticoagulation: Aspirin (chewable preferred). Clopidogrel is an alternative for those with true aspirin allergy.
- *Note:* Morphine helps with pain control but does not affect outcome.
- Other possible additions:
  - Either unfractionated heparin or low-molecular-weight heparin can be used. The rationale behind using both aspirin and heparin is that they act at different sites.
  - GP IIb/IIIa inhibitors have shown to be beneficial for high-risk patients.
  - *Note:* Thrombolytics are not used in unstable angina or non-ST-elevation MI because 60–80% of the time the infarcted artery is not occluded.
- **MONA + beta blocker for all ACS patients, but additional treatment depending on type of ACS.** ACS is divided into two major types:
  1. **ST-elevation MI (STEMI):** This is the most dangerous type of ACS. (This group also includes those with a new left bundle branch block [LBBB] on ECG).
     - **Treatment:** These patients need aggressive treatment in addition to MONA + beta blocker. They need urgent opening of blockage (revascularization). This can be done with (1) thrombolytics (medicines that break up clots) and/or (2) cardiac catheterization and stent (percutaneous transluminal coronary angioplasty [PTCA]) (see section on cardiac catheterization above). Cardiac catheterization is generally considered superior to thrombolytics in STEMI. **Thrombolytics:** Examples include streptokinase, urokinase, anistreplase, alteplase, and reteplase. Contraindications are risks of bleeding, particularly in the brain: prior intracranial hemorrhage, stroke within 1 year, brain tumor, active internal bleeding, or suspected aortic dissection.
  2. **Unstable angina** and **non-ST-elevation MI (NSTEMI):** These two have similar pathogenesis. Non-ST-elevation MI differs from unstable angina in that the lack of oxygen is severe enough to cause myocardial damage and enzyme leakage (unlike unstable angina, where there is no enzyme leakage).
     - **Treatment:** MONA + beta blocker as described above. Can treat with invasive treatment (cardiac catheterization) or conservatively (medications). Ongoing chest pain and signs of cardiac dysfunction would prompt intervention.

Heparin does not dissolve already-present clots; rather, it prevents future ones from forming.

What is a TIMI score?
Scoring system used to evaluate risks of patients with NSTEMI and determine if early invasive management (ie, cardiac cath) is warranted. Each item is worth a point:
- Age > 65
- ≥ 3 CAD risk factors
- Prior coronary stenosis > 50%
- ST changes on ECG
- ≥ 2 anginal episodes in 24 hours
- Use of aspirin in prior week
- Positive serum markers
TIMI > 4: Patient should get invasive management.

- Cocaine can cause MI without a clot, rather vasospasm, or simply drug-induced heart strain in which the oxygen supply cannot keep up (do urine drug screen if suspicious).
- **Inferior wall MI—a special case:** Inferior wall MI (ECG changes in II, III, and aVF) affects the right ventricle. Therefore, there is a *major danger of dropping preload.* Treatment must maintain preload with aggressive fluids and *avoid nitrates* (will drop preload).

Cardiac output = stroke volume × heart rate.

Typical ECG Findings in MI

Location of ECG abnormalities tells which vessel in the heart is infected.

- **Inferior wall MI:** ST elevation in II, III, aVF (cor pulmonale: ST *depression* in II, III, aVF) (see Figure 2.1-1).
- **Anteroseptal MI:** ST elevation in V_1, V_2, V_3 (see Figure 2.1-2).
- **Lateral wall MI:** ST elevation in V_5, V_6, I, aVL.
- **Posterior wall MI:** Tall ST elevation in II, III, AVF, tall R with ST depression in V1, V2, and ST elevation in V4R.

Causes of ST elevation:
- MI
- Pericarditis
- Left ventricular (LV) aneurysm
- Early repolarization (young people)

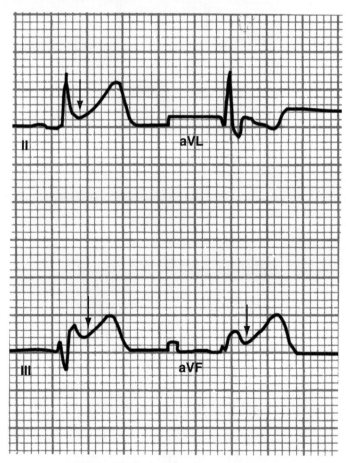

FIGURE 2.1-1. **ECG of inferior wall MI demonstrating ST elevation in leads II, III, and aVF.**

CARDIOLOGY

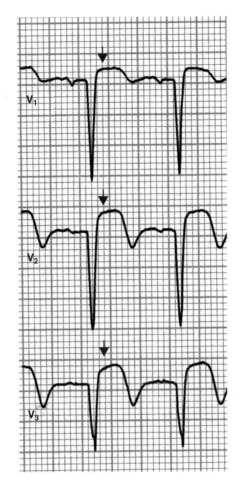

FIGURE 2.1-2. ECG of anteroseptal MI demonstrating ST elevation in leads V₁, V₂, and V₃.

FIGURE 2.1-3. Right bundle branch block.

Medications at Discharge for Patients with ACS

- Aspirin indefinitely.
- Beta blocker indefinitely.
- Angiotensin-converting enzyme (ACE) inhibitor indefinitely; can particularly help patients with resulting low cardiac function (congestive heart failure [CHF]).
- Statin (hydroxymethylglutaryl coenzyme A [HMG CoA] reductase inhibitor) to maintain LDL < 70.
- Clopidogrel (Plavix) if a stent was placed.

Secondary Prevention of MI

- Smoking cessation
- Diabetes control
- Hypertension control
- Control of hyperlipidemia

 A 65-year-old woman with a history of CAD and drug-eluting stent (DES) placed 6 months ago presents with acute crushing chest pain. She says that she had stopped taking her Plavix 1 week ago for a dental procedure. *Think: Acute in-stent thrombosis.*

Next step: ECG (may show ST elevation; send for urgent cardiac catheterization).

Post-MI patient upon discharge: aspirin, beta blocker, angiotensin-converting enzyme (ACE) inhibitor, and statin (and Plavix if a stent was placed).

Postinfarction Complications

- **Ruptures** (usually occur within 4–5 days of a large MI). These can be in the free wall of the heart, the intraventricular septum, or the papillary muscle, which causes acute mitral regurgitation.
- **Arrhythmias:** Ventricular tachycardia (usually within 48 hours, when the myocardium reperfuses), bradycardia (usually from inferior wall MI), atrioventricular block (can be from anterior wall or inferior wall MI).
- **Dressler's syndrome:** Usually occurs 1 or 2 weeks after cardiac injury (MI or cardiac surgery). It is associated with fever, pericarditis, and sometimes pericardial or pleural effusions; likely a hypersensitivity process. Treat with nonsteroidal anti-inflammatory drugs (NSAIDs) and steroids.

A patient presents with a known history of CHF with a low EF. What is the most likely cause of death? Arrhythmia.

 A 58-year-old man who was discharged from the hospital after an MI 2 weeks ago presents with fever, chest pain, and generalized malaise. ECG shows diffuse ST-T wave changes. *Think: Dressler's syndrome.* Treat with NSAIDs.

Congestive heart failure (CHF) is the failure of the heart to pump blood effectively to the tissues. Left heart failure (LHF) causes pulmonary venous congestion (blood flow back-up into the lungs) and compromised systemic circulation. Right heart failure (RHF) causes systemic venous congestion.

Most Common Causes of Right- and Left-Sided Heart Failure

Right Heart Failure	Left Heart Failure
CAD (MI that has damaged the right ventricle)	CAD (MI that has damaged the left ventricle)
2° to LHF (then further "backup" of blood)	Hypertension
Pulmonary hypertension (right ventricle has to push against a higher pressure and gets hypertrophied and damaged)	Mitral and aortic valve disease
Endocarditis damaging triscuspid valve	Endocarditis
Ventricular septal defect (VSD)	Dilated cardiomyopathy

Decompensated Heart Failure

Refers to the worsening or exacerbation of an underlying CHF. It can be precipitated by:

- Ischemia (most common).
- Noncompliance with meds (eg, skipped diuretic).
- Dysrhythmias.
- Other noncardiac causes (pulmonary embolism, EtOH, thyrotoxicosis, wet beriberi, viruses).

SIGNS AND SYMPTOMS OF HEART FAILURE

Left Heart Failure
- Symptoms:
  - Shortness of breath (SOB).
  - Orthopnea.
  - Paroxysmal nocturnal dyspnea (PND)—SOB when lying down.
  - Dyspnea on exertion (DOE).
  - Cough.
  - Diaphoresis.
  - Nocturia.
- Signs:
  - Rales.
  - S3 gallop.
  - Tachycardia.
  - Peripheral edema.

Right Heart Failure
- Symptoms:
  - RUQ pain (due to hepatic congestion).
  - SOB.
  - Abdominal swelling (ascites).
  - Weight gain (fluid retention).

The most common cause of right heart failure is left heart failure.

- **Signs:**
  - Hepatomegaly.
  - Hepatojugular reflex.
  - Jugular venous distention (JVD).
  - Ascites.
  - Cirrhosis.
  - Abnormal LFTs (congestive hepatopathy).
  - Peripheral edema.
  - Cyanosis.

DIAGNOSIS

- Chest x-ray can show enlargement of cardiac silhouette, pulmonary vascular congestion with redistribution to upper lobes, and effusion.
- Echocardiogram can show ↓ cardiac function.
- Brain natriuretic peptide (BNP) is elevated in CHF.

TREATMENT

- **Nonpharmacologic**: Sodium and water restriction, exercise, education, and avoidance of alcohol.
- **Pharmacologic:**
  - First-line therapy:
    - **ACE inhibitors:** ↓ afterload; ↓ symptoms, mortality, incidence of heart failure symptoms, and hospitalization.
    - **Diuretics:** Use in NHYA class II–IV for fluid retention. Helps to reduce preload. Thiazides and loop diuretics (furosemide) are examples.
    - **Beta blockers:** For NYHA class II–III (↓ symptoms, improve survival).
    - **Digoxin:** Add for NYHA class III–IV (for symptomatic relief only; **does not** improve survival but reduces hospitalization).
    - **Spironolactone (potassium-sparing diuretics):** Low dose, use in New York Heart Association (NYHA) class III–IV. ↓ mortality. Monitor potassium closely. Concomitant use of ACE inhibitors can make potassium go very high, so monitor closely.
    - **Eplerenone:** Similar to spironolactone, but fewer side effects (namely gynecomastia).
  - Second-line therapy:
    - **Angiotensin receptor blockers (ARBs):** If ACE inhibitors are not well tolerated (eg, cough).
    - **Nitrate-hydralazine combination:** Improve symptoms and survival. High rate of intolerance and lower effect on mortality make this therapy a second line to ACE inhibitors.
    - **Cardiac resynchronization therapy:** Reserved for patients who are in Class III HF despite maximal therapy. Essentially a pacemaker that times the contractions of atria and ventricles for maximum efficiency.

Acute Cardiogenic Pulmonary Edema

- **Acute pulmonary edema (APE)** is caused by rapid decompensation of LV function due to dysrhythmias (atrial fibrillation, ventricular tachycardia [VT], supraventricular tachycardia [SVT]), MI, ↑ sodium intake, noncompliance with medications (ie, diuretics), drugs, infection (less common).

Diastolic Dysfunction
CHF that may have a normal ejection fraction; the problem occurs during filling (diastole) due to cardiac wall stiffness.
- Accounts for 40–60% of heart failure.
- Signs/symptoms of heart failure with normal ejection fraction (> 50%).
- More common in women.
- Associated with hypertension, left ventricular hypertrophy (LVH), dilated cardiomyopathy, and ischemia.
- Treat the hypertension, use diuretics for congestion and edema, and control rate if atrial fibrillation.

New York Heart Association Functional Classification of Heart Failure
Class I: No limitation
Class II: Slight limitations (symptoms at ordinary efforts)
Class III: Marked limitation (comfortable at rest, symptoms at minimal efforts)
Class IV: Symptomatic at rest

In pregnancy there is ↑ cardiac output, ↓ vascular resistance, and ↑ plasma volume. These cause ↑ shortness of breath! And the plasma volume ↑ causes a drop in hemoglobin (dilutes blood!).

- First-line therapy: **NOMAD**
  - Nitroglycerin
  - Oxygen
  - Morphine
  - Aspirin
  - Diuretic
- Other therapy: **MDDN**
  - Milrinone ↑ inotropy with vasodilation.
  - Dobutamine ↑ inotropy without vasoconstriction.
  - Dopamine ↑ inotropy with vasoconstriction.
  - Nesiritide is basic natriuretic peptide—causes smooth muscle to relax and diuresis.

Paroxysmal Nocturnal Dyspnea (PND)

A brief episode of breathlessness that awakens patient from sleep. Also called cardiac asthma.

ETIOLOGY

Due to ↑ volume load on the heart when lying in the horizontal position or sudden ↓ in myocardial contractility, which results in pulmonary edema, impairing the exchange of oxygen.

DIAGNOSIS

Distinguished from true asthma by improvement with sitting upright, walking a few steps, and lack of improvement with bronchodilators.

TREATMENT

Nitroglycerin, oxygen, diuretic (NOD).

CARDIOMYOPATHIES

Dilated Cardiomyopathy

Left or right ventricular enlargement with loss of contractile function resulting in congestive heart failure, dysrhythmias, or thrombus formation.

ETIOLOGY

ITEMM:

- Infectious: Viral myocarditis (one-third improve, one-third stay the same, one-third get worse).
- Toxic: Reversible—prolonged EtOH abuse.
- Endocrine: Reversible—thyroid disease (hypo or hyper). Irreversible—acromegaly, pheochromocytoma.
- Metabolic: Reversible—hypocalcemia, hypophosphatemia, thiamine deficiency (wet beriberi), selenium deficiency. Irreversible—genetic: 20% of cases have positive family histories; pregnancy (postpartum cardiomyopathy, 1–9 months after delivery—similar prognosis as viral); neuromuscular; idiopathic.
- Mechanical: Dysrhythmias (tachycardia induced cardiomyopathy); valvular disease.

A 26-year-old man presents with SOB, PND, orthopnea, and pleuritic chest pain for 1 week. He had an upper respiratory infection (URI) 1 week prior to onset of symptoms. *Think: Viral myocarditis.*

Next step: ECG shows diffuse ST-segment elevation and PR-segment depression. Treat with NSAIDs and steroids if severe.

A known alcoholic presents with orthopnea and swelling of legs, but no ascites. *Think: Alcohol-induced cardiomyopathy.*

A patient with multiple myeloma has SOB and a chest x-ray showing pulmonary edema. An echo shows a "speckled" appearance. Diagnosis? Cardiac amyloidosis. Type of cardiomyopathy? Restrictive.

SIGNS AND SYMPTOMS

- Symptoms of heart failure.
- Angina due to $\uparrow O_2$ demands of enlarged ventricles.
- Sudden death from arrhythmias.

DIAGNOSIS

Echocardiography shows dilated ventricles/atria, regurgitant valves, low ejection fraction.

TREATMENT

- Address any reversible causes (eg, discontinue toxic agent).
- Supportive care—medical management of heart failure (ACE inhibitors and diuretics reduce mortality).
- Anticoagulation with Coumadin (with severe LV dysfunction, even if no evidence of thrombus).
- Implanted automatic defibrillator for patients with life-threatening dysrhythmias or EF < 30% despite maximal therapy at 3 months.
- Heart transplant.

Stress-Induced Cardiomyopathy (Takotsubo Cardiomyopathy)

ETIOLOGY

- Rare form of cardiomyopathy that is precipitated by emotional and physical stress. More commonly seen in female patients in postmenopausal age group.
- It may happen in situations with sudden sympathetic surge (eg, subjects undergoing dobutamine stress test).
- Pathophysiology thought to be combination of sympathetic overactivation, coronary microcirculation dysregulation, and hormonal effects.

SYMPTOMS

Chest pain and/or SOB.

MANAGEMENT

- Supportive care with cardiac monitoring, serial echocardiograms, treatment of heart failure, and arrhythmias.
- Beta blockers have important role in management as sympathetic stimulation seems to play a central role.

PROGNOSIS

Usually good, with recovery within 1–3 months.

Restrictive Cardiomyopathy

Scarring and infiltration of the myocardium causing ↓ right or LV filling.

ETIOLOGY

Amyloidosis; endomyocardial fibrosis; hemochromatosis; sarcoidosis; carcinoid heart disease; congenital (Gaucher's, Hurler's, glycogen storage disease).

SIGNS AND SYMPTOMS

- Signs of LHF/RHF; RHF usually predominates.
- Exercise intolerance is a common presenting symptom.

DIAGNOSIS

- Endomyocardial biopsy may detect eosinophilic infiltration or myocardial fibrosis or amyloid.
- Echocardiography—normal-sized ventricles, large atria, thickened ventricular walls, mitral/tricuspid regurgitation; typically has a speckled appearance if amyloid is cause. *Ejection fraction is normal or ↑.*
- **Other findings:**
  - **Auscultation:** S3 and/or S4 gallop murmurs, occasional mitral or tricuspid regurgitation.
  - **ECG:** Low voltages, conduction abnormalities, nonspecific ST segment/T wave changes, left bundle branch block.
  - **CXR:** Normal cardiac silhouette or enlarged atria, pulmonary venous congestion.

TREATMENT

Treat underlying cause; treat the resulting heart failure; heart transplant if candidate.

Hypertrophic Cardiomyopathy (HCM)

Hypertrophy of the interventricular septum narrows the LV outflow tract. High-velocity systolic flow draws the anterior leaflet of the mitral valve into the tract (via the Bernoulli effect) causing a dynamic LV outflow tract obstruction. **Put simply,** thick intraventricular septum obstructs blood flow out of the heart and can cause sudden death by arrhythmia.

Restrictive cardiomyopathy is often difficult to distinguish from constrictive pericarditis—biopsy can usually confirm.

Hypertrophic cardiomyopathy used to be called idiopathic hypertrophic subaortic stenosis, or IHSS. Don't get this confused with ventricular hypertrophy.

In HCM, symptoms prior to 30 years of age correlate with ↑ risk of sudden death, but severity of symptoms (whenever they occur) does not correlate with risk of death.

CARDIOLOGY

ETIOLOGY

~ 50% idiopathic, ~ 50% familial (autosomal dominant, with variable penetrance).

CLINICAL SEQUELAE

These are the young patients with sudden death!!

- Conditions that ↓ the LV end-diastolic volume ↑ the obstruction and make it worse (and make murmur more pronounced (eg, inotropic drugs, afterload reduction, Valsalva).
- Outflow obstruction can result in left atrial dilatation, atrial fibrillation, CHF, right heart failure.
- May have angina for reasons poorly understood, also syncope, or arrhythmias.
- **Sudden death due to arrhythmia.**
- **Diagnosis:** Echocardiography: Septal hypertrophy and LVH.
- **Other findings:** The murmur changes with position—systolic ejection murmur heard best along the left sternal border, ↓ with ↑ LV blood volume (squatting), ↑ with ↑ blood velocities (exercise), and ↓ LV end-diastolic volume (Valsalva) and standing. Paradoxical splitting of S2.
- **Treatment: Counseling** and **screening** should be offered to immediate family members. Patient should refrain from vigorous exercise. Beta blockers reduce heart rate, ↑ LV filling time and ↓ inotropy; calcium channel blockers are considered second-line agents. Septal myomectomy (not always effective); implantable cardioverter defibrillator (ICD) for primary prevention as well as secondary prevention; avoid anything that ↓ preload (nitrates, diuretics, volume depletion) as this will worsen obstruction by allowing LV collapse.

 A 25-year-old man becomes severely dyspneic and collapses while running laps. His father died suddenly at an early age. *Think: Hypertrophic cardiomyopathy.*
Very few murmurs ↓ with squatting (HCM does).

MYOCARDITIS

Inflammation of the myocardium.

ETIOLOGY

- **Viral:** Coxsackie A or B, echovirus, HIV, cytomegalovirus (CMV), influenza, Epstein–Barr (EBV), hepatitis B virus (HBV), adenovirus.
- **Bacterial:** Group A beta-hemolytic strep (rheumatic fever), *Corynebacterium, meningococcus, Borrelia burgdorferi* (Lyme), *Mycoplasma pneumoniae.*
- **Parasitic:** *Trypanosoma cruzi* (Chagas'), *Toxoplasma, Trichinella, Echinococcus.*

Causes of paradoxical splitting of S2:
- Hypertrophic cardiomyopathy
- Aortic stenosis
- LBBB (left bundle branch block)

Splitting of S2: Normal physiologic: Aortic before pulmonic valve closure. Split widened by inspiration as increasingly negative intrathoracic pressure augments right heart filling, resulting in longer ventricular emptying times. **Paradoxical:** Pulmonic before aortic valve due to a delay in aortic valve closure. Inspiration still delays pulmonic closure but now brings it closer to aortic closure, *paradoxically* narrowing the split.

Coxsackie B is the most common viral cause of myocarditis.

- **Systemic disease:** Kawasaki's, systemic lupus erythematosus (SLE), sarcoidosis, inflammatory conditions.
- **Drugs:** Cocaine, ephedra.
- Idiopathic.

SIGNS AND SYMPTOMS

- Spectrum of disease ranges from asymptomatic to fulminant cardiac failure and death.
- Findings may include: chest pain, fever, recent upper respiratory infection, fatigue, signs of CHF.

DIAGNOSIS

- Myocardial biopsy.
- Echocardiography shows hypokinetic wall movement, dilated ventricles/atria and sometimes pericardial effusion.
- **Other findings:**
  - **Auscultation:** S3/S4, mitral or tricuspid regurgitation, friction rub (if pericardium involved.
  - **ECG:** Nonspecific changes, low voltage, dysrhythmias.
  - **Labs:** Leukocytosis, elevated ESR, elevated cardiac enzymes (slower rise and fall than acute MI, troponin I is most sensitive).

TREATMENT

- Primarily supportive.
- Limit activity.
- Treat CHF and dysrhythmias.
- Address etiology if known/applicable (eg, antivirals, antibiotics, diphtheria—antitoxin, discontinue drug use); intravenous immunoglobulin G (IVIG) may be of benefit.

PERICARDITIS

Inflammation of the pericardium.

ETIOLOGY

- **Viral:** Recent viral URI, though a definitive cause is not known.
- **Bacterial:** Tuberculosis (TB), streptococci, staphylococci (rheumatic fever causes pancarditis).
- **Metastases:** 1° tumors usually breast, lung, or melanoma.
- **Immediate post MI:** Pericarditis occurs within 24 hours of a *transmural* infarction due to direct pericardial irritation from injured myocardium.
- **Dressler's syndrome:** Pericarditis occurring 1 week to months after an MI due to an autoimmune response to infarcted myocardium.
- Uremia.
- Rheumatologic condition (SLE, scleroderma).
- Drug reaction.
- Myxedema.
- Trauma.

SIGNS AND SYMPTOMS

Chest pain, often pleuritic, radiating to left shoulder; often relieved by leaning forward; does not respond to nitroglycerin.

DIAGNOSIS

- **Auscultation:** Pericardial friction rub on expiration, pathognomonic but variably present.
- **ECG:** *Diffuse* ST elevations and PR depressions (no discreet pattern of infarction) (see Figure 2.1-4).

TREATMENT

- Address **underlying cause** if known/applicable (eg, hemodialysis for uremia).
- **NSAIDs** to relieve pain and reduce inflammation (aspirin, indomethacin, ibuprofen).
- **Steroids** for intractable cases (eg, Dressler's), generally not used < 10 days post MI.

PERICARDIAL TAMPONADE

Tamponade is the physiologic result of rapid accumulation of fluid within the relatively inelastic pericardial sac. Pericardial tamponade impairs cardiac filling and reduces cardiac output.

ETIOLOGY

- Pericarditis.
- Trauma (accidental or iatrogenic).
- Ruptured ventricular wall (post MI).
- Aortic dissection with rupture into pericardium.
- Malignancy.

SIGNS AND SYMPTOMS

In addition to dyspnea and tachycardia:

- **Beck's triad:** (1) Hypotension, (2) muffled heart sounds, (3) JVD.
- **Pulsus paradoxus:** Systolic blood pressure ↓ by > 10 mm Hg with inspiration.
- **Narrow pulse pressure:** Only a small difference between systolic and diastolic blood pressure.

DIAGNOSIS

- Echocardiogram will show large pericardial effusion and ↓ filling.
- **Other findings:**
  - ECG: May show low voltage or electrical alternans.
  - CXR: Enlarged cardiac silhouette.
  - Auscultation: Distant heart sounds.

TREATMENT

- Immediate pericardiocentesis (aspirate fluid from pericardial sac) for unstable patients.
- Infuse fluids to expand volume.
- Pericardial window (surgery) for stable patients and recurrent effusions.

Always suspect a patient with lupus (or any rheumatologic condition) who presents with shortness of breath of having cardiac tamponade. These patients get pericardial effusions. JVD would be a tip off. **Next step:** Give IV fluid to ↑ preload, then immediately do a pericardiocentesis.

Pulsus paradoxus is a transient fall in measured blood pressure > 10 mm Hg associated with inspiration (due to reduced stroke volume during inspiration).

Tamponade physiology: During inspiration, venous return to the right atrium ↑ because of greater negative pressure. In tamponade, the transiently enlarged right atrium bulges leftward, reducing left ventricular volume and output, causing BP to fall with inspiration. Pericardiocentesis yielding *clotted* blood probably came from the right ventricle, not the pericardial sac. Fluid in the pericardium usually is not entirely blood (ie, usually other fluid, too) and therefore won't clot.

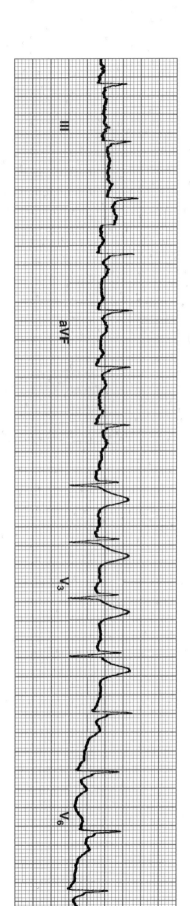

FIGURE 2.1-4. Pericarditis.

Note diffuse ST segment elevation and PR depression.

Granulation and scarring of the pericardium secondary to acute pericarditis. Cardiac output is diminished.

SIGNS AND SYMPTOMS

- Dyspnea.
- Fatigue.
- Tachycardia.
- JVD with patient upright.
- Kussmaul's sign: Paradoxic rise in JVD during inspiration.
- LV failure.
- Peripheral edema.

DIAGNOSIS

- Echocardiogram will show *normal left ventricular function* and may show pericardial thickening.
- **Other findings:**
    - Auscultation may demonstrate distant heart sounds. Pericardial "knock" may be heard.
    - CXR may show pericardial calcification.
    - ECG may show low voltage, T wave flattening or inversion in V_1 and V_2, notched P waves.

TREATMENT

Pericardiectomy.

VALVULAR HEART DISEASE (VHD)

Mitral Stenosis

ETIOLOGY

Rheumatic heart disease (most common), congenital (rare).

EPIDEMIOLOGY

Most cases occur in women.

SIGNS AND SYMPTOMS

These are due to resulting decompensation of cardiac function; from the left atrium backing up into the lungs and then the right heart: symptoms of CHF and right-sided failure (dyspnea on exertion, rales, cough). See Table 2.1-3 for classic signs and symptoms of valvular diseases.

DIAGNOSIS

- Echocardiography demonstrates diseased valve.
- **Other findings:**
    - Murmur is mid-diastolic with opening snap, low-pitched rumble best heard over left sternal border between 2nd and 4th interspace (see Figure 2.1-5).

Any disorder that causes dilation of the atria can → atrial fibrillation. Also any disorder that causes dilation can → thrombus in the ventricle and emboli.

TABLE 2.1-3. Classic Signs and Symptoms of Valvular Diseases

	ETIOLOGY	SYMPTOMS	SIGNS/MURMUR
Mitral stenosis	▪ Rheumatic heart disease ▪ Congenital ▪ Degenerative	▪ Right heart failure ▪ SOB (orthopnea, PND) ▪ Cough/hemoptysis ▪ Atrial fibrillation	▪ Loud S2/tapping apex ▪ Opening snap followed by mid-diastolic rumbling murmur
Mitral regurgitation	▪ Rheumatic heart disease ▪ Papillary muscle rupture (post MI) ▪ Physiologic ▪ Dilated cardiomyopathy ▪ Ischemia ▪ Endocarditis	▪ SOB, orthopnea, PND ▪ Pulmonary edema ▪ Right heart failure	▪ Holosystolic murmur best heard at the apex with radiation to the axilla
Aortic stenosis	▪ Congenital ▪ Degenerative ▪ Bicuspid valve ▪ Rheumatic heart disease	▪ SOB ▪ Chest pain ▪ Syncope	▪ Systolic ejection murmur, crescendo/decrescendo, radiating to the carotids ▪ Low-volume pulse, slow rising (pulsus parvus et tardus)
Aortic regurgitation	▪ Rheumatic heart disease ▪ Congenital bicuspid valve ▪ Endocarditis ▪ 2° aortic root dilatation (eg, syphilis, ankylosing spondylitis)	▪ SOB, orthopnea, PND	▪ Early diastolic decrescendo murmur best heard at left 3rd/4th intercostal space
Tricuspid regurgitation	▪ Endocarditis ▪ 2° left heart failure ▪ Pulmonary hypertension ▪ Carcinoid	▪ Pedal edema ▪ Ascites ▪ Fatigue	▪ Holosystolic murmur left sternal border, ↑ by inspiration (Carvallo's sign) ▪ Hepatomegaly (may be pulsatile)
Tricuspid stenosis	▪ Rheumatic heart disease ▪ Congenital ▪ Carcinoid	▪ Fatigue ▪ Abdominal discomfort (2° hepatomegaly) ▪ Pedal edema	▪ Diastolic murmur left sternal edge ▪ Hepatomegaly ▪ Icterus, edema

- CXR may show straight left heart border due to enlarged left atrium and Kerley B lines from pulmonary effusion.

TREATMENT

- Surgical repair or balloon valvuloplasty in symptomatic patients with severe stenosis.
- Endocarditis prophylaxis.
- Treat for heart failure (diuretics, digitalis) and dysrhythmias as needed.

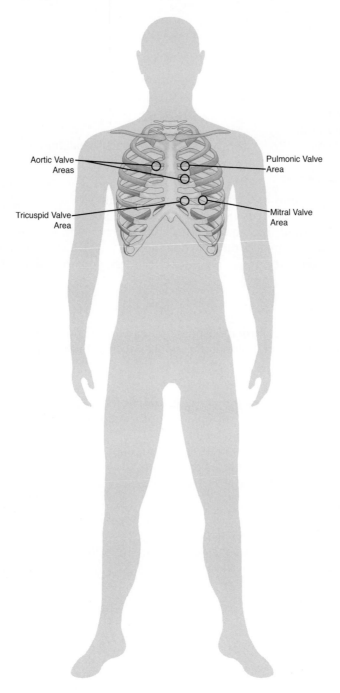

Aortic Valve
Areas

Pulmonic Valve
Area

Tricuspid Valve
Area

Mitral Valve
Area

FIGURE 2.1-5. **Cardiac auscultation sites.**

(Reproduced, with permission, from DeGowin RL. *DeGowin & DeGowin's Diagnostic Examination*, 6th ed. New York: McGraw-Hill, 1994: 359.)

Mitral Regurgitation

ETIOLOGY

Acute	Chronic
▪ MI with papillary muscle rupture	▪ Rheumatic fever
▪ Endocarditis	▪ Mitral prolapse that evolves into regurgitation
▪ Ischemia	▪ Left ventricular dilation

SIGNS AND SYMPTOMS

These are symptoms of CHF—back up from mitral valve through lungs and right heart. When left ventricle contracts, blood goes both backward into left atrium and forward into aorta. At first this can be asymptomatic in chronic cases, and then progress as the left ventricle and left atrium dilate and fail, and pulmonary artery pressure ↑. Dyspnea, weakness, and atrial fibrillation develops.

DIAGNOSIS/SIGNS

- Echocardiography demonstrating diseased/prolapsed valve.
- **Murmur** is loud, holosystolic, apical radiating to the axilla.

TREATMENT

- Medical therapy (diuretics, ACE inhibitors).
- Surgical therapy (valve replacement or repair) is definitive therapy if signs of LV dysfunction begin.
- Acute mitral regurgitation (from papillary muscle rupture from MI) usually results in severe CHF and requires emergent surgery.

Patient with mitral regurgitation has a good prognosis if LV function is preserved.

Mitral Valve Prolapse

ETIOLOGY

- Most common valvular disorder (women are 90% of cases).
- Idiopathic.
- Rheumatic heart disease.
- Ischemic heart disease.
- Atrial septal defect.
- Marfan's syndrome.
- Genetic (can be inherited as an autosomal dominant trait).

SIGNS AND SYMPTOMS

Mostly asymptomatic, but can rarely have chest pain and shortness of breath.

A young woman presents with atypical chest pain and mid-systolic click. *Think: Mitral valve prolapse.*

DIAGNOSIS/SIGNS

- Echocardiography.
- **Murmur:**
  - *Mid-systolic click* (that's what you get on exams); followed by late systolic, high-pitched murmur (*if mild regurgitation is present also*).
  - Best heard at apex.
  - Wide splitting of S2.

TREATMENT

None.

Aortic Stenosis (AS)

ETIOLOGY

Degenerative calcific (calcification) disease (idiopathic, older population); also bicuspid aortic valve (most common *congenital* valve abnormality) can result in aortic stenosis around age 40.

SYMPTOMS

Classic triad: (1) angina, (2) syncope, (3) CHF.

PATHOPHYSIOLOGY

- **Asymptomatic** early in course.
- Then develop **angina and syncope**, particularly during exercise. Exertion increases heart rate, which results in less filling time and decreased flow across the stenotic valve. Syncope results from decreased blood flow to the brain. Angina results from subendocardial ischemia as a result of LVH.
- With longstanding severe aortic stenosis, the left ventricle ultimately fails and CHF develops.

PROGNOSIS

- Mean survival for patients with AS correlates with symptoms:
  - Angina: 5 years
  - Syncope: 2–3 years
  - Heart failure: 1–2 years
- **Murmur:** Loud systolic ejection murmur, crescendo–decrescendo, medium pitched loudest at second right intercostal space, radiates to carotids.

DIAGNOSIS

- Echocardiography.
- **Other possible findings:**
  - Narrow pulse pressure.
  - Paradoxical splitting of S2.
  - Calcification of aortic valve may be seen on CXR.
  - Carotid pulse is "parvus and tardus" (weak and slow).

TREATMENT

- Avoid strenuous activity.
- Valvuloplasty produces only temporary improvement as rate of restenosis is very high.
- Valve replacement is definitive therapy.

Conditions with narrow pulse pressure (small difference between systolic and diastolic blood pressure):
- Aortic stenosis
- Cardiac tamponade
- Heart failure
- Hypovolemia
- Shock/Anaphylaxis

Left ventricular strain pattern is ST segment depression and T wave inversion in I, aVL, and left precordial leads.

When to go for valve replacement surgery?
- Persistent symptoms
- Aortic orifice < 0.7 cm^2
- Gradient > 70 mm Hg across valve

Acute valvular disorders (eg, acute MR or AR) result in severe decompensation into CHF due to the absence of hemodynamic compensation. Emergent surgery is required.

Aortic Regurgitation

ETIOLOGY

- Can be caused by a dilation of the aortic root causing the valve not to work, or a problem with the aortic valve itself.
- **Causes of aortic root dilatation:** Idiopathic, Marfan's, collagen vascular disease.
- **Causes of aortic valve problem:** Rheumatic heart disease, endocarditis, syphilis, Marfan's, Ehlers-Danlos syndrome, Turner's syndrome, trauma.

DIAGNOSIS

- Echocardiography.
- **Murmur:**
  - High-pitched, blowing, decrescendo diastolic murmur best heard over second right interspace or third left interspace, accentuated by leaning forward.
  - **Austin Flint murmur:** Observed in severe regurgitation, low-pitched diastolic rumble due to regurgitated blood striking the anterior mitral leaflet (similar sound to mitral stenosis).
- **Other findings:**
  - Hyperdynamic, down and laterally displaced point of maximum impulse (PMI) due to LV enlargement.
  - ECG shows LVH (see Figure 2.1-6).
  - Wide pulse pressure.

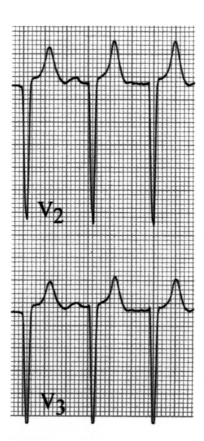

FIGURE 2.1-6. Left ventricular hypertrophy.

- Dyspnea, orthopnea, PND.
- Angina (due to reduced diastolic coronary blood flow due to low pressure in aortic root).
- LV failure.
- **Other signs with fancy names:**
  - Bounding "Corrigan" pulse, "pistol shot" femorals, pulsus bisferiens (dicrotic pulse with two palpable waves in systole).
  - **Duroziez sign:** Presence of diastolic femoral bruit when femoral artery is compressed enough to hear a systolic bruit.
  - **Hill's sign:** Systolic pressure in the legs > 20 mm Hg higher than in the arms.
  - **Quincke's sign:** Alternating blushing and blanching of the fingernails when gentle pressure is applied.
  - **De Musset's sign:** Bobbing of head with heartbeat.

TREATMENT

- Treat LV failure.
- Endocarditis prophylaxis.
- Valve replacement is necessary for severe cases and is the only definitive treatment.

Tricuspid Stenosis

ETIOLOGY

- Rheumatic heart disease, congenital, carcinoid.
- Rare.

SIGNS AND SYMPTOMS

Right-sided heart failure (peripheral edema, JVD, hepatomegaly, ascites, jaundice).

DIAGNOSIS

- Echocardiography demonstrates diseased valve.
- **Murmur** is diastolic, rumbling, low pitched accentuated with inspiration. Best heard over left sternal border between fourth and fifth interspace.

TREATMENT

Surgical repair.

Tricuspid Regurgitation

ETIOLOGY

- ↑ pulmonary artery pressure (eg, from left-sided failure or mitral regurgitation/stenosis).
- Right ventricular dilation stretching the outflow tract (eg, from right heart failure, infarction, or tricuspid regurgitation itself).
- Right papillary muscle rupture from infarction.
- Tricuspid valvular lesions (eg, from rheumatic heart disease or bacterial endocarditis).

Acute valvular disorders (eg, acute MR or AR) result in severe decompensation into CHF due to the absence of hemodynamic compensation. Emergent surgery is required.

Conditions with wide pulse pressure:
- Aortic regurgitation
- Hyperthyroidism
- Anemia
- Wet beriberi
- Hypertrophic subaortic stenosis
- Hypertension

CARDIOLOGY

SIGNS AND SYMPTOMS

Signs of right heart failure: Prominent JVD, pulsatile liver.

DIAGNOSIS

- Echocardiography.
- **Murmur:** Holosystolic, blowing, medium-pitched murmur heard best along the left sternal border in the fifth interspace, accentuated with inspiration.
- **Other findings:**
  - ECG shows right ventricular enlargement.
  - Atrial fibrillation is common.

TREATMENT

- Treat left heart failure, if applicable.
- Diuresis to reduce volume load.
- Endocarditis prophylaxis.
- Surgical repair.

Right-sided bacterial endocarditis (ie, tricuspid or pulmonary valve vegetations) is most frequently associated with nonsterile technique in IV drug abusers.

DYSRHYTHMIAS

Ventricular Fibrillation and Pulseless Ventricular Tachycardia

- **Ventricular fibrillation** (see Figure 2.1-7) is disorganized electrical activity of the ventricular myocardium. Because the myocardium depolarizes in an irregular, disorganized fashion, regular myocardial contraction does not occur (looks like a "bag of worms").
- **Pulseless ventricular tachycardia:** Organized rapid contraction of myocardium, with insufficient filling time and lack of forward flow resulting in loss of pulse. It may degenerate into ventricular fibrillation. Both of these conditions are medical emergencies and require immediate cardioversion (shocking) and IV administration of amiodarone or lidocaine.

ETIOLOGY

- Can be caused by many things, but MI is the most common.
- Prolonged QT syndrome.
- Torsades de pointes.
- Wolff-Parkinson-White (WPW) with atrial fibrillaton and rapid ventricular response.
- Drugs (usually antidysrhythmic drugs!).

Ventricular fibrillation usually occurs after ventricular tachycardia.

FIGURE 2.1-7.   Ventricular fibrillation.

SIGNS AND SYMPTOMS

Ventricular fibrillation is not compatible with life. A patient with V-fib lasting more than 5–6 seconds will lose consciousness.

TREATMENT

- Emergent electrical cardioversion (shocking).
- Medications: Amiodarone/lidocaine as per ACLS protocol.
- **For prevention:**
  - Implanted cardioverter/defibrillator (ICD) in patients who have underlying conditions that predispose to VT/VF or survivors of cardiac arrest 2° to VT/VF (this does not prevent the rhythm, but treats it if it comes about).
  - Electrophysiologic testing and radiofrequency ablation for accessory bypass tracts, AV nodal re-entrant SVT, and others (basically you find the abnormal electrical tract in the myocardium and ablate it).

Torsades de Pointes

Wide-complex arrhythmia with rotating axis and prolonged QT (see Figure 2.1-8). Emergency—usually degenerates into ventricular fibrillation!

TREATMENT

- Magnesium IV
- Overdrive pacing
- Beta blockers for prolonged QT syndrome

Atrial Fibrillation

Disorganized electrical activity of the atrial myocardium, causing ineffective atrial contractions.

ETIOLOGY

Seen often in patients with dilated atria, related to heart failure or valvular disease.

> **Etiology of Torsades—**
>
> **POINTES**
>
> **P**henothiazines
> **O**ther meds (tricyclic antidepressants)
> **I**ntracranial bleed
> **N**o known cause (idiopathic)
> **T**ype I antidysrhythmics (quinidine and procainamide)
> **E**lectrolyte abnormalities (low K+ or Mg+)
> **S**yndrome of prolonged QT

> Rapid atrial fibrillation with a low blood pressure and symptoms. **Next step:** Cardioversion (key is that the patient is unstable).

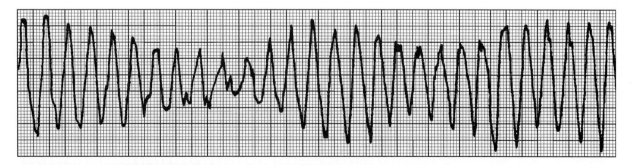

FIGURE 2.1-8. Torsades de pointes.

Note bizarre, twisted point of QRS complexes and varying amplitude.

Etiology of Atrial Fibrillation—

PIRATES

Pulmonary disease
Ischemia
Rheumatic heart disease
Anemia, atrial myxoma
Thyrotoxicosis
Ethanol
Sepsis

Atrial flutter may be confused with atrial fibrillation at high rates. Atrial flutter is distinguished by regular, distinct P waves in a sawtooth pattern.

Rapid atrial fibrillation is often difficult to identify. Adenosine can be used to temporarily slow a rapid supraventricular rhythm.

SIGNS AND SYMPTOMS

- Sensation of **palpitations** or skipped beats.
- **Light-headedness**, fatigue comes from the fact that without the "atrial kick" that the atrial contraction provides, the cardiac output falls.
- May develop chest pain.
- **Thrombus** can develop in dyskinetic atrium and then subsequently embolize to cause transient ischemic attack (**TIA**) **or stroke.**

DIAGNOSIS

- **ECG:** Absent P waves. Wavy undulating baseline: R-R interval is variable (see Figure 2.1-9).
- **Other findings:**
  - Pulse is irregularly irregular.
  - Echo: May be used to identify presence of clot in the left atrium.

TREATMENT

- **Rate control:** Slow rate with digoxin, calcium channel blocker (diltiazem), or beta blocker. Often just controlling rate but not changing rhythm can control symptoms. For these patients who stay in A-fib (or flip in and out [paroxysmal A-fib]), anticoagulation is necessary to prevent stroke.
- **Rhythm control:** In some cases the goal is to convert back to sinus rhythm. If patient has been in A-fib < 48 hours and no evidence of ischemia, synchronized cardioversion can be considered (shocking), and amiodarone and beta blockers can help maintain in sinus rhythm after conversion.
- **For unstable patients with any rate or duration of rhythm:** Immediate synchronized cardioversion (shock).

Wolff-Parkinson-White Syndrome (WPW)

WPW is a syndrome in which there is an "accessory pathway" that allows the electrical signal to travel from sinus node to ventricle bypassing the A-V node (this is called a "pre-excitation syndrome"), and then back up the normal His-Purkinje system. This results in an abnormal finding on ECG (delta wave—see below) and a risk for certain arrhythmias. *Anti-arrhythmia meds that block the AV-node (adenosine, beta blockers, calcium channel blockers, and digoxin) are contraindicated—will make it worse!*

FIGURE 2.1-9. Atrial fibrillation.

Note lack of P wave.

- ECG: Shows a "delta" wave, a slurred upstroke of the QRS complex (see Figure 2.1-10).
- Patients with suspected WPW should have electrophysiologic testing (test that finds the abnormal electrical tract) in the cardiac catheterization lab and radiofrequency ablation of the detected bypass tract.

TREATMENT

- **Unstable patients** with WPW and rapid atrial fibrillation with rapid ventricular response require emergent synchronized cardioversion.
- **Stable patients** with WPW and atrial fibrillation or wide-complex SVT are treated with procainamide, amiodarone, or sotalol.

Heart Block

- **First-degree** (see Figure 2.1-11):
  - Prolonged PR interval (> 0.20 s).
  - No treatment required, not usually a problem!
- **Second-degree** (two types—Mobitz I and II):
  - **Mobitz I (Wenckebach),** less dangerous (see Figure 2.1-12).
    - Progressive PR prolongation with progressive shortening of the R-R interval until a beat is dropped.
    - **Only if symptoms,** treat with atropine or temporary pacing.
  - **Mobitz II,** more dangerous (see Figure 2.1-13).
    - Fixed prolonged PR interval followed by a nonconducted beat at a regular interval.
    - Treat with atropine, temporary pacing, and permanent pacemaker.
    - **Dangerous**—always place pacemaker!
    - Important to treat quickly, as this can rapidly degenerate into complete heart block.
- **Third-degree** (complete heart block):
  - Independent atrial and ventricular activity (see Figure 2.1-14) (total asynchrony).
  - **Emergency**—treat symptomatic patients with atropine and temporary pacing, followed by permanent pacemaker.
  - Always needs pacemaker (dangerous rhythm).

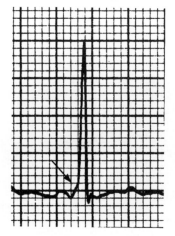

FIGURE 2.1-10. **Wolff-Parkinson-White syndrome.**

Note slurred upstroke of QRS (arrow) known as the "delta" wave.

Cardioversion in A-fib: The ineffective atrial contractions of A-fib permit clot formation in the left atrium, which may embolize to the systemic circulation. Unless a patient is unstable, anticoagulate prior to cardioversion.

Don't give ABCD (adenosine, beta blockers, calcium channel blocker, or digoxin) to someone with WPW. *Procainamide* is the classic choice.

Causes of Mobitz I:
- Inferior wall MI
- Digitalis toxicity
- ↑ vagal tone

Causes of Mobitz II:
- Inferior wall or septal MI
- Conduction system disease

Causes of third-degree heart block:
- Inferior wall MI
- Digitalis toxicity
- Conduction system disease

FIGURE 2.1-11. **First-degree AV block.**

Note pause (arrow) before QRS complex.

FIGURE 2.1-12. **Wenckebach second-degree AV block (Mobitz I).**

Note progressive lengthening of PR segment until a QRS complex is dropped. Arrow denotes nonconducted P wave.

FIGURE 2.1-13. **Mobitz II second-degree AV block.**

Note constant PR interval followed by a nonconducted P at a regular interval.

FIGURE 2.1-14. **Complete (third-degree) AV block.**

Note dissociation between atrial and ventricular rhythms. Arrows denote P waves.

CARDIOLOGY

Sinus Bradycardia

- Heart rate < 60.
- Normal P waves and PR intervals.

ETIOLOGY

- Medication (beta blocker, calcium channel blocker, digoxin).
- Inferior wall MI.
- ↑ intracranial pressure.
- Normal variant: Well-trained athletes can have very low resting heart rates.
- Carotid sinus hypersensitivity.
- Hypothyroidism.

SIGNS AND SYMPTOMS

Often asymptomatic; light-headedness and/or syncope can occur.

TREATMENT

- **Asymptomatic patients** do not require immediate treatment: Look for underlying cause.
- **Symptomatic patients:** Atropine +/– pacing.

Causes of Bradycardia—

"One INCH"

If the R-R distance is at least one inch, consider:
Overmedication
Inferior wall MI/ Increased intracranial pressure
Normal variant
Carotid sinus hypersensitivity
Hypothyroidism

HYPERTENSION

Defined as systolic BP > 140 or diastolic BP > 90 on two separate occasions (see Table 2.1-4).

EPIDEMIOLOGY

Twenty-five to thirty-five percent of adults have hypertension.

ETIOLOGY

- **Primary:** Essential hypertension (primary, idiopathic)—90% is this!
- **Secondary causes:**
  - Renal parenchymal disease (chronic pyelonephritis).
  - Renal artery stenosis.
  - Primary hyperaldosteronism (Cushing's and Conn's syndromes).
  - Pheochromocytoma.
  - Eclampsia and preeclampsia.
  - Coarctation of the aorta (congenital).

TABLE 2.1-4. Definition of Hypertension (JNC-7).

HYPERTENSION	SYSTOLIC BLOOD PRESSURE	DIASTOLIC BLOOD PRESSURE
Normal	< 120	< 80
Prehypertension	120–139	80–89
Stage 1	140–159	90–99
Stage 2	> 160	> 100

If patients do not fit into a discrete category, use the highest (worst) one.

CARDIOLOGY

43

PATHOPHYSIOLOGY

For primary, it is simply due to normal cardiac output with ↑ peripheral vascular resistance.

RISK FACTORS

- Diabetes
- High-sodium diet
- Obesity
- Tobacco use
- Family history of hypertension
- Black race
- Male gender

SIGNS AND SYMPTOMS

- Most patients with hypertension have no symptoms.
- Severe hypertension may present with:
  - Light-headedness.
  - Morning occipital headaches.
  - Epistaxis.
  - Hematuria.
  - Blurred vision.
  - Angina.
  - Congestive heart failure.

EVALUATION

- Blood pressure in both arms, repeated if abnormal.
- Funduscopic examination to look for AV nicking, retinal hemorrhage, papilledema.
- Auscultation for renal artery bruits.
- ECG may show LVH or left ventricular strain.
- Urinalysis to look for active sediment, hematuria.
- Blood urea nitrogen (BUN)/creatinine, serum potassium (evidence of renal insufficiency).

TREATMENT

For repeated elevated blood pressure measurements:

- **Nonpharmaceutical:**
  - Dietary changes: High fruits, vegetables, and low-fat dairy products, low total and saturated fats, low salt.
  - Weight loss, physical exercise.
- **Drug therapy:**
  - Low-dose thiazide diuretics are first choice for stage 1 hypertension.
  - Low-dose ACE inhibitor, calcium channel blockers, or beta blockers are also effective.
  - Two- or three-drug therapy for patients not initially controlled.

COMPLICATIONS

Hypertension ↑ risk of:

- Stroke
- MI
- Atrial fibrillation
- Heart failure

Hypertension due to **pheochromocytoma** is characterized by ectopic production of epinephrine and norepinephrine, causing wide swings in blood pressure.

What drug do you use for a diabetic patient with hypertension? ACE inhibitor (it will protect the kidneys also).

- Peripheral vascular disease
- Renal disease
- Retinopathy

> A 24-year-old woman with preeclampsia treated with IV drip of magnesium complains of difficulty breathing and has diminished reflexes. **Next step?** Stop magnesium and give IV calcium. (High magnesium levels result in cardiac suppression)

Hypertensive Emergency

Malignant hypertension is characterized by severely elevated blood pressure accompanied by end-organ damage. New-onset neurologic signs, papilledema, chest pain or heart failure, and renal failure should alert the physician to the need for rapid blood pressure reduction.

DIAGNOSIS

Presence of end-organ damage (ECG changes, new-onset renal failure, active urinary sediment, intracranial bleed, etc.).

TREATMENT

ICU monitoring is required. Reduce the mean arterial pressure by no more than 20%. Common intravenous agents include:

- Labetalol.
- Nitroprusside.
- If pheochromocytoma is the cause, use phentolamine.
- For preeclampsia-related hypertension, use magnesium or hydralazine.

Aortic Dissection

- Usually associated with a transverse tear through the intima and internal media of the aortic wall.
- Can → death by extension of the intimal tear to a full-thickness tear with hemorrhage into the extravascular space, dissection into the pericardium with tamponade, or extension into the branch arteries, including coronary arteries, carotids, mesenteric, renal, and iliac arteries.

CLASSIFICATION

- **DeBakey classification:**
  - Type I: Ascending plus part of distal aorta (most common).
  - Type II: Ascending aorta only.
  - Type III: Distal aorta only.
- **Stanford classification:**
  - Type A: Ascending aorta or both ascending and descending.
  - Type B: Descending aorta only.

ETIOLOGY

- **Hypertension.**
- Connective tissue disease: **Marfan's** (classic test question!) and Ehlers–Danlos syndromes.

An active urinary sediment contains blood, protein, and red and white cell casts.

The **mean arterial pressure (MAP)** is: (2dBP + sBP) / 3.

Use parenteral blood pressure–lowering agents only if end-organ damage is found, due to the risk of rapid reduction in coronary and cerebral perfusion with rapidly lowered blood pressure.

A patient presenting to the ER with tearing chest pain and has different blood pressures in each arm. **Next step?** Start an IV beta blocker ASAP (with or without nitrates). **Think:** Aortic dissection and order emergency CT angiogram to confirm.

Aortic dissection due to syphilis occurs because the *Treponema* infects the vasa vasorum of the aorta.

- Congenital heart disease.
- Trauma.
- Pregnancy (third trimester).
- Aortic coarctation: Turner's syndrome, idiopathic.
- Cocaine use (hypertension), syphilis.

SIGNS AND SYMPTOMS

- Severe *"tearing"* chest pain, may radiate to back.
- Unequal pulses distally for descending aortic dissection.
- Aortic regurgitation murmur transmitted down right sternal border with ascending aortic dissection.

 A middle-aged man comes to the ER with severe hypertension and a tearing pain in his back. **What do you do?** Control hypertension with labetolol and do a CT-dissection study to rule out aortic dissection.

DIAGNOSIS

- If aortic dissection is strongly suspected despite negative studies, the gold standard is aortic angiogram.
- **Other findings with other tests:** Helical CT with IV contrast or transesophageal echocardiography can also diagnose; may show dissection with extravasation of blood, intimal flap.
- **CXR:** Can be normal but often shows **widened mediastinum**, apical pleural capping, and loss of the aortic knob.

TREATMENT

- Blood pressure control is crucial! Use beta blocker + nitroprusside to keep SBP below 120, as long as the patient can maintain organ perfusion.
- Immediate surgical repair for type A dissection (ascending aorta).
- Medical stabilization for type B dissection (descending aorta).

COMPLICATIONS

- MI: Dissection or obstruction of coronary arteries.
- Stroke: Dissection or obstruction of carotids.
- Aortic regurgitation: Dissection through aortic root.
- Cardiac tamponade: Dissection into pericardium which fills with blood and compresses heart.

BACTERIAL ENDOCARDITIS

Localized infection of the endocardium characterized by vegetations involving the valve leaflets or walls. It is best categorized by the infecting organism, which determines the course of the disease. It can also be classified as acute or subacute.

- **Acute bacterial endocarditis (ABE):**
  - Infection of **healthy valves** by high-virulence organisms.
  - Produces metastatic foci (embolizes).

Causes of aortic dissection—

PATC³H

Pregnancy
Aortic coarctation
Trauma
Cocaine, **C**ongenital, **C**onnective tissue
Hypertension

 Always get a chest film when you suspect MI—some of these patients will have aortic dissection, and thrombolysis may kill them. If there is a widened mediastinum, do not give lytics!

Staphylococcus lugdunensis is the organism that most often causes aggressive endocarditis requiring surgical intervention.

- Usually fatal if not treated within 6 weeks.
- Most common organism is *Staphylococcus aureus*.
- **Subacute bacterial endocarditis (SBE):**
  - Seeding of **previously damaged valves or abnormal** (rheumatic heart disease, congenital valve defects: mitral valve prolapse) by low-virulence organisms.
  - May not *always* result in embolic phenomena.
  - Most common organism is *Streptococcus viridans*.
  - Mitral valve is most often affected.

ETIOLOGY

- **Acute**: *S aureus*, gram-negative organisms.
- **Subacute**: *S viridans*, other oral flora, group A beta-hemolytic strep, enterococci, *Staphylococcus epidermidis*.
- **Special conditions:**
  - **IV drug users**: *S aureus*, streptococci, enterococci, *Candida*.
  - **Prosthetic valves** (10–20% of cases): *S aureus*, *S viridans*, gram-negative bacilli, fungi.
  - **Nosocomial infections:** Indwelling venous catheters, hemodialysis, CT surgery.

SIGNS AND SYMPTOMS

- **ABE:**
  - Acute onset of fever, chills, rigors.
  - New cardiac murmur.
  - Metastatic infections—meningitis, pneumonia.
- **SBE:**
  - Gradual onset of fever, sweats, weakness, arthralgia, anorexia, weight loss, and cutaneous lesions.
  - New cardiac murmur.
  - Splenomegaly.
  - Petechiae: Multiple nonblanching red macules on upper chest and mucous membranes.
- **Other findings:**
  - **Osler's nodes:** *Tender* violaceous subcutaneous nodules on fingers and toes (see Figure 2.1-15).
  - **Splinter hemorrhages:** Fine linear hemorrhages in middle of nail bed (see Figure 2.1-16).
  - **Janeway lesions:** Multiple hemorrhagic *nontender* macules or nodules on palms and soles (see Figure 2.1-17).
- **Roth's spots:** Retinal hemorrhages seen on funduscopy.
- Conjunctival hemorrhages.

DIAGNOSIS

Duke's criteria (patient must have 2 major, 1 major + 3 minor, or 5 minor criteria for diagnosis):

- **Major criteria:**
  - Two positive blood cultures taken at least 12 hours apart, or 3+ positive cultures taken at least 1 hour apart with typical organisms.
  - Echocardiography—vegetations are pathognomonic, but their absence does not rule out endocarditis; transesophageal echo is more sensitive.

The organism that most often causes endocarditis in IV drug users? *Staph aureus.*

Right-sided acute bacterial endocarditis often affects the tricuspid valve and septic pulmonary emboli are common. *Think: IV drug users.*

There is a strong association between *Streptococcus bovis* endocarditis and colonic neoplasms.

FIGURE 2.1-15.   Osler's node.

(Photo contributor: Armed Forces Institute of Pathology, Bethesda, Maryland. Reproduced, with permission, from Knoop KJ, Stack LB, Storrow AB. *Atlas of Emergency Medicine*. 3rd ed. New York: McGraw-Hill, 2010: 375.)

- **Minor criteria:**
  - Predisposing lesion on valve or IV drug use.
  - Fever > 38°C.
  - Arterial emboli (Janeway lesions).
  - Osler's nodes, Roth's spots.
  - Positive blood cultures not meeting major criteria.
  - Echocardiogram suspicious for endocarditis but not meeting major criteria.

FIGURE 2.1-16.   Splinter hemorrhage.

(Photo contributor: Armed Forces Institute of Pathology, Bethesda, Maryland. Reproduced, with permission, from Knoop KJ, Stack LB, Storrow AB. *Atlas of Emergency Medicine*. 3rd ed. New York: McGraw-Hill, 2010: 375.)

FIGURE 2.1-17. Janeway lesion.

(Photo contributor: Department of Dermatology, Wilford Hall USAF Medical Center and Brooke Army Medical Center, San Antonio, Texas. Reproduced, with permission, from Knoop KJ, Stack LB, Storrow AB. *Atlas of Emergency Medicine.* 3rd ed. New York: McGraw-Hill, 2010: 374.)

TREATMENT

- Streptococci: Penicillin G or ceftriaxone × 4 weeks.
- Staphylococci: Nafcillin or oxacillin × 4 weeks.
- MRSA: Vancomycin × 4 weeks.

RHEUMATIC FEVER

- **Rheumatic fever (RF)** is a systemic immune process that usually occurs secondary to pharyngeal streptococcal infection.
- **Rheumatic heart disease (RHD)** is the occurrence of valvular abnormalities due to immune complex deposition in valve leaflets generated by rheumatic fever.

ETIOLOGY

Recent streptococcal infection of pharynx.

Most common valve affected by RHD is mitral, followed by aortic, then tricuspid.

DIAGNOSIS

- **Laboratory findings:**
  - Positive antistreptolysin-O (ASLO) antibody titers.
  - Elevated ESR.
- Diagnosis of rheumatic fever requires presence of two major criteria or one major and two minor criteria.
  - **Major criteria:**
    - Arthritis (migratory, multiple joints).
    - Carditis (endo-, myo-, peri-).
    - Erythema marginatum rash.
    - Subcutaneous nodules.
    - Sydenham's chorea.
  - **Minor criteria:**
    - Fever.
    - Arthralgias.
    - Elevated ESR.
    - Prolonged PR interval.
    - Recent streptococcal pharyngitis.

TREATMENT

- **Acute:**
  - Course of penicillin to eradicate throat carriage of group A streptococci.
  - Aspirin for arthritis.
  - Steroids for carditis.
- **Chronic:**
  - Monthly doses of benzathine penicillin to prevent recurrences.
  - Follow-up with cardiologist in severe cases.

The reason for treating strep throat is to prevent the complication of rheumatic fever, not due to worry of the pharyngitis itself, which would resolve without antibiotics.

DYSLIPIDEMIA

About half of all cases of coronary artery disease are associated with disorders of lipid metabolism. Formulas for calculating lipid levels:

- LDL = TC – HDL – VLDL
- VLDL = Trig/5
- Total cholesterol (TC):
  - Normal: < 200
  - Borderline: 200–240
  - High: > 240
- Normal HDL: 30–100

Major Lipoproteins

A level of HDL > 60 is cardioprotective.

- Chylomicrons: Transport cholesterol from the gut in the bloodstream.
- Chylomicron remnants: Left over after lipoprotein lipase liberates free fatty acids from chylomicrons for use in tissues.
- Very low-density lipoprotein (VLDL): Secreted from the liver; carries cholesterol in the bloodstream.
- Intermediate-density lipoprotein (IDL): Metabolized from VLDL.

- LDL: Metabolized from IDL, it carries cholesterol in the bloodstream to tissues.
- HDL: Uptakes free cholesterol secreted by tissues and transports it to the liver.

Isolated Hypercholesterolemia

- Familial hypercholesterolemia: Elevated LDL (type IIa).
- Familial defective apo B100: Elevated LDL (type IIa).
- Polygenic hypercholesterolemia: Elevated LDL (type IIa).

Isolated Hypertriglyceridemia

- Familial hypertriglyceridemia: Elevated VLDL (type IV).
- Familial lipoprotein lipase deficiency: Elevated chylomicrons (type I, V).
- Familial apo CII deficiency: Elevated chylomicrons (type I, V).

Combined Hypertriglyceridemia and Hypercholesterolemia

- Combined hyperlipidemia: Elevated VLDL, LDL (type IIb).
- Dysbetalipoproteinemia: Elevated VLDL, IDL (type III).

PHYSICAL FINDINGS

- Xanthelasma: Painless, nonpruritic raised yellow plaques that occur on eyelids near inner canthi.
- Xanthoma: Reddish brown papules on scalp, face, trunk, and flexor surfaces of limbs.

DIAGNOSIS

- Serum lipoprotein analysis is done after a 12-hour fast.
- One-time sample cholesterol levels may not represent true levels in the following circumstances:
  - Weight loss
  - Pregnancy
  - Major surgery
  - Severe illness
- *Note:* In patients who have MI, lipoprotein levels obtained within the first 24 hours will more closely approximate true pre-MI levels than later levels, which may not return to baseline for several weeks.
- For cholesterol levels, see Table 2.1-5.

TREATMENT OF HYPERCHOLESTEROLEMIA

Goals of treatment:

- For a patient with 0–1 risk factors (low risk), keep LDL ≤ 160.
- For a patient with 1–2 risk factors (moderate risk), keep LDL ≤ 130.
- For a patient with known atherosclerotic heart disease (high risk), keep LDL ≤ 70.
- For treatment strategies, see Table 2.1-6.

A high-risk cardiac patient who is on a statin and has a good LDL but a low HDL should be started on fibrate.

Patients with very high triglyceride levels (> 1,000) are at risk of developing pancreatitis.

TABLE 2.1-5. Cholesterol Levels Associated with Familial Disease

	TYPE	TOTAL CHOLESTEROL LEVEL (mg/dL)	LDL LEVEL	VLDL	CHYLOMICRONS
Familial hypercholesterolemia	IIa	275–500	High	Normal	Normal
Familial defective apo B100	IIa	275–500	High	Normal	Normal
Polygenic hypercholesterolemia	IIa	240–350	High	Normal	Normal
Familial hypertriglyceridemia	IV	250–750	Normal/High	High	Normal/High
Familial lipoprotein lipase deficiency	I, (I,V)	> 750	Normal/High	Normal/High	High
Familial apoprotein CII deficiency	I, (I,V)	> 750	Normal/High	Normal/High	High
Familial combined hyperlipidemia	IIb	250–500	High	High	Normal/High
Dysbetalipoproteinemia	III	250–500	Normal	High	Normal/High

TABLE 2.1-6. Treatment of Hypercholesterolemia

TREATMENT	MECHANISM	RESULTS
Diet therapy	Therapeutic Lifestyle Changes (TLC) diet ■ Total fat 25–30% total calories ■ Polyunsaturated fat < 10% ■ Monounsaturated fat < 20% ■ Carbohydrate 50–60% ■ Fiber 20–30 g/day ■ Protein 15% total calories ■ Saturated fat < 10% ■ Dietary cholesterol < 300 mg/day	Step 2 diet reduces total cholesterol by 10–12%. Exercise variably raises HDL. If diet therapy and exercise fail by 6 weeks, progress to medications.
Statins	Statins are HMG-CoA reductase inhibitors and act to ↓ LDL and ↑ HDL.	Can lower LDL cholesterol by 35% and raise HDL by −8%.
Bile acid sequestrants	Cholestyramine and colestipol bind bile acids in the gut.	Reduces LDL cholesterol by 15–20%.
Nicotinic acid	Reduces lipolysis in adipose tissue, inhibits hepatic synthesis of cholesterol.	Can reduce LDL cholesterol by −20% over 6 months. Side effects include cutaneous flushing, abdominal pain, nausea.
Fibrinates	Best for reducing triglycerides (in VLDL and chylomicrons).	↑ HDL by 5–30%.

	MEDICATION	MAIN CLINICAL USES	ADVERSE EFFECTS
Class I: Sodium channel blockers	Lidocaine	Suppresses ventricular dysrhythmias.	Mild: drowsiness, confusion, ataxia. Severe: psychosis, seizures, AV block, respiratory depression.
	Quinidine	Suppresses ventricular dysrhythmias, atrial premature beats, A-fib.	Cinchonism: tinnitus, hearing loss, visual changes, delirium, psychosis. Also causes GI upset, promotes torsades de pointes (prodysrhythmic). Potentiates many other medications.
	Procainamide	Suppresses ventricular dysrhythmias and A-fib, A-flutter, WPW.	Myocardial depression, prolonged QT and QRS, torsades de pointes, V-fib.
Class II: Beta blockers	Propranolol	SVT, thyrotoxicosis, acute MI, hypertension.	All beta blockers can cause bronchoconstriction; use with caution in asthmatics. Hypotension, light-headedness, fatigue, depression, and elevation of triglycerides can occur.
	Metoprolol	SVT, acute MI, hypertension.	
	Esmolol	SVT, thyrotoxicosis.	
	Labetalol	Hypertension.	
Class III: Prolongs action potentials	Amiodarone	VT, VF, A-fib, WPW.	Bradycardia, AV block, peripheral neuropathy, pulmonary fibrosis, corneal deposits, skin discoloration, hepatotoxicity. Due to high iodine content, can cause hypo- or hyperthyroidism.
	Bretylium	Ventricular dysrhythmias.	Transient hypertension, hypotension.
	Sotalol	AV reentry SVT, WPW	Bradycardia, CHF, peripheral edema.

	MEDICATION	MAIN CLINICAL USES	ADVERSE EFFECTS
Class IV: Calcium channel blockers	Verapamil	Mild to moderate hypertension.	Calcium channel blockers reduce inotropy and are contraindicated in patients with heart failure, 2nd- or 3rd-degree heart block.
	Diltiazem	Mild to moderate hypertension.	
	Amlodipine, nifedipine	Mild to moderate hypertension.	
Other antidysrhythmic agents	Adenosine	Supraventricular tachycardia.	Transient asystole, hypotension, flushing.
	Digoxin	Rate control of atrial tachydysrhythmia, increased inotropy for CHF.	Toxicity can occur in therapeutic range. Vomiting, anorexia, confusion, visual changes, AV block, PVCs, VT, VF. Hyperkalemia is seen with acute poisoning. Hypokalemia lowers threshold for toxicity (remember, many drugs used for CHF can cause hypokalemia). Chronic therapy can cause gynecomastia.
	Magnesium	Torsades de pointes, hypertension due to preeclampsia.	Hypotension, flushing, CNS changes, decreased reflexes, respiratory collapse.
	Epinephrine	Asystole, anaphylaxis, pressor.	May cause ischemia.
Inotropic agents	Dopamine	Increases inotropy, chronotropic, pressor.	Increases peripheral vasoconstriction at doses > 5–10 µg/kg/min.
	Dobutamine	Increases inotropy.	Associated with reflex arterial vasodilatation and tachycardia.
Chronotropic agents	Atropine	Asystole, symptomatic bradycardia.	Anticholinergic.
Venous/coronary dilators	Nitroglycerin	Venous and coronary artery dilator, can be used for malignant hypertension.	Hypotension, headache.
Antihypertensive agents	Nitroprusside	Malignant hypertension.	Can cause hypotension, cyanide toxicity, methemoglobinemia.
	Minoxidil	Severe hypertension.	Can cause hypotension, tachycardia, hair growth.

MEDICATION	MAIN CLINICAL USES	ADVERSE EFFECTS
Hydralazine	Moderate to severe hypertension, particularly in the setting of preeclampsia and eclampsia. Hydralazine is a direct vasodilator.	Can cause tachycardia, angina, lupus-like syndrome with a malar rash that disappears after discontinuing the drug.
Clonidine	Central-acting agent for hypertension.	Hypotension, rebound hypertension after halting medication.
Phentolamine	Parenteral alpha blocker used for hypertension due to pheochromocytoma, cocaine.	Hypotension, tachycardia, light-headedness.
Prazosin	PO alpha-blocker used for mild to moderate hypertension.	
ACE inhibitors	Hypertension (decrease preload and afterload), nephroprotective CHF. Decrease cardiovascular events and mortality in high-risk patients > 55 years old.	All ACE inhibitors are variably associated with cough and angioedema and can cause acute renal failure in patients with bilateral renal artery stenosis. Hyperkalemia.
Angiotensin receptor blockers	Hypertension. Unclear magnitude of renal protection compared to ACE inhibitors.	Side effects similar to ACE inhibitors but less cough.
Antiplatelet agents — Aspirin	Used to prevent MI in patients with risk factors, can improve mortality from MI by about 25%.	Associated with GI bleed. Some patients can have hypersensitivity reaction to aspirin.
2b,3a inhibitors	Intravenous adjunct to heparin and thrombolysis in setting of acute MI; best use still being investigated.	Can be associated with excessive bleeding.
Antithrombotic agents — Warfarins	Long-term prevention of clots in deep vein thrombosis (DVT), A-fib, stroke, and others.	Warfarins have an initial procoagulant effect. When anticoagulating as an inpatient, use heparin coverage initially. For outpatients, start at very low doses and raise gradually.
Heparins	Myocardial infarction, pulmonary embolism, deep venous thrombosis.	Both low-molecular-weight and unfractionated heparins can be associated with excessive bleeding.

CARDIOLOGY

MEDICATION		MAIN CLINICAL USES	ADVERSE EFFECTS
Thrombolytic agents	Streptokinase	Myocardial infarction, pulmonary embolism, embolic cerebrovascular accident (CVA).	Relatively low cost. Cannot be used more than once within a 6-month period. Associated with hemorrhage at various sites.
	Tissue plasminogen activator	Myocardial infarction, pulmonary embolism, embolic CVA.	High cost. Associated with hemorrhage at various sites.

HOW TO PRESENT AN ELECTROCARDIOGRAM (ECG)

First, confirm that the ECG belongs to your patient. If possible, compare to a previous tracing. Then, present in a systematic manner:

1. *Rate* (see Figure 2.1-18): The rate is [number of] beats per minute (bpm):
   - The ECG paper is scored so that one big box is 0.20 seconds. These big boxes consist of five little boxes, each of which is 0.04 seconds.
   - A quick way to calculate rate when the rhythm is regular is the mantra: **300, 150, 100, 75, 60, 50** (= 300 / # large boxes), which is measured as the number of large boxes between two QRS complexes. Therefore, a distance of one large box between two adjacent QRS complexes would be a rate of 300, while a distance of five large boxes between two adjacent QRS complexes would be a rate of 60.
   - For irregular rhythms, count the number of complexes that occur in a 6-second interval (30 large boxes) and multiply by 10 to get a rate in bpm.
2. *Rhythm:* The rhythm is [sinus]/[atrial fibrillation]/[atrial flutter] or other:
   - If p waves are present in all leads and upright in lead I and inverted in lead AVR, then the rhythm is sinus. Lack of p waves suggests a disorganized atrial rhythm, a junctional rhythm, or a ventricular rhythm. A ventricular rhythm (V-fib or V-tach) is an unstable one

FIGURE 2.1-18. Calculating rate.

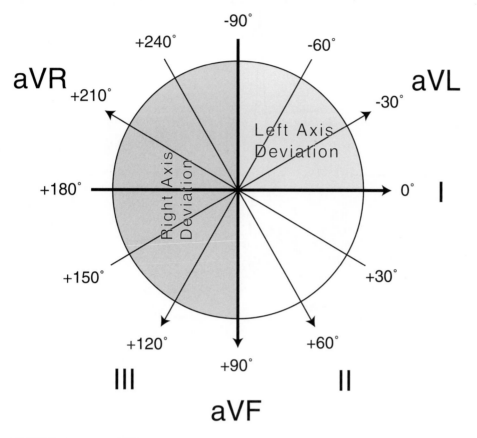

FIGURE 2.1-19. **ECG axes.**

(could spell imminent death), and you should be getting ready for advanced cardiac life support (ACLS).

- Normal sinus rhythm is usually a regular narrow-complex rhythm with each QRS complex preceded by a p wave.

3. *Axis* (see Figure 2.1-19): The axis is [normal]/[deviated to the right]/[deviated to the left]:
    - If I and aVF are both upright or positive, then the axis is normal.
    - If I is upright and aVF is upside down, then there is left axis deviation (LAD).
    - If I is upside down and aVF is upright, then there is right axis deviation (RAD).
    - If I and aVF are both upside down or negative, then there is extreme RAD.

4. *Intervals* (see Figure 2.1-20): The [PR]/[QRS] intervals are [normal]/[short-ened]/[widened]:
    - Normal PR interval = 0.12 to 0.20 seconds:
    - Short PR is associated with Wolff-Parkinson-White syndrome (WPW).
    - WPW syndrome is characterized by a "delta" wave, or slurred upstroke of QRS complex.
    - Long PR interval is associated with heart block, of which there are three types:
        - First-degree block: PR interval > 0.20 seconds (one big box).

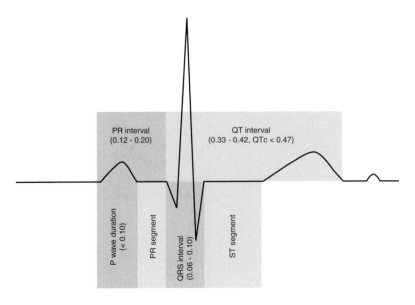

FIGURE 2.1-20. **ECG intervals.**

■ Second-degree (Mobitz type I or Wenckebach) block: PR interval lengthens progressively until a QRS is dropped.
■ Second-degree (Mobitz type II) block: PR interval is constant, but one QRS is dropped at a fixed interval.
■ Third-degree heart block: P waves and QRS complexes have independent rates, no association is noted between P waves and QRS complexes.

■ Normal QRS interval ≤ 0.12 seconds: Prolonged QRS is seen when the beat is initiated in the ventricle rather than the sinoatrial node, when there is a bundle branch block, and when the heart is artificially paced with longer QRS intervals. Prolonged QRS is also noted in tricyclic overdose and Wolff-Parkinson-White syndrome.

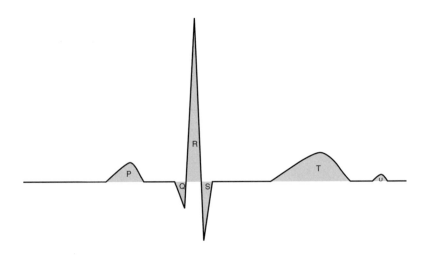

FIGURE 2.1-21. **ECG wave morphology.**

5. *Wave morphology* (see Figure 2.1-21):
   a. *Ventricular hypertrophy*: There [is/is no] [left/right] [ventricular/ atrial] hypertrophy. There are multiple criteria for determining right (RVH) and left ventricular hypertrophy (LVH). A few are listed here:
      - *Clues for LVH:*
         - $R_I > 15$ mm
         - $R_{I, II \text{ or } aVF} > 20$ mm
         - $R_{aVL} > 11$ mm
         - R_{V5} or $R_{V6} > 26$ mm
         - $R_I + S_{III} > 25$ mm
         - R + S in V lead > 45 mm
         - $S_{V1} + R_{V5}$ or $R_{V6} > 35$ mm
      - *Clues for RVH:*
         - $R_{V1} > 7$ mm
         - $S_{V1} < 2$ mm
         - R/S ratio in $V_1 > 1$
         - RAD of 110° or more
   b. *Atrial hypertrophy*:
      - Right atrial hypertrophy: Tall or peaked p waves in limb or precordial leads.
      - Left atrial hypertrophy: Broad or notched p waves in limb leads.
   c. *Ischemic changes*: There [are/are no] S-T wave [depressions/elevations] or [flattened/inverted] T waves. Presence of Q wave indicates an old infarct.
   d. *Bundle branch block*: There [is/is no] [left/right] bundle branch block. Clues:
      - Presence of RSR′ wave in leads V_1–V_3 with ST depression and T wave inversion goes with RBBB.
      - Presence of notched R wave in leads I, aVL, and V_4–V_6 goes with LBBB.

Endocrinology

Type 1 Diabetes Mellitus

- Type 1 diabetes is characterized by absolute insulin deficiency from selective autoimmune destruction of the pancreatic beta cells, which are responsible for producing insulin.
- It accounts for < 10% of all diabetes cases and mainly affects lean children, teenagers, and young adults. Usually diagnosed before age 30.

ETIOLOGY

- **Type 1A diabetes:** Autoimmune-mediated diabetes. There are strong genetic associations with linkage to the HLA DQA and DQB genes. Several autoantibodies directly against the beta cells or their products are usually detectable:
  - Anti–islet cell autoantigen (anti-ICA).
  - Anti–glutamic acid decarboxylase (anti-GAD).
  - Anti-insulin antibodies.
  - Antibody to the tyrosine phosphatase IA-2.
- **Type 1B diabetes:** Idiopathic, with no autoimmune markers, occurs more commonly in Asian or African ancestry.

HbA$_{1c}$ and corresponding average blood glucose levels:

HbA$_{1c}$	Blood glucose
6	120
7	150
8	180
9	210

(Increments of 30)

 A woman presents with a recurrent vaginal candidiasis that is refractory to treatment. *Think: Diabetes mellitus.* **Next step:** Get a finger stick for blood glucose.

SIGNS AND SYMPTOMS

Usually presents with symptomatic hyperglycemia or diabetic ketoacidosis (discussed later).

- Polyuria.
- Polydipsia.
- Weight loss.
- Dehydration.
- Blurred vision.
- Fatigue.
- Foot ulcers.
- Can get restrictive cardiomyopathy without coronary artery disease.

DIAGNOSIS

- Confirmed with a fasting serum glucose of > 126 mg/dL.
- Glycosuria (causes an osmotic diuresis that leads to dehydration).
- HbA$_{1c}$ is a measure of glucose control over the past 3 months. Most complications can be prevented if the HbA$_{1c}$ level is kept below 7%.

TREATMENT

Treated solely with insulin (see Table 2.2-1 for types); oral agents have no role in its management.

The only treatment for Type 1 DM patients is insulin (both long and short acting), administered by subcutaneous injection. Oral hypoglycemics have no role in management because these patients have no functioning pancreatic beta cells.

ENDOCRINOLOGY

TABLE 2.2-1. Insulin Preparations and Their Pharmacokinetic Properties

PREPARATION	ONSET	PEAK (HR)	DURATION (HR)
Rapid-acting			
Insulin lispro	10–15 min	1–2	3–5
Insulin aspart	10–15 min	1–2	3–5
Short-acting			
Regular	30–60 min	2–4	4–8
Intermediate-acting			
Neutral Protamine Hagedorn (NPH)	1–3 hrs	4–10	10–18
Lente	2–4 hrs	4–12	10–20
Long-acting			
Insulin detemir	2–3 hrs	No peak	Up to 24 hrs
Insulin glargine	2–3 hrs	No peak	24 hrs

Measure finger-stick glucose levels 5×/day:
- Morning fasting
- Breakfast postprandial
- Lunch postprandial
- Dinner postprandial
- Before bed

Postprandial is 2 hours after the meal.

 A 60-year-old diabetic who was recently started on insulin came back with complaints of high finger sticks in the early morning with recurrent nightmares. *Think: Somogyi effect.* **What will you do?** Change to longer acting insulin at night to avoid 3 AM hypoglycemia.

Initiating Therapy
- Patients are usually hospitalized at the time of initial diagnosis (because often present with DKA which is dangerous) and are treated with regular insulin.
- The average total daily dose of regular insulin is used as the initial dose of outpatient insulin therapy (be conservative so as not to induce hypoglycemic episodes).
- Divide the total daily dose to give two-thirds before breakfast and one-third before dinner if using NPH or 70/30 preparations.
- Initially, the patient should monitor finger-stick glucose levels five times a day and keep a record of the levels:
  - Choose the regimen that is easiest for the patient to follow while maintaining good blood glucose control.
  - **Type I DM patients must always take insulin to avoid ketosis, even if fasting** (may decrease dose).

ENDOCRINOLOGY

DAWN PHENOMENON

An exaggeration of the normal tendency of the plasma glucose to rise in the early morning hours before breakfast, probably secondary to an increase in growth hormone (GH) secretion.

SOMOGYI EFFECT

- Characterized by nighttime hypoglycemia followed by a dramatic increase in fasting glucose levels and increased plasma ketones.
- If Somogyi phenomenon is suspected, patients should check their blood glucose around 3 AM Hypoglycemia at this time confirms diagnosis.
- **The morning hyperglycemia is a rebound effect.**
- Replacement of intermediate-acting insulin with long-acting insulin at bedtime can prevent this effect (want to try to avoid peaking of insulin effect in the middle of the night).

If a patient has hypoglycemic finger sticks in AM, decrease the bedtime NPH, even if the bedtime finger sticks are high.

Type 2 Diabetes Mellitus

- Type 2 diabetes is characterized by variable degrees of **insulin deficiency and insulin resistance.**
- It accounts for > 90% of diabetes cases in the United States. Usually diagnosed after age 30, but increasingly seen in adolescents and children due to rising incidence of obesity and sedentary lifestyle.
- Concordance rate for type 2 DM in monozygotic twins is > 90% (< 50% in type 1).
- Commonly associated with obesity, and often presents after period of weight gain.

> A patient presents with persistent morning hyperglycemia, despite steadily increasing his nighttime NPH insulin dose. He also complains of frequent nightmares. His wife brings him in because she witnessed him having a seizure in the middle of the night. *Think: Somogyi effect.* **Next step:** Check 3 AM blood glucose.

ETIOLOGY

- Hyperglycemia is caused by:
  - Impaired secretion of insulin.
  - Decreased cellular responsiveness to insulin.
  - Impaired inhibition of hepatic gluconeogenesis.
- The syndrome of insulin resistance (**metabolic syndrome**—see below) associated with hyperglycemia leading to obesity, hypertension, hyperlipidemia, and coronary artery disease.
- Glucose toxicity: Hyperglycemia itself can induce impaired glucose tolerance and increased hepatic glucoseogenesis.

SIGNS AND SYMPTOMS

- Patients may be asymptomatic.
- Presenting complaint is often a complication of their diabetes, such as a soft tissue infection. Can also present with signs of hyperglycemia.

It is important for diabetics to have their feet frequently inspected to look for small cuts that may develop into ulcers. Due to neuropathy, diabetics can often have significant foot pathology and not feel anything.

Diabetics have increased susceptibility to infections due to decreased efficacy of granulocytes despite normal number:

- *Pseudomonas*
- Mucormycoses
- Actinomycoses
- Aspergillosis (eosinophilic pneumonia with asthma; treat with steroids)
- Renal abscesses (with urinary tract infections)

Metformin and thiazolidinediones are contraindicated in patients with advanced heart failure.

- Increased susceptibility to fungal infections (cell-mediated immunity is impaired by acute hyperglycemia).
- Patients with type 2 DM will suffer from DKA only in rare instances (called ketosis-prone or atypical type 2 diabetes).
- The nonketotic hyperglycemic-hyperosmolar coma (NKHC) is more common in type 2 DM, but still rare.

DIAGNOSIS

Requires any one of the following:

- Random glucose > 200 mg/dL in the presence of symptoms.
- Asymptomatic patients require a fasting glucose of > 126 mg/dL on two separate occasions.
- If patients have fasting glucose levels of > 100 mg/dL and < 126 mg/dL, an oral glucose tolerance test is indicated.
- Positive oral glucose tolerance test is a plasma glucose > 200 mg/dL at 2 hours after ingesting 75 g of glucose in solution.

TREATMENT

- Initial management should consist of **education,** diet, and exercise to achieve weight control.
- Patient education increases compliance with diet, exercise, and medication therapy. Discussions should involve when to seek medical attention, side effects of medications, proper foot care, ophthalmology visits, and symptoms of hyper- and hypoglycemia.
- If glycemic control cannot be obtained with diet and exercise, start oral hypoglycemic.
- Combination of low-dose insulin secretogogues (Glyburide) plus low-dose insulin sensitizers (metformin) may improve HbA_{1c} with few side effects but DPP-4 inhibitors are also being increasingly used in the initial therapeutic regimen.
- Patients not controlled with oral hypoglycemics alone may require insulin.
- Glucose-lowering drugs: See Table 2.2-2.

Metabolic Syndrome

A constellation of findings that lead to increased risk of cardiovascular disease such as myocardial infarction, stroke, and death. With the growing epidemic of obesity, the prevalence of metabolic syndrome is rapidly increasing even among adolescents and children. The definition of metabolic syndrome in adults includes at least three of the following:

1. Fasting plasma glucose ≥ 100 mg/dL (6.1 mmol/L).
2. Abdominal obesity: waist girth > 102 cm (> 40 in) for men and > 88 cm (> 35 in) for women.
3. Serum TG > 150 mg/dL (1.7 mmol/L).
4. HDL-C < 40 mg/dL (1 mmol/L) for men; < 50 mg/dL (1.3 mmol/L) for women.
5. Blood pressure ≥ 130/85 mm Hg or on medications.

TABLE 2.2-2. Glucose-Lowering Drugs

Sulfonylureas: glimepiride, glyburide, glipizide	▪ HgA$_{1C}$ change: Moderately effective, lower blood glucose by 20% and A$_{1C}$ by 1–2%. ▪ Mechanism: Stimulates insulin secretion from the pancreas. ▪ Benefits: Extensive experience; low cost; daily dosing. ▪ Risks/Concerns: Hypoglycemia especially with renal disease; weight gain; may impede ischemic preconditioning.
Meglitinides: repaglinide (Prandin), nateglinide (Starlix)	▪ HgA$_{1C}$ change: Reduce A$_{1C}$ by 1–2%. ▪ Mechanism: Increase insulin production by the pancreas. ▪ Benefits: Less hypoglycemia, targets postprandial glucose, mimics physiological insulin secretion. ▪ Risks/Concerns: Short-acting glucose lowering drugs, should be taken before each meal; slightly less effective compared to sulfonylureas.
Biguanides: metformin	▪ HgA$_{1C}$ change: Reduce A$_{1C}$ by 1–2%. ▪ Mechanism: Decreases liver's glucose production and slightly increases muscle glucose uptake. ▪ Benefits: No weight gain; no hypoglycemia when used alone (it may even lead to initial weight loss). ▪ Risks/Concerns: Major side effects are GI symptoms; most serious side effect is lactic acidosis (50% mortality). ▪ Contraindications: Within 24–48 hours of injection of radiographic contrast material; renal disease with GFR < 60 mL/min or creatinine > 1.5 (increased risk of lactic acidosis); liver disease; CHF; excessive alcohol intake. ▪ *Note: Unless contraindicated, it is the first choice for an oral hypoglycemic agent.*
Thiazolidinediones: troglitazone, rosiglitazone, pioglitazone	▪ HgA$_{1C}$ change: Reduce A$_{1C}$ by 0.5–1.4%. ▪ Mechanism: Decreases insulin resistance at the muscle and liver. ▪ Benefits: No hypoglycemia; may improve HDL cholesterol and triglycerides. ▪ Risks/Concerns: Slow onset of action (take 4–6 weeks to see an effect on blood glucose); weight gain (subcutaneous insulin-sensitive fat); fluid retention; major side effects is hepatotoxicity, which requires liver monitoring; expensive. ▪ Contraindications: Class III and IV heart failure and liver disease. Recently, there has been a concern for increased cardiovascular disease that lead to FDA warning.
Alpha-glucosidase inhibitors: acarbose, miglitol	▪ HgA$_{1C}$ change: Reduce A$_{1C}$ by 0.5–1.0%. ▪ Mechanism: Slows the digestion of carbohydrates. ▪ Benefits: No weight gain; no hypoglycemia when used alone. ▪ Risks/Concerns: Major side effects are GI symptoms (transient diarrhea, nausea, and abdominal pain); caution use with IBD, intestinal obstructions; expensive.
DPP-4 Inhibitors: sitagliptin (Januvia)	▪ HgA$_{1C}$ change: Reduce A$_{1C}$ by 0.5–1.0%. ▪ Mechanism: Increases insulin production and decreases the liver's production of glucose. ▪ Benefits: No weight gain; less hypoglycemia. ▪ Risks/Concerns: Low side effect profile—URI symptoms, nausea, and diarrhea; require dose adjustment in renal insufficiency; expensive.

ENDOCRINOLOGY

(continues)

TABLE 2.2-2. **Glucose-Lowering Drugs** *(continued)*

GLP-1 analog:	• HgA$_{1C}$ change: Reduce A$_{1C}$ about 0.8%.
exenatide (Byetta)	• Mechanism: Enhances insulin secretion, decreases liver's glucose output, and may suppress appetite.
	• Benefits: Weight loss; less hypoglycemia.
	• Risks/Concerns: Nausea and vomiting; hypoglycemia risk increased when combined with sulfonylurea; hypertriglyceridemia.
Pramlintide (Symlin):	• Synthetic analog of the human hormone amylin that is cosecreted normally with insulin.
	• New class of agents, was approved as adjunctive therapy in patients with type 1 or 2 diabetes mellitus.
	• It is used in patients who fail to achieve good glycemic control, despite intensive insulin therapy, with or without metformin and/or sulfonylureas.
	• Its use is associated with weight loss.

DKA is a complication mostly associated with type 1 DM, while nonketotic hyperglycemic hyperosmolar syndrome (HHS) is associated with type 2 DM. However, there is some overlap between type 1 and type 2.

DKA is the most life-threatening acute complication of diabetes, and is often the presenting syndrome of type 1 DM, but can also occur in type 2 DM, especially in people of color.

When calculating the anion gap in DKA, use the actual Na, not the corrected Na.

Acute Complications of Diabetes Mellitus

The major acute complications of diabetes are the hyperglycemic and hypoglycemic emergencies. Hyperglycemic emergencies include diabetic ketoacidosis (DKA) and hyperglycemic hyperosmolar syndrome (HHS).

DIABETIC KETOACIDOSIS

Metabolic acidosis due to ketoacid accumulation secondary to severely depressed insulin levels.

ETIOLOGY

- Severe insulin deficiency causes the body to switch from metabolizing carbohydrates to metabolizing and oxidizing lipids.
- Usually precipitated by lapse in insulin treatment, acute infection, major trauma, or stress.

PATHOPHYSIOLOGY

- Insulin deficiency causes hyperglycemia, which induces an osmotic diuresis (**severe dehydration**).
- Profound dehydration, sodium loss, and potassium loss occurs.
- The body believes there is no glucose because the cells aren't getting any, which triggers the oxidation of free fatty acids from adipose tissue. The liver converts these free fatty acids into an alternative energy source: **ketones** (acetoacetic acid and beta-hydroxybutyric acid), which causes the metabolic ketoacidosis.
- There is respiratory compensation for this metabolic acidosis (fast breathing [ie, Kussmaul], blowing off CO_2).
- Other findings:
  - Acetone is produced from spontaneous decarboxylation of acetoacetic acid. The acetone is disposed of by respiration and its odor is present on the patient's breath (fruity odor).
  - *Pseudohyponatremia* (not real hyponatremia) is due to a normal response to the osmotic shifts of severe hyperglycemia. The sodium reading in the lab value does not accurately represent what the true sodium is. The "corrected" sodium concentration is obtained by adding 1.6 mEq of sodium for each 100 mg/dL of glucose above normal.

ENDOCRINOLOGY

- **Polyuria** and **polydypsia**, nausea, vomiting and vague abdominal pain.
- Lethargy and fatigue are later components.
- May progress to coma.
- Signs of dehydration are present, and patients may be hypotensive and tachycardic.
- Kussmaul respirations (rapid deep breaths) may be present.
- Acetone (fruity) odor may be present on the patient's breath.

DIAGNOSIS

- Anion gap metabolic acidosis (ketones are unmeasured ions) serum pH < 7.30.
- Hyperglycemia.
- Hyperketonemia.
- Usually, the diagnosis can be presumed at the bedside if patient's urine is strongly positive for ketones and the finger-stick glucose is high.
- Glucose is usually between 400 and 800 mg/dL.
- Initially, potassium is high due to acidosis, but drops with treatment (insulin drives K^+ into cells).

TREATMENT

- Goals of treatment are to remove ketones and correct the acidosis.
  - You must follow the anion gap as a measure; correction of acidosis is a critical endpoint (correction of high glucose does not mean DKA is over!). Stopping insulin and fluids when glucose is normal but acidosis is still present is a critical mistake!).
  - Can give bicarbonate in fluid to help when severe acidosis, but controversial.
- Aggressive fluid resuscitation to correct volume deficit.
- Correct hyperglycemia with insulin drip. Insulin is required in DKA even after blood glucose returns to normal range. Continue to give insulin and glucose-containing IV fluids.
- Correct underlying causes (eg, infection).
- Bicarbonate may be used to correct severe acidosis (rarely necessary).
- This is a critical patient—usually requires admission to intensive care unit (ICU).

PROGNOSIS

- Mortality rate is approximately 10%.
- Hypotension or coma present at admission are negative prognostic indicators.
- Major causes of death are circulatory failure, hypokalemia, and infection.

HYPERGLYCEMIC HYPEROSMOLAR SYNDROME

- Hyperglycemic hyperosmolar syndrome (HHS) is defined by a plasma osmolarity > 320 mOsm/L and a plasma glucose level > 600 mg/dL but a **normal bicarbonate level, normal PH,** and no significant evidence of ketosis.
- Occurs in patients with **type 2 DM.** The diagnosis is considered in any elderly patient with altered mental status and dehydration, particularly with known diabetes.

DKA is a life-threatening condition and must be recognized early and treated correctly.

PATHOPHYSIOLOGY

- Patients usually have a period of symptomatic hyperglycemia before the syndrome develops.
- When fluid intake becomes insufficient, **extreme dehydration** ensues because of the hyperglycemia-induced osmotic diuresis.

ETIOLOGY

- Medication noncompliance.
- Severe infection or sepsis.
- Dehydration.
- Diuretics.
- Glucocorticoids.

SIGNS AND SYMPTOMS

- Altered mental status.
- Signs of profound dehydration.
- Seizures and transient neurologic deficits may occur.

DIAGNOSIS

- Serum glucose levels are usually > 1,000 mg/dL (much higher than in DKA).
- Serum osmolarity is usually around 385 mOsm/kg.
- Blood urea nitrogen (BUN)/creatinine levels are markedly increased from prerenal azotemia.

TREATMENT

Goal of treatment is to expand the intravascular volume to stabilize vital signs and improve circulation and urine output:

- **Aggressive hydration**! Infuse 2–3 L of normal saline over 1–2 hours.
- Once vital signs have stabilized, change fluid to D_5 ½ NS and monitor vital signs, urine output, serum electrolytes, and BUN/creatinine carefully.
- Electrolytes should be monitored, especially potassium because the concentration may fall as urine output is restored and renal function improves. Begin potassium replacement with the initial infusion of D_5 ½ NS, and keep serum potassium at 4 mEq/L or more.
- Insulin should be administered only after plasma expansion has been initiated. If insulin is given before plasma expansion, it drives glucose into the cells, exacerbating volume depletion.
- Monitor patient for signs and symptoms of cerebral edema, which may occur if the osmolarity is corrected too quickly.
- If insulin is deemed necessary in the initial resuscitation, 5% glucose should be added to the infusion to prevent hypoglycemia when the serum glucose reaches 250 mg/dL.

HYPOGLYCEMIA

Abnormally low serum glucose level that causes sympathetic stimulation followed by altered mental status.

HHS most commonly occurs in patients unable to affect their own environment (eg, nursing home residents) or in elderly residents with impaired thirst mechanism and lack of access to water.

In hyperglycemic hyperosmolar syndrome, the preservation of vascular volume is critical. Normal saline is the initial fluid of choice and it should be initiated even before insulin.

Hypoglycemia is the most common cause of altered mental status in hospitalized patients.

ENDOCRINOLOGY

ETIOLOGY

- **Drug-induced** (most common cause): Insulin, sulfonylureas.
- **Alcohol.**
- Insulinomas.
- Adrenal insufficiency.
- Insulin receptor antibodies.
- Severe liver or renal disease.
- Endotoxic shock.
- Hypopituitarism with deficiency of both GH and cortisol.

PATHOPHYSIOLOGY

- Glucose transport across the blood-brain barrier is regulated by adrenergic nervous system activity (resulting in ↑ GH and cortisol secretion and ↓ insulin secretion).
- Glucagon is secreted by the pancreatic alpha cells. It increases plasma glucose levels and stimulates gluconeogenesis in the liver.
- The adrenergic outflow causes the typical sympathetic stimulatory symptoms of hypoglycemia and the lack of glucose to the brain results in altered mental status.

SIGNS AND SYMPTOMS

- History of insulin or sulfonylurea treatment.
- Adrenergic symptoms: Diaphoresis, anxiety, tremor, feeling faint, palpitations, and hunger.
- Central nervous system (CNS) manifestations: Confusion, inappropriate behavior (sometimes mistaken for alcohol intoxication), visual problems, stupor, and coma.

DIAGNOSIS

- Abnormally low serum glucose is < 50 mg/dL.
- Distinguish medication-induced vs. endogenous cause: Send C-peptide level to distinguish between endogenous (high C-peptide) and exogenous (low C-peptide) insulin because synthetic insulin has no C-peptide.

TREATMENT

- Once hypoglycemia is confirmed or if serum glucose level is not immediately available, obtain IV access and administer IV fluids with glucose.
- Only if patient's mental status is okay should you try giving food (PO); otherwise, they may aspirate.
- Whenever dextrose is administered for hypoglycemia, and alcoholism or nutritional deficiency is suspected, administer **thiamine** prior to glucose to prevent **Wernicke's encephalopathy.**
- Continue checking glucose levels, as they can drop again quickly (rebound hypoglycemia), or if from a medication, it may have a long half-life and still be on board.
- If hypoglycemia is refractory to glucose administration, consider adrenal insufficiency and give steroids.

Hypoglycemia due to oral hypoglycemic agents lasts about 24 hours. Patients with sulfonylurea (and/or long-acting insulin analogues) overdose should be admitted to the hospital for 24 hours for monitoring and continuous glucose administration.

For alcoholics and people with malnutrition, always give thiamine prior to glucose to prevent Wernicke's encephalopathy.

Whipple's triad of hypoglycemia:
1. Plasma glucose < 60 mg/dL
2. Symptoms of hypoglycemia
3. Improvement of the symptoms with administration of glucose

Chronic Complications of Diabetes Mellitus

DIABETIC RETINOPATHY

ETIOLOGY

The highly vascular retina is commonly involved in long standing diabetes. Diabetes is responsible for most cases of legal blindness in adults in the United States.

PROGRESSION

1. **Background diabetic retinopathy:** Early changes, include hard exudates, microaneurysms, and minor hemorrhages on funduscopic examination.
2. **Preproliferative retinopathy:** Presence of "cotton-wool spots," which are indicative of retinal infarcts.
3. **Neovascularization/proliferative retinopathy:** Abnormal vessels form on the retina can cause damage. They are abnormal in both appearance and structure and are prone to hemorrhage (retinal and vitreous hemorrhage).

DIAGNOSIS

Regular and careful screening by opthalmologist is necessary to detect the early changes of diabetic retinopathy.

TREATMENT

- Control blood glucose level.
- Blood pressure reduction is beneficial.
- Controlling plasma lipids may also slow the progression of eye disease.
- Ophthalmologist can do laser ablation of abnormal vessels.

DIABETIC NEPHROPATHY

ETIOLOGY

Diabetes is the most common cause of renal failure in the United States. Diabetic nephropathy begins with a period of glomerular hyperfiltration and intraglomerular hypertension. Subsequently, glomerular injury develops with the eventual loss of filtration capacity, leading to azotemia.

PROGRESSION

Progresses from a small amount of a small protein (microalbumin) to large amounts of a large protein.

1. Microalbuminuria (30–300 mg/d).
2. Macroalbuminuria (> 300 mg/d).
3. Frank nephrotic syndrome (> 3.5 g/d).

DIAGNOSIS

Annual measurement of microalbumin-to-creatinine ratios on spot urine samples, and serum creatinine concentrations to screen for diabetic kidney disease.

TREATMENT

- Aggressive blood pressure control, particularly with ACE inhibitor or angiotensin II receptor blockers.
- Control glucose level.

ACE inhibitors reduce albuminuria and slow the progression of renal disease in diabetic patients with and without hypertension.

ENDOCRINOLOGY

DIABETIC FOOT

ETIOLOGY

Diabetic patients frequently have peripheral vascular disease and peripheral neuropathy. These place the diabetic foot at extreme risk for ulceration, infection, and, ultimately, possible amputation.

SIGNS AND SYMPTOMS

- Cold feet.
- Claudication, leg discomfort on ambulation (relieved with rest).
- Numbness, burning, or tingling sensation of the hands and feet, in a glove and stocking distribution.

DIAGNOSIS

- Frequent, careful examination of the feet.
- Detect sensory deficits in the foot (Monofilament test).

TREATMENT

- Glucose control is critical.
- Use comfortable, protective, and well-fitting shoes and plain cotton socks.
- Ongoing foot care by a podiatrist is important.
- Aggressive treatment of the diabetic foot ulcer or infection with broad-spectrum antibiotics, often for longer periods of time. Debridement if necessary.

Counterregulatory Hormones

Counterregulatory hormones are hormones that counteract insulin action. Therefore, they can cause insulin resistance and diabetes if there is too much of them, or they can rise in response to hypoglycemia (too much insulin). High-yield facts and potential questions include:

- **Glucagon:**
  - The most important and fastest to act. It acts on the liver to increase gluconeogenesis and glycogenolysis.
  - Glucagon (1 mg IM) is used to resuscitate hypoglycemic coma if you cannot get IV access. (Never give anything by mouth, including glucose gel.)
  - Will not work in a patient who is alcoholic with liver failure. Alcohol will suppress gluconeogenesis, and glycogen stores are impaired in severe liver disease.
  - Loss of the glucagon response to hypoglycemia occurs after a long period of diabetes, especially type 1, leading to hypoglycemia unawareness.
  - Too much glucagon (glucagonoma) will present with new-onset diabetes, weight loss and characteristic rash (necrolytic migratory erythema).
- **Catecholamine:**
  - Too much insulin leads to hypoglycemia; catecholamines rise, giving the signs and symptoms of hypoglycemia such as tachycardia, sweating, and anxiety.
  - Pheochromocytoma patients (too much catecholamine) have an ↑ risk of hyperglycemia and diabetes.

- **Cortisol:**
  - Too much cortisol, as in Cushing's syndrome or in treatment of various diseases such as asthma, leads to hyperglycemia and diabetes.
  - Too little cortisol, as in Addison's disease, leads to hypoglycemia.
- **Growth hormone:**
  - A high level of GH in the early morning leads to hyperglycemia (dawn phenomenon).
  - A high level of GH in acromegaly is associated with hyperglycemia and diabetes in nearly half of cases.
  - In addition to measuring IGF_1, screen for acromegaly by conducting an oral glucose tolerance test to see if the GH will be suppressed in response to insulin release by the glucose given. If there is no suppression, the test is positive for acromegaly.
  - Neonatal hypoglycemia is a cardinal sign of GH deficiency.
- **Placental secretion hormones,** including GH, corticotropin-releasing hormone, progesterone, and human placental lactogen, could lead to gestational diabetes in susceptible individuals, which is why diabetes screening during pregnancy is conducted when these hormone levels are at their peak—around the 24th week of gestation.

Counterregulatory Hormones

Glucagon — Insulin
Catecholamines
Hydrocortisone
Growth hormone
Human placental
lactogen
Progesterone

DISORDERS OF THE PITUITARY GLAND

Pituitary Tumors

- Anterior pituitary (adenohypophysis): Derivative of Rathke's pouch.
- Posterior pituitary (neurohypophysis): Composed of hypothalamic neuronal axon terminals, storage and release site for hormones produced by these neurons.
- For specific hormones, see Table 2.2-3.

PATHOLOGY

- Constitute ~ 10% of intracranial tumors.
- Most are benign, slow growing.
- Anterior pituitary: Craniopharyngiomas, adenomas.
- Posterior pituitary: No primary tumors.
- Metastases and meningiomas are occasionally seen.
- Pathology/manifestations arises from:
  - Excess hormone production.
  - Compression of suprasellar structures.
  - Destruction of normal pituitary parenchyma.
  - Compression of pituitary stalk → ↑ prolactin due to loss of inhibition by dopamine.

Pituitary adenomas are part of multiple endocrine neoplasia (MEN) type I (pituitary, pancreas, parathyroid).

TABLE 2.2-3. Pituitary Hormones and Their Functions

ANTERIOR LOBE	MAIN STIMULATORY ACTIONS	HYPOTHALAMIC STIMULUS
Adrenocorticotropic hormone (ACTH, corticotropin)	▪ Growth and secretion of adrenal cortex to make cortisol and sex hormones	▪ CRH
Growth hormone (GH, somatotropin)	▪ Secretion of somatomedin C (insulin-like growth factor) ▪ Body growth	▪ GRH
Thyroid-stimulating hormone (TSH, thyrotropin)	▪ Growth of thyroid gland ▪ Production of T_3 and T_4	▪ TRH
Follicle-stimulating hormone (FSH)	▪ Spermatogenesis in the male ▪ Ovarian follicle growth in the female	▪ GnRH
Luteinizing hormone (LH)	▪ Testosterone secretion in the male ▪ Ovulation in the female	▪ GnRH
Prolactin	▪ Milk production ▪ Maternal behavior	▪ PRH (stimulates) ▪ Dopamine (inhibits)
Melanocyte-stimulating hormone (MSH)	▪ Skin pigmentation	

POSTERIOR LOBE		RELEASING STIMULUS
Antidiuretic hormone (ADH; vasopressin, AVP)	▪ Retains sodium and water, producing concentrated urine	▪ Osmoreceptors
Oxytocin	▪ Milk letdown ▪ Contractions of labor	▪ Touch receptors in uterus, genitalia, and breast

Pituitary Adenomas

- **Prolactinoma** is the most common pituitary tumor. It can present with galactorrhea or amenorrhea. Women usually present earlier than men. Prolactin levels correlate with tumor size. Treat with dopamine agonists (bromocriptine).
- **Nonfunctioning tumors** are the second most common pituitary tumors. Symptoms include visual changes or slightly high prolactin levels due to mass effect, which disrupts the inhibitor signal that dopamine has on prolactin-producing cells. Treat with surgery.
- Less common pituitary adenomas include **somatotrophs** (GH; see Acromegaly), **corticotrophs** (ACTH), and **thyrotrophs** (TSH).
- **Pituitary microadenomas** (< 10 mm) are found in ~15% of asymptomatic women by MRI; in the absence of progression (assessed by follow-up MRI), they are clinically insignificant.

Craniopharyngiomas

- Arise from embryologic remnants of Rathke's pouch.
- Most common tumors of suprasellar region in children.
- Solid or cystic; usually calcified.

NEUROLOGIC SYMPTOMS

- Headache.
- Compression of optic chiasm:
  - Superior bitemporal quadrantanopsia: Early visual defect, since compression begins on inferior surface of chiasm.
  - Bitemporal hemianopsia ("tunnel vision"): Classic finding, occurs when tumor has reached significant size.
- Signs of increased intracranial pressure (ICP) are rare, as tumors are usually diagnosed before they reach the requisite dimensions.

DIAGNOSIS OF PITUITARY ADENOMAS/CRANIOPHARYNGIOMAS

- **Magnetic resonance imaging (MRI):** More sensitive than CT, can detect microadenomas; use with gadolinium contrast.
- **Computed tomography (CT):** More sensitive than x-ray.
- **X-ray:** May show enlargement of sella; craniopharyngiomas may show calcifications in suprasellar regions.
- **Hormone studies:** Detect excesses or deficiencies, give information about type of tumor; useful when tumor cannot be detected radiographically.
- If a patient presents with manifestations of a specific disease (such as acromegaly, Cushing's, etc.), always start with hormonal workup prior to diagnostic imaging. That is because of the high prevalence of incidentalomas in the general population.

TREATMENT OF PITUITARY ADENOMAS/CRANIOPHARYNGIOMAS

- Dopamine agonists for prolactinomas (dopamine inhibits prolactin).
- Surgery: Indicated whenever there are neurologic symptoms.
- Radiotherapy: Can reduce size of tumor without surgery, sometimes used as surgical adjunct.
- Hormone replacement for hypopituitarism.

Acromegaly

- Type of pituitary adenoma also, but diagnosis and treatment are somewhat specific.
- Disorder marked by progressive enlargement (megaly) of peripheral (acral) body parts resulting from excess GH production.

ETIOLOGY

- Pituitary somatotroph (cells that make GH, or somatotropin) adenoma is by far the most common cause.
- Ectopic GH secretion; hypothalamic tumors secreting growth hormone–releasing hormone (GHRH) are rare.

SIGNS AND SYMPTOMS

- Progressive enlargement of peripheral body parts, particularly head, hands, and feet.
- Progressive and irreversible organomegaly, especially cardiomegaly.

Patients rarely complain of "tunnel vision" (bitemporal hemianopsia) or a deficit when the defect is confined to the temporal visual fields. They more typically just report increased clumsiness or bumping into things.

Acromegaly: The changes in a patient's appearance occur over many years and may not be apparent to the patient or his family. Old photos may suggest the diagnosis.

ENDOCRINOLOGY

- Often, patients present with decompensated heart failure prior to diagnosis.
- Impaired glucose tolerance due to the anti-insulin actions of GH.
- Hyperphosphatemia due to GH's influence on tubular resorption of phosphate.
- Gigantism in children due to excess linear growth prior to epiphyseal closure.

DIAGNOSIS

- Lack of GH suppression by glucose load.
- **Serum insulin-like growth factor I (IGF-I) levels** is the best single test for diagnosis of acromegaly. It is made by the liver under stimulation by GH, elevated in acromegalics and does not fluctuate as does GH itself.
- **GH levels** are highly variable so testing will yield inaccurate results. Always check IGF-I if acromegally is suspected.

TREATMENT

- Surgery (transsphenoidal or transfrontal adenectomy, depending on the size and location of the tumor).
- Radiation therapy (takes 6–10 years to work).
- Dopamine agonist such as bromocriptine (preferred because of lower cost) or somatostatin analog such as octreotide.
- GH receptor blocker such as pegvisomant (Somavert).

Hypopituitarism

- **Tumors** causing dysfunction either by invasion, replacement, or compression. It can affect normal pituitary parenchyma, pituitary stalk, and hypothalamic parenchyma.
- **Surgical destruction** of pituitary or hypothalamus: Either therapeutic or as a result of an unrelated neurosurgical procedure.
- **Sheehan's syndrome:** Pituitary gland enlarges during pregnancy due to hyperplasia of lactotrophs without commensurate increase in blood supply; if hypotension occurs during childbirth, pituitary infarction can result.
- **Systemic** (rare): Hemochromatosis, sarcoid, lymphocytic hypophysitis (more common in women in late pregnancy and postpartum).
- **Infectious** (rare): Tuberculosis (TB), neurosyphilis.

> A 29-year-old woman presents with inability to lactate after childbirth. Delivery was complicated by blood loss and hypotension. *Think: Sheehan's syndrome.* **Next step:** Check prolactin level and MRI with contrast of head.

SIGNS AND SYMPTOMS

- **ACTH deficiency:** See Adrenal Insufficiency section.
- **GH deficiency:** Growth retardation in children.
- **Prolactin:**
  - Deficiency: Failure to lactate after childbirth.
  - Excess: Amenorrhea and galactorrhea in women, ↓ libido and gynecomastia in men.

- **TSH deficiency:** See Hypothyroidism section.
- **Luteinizing hormone (LH)** and **follicle-stimulating hormone (FSH) deficiency:** Amenorrhea and genital atrophy in women, ↓ libido in men.
- In slow-growing tumors, GH, FSH, and LH levels are affected early; ACTH and prolactin levels decline only with advanced disease.
- **Antidiuretic hormone (ADH) deficiency:** known as diabetes insipidus (discussed in separate section below).

> A 36-year-old woman complains of amenorrhea for 1 year, increasingly bad headaches, clumsiness, and sporadic nipple discharge; beta-hCG levels are normal. *Think: Prolactinoma.* **Next step:** Check serum prolactin level, MRI brain.

Drugs that inhibit dopamine activity also cause hyperprolactinemia: tricyclic antidepressants, prochlorperazine, haloperidol, methyldopa, metoclopramide, cimetidine.

DIAGNOSIS

The following circumstances must be considered when interpreting pituitary hormone levels:

- ACTH levels must be taken with serum cortisol levels; if cortisol is high, ACTH is probably low due to feedback inhibition. Insulin-induced hypoglycemia stimulates ACTH secretion and is an effective test of the entire hypothalamic-pituitary-adrenal axis. Test is administered similarly to GH provocation described below.
- Prolactin levels are normally elevated in the third trimester and in breast-feeding mothers.
- GH levels are pulsatile and decline to minimal levels by age 30. Evaluation requires stimulation testing: Insulin or levodopa stimulate a burst in serum GH, serum levels are drawn at 30, 60, and 90 minutes post stimulus and compared to normal values.
- Thyroid-stimulating hormone (TSH) must be taken with serum tri-iodothyronine (T_3) and thyroxine (T_4); if they are normal or high, TSH is probably low due to feedback inhibition.
- In women, LH and FSH levels vary with the menstrual cycle, so the timing of the levels is important; postmenopausal women have high LH and FSH levels normally.
- ADH levels normally vary according to plasma osmolality; testing is discussed in Diabetes Insipidus section.
- Evaluation of target organ function is usually required: Tests include imaging studies, hormone levels, and response to exogenous pituitary hormones.

TREATMENT

- Address underlying cause: Tumor, infection, systemic disease.
- **Hormone replacement:**
  - Cortisol for ACTH deficiency.
  - Prolactin:
    - No treatment for deficiency.
    - Bromocriptine (dopamine agonist; dopamine suppresses prolactin production).
    - Surgery, or radiation for large tumors not responding to dopamine agonists.

- GH for GH deficiency in children.
- Thyroxine for TSH deficiency.
- FSH and LH deficiency can be treated with estrogen/progesterone replacements in women (fertility is usually not restored unless GNRH is given in a pulsatile fashion, via pump) and testosterone replacements in men.
- DDAVP for ADH deficiency.

ANTIDIURETIC HORMONE (ADH) DISORDERS

Diabetes Insipidus (DI)

- Central DI: Inadequate pituitary release of ADH.
- Nephrogenic DI: Lack of renal response to ADH.

ETIOLOGY

- **Central DI:**
  - Idiopathic: Accounts for 50% of cases.
  - Posterior pituitary or hypothalamic damage (tumor, trauma, neurosurgery).
  - Systemic: Sarcoidosis, neurosyphilis, encephalitis.
- **Nephrogenic DI:**
  - Familial.
  - Chronic renal disease.
  - Sickle cell anemia (renal papillary necrosis).
  - Hypokalemia.
  - Hypercalcemia.
  - Drugs: Lithium, demeclocycline, methoxyflurane.

Psychogenic polydipsia:
Psychiatric disorder of compulsive water drinking most common in young to middle-aged women. Presents with polyuria and dilute urine, distinguished from DI by *low* plasma osmolality.

SIGNS AND SYMPTOMS

- Polyuria (3–15 L/day).
- Thirst.
- Dilute urine (specific gravity < 1.005).

DIAGNOSIS

- High plasma osmolality (280–310 mOsm/L) due to incomplete compensation for the inability to resorb free water.
- Water deprivation followed by exogenous ADH:
  - Central DI: Low urine Osm → high urine Osm
  - Nephrogenic DI: Low urine Osm → low urine Osm
  - Normal: High urine Osm → high urine Osm
- Infusion of hypertonic saline normally results in a sharp ↓ in urine output; patients with DI do not respond.

TREATMENT

- **Desmopressin (DDAVP):** Analog of ADH, useful in **central DI.**
- **Thiazide diuretics:** Paradoxically ↓ urine output in patients with DI by increasing sodium and water resorption in the proximal tubule leading to ↓ water delivery to the ADH responsive sites in the collecting ducts. They are the only therapy useful in **nephrogenic DI.**

- **Chlorpropamide:** Oral hypoglycemic with side effect of potentiating secretion and action of endogenous ADH. Partial function must exist for this therapy to be of use.

Syndrome of Inappropriate Antidiuretic Hormone Secretion (SIADH)

Excess production of ADH.

ETIOLOGY

- Idiopathic overproduction via the hypothalamic–posterior pituitary axis: Often associated with disorders of the central nervous system (encephalitis, stroke, head trauma) and pulmonary disease (TB, pneumonia).
- Ectopic production by malignant tumors, particularly small cell lung cancer and pancreatic carcinoma.
- Pharmacologic stimulation of the hypothalamic-pituitary axis: Carbamazepine, chlorpropamide, clofibrate, vincristine.

SIGNS AND SYMPTOMS

Attributable to hyponatremia—see chapter on fluid and electrolytes.

DIAGNOSIS

- Hyponatremia.
- Low serum osmolality.
- High urinary sodium.
- Osmolality of urine > serum.
- Normal adrenal and thyroid functions.

TREATMENT

- Fluid restriction.
- Hypertonic saline in severe hyponatremia.
- Demeclocycline: Due to causing nephrogenic DI, reserved for cases not responding to fluid restriction.
- Newer agents are direct vasopressin (V2) receptor antagonists: **the vaptans.**
  - IV conivaptan approved for use in volume overloaded hyponatremic states.
  - New oral agent **tolvaptan** recently received FDA approval for treatment of hyponatremia.

THYROID DISORDERS

Hyperthyroidism

Increased synthesis and secretion of free thyroid hormones resulting in hypermetabolism.

EPIDEMIOLOGY

- Ten times more common in women than in men.
- Annual incidence is 1 in 1000 women.

Causes of large tongue (macroglossia):
- Acromegaly
- Myxedema
- Amyloidosis

ENDOCRINOLOGY

- Graves' disease (most common cause, 80% of cases in the United States).
- Toxic multinodular goiter.
- Toxic adenoma (Plummer's disease).
- Iatrogenic (lithium therapy), inadvertent toxic ingestion, or factitious (thyrotoxicosis factitia).
- Transient hyperthyroidism (subacute thyroiditis).
- Ectopic thyroid hormone secretion (struma ovarii).

PATHOPHYSIOLOGY

High levels of free thyroid hormones increase levels of cellular metabolism and cause multiple effects, resulting in a general state of hypermetabolism.

SIGNS AND SYMPTOMS

- Heat intolerance, sweating.
- Palpitations (hyperthyroidism is a common cause of atrial fibrillation).
- Weight loss.
- Tremor.
- Nervousness and anxiety.
- Weakness and fatigue.
- Diarrhea/hyperdefecation.

DIAGNOSIS

Measure TSH, free T_4, and free T_3 (if the T_4 level is normal) (see Table 2.2-4).

Serum TSH is the most sensitive test for thyroid dysfunction.

TABLE 2.2-4. Laboratory Evaluation of Thyroid

THYROID STATE	T_4	FT_4	T_3	FT_3	TSH	TRH
Hypothyroidism						
1°	↓	↓	↓	↓	↑	↑
2°	↓	↓	↓	↓	↓	N
3°	↓	↓	↓	↓	↓/N	↓
Peripheral unresponsiveness	↑/N	↑/N	↑/N	↑	↓/N	↑/N
Hyperthyroidism						
Pituitary tumor (secretes TSH)	↑	↑	↑	↑	↑	↓
Graves' disease	↑	↑	↑	↑	↓	↓
T_3 thyrotoxicosis	N	N	↑	↑	↓	↓
T_4 thyrotoxicosis	↑	↑	N	N	↓	↓
Toxic nodular goiter	↑	↑	↑	↑	↓	↓

ENDOCRINOLOGY

TREATMENT

Depends on underlying disorder (see below for specifics).

Thyroid Storm

- Exaggerated manifestation of hyperthyroidism with fever, CNS, CV, and GI dysfunction.
- Mortality is high (20–50%) even with the correct treatment.

ETIOLOGY

- Infection.
- Trauma and major surgical procedures.
- DKA.
- MI, cerebrovascular accident (CVA), pulmonary embolism (PE).
- Withdrawal of antihyperthyroid medications, iodine administration, thyroid hormone ingestion.
- Idiopathic.

Thyroid storm and myxedema coma are life-threatening medical emergencies.

SIGNS AND SYMPTOMS

Overactivated sympathetic nervous system causes most of the signs and symptoms of this syndrome:

- Fever > 101°F.
- Tachycardia (out of proportion to fever).
- High-output congestive heart failure (CHF) and volume depletion.
- Exhaustion.
- GI manifestations: Diarrhea, abdominal pain.
- Continuum of CNS alterations (from agitation to confusion when moderate, to stupor or coma with or without seizures when most severe).
- Jaundice is a late and ominous manifestation.

DIAGNOSIS

- This is a clinical diagnosis, and since most patients present in need of emergent stabilization, treatment is initiated empirically.
- Patients may have inadequately treated hyperthyroidism.
- May also occur in the setting of unintentional or intentional toxic ingestion of synthetic thyroid hormone in the hypothyroid patient.

TREATMENT

- **Treat the manifestations.**
- **Primary stabilization:**
  - **Airway protection.**
  - Oxygenation.
  - Assess circulation (pulse/BP) and continuous cardiac monitoring.
  - IV hydration.
  - Beta-blocker therapy (eg, propranolol) to block adrenergic effects and block peripheral conversion of T_4 to T_3.
  - Treat fever with acetaminophen and cooling blanket (not aspirin, which displaces T_4 from thyroid binding protein).
- **Addressing the thyroid hormone itself:**
  - **Propylthiouracil (PTU)** or **methimazole** to block synthesis of new thyroid hormone.

Never send any thyroid storm patient for a procedure involving iodine contrast before giving **propylthiouracil.**

- **Iodine** to decrease release of preformed thyroid hormone. Do not give iodine until the PTU has taken effect (1.5 hours) because more thyroid hormone will otherwise be produced using the iodine given.
- **Corticosteroids** also given to prevent peripheral conversion of T_4 to T_3 and to treat "relative" adrenal failure occurring due to high metabolic rate.
- Treat any possible precipitating factors that may be present (eg, MI, infection, etc.).

Graves' Disease

Autoimmune disease causing hyperthyroidism due to antibody which stimulates TSH receptor.

PATHOPHYSIOLOGY

- Antibody is produced that interacts with the receptor for TSH resulting in continuous excess secretion.
- Cause of the exophthalmos (infiltrative opthalmopathy) in Graves' is unknown, but is thought to be due to immunoglobulins that interact with self-antigens in the extraocular muscles and on orbital fibroblasts.

SIGNS AND SYMPTOMS

- Diffusely enlarged thyroid.
- Exophthalmos.
- Pretibial myxedema.
- Tachycardia, palpitations.
- In elderly patients the presentation is less classic. Apathy can be present without the common hyperactivity signs (apathetic hyperthyroidism). Cardiovascular features may be prominent and hyperthyroidism may not be suspected initially.

DIAGNOSIS

- High radioactive iodine uptake on a radionuclide scan. (If uptake is present but low, then diagnosis is thyroiditis or factitious hyperthyroidism.)
- Elevated free thyroid hormones (T_3, T_4).
- Undetectable TSH levels.
- High TSH receptor antibodies to confirm diagnosis and assess severity.

TREATMENT

- **Long-term antithyroid therapy:**
  - Usually accomplished with **propylthiouracil (PTU)**.
  - Methimazole is as effective as PTU when administered at one-tenth of the PTU dosage.
  - PTU has the advantage of inhibiting the peripheral conversion of T_4 to T_3, thus there is usually a more rapid symptomatic improvement. However, euthyroid state is achieved more quickly with methimazole.
  - *Complications*: Leukopenia (check CBC before initiating therapy). Stop medication if absolute PMN drops below 1500 cells/μL. If patient develops fever or sore throat, he or she should be instructed to seek medical care.
- **Methimazole is contraindicated in pregnancy—use PTU.**

Graves' disease is the most common cause of hyperthyroidism.

Graves' (and Hashimoto's thyroiditis) are sometimes associated with other autoimmune diseases (type I diabetes mellitus, vitiligo, myasthenia, pernicious anemia, collagen diseases).

ENDOCRINOLOGY

- **Radioactive iodine ablation therapy:**
  - Can produce the same effects as surgery without the surgical complications.
  - Commonly results in hypothyroidism over time.
  - **Complications:** Radiation thyroiditis commonly appears within 7–10 days after therapy and is associated with accelerated release of thyroid hormone into the blood. Rarely, this results in thyrotoxic crisis.
- **Beta blockers:**
  - Propranolol is the most commonly used. Atenolol could also be used in once a day dosage.
  - Should be used only as adjunctive therapy because it does not treat the underlying problem.
- **Subtotal thyroidectomy:**
  - Still used for younger patients or when ablation therapy is unsuccessful.
  - Delayed complications include hypoparathyroidism (can be life threatening) and hypothyroidism.

Hypothyroidism

- TSH levels greater than twice the upper limit of normal in primary hypothyroidism.
- Can be (1) clinically evident hypothyroidism with classic physical findings or (2) subclinical hypothyroidism detectable only upon laboratory analysis.

EPIDEMIOLOGY

- Clinically evident hypothyroidism occurs in 2% of women and in 0.2% of men.
- The incidence increases with age, usually between 40 and 60.

ETIOLOGY

- **Primary hypothyroidism** (thyroid gland dysfunction):
  - Hashimoto's thyroiditis.
  - Previous treatment for hyperthyroidism.
  - Painless thyroiditis.
  - Radiation therapy to the neck (for other malignancy).
  - Iodine deficiency or excess.
  - Medications (lithium is the most common).
  - Prolonged treatment with iodine-containing substances.
- **Secondary hypothyroidism** (pituitary dysfunction):
  - Postpartum necrosis (Sheehan's syndrome).
  - Space-occupying pituitary neoplasm.
  - Infiltrating disease (TB) causing TSH deficiency.
- **Tertiary hypothyroidism** (deficiency in TRH secretion; hypothalamic dysfunction):
  - Granuloma.
  - Neoplasm.
  - Hypothalamic radiation.

SIGNS AND SYMPTOMS

- Fatigue, lethargy, weakness.
- Constipation, weight gain (usually > 15 pounds).

Hashimoto's thyroiditis (chronic lymphocytic thyroiditis) is the most common cause of hypothyroidism in North America.

Muscle weakness and cramps occur in both hyper- and hypothyroidism. In hyperthyroidism, CPK will be normal. In hypothyroidism, it will be elevated.

- Muscle weakness, cramps, arthralgias.
- Cold intolerance.
- Slow speech with hoarse voice (from myxedematous changes in vocal cords).
- Slow thinking with poor memory.
- Skin: Dry, coarse, thick, and cool; nonpitting edema of the skin and eyelids.
- Hair: Brittle and coarse; loss of outer one-third of eyebrows.
- Thyroid gland: May or may not be palpable (depending on the etiology of the hypothyroidism).
- Heart: Distant heart sounds may be present if pericardial effusion is present. Bradycardia may occur.
- **Neurologic: Delayed relaxation phase of deep tendon reflexes** (very specific). Cerebellar ataxia can be present. Peripheral neuropathies with paresthesias; carpal tunnel syndrome.
- Musculoskeletal: Muscular stiffness and weakness.

Consider evaluating thyroid function tests in any patient with hypercholesterolemia.

DIAGNOSIS

- See Table 2.2-4 for results of thyroid tests.
- Also, **in Hashimoto's thyroiditis:** May show **increased antithyroglobulin and antimicrosomal antibody titers.**
- The TRH stimulation test is useful in distinguishing secondary from tertiary hypothyroidism.

Thyroid peroxidase autoantibodies (TPO Ab) are indicative of autoimmune thyroid disease and have predictive value for progression to overt hypothyroidism or development of drug-induced thyroid dysfunction.

TREATMENT

- Start therapy with low-dose levothyroxine and increase dose every 6–8 weeks, depending on the patient's response (*start low, go slow*).
- Elderly patients and patients with coronary artery disease should be started on a low dose of levothyroxine because high doses may precipitate angina pectoris.
- **Monitoring therapy:**
  - In 1° hypothyroidism, it is adequate to measure the TSH level, which should fall well within the normal range.
  - In 2° hypothyroidism, measure the T_4 level, which should fall well within the normal range.

Hypothermia is often missed by tympanic thermometers. Use a rectal probe if hypothermia is suspected.

Subclinical Hypothyroidism

Elevated TSH level with normal thyroid hormone levels in the absence of overt clinical symptoms.

CLINICAL COURSE

This is not usually a precursor to 1° hypothyroidism. There are usually two distinct patterns:

- Patients who will eventually develop 1° hypothyroidism: Patients with both elevated TSH and detectable antithyroid antibodies often progress to clinically evident hypothyroidism.
- Euthyroidism with reset thyrostat: Permanent state without definitive progression to 1° hypothyroidism. Probably due to subtle damage to the thyroid gland from another cause.

Infection is a common precipitant of myxedema coma; pan-culture and empiric antibiotic therapy with broad-spectrum antibiotics is recommended for all affected patients.

TREATMENT

Thyroid replacement therapy is necessary only in the following circumstances:

- All patients with TSH > 10.
- Patients with TSH > 5 and goiter or antithyroid antibody.

Myxedema Coma

Life-threatening complication of hypothyroidism with profound lethargy or coma usually accompanied by hypothermia. Mortality is 20–50% even if treated early.

ETIOLOGY (PRECIPITATING FACTORS)

- Sepsis.
- Prolonged exposure to cold weather.
- CNS depressants (sedatives, narcotics).
- Trauma or surgery.

SIGNS AND SYMPTOMS

- Profound lethargy or coma is obvious.
- Hypothermia: Rectal T < 35°C (95°F).
- Bradycardia or circulatory collapse.
- Hypoventilation with respiratory acidosis.
- Delayed relaxation phase of deep tendon reflexes, areflexia if severe (this is important clue).

Differential diagnosis of myxedema coma:
Severe depression or primary psychosis
Drug overdose or toxic exposure
CVA
Liver failure
Hypoglycemia
CO_2 narcosis
CNS infection

 A 75-year-old female presents with progressive obtundation and nonarousal. Core temperature is 35°C; cold, doughy skin; delayed deep tendon reflex relaxation phase. Urine analysis with many leukocytes and gram-negative rods. *Think: Myxedema coma.*

DIAGNOSIS

Lab tests for the patient presenting with signs and symptoms of myxedema coma (in descending order):

- TSH, T_3, T_4, free thyroxine (FT_4).
- Cortisol level.
- Complete blood count (CBC) with differential.
- Serum electrolytes.
- Blood urea nitrogen (BUN) and creatinine.
- Blood glucose.
- Blood and urine cultures.
- Urine toxicology screen.
- Serum transaminases and lactic dehydrogenase (LDH), creatine phosphokinase (CPK).
- Arterial blood gas (ABG) to rule out hypoxemia and CO_2 retention.
- Carboxyhemoglobin.
- Chest radiograph.
- Brain CT.

TREATMENT

- Airway management with mechanical ventilation if necessary (ABCs, etc).
- Pharmacologic therapy:
  - Intravenous levothyroxine.
  - Glucocorticoids (until coexisting adrenal insufficiency is excluded).
- Prevent further heat loss.
- Monitor patient in intensive care unit.
- IV hydration (D_5 ½ NS).
- Rule out and treat any precipitating causes (antibiotics for suspected infection).

Thyroiditis

- Inflammation of the thyroid.
- Can be divided into three common types (Hashimoto's, subacute, and silent) and two rarer forms (suppurative and Riedel's).

ETIOLOGY

- **Hashimoto's thyroiditis:** Autoimmune disorder that involves CD4 lymphocyte-mediated destruction of the thyroid. The lymphocytes are specific for thyroid antigens. Cause for activation of these cells is unknown.
- **Subacute thyroiditis:** Possibly a postviral condition because it usually follows a viral upper respiratory infection (URI). Not considered an autoimmune reaction.
- **Silent thyroiditis:** Usually occurs **postpartum** and is thought to be autoimmune mediated.
- **Suppurative thyroiditis:** Usually a bacterial infection, but fungi and parasites have also been implicated in some cases. Commonly seen in HIV-positive patients with *Pneumocystis jiroveci* pneumonia (PCP).
- **Riedel's thyroiditis:** Fibrous infiltration of the thyroid of unknown etiology; also called fibrous thyroiditis.

SIGNS AND SYMPTOMS

- **Hashimoto's:** There may be signs of hyper- or hypothyroidism depending on the stage. Usually, there is diffuse, firm enlargement of the gland, but it may be of normal size if the disease has progressed.
- **Subacute:** Tender, enlarged gland, severe neck pain, often mistaken for pharyngitis. Fever and signs of hyperthyroidism are initially present. Hypothyroidism may develop. Very high erythrocyte sedimentation rate (ESR).
- **Silent:** Similar to subacute except there is no tenderness of the gland (painless thyroiditis).
- **Suppurative:** Fever with severe neck pain. Focal tenderness of involved portion of the gland.
- **Riedel's:** Slowly enlarging rock-hard mass in the anterior neck. Tight, stiff neck. Must differentiate from thyroid cancer. Hypothyroidism may occur if advanced. Fibrosis may involve mediastinum.

Corticosteroids are given empirically in myxedema coma before T_4 is given due to concern that associated Addison's disease exists. Giving only T_4 could precipitate an addisonian crisis.

A patient who comes in with fever, anxiety, and a painful neck should be worked up for thyroiditis (pain!). Thyroid function tests will show decreased TSH with increased T_4 but decreased uptake on iodine scan. **Next step?** *Prescribe an NSAID or steroid.*

Workup of someone with recent onset of hyperthyroid symptoms (anxiety, heat intolerance) and a painful neck shows: decreased TSH and increased free T_4 and decreased uptake on iodine scan. *Next step: NSAID/ steroid (this is thyroiditis).*

The thyroid in Hashimoto's is nontender, which distinguishes it from other forms of thyroiditis.

A 35-year-old female with a history of hyperthyroidism and a recent flu presents with neck pain and an elevated ESR. *Think: Subacute thyroiditis.* **Next step:** Check thyroid function tests.

DIAGNOSIS

- **History:**
  - Presentation following viral URI is suggestive of subacute thyroiditis.
  - Presentation after penetrating injury to the neck is suggestive of suppurative processes.
  - Postpartum presentation is suggestive of silent thyroiditis.
- **Laboratory examination:**
  - TSH and FT_4 may be normal or indicative of hypo- or hyperthyroidism.
  - White blood count (WBC) with differential should be obtained to look for leukocytosis and left shift (subacute and suppurative).
  - Antimicrosomal antibodies are present in > 90% with Hashimoto's and 50–80% with silent thyroiditis.
  - Serum thyroglobulin levels are elevated in subacute and silent thyroiditis (test is very nonspecific).
- **Imaging studies:** Radioactive iodine uptake (RAIU) can be useful to distinguish Graves' disease (increased RAIU) from subacute thyroiditis (decreased RAIU), in a hypothyroid patient.

Differential diagnosis of thyroiditis:

The hyperthyroid stage of Hashimoto's, subacute, or silent thyroiditis, may mimic Graves' disease.

Riedel's must be differentiated from thyroid cancer.

Subacute thyroiditis can be mistaken for oropharyngeal, tracheal infections, or for suppurative thyroiditis.

TREATMENT

- Treat hypothyroidism, if present, with levothyroxine for 6–8 weeks. Re-evaluate the TSH level, particularly in postpartum thyroiditis that might be manifested as depression.
- Control symptoms of hyperthyroidism, if present, with propranolol.
- Pain management in patients with subacute thyroiditis should be accomplished with nonsteroidal anti-inflamatory drugs (NSAIDs). If ineffective, begin a tapering course of steroids.
- IV antibiotics and abscess drainage, if present, should be performed in suppurative thyroiditis.
- **Do not** give PTU or methimazole in thyroiditis—the mechanism is release of preformed hormone from inflamed gland, *not* overproduction of hormone by the gland.

PROGNOSIS

- **Hashimoto's:** Most patients do not completely recover their total thyroid function.
- **Subacute:** Hypothyroidism persists in 10%.
- **Silent:** Hypothyroidism persists in 6%.
- **Suppurative:** Full recovery is common.
- **Riedel's thyroiditis:** Hypothyroidism occurs when the entire gland undergoes fibrosis.

Evaluation of a Thyroid Nodule

EPIDEMIOLOGY

- Common (1% of men and 5% of women).
- Incidence ↑ after age 45.
- History of neck irradiation (increased CA risk).
- Family history of pheochromocytoma, thyroid CA, or hyperparathyroidism (MEN II) increases suspicious for cancer.

SIGNS AND SYMPTOMS

- Dysphagia, hoarseness (indicative of malignant infiltration).
- Physical exam: Likelihood of malignancy increases with nodule > 2 cm, regional lymphadenopathy, fixation to tissues, age < 40, male sex, family history of thyroid cancer, history of head and neck irradiation.

DIAGNOSIS (SEE FIGURE 2.2-1)

- Fine-needle aspiration is the best initial study. Accuracy can be > 90%.
- Thyroid ultrasound is performed to evaluate the size and number of thyroid nodules. It also evaluates whether the nodules are cystic or solid.
- Thyroid scan with technetium 99m–labeled iodine (RAIU) classifies nodules as hyperfunctioning (hot nodules, less likely to be malignant) or hypofunctioning (cold nodules, more likely to be malignant).

Thyroid Cancer

EPIDEMIOLOGY

- Incidence ~ 9/100,000.
- 2:1 female predominance.
- Increases with age and plateaus after age 50.
- Worse prognosis if < 20 years old or > 65 years old.

RISK FACTORS

- History of childhood head or neck irradiation.
- Large nodule (> 4 cm).
- Enlarging neck mass.
- Family history.

CLASSIFICATION

Two types—follicular (epithelial) and parafollicular:

- **Epithelial** (three histologic types):
  - Papillary: Most common, has best prognosis.
  - Follicular: Early metastasis.
  - Anaplastic: Rare, worst prognosis.

If thyroidectomy is planned, obtain a thyroglobulin level after surgery. A return to normal following thyroidectomy suggests the absence of metastatic thyroid tissue.

Measurement of serum thyroglobulin is useful for following thyroid cancers in response to treatment, but a serum thyroglobulin level is not useful in distinguishing benign from malignant nodules.

ENDOCRINOLOGY

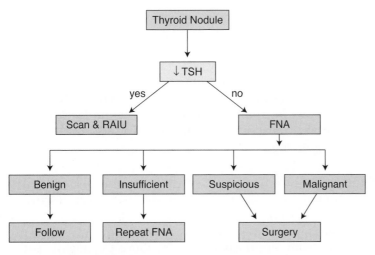

FIGURE 2.2-1. Initial approach to the thyroid nodule.

Causes of hypercalcemia:
Hyperparathyroidism
Bone metastases
Sarcoidosis
Hyperthyroidism
Thiazide diuretics
Immobilization
Paget's disease (only if patient is immobilized)

A patient who is post thyroid surgery has symptoms of muscle aches, weakness, and perioral parasthesias. *Think: Hypocalcemia from hypoparathyroid (either damaged by clamping off thyroid vessels or accidentally excised).*

Before you send a patient with 1° hyperparathyroidism to surgery, make sure you are not dealing with familial benign hypocalciuric hypercalcemia (FBHH). Urine calcium is usually < 50 mg/24 hr. It is autosomal dominant with 100% penetrance and is benign. No treatment, only reassurance, of patient and family members. Family history of kidney stones may be a tip-off.

ENDOCRINOLOGY

- **Parafollicular** (also called medullary thyroid cancer):
  - Calcitonin is increased from parafollicular C-cells.
  - Seen in MEN IIa and IIb.

TREATMENT

- Thyroidectomy.
- Radioiodine ablation of residual cancer and micrometastasis.
- Oral T_4 suppressive therapy after surgery, to suppress TSH that is thought to promote thyroid growth.
- Careful monitoring of TSH and thyroglobulin levels (a rise indicates recurrence of the cancer).

PARATHYROID DISORDERS

Hyperparathyroidism

- **Primary:** Hypersecretion of parathyroid hormone (PTH) by the parathyroid glands (*the rest of the section refers to 1° only*).
- **Secondary:** Glandular hyperplasia and elevated PTH in an appropriate response to hypocalcemia (due to renal failure, GI disturbances, etc.).
- **Tertiary:** Continued elevation of PTH after the disturbance causing 2° hyperparathyroidism has been corrected.

EPIDEMIOLOGY

- Most common in middle-aged and elderly women.
- Common: Present in 0.1% of the population.

ETIOLOGY

- Parathyroid adenoma: 85%, 1 gland involved.
- Parathyroid hyperplasia: 14%, all four glands involved.
- Parathyroid carcinoma: 1%, 1 gland involved.
- Associated with MEN I and IIa (10% of cases).
- Neck irradiation increases risk.

PATHOPHYSIOLOGY

Parathyroid hormone (PTH) increases serum Ca^{2+} levels:

- Stimulates renal hydroxylation of vitamin D (necessary for GI absorption of Ca^{2+}).
- Increases renal resorption of Ca^{2+}.
- Decreases renal resorption of PO_4^-.
- Increases resorption of bone (increases osteoclastic activity).
- PTH secretion is stimulated by decreased serum levels of Ca^{2+} and inhibited by high levels, except in adenomas and carcinomas in which feedback inhibition is lost.

SIGNS AND SYMPTOMS

- Most patients are asymptomatic and the disease gets discovered during routine blood work.
- Symptoms range from mild to severe.
- Generally, with **serum calcium** levels above 13.5 mg/dL, patients experience fatigue, polyuria, weakness, nausea, vomiting, abdominal pain,

and changes in mental status from confusion to lethargy to obtundation and coma.

- Milder elevations in calcium can result in mild neurocognitive impairment.

DIAGNOSIS

- Elevated serum Ca^{2+}, low serum PO_4^-.
- High serum PTH.

TREATMENT

- Older asymptomatic patients with serum $Ca^{2+} < 12$ should just be followed for progression.
- **Surgery:**
  - Adenomas should be excised.
  - In hyperplasia, all four glands are removed and a small portion is re-inserted in an easily accessible place such as the forearm, so that it can function, but if hyperplasia recurs, subsequent surgical intervention is simplified.
- **Emergency measures:**
  - Hydration with normal saline (salt leads to increased urinary calcium excretion), followed by furosemide diuresis.
  - Bisphosphonates to block bone resorption (IV pamidronate).
  - Calcitonin acts rapidly but loses its efficacy after several days.

Hypoparathyroidism

Condition characterized by PTH deficiency.

ETIOLOGY

- Idiopathic.
- DiGeorge syndrome: Congenital aplasia or hypoplasia of thymus caused by missing gene on chromosome 22. Findings include hypoparathyroidism (parathyroid hypoplasia, heart defects, and deficiency of T cells and cell-mediated immunity (CMI).
- Postsurgical (ie, thyroidectomy).
- Infiltrative carcinoma.
- Irradiation.
- Hypomagnesemia (magnesium is necessary for parathyroid gland to secrete PTH).

EPIDEMIOLOGY

Equal incidence in men and women.

A 30-year-old woman presents with perioral paresthesias and a long QT interval on electrocardiogram (ECG). She recently had surgery for a thyroid goiter. *Think: Hypoparathyroidism* (due to neck surgery with probable accidental resection of the parathyroids). **Next step:** Check serum calcium, PTH, and vitamin D levels.

Vitamin D acts on the intestines to increase absorption of calcium and phosphate. It is formed in the skin via sunlight as a previtamin and is converted to an inactive intermediate (25-OH vitamin D) in the liver before being converted to its active form $1,25\text{-}(OH)_2$ vitamin D (calcitriol) in the kidney.

Pseudohypoparathyroidism presents the same as hypoparathyroidism, except that the pathophysiology in pseudohypoparathyroidism is tissue resistance to PTH, so that PTH is high (distinguishing feature). Pseudohypoparathyroidism is associated with Albright's hereditary osteodystrophy (round facies, short stature, short fourth metacarpal bone, and subcutaneous calcification).

Addisonian or adrenal crisis is an acute complication of adrenal insufficiency characterized by shock, dehydration, confusion, vomiting, hyponatremia, hyperkalemia, and hypoglycemia. It is precipitated by sepsis, hemorrhage, trauma, and other stressors.

ENDOCRINOLOGY

SIGNS AND SYMPTOMS

Signs and symptoms of hypocalcemia (see also chapter on nephrology and acid-base disorders):

- Seizures.
- Perioral paresthesia.
- Fasciculations, tetany, and muscle weakness.
- CNS irritability, confusion and seizure.
- Chvostek's and Trousseau's signs.
- Bronchospasm.
- Anxiety, psychosis.

DIAGNOSIS

- Low serum calcium.
- High serum phosphorus.
- Normal or low PTH.
- Normal 25-OH vitamin D.
- Low $1,25\text{-}(OH)_2$ vitamin D.
- QT prolongation on ECG.

TREATMENT

- Treat severe, life-threatening hypocalcemia with intravenous calcium.
- Maintenance therapy with calcitriol and oral calcium supplementation.

ADRENAL DISORDERS

Adrenal Insufficiency

- Primary insufficiency (Addison's disease) is due to a problem with the adrenal gland itself, in which it does not produce hormones.
- In secondary insufficiency, the adrenal gland is intact, but the pituitary does not produce ACTH, so that there is no stimulus for the adrenal gland to secrete its hormones.
- Tertiary insufficiency is due to hypothalamic failure.

EPIDEMIOLOGY

More common in women (2:1), in its autoimmune form.

ETIOLOGY

- **Primary insufficiency (Addison's disease):**
  - Autoimmune (80%).
  - Tuberculosis (15%).
  - Neoplastic disease.
  - Sarcoidosis.
  - Amyloidosis.
  - Blastomycosis.
  - Hemochromatosis.
  - AIDS.
  - Adrenal hemorrhage due to trauma, anticoagulants, or coagulopathies.
  - Waterhouse-Friederichsen syndrome (fulminant septicemia).
  - Adrenalectomy.
- **Secondary insufficiency:**
  - Suppression of hypothalamic-pituitary-adrenal axis by exogenous steroids (most common).

- Sheehan's syndrome (postpartum pituitary necrosis).
- Pituitary infarct/tumor.
- Autoimmune destruction of pituitary.

ANATOMY

- The adrenal cortex consists of three zones (GFR):
  - Outer—**zona glomerulosa:** Produces aldosterone (mineralocorticoids).
  - Middle—**zona fasciculata:** Produces cortisol (glucocorticoids).
  - Inner—**zona reticularis:** Produces androgens and estrogens (sex hormones).
- The adrenal medulla produces catecholamines.

PATHOPHYSIOLOGY

- **Aldosterone:**
  - Produced when angiotensin II (stimulated by renin secretion from the kidney), acts on the zona glomerulosa to convert corticosterone to aldosterone.
  - Principal function is to increase renal sodium reabsorption in the distal tubule and collecting ducts, causing secretion of potassium and hydrogen ions.
  - Deficiency results in hyperkalemia and hyponatremia.
- **Cortisol:**
  - Stimulates gluconeogenesis by increasing protein and fat catabolism and decreasing utilization of glucose and tissue sensitivity to insulin.
  - Promotes anti-inflammatory state via inhibition of arachidonic acid, inhibition of interleukin-2 production, and inhibiting release of histamine from mast cells.
  - Has widespread effects on carbohydrate and protein metabolism.
  - Acts to counteract the effects of insulin and maintain blood glucose levels.
  - Governs body water distribution.
  - Enhances the pressor effects of catecholamine on heart muscle and blood vessels.
  - Inhibits inflammatory and allergic reactions.
  - Deficiency results in impairment of body's ability to handle stress.

Primary adrenal insufficiency results in increased levels of ACTH. Melanocyte-stimulating hormone (MSH) and ACTH are cleaved from the same propeptide, so elevated ACTH results in increased skin pigmentation.

SIGNS AND SYMPTOMS

- Hyperpigmentation of mucosa, areolae, hand creases, knees, elbows, and knuckles (1° only).
- Salt craving (1° only).
- Orthostatic hypotension.
- Weakness.
- Anorexia.
- Weight loss.
- Abdominal pain.

An 18-year-old man with hemophilia A who was recently mugged (receiving multiple blows to the back and abdomen) is now complaining of dizziness, abdominal pain, dark patches on his elbows and knees, and uncontrollable cravings for pizza and French fries. *Think: 1° adrenal insufficiency.* **Next step:** ACTH stimulation test.

ENDOCRINOLOGY

Secondary adrenal insufficiency can be distinguished from Addison's disease by:
- Absence of hyperpigmentation
- Normal aldosterone secretion
- Other signs of hypopituitarism such as hypothyroidism and hypogonadism suggest presence of pituitary lesion or tumor

The most common source of glucocorticoid excess is exogenous corticosteroid therapy.

DIAGNOSIS

- **ACTH (Cortrosyn) test:**
  - Give test dose of ACTH and measure serum cortisol levels at 0, 30, and 60 minutes. A peak level < 18–20 µg/dL suggests adrenal insufficiency.
  - Measuring the plasma ACTH after test will tell you whether it is primary adrenal insufficiency (high ACTH) or secondary adrenal insufficiency (low or normal ACTH).
- Hyperkalemia, hyponatremia, extracellular fluid (ECF) volume contraction and metabolic acidosis due to aldosterone deficiency (1° only).
- Hypoglycemia (more common in 2° adrenal failure due to GH deficiency as well).
- Anemia.
- Elevated BUN and creatinine.
- Elevated ACTH, low serum cortisol.

TREATMENT

- Glucocorticoid replacement for all patients.
- Instruct patients to increase their glucocorticoid dose in times of stress and infection.
- Patients with Addison's disease should also receive mineralocorticoid replacement therapy.

Adrenal Excess: Cushing's Syndrome

- **Cushing's syndrome:** Symptoms caused by excess cortisol production.
- **Cushing's disease:** Cushing's syndrome caused by excess ACTH secretion by pituitary.

ADDISON'S DISEASE	CUSHING'S DISEASE
Cortisol deficiency	Cortisol excess
Patient is thin	Patient is obese
Hyponatremia	Hypernatremia
Hyperkalemia	Hypokalemia
Metabolic acidosis	Metabolic alkalosis
Hypotension	Hypertension
Hypoglycemia	Hyperglycemia (or diabetes)
Lymphocytosis	Lymphopenia
Eosinophilia	No eosinophilia

EPIDEMIOLOGY

More common in females.

ETIOLOGY

- Exogenous corticosteroid therapy.
- Pituitary tumors (Cushing's disease).
- Adrenal adenomas.
- Ectopic ACTH production (such as small cell lung carcinoma, pheochromocytoma, medullary thyroid carcinoma, and carcinoids).

Small cell lung carcinoma is frequently associated with ectopic ACTH production.

SIGNS AND SYMPTOMS

- Hypertension.
- Facial plethora.
- Hair loss.
- Central obesity (apple-shaped habitus, moon facies, thin extremities).
- Hump on back of neck (Buffalo's hump).
- Fragile, easily bruised skin.
- Abdominal purplish striae.
- Proximal muscle weakness.
- Hirsutism.
- Emotional lability.
- Osteoporosis.

Patients with ectopic ACTH production often do not have all the mentioned symptoms; they usually have only hypertension and muscle weakness due to hypokalemia.

DIAGNOSIS

Twenty-four-hour urinary free cortisol is a reliable test for screening and should be done twice and be three times higher than the upper limit of normal for confirmation.

- **Overnight dexamethasone suppression test:**
  - Dexamethasone 1 mg is given at midnight, plasma cortisol measured at 8 AM.
  - If < 2 μg/100 mL, excludes Cushing's as a diagnosis.
- **High-dose dexamethasone suppression test:**
  - Give 8 mg dexamethasone at midnight, then measure serum cortisol and at 8 AM.
  - If ACTH is undetectable or decreased and there is no cortisol suppression, likely adrenal etiology.
  - If ACTH is normal or increased and there is no cortisol suppression, likely ectopic ACTH etiology.
  - If ACTH is high with partial cortisol suppression, likely pituitary etiology (Cushing's syndrome) where the pituitary is only relatively resistant to negative feedback.
- **Other findings:**
  - Increased 24-hour urinary free cortisol (> 100 μg/24 hr).
  - Hypokalemia, hypochloremia, metabolic alkalosis.
  - Hyperglycemia, hypercholesterolemia.
  - CT of adrenals to look for mass.
  - MRI of pituitary to look for mass.
  - Malignancy workup if ectopic ACTH production is suspected.
  - In equivocal cases, petrosal venous sampling will be needed to demonstrate pituitary ACTH hypersecretion.

Screening tests for Cushing's syndrome in clinically suspect patients include the 24-hour urine free cortisol test and the overnight dexamethasone-suppression test.

Cushing's disease can be distinguished from Cushing's syndrome by the presence of hyperpigmentation (only in Cushing's disease).

The most sensitive screening test for primary aldosteronism is the plasma aldosterone-plasma renin activity ratio.

A 42-year-old woman on long-term steroids for asthma has excess adipose tissue in her neck and upper trunk, a wide "moon face," and very fine hair. *Think: Cushing's syndrome* (due to exogenous steroids).

ENDOCRINOLOGY

A 44-year-old woman has hypertension, muscle cramps, and excessive thirst. *Think: Hyperaldosteronism.*

Secondary causes of hypertension:
Renovascular hypertension
Primary aldosteronism
Pheochromocytoma
Cushing's syndrome
Renal disease
Acromegaly

TREATMENT

- **Pituitary adenomas** (see Figure 2.2-2):
  - Transsphenoidal surgery.
  - Pituitary irradiation for children and cases refractory to surgery.
- **Adrenal adenoma:** Unilateral resection, followed by 3–12 months of glucocorticoid replacement (normal adrenal needs time to come out of suppression).
- **Bilateral adrenal hyperplasia:** Bilateral resection with lifelong replacement of glucocorticoids and mineralocorticoids.
- **Ectopic ACTH production:**
  - Treat underlying disease.
  - Remove source of neoplasm if possible.

Hyperaldosteronism

- Isolated excess production of aldosterone.
- Also called Conn's syndrome.

EPIDEMIOLOGY

- One to two percent of all patients with hypertension.
- Most frequent in ages 30–60.
- Adrenal tumor more common in women.

FIGURE 2.2-2. Pituitary adenoma (arrow).

(Reproduced, with permission, from Lee SH, Rao K, Zimmerman RA. *Cranial MRI and CT,* 4th ed. New York: McGraw-Hill, 1999: 653.)

ENDOCRINOLOGY

A young man is evaluated with persistent hypertension. He was diagnosed at a routine examination. His blood pressure has remained high despite diet, weight loss, and compliance with therapy, which includes four BP medications. *Think: Secondary hypertension.*

ETIOLOGY

- Unilateral aldosterone producing adenoma (most common cause).
- Bilateral hyperplasia of zona glomerulosa (idiopathic).

SIGNS AND SYMPTOMS

- Usually asymptomatic.
- Hypertension.
- May see signs of hypokalemia (muscle cramps, palpitations).

DIAGNOSIS

- Measure plasma aldosterone to plasma renin activity ratio; a ratio > 20 suggests hyperaldosteronism.
- **Other findings:**
  - Hypokalemia, hypernatremia, and metabolic alkalosis.
  - High serum aldosterone, low renin levels.
  - Twenty-four-hour urine high in potassium and aldosterone.
  - Evidence of adrenal mass on abdominal CT.
  - Aldosterone escape: After initial edema and weight gain, patients usually diurese and shed the edema.

> **Pheochromo-cytoma—**
>
> **Rule of 10s**
>
> 10% are extra-adrenal
> 10% are bilateral
> 10% are malignant
> 10% are familial
> 10% are pediatric
> 10% calcify
> 10% recur after resection

TREATMENT

- Adrenalectomy for tumor.
- Medical management for hyperplasia:
  - Spironolactone (potassium sparing) or ACE inhibitors to control blood pressure.
  - Low-sodium diet.
  - Maintenance of ideal body weight, regular exercise, smoking cessation.

Pheochromocytoma

Tumor of the adrenal medulla resulting in catecholamine excess.

> **Multiple endocrine neoplasia type I: (3Ps)**
>
> Pituitary tumors
> Pancreatic islet tumors
> Hyperparathyroidism due to Parathyroid hyperplasia

EPIDEMIOLOGY

Equal incidence in men and women. Tumors in women are three times as likely to be malignant.

ETIOLOGY

- MEN types IIa and IIb.
  - MEN IIa: Pheochromocytoma, parathyroid hyperplasia, and medullary thyroid cancer.
  - MEN IIb: Pheochromocytoma, medullary thyroid CA, and mucosal neuromas.

> **5H's**
>
> Headache
> Hypertension
> Hot (diaphoretic)
> Heart (palpitations)
> Hyperhidrosis

- Neurofibromatosis.
- Von Hippel–Lindau disease: Pheochromocytoma, retinal angiomas, CNS hemangioblastomas, renal cell carcinoma, pancreatic pseudo-cysts, ependymal cystadenoma.

SIGNS AND SYMPTOMS

- Patients experience "paroxysmal attacks" of high blood pressure.
- Physical exam usually normal outside of an attack.
- Symptoms of catecholamine (sympathetic) excess will predominate during an attack.
- Tremor.
- Anxiety.
- Weight loss.

> A 38-year-old woman on labetalol presents with poorly controlled hypertension, frequent headaches, and palpitations. *Think: Pheochomocytoma.* **Next step:** Stop labetalol and check urine catecholamines and serum metanephrines.
>
> The classic triad of symptoms for pheochromocytoma consists of hypertension with the triad of headaches, palpitations, and diaphoresis.

Patients with pheochromocytoma may carry an incorrect diagnosis of anxiety disorder.

DIAGNOSIS

- Elevated 24-hour urine catecholamines and metanephrines.
- Fractionated plasma free metanephrines.
- CT or MRI to look for adrenal mass, if negative with clinical impression and biochemical tests being positive, obtain MIBG scan. MIBG is a compound that resembles metanephrine and is taken up by phochromocytoma tissue.

TREATMENT

- Surgical resection.
- Alpha-adrenergic blockade (may also add beta blocker).

BONE DISORDERS

Osteomalacia

- Disease of impaired bone mineralization.
- Termed *rickets* in the pediatric population.

ETIOLOGY

Urinary excretion of metanephrine, normetanephrine, and catecholamines may be used to confirm the presence of excess catecholamine production.

- Decreased Ca^{2+} absorption.
- Dietary calcium deficiency: Rare, avoidance of dairy products.
- GI disorders: Malabsorption syndromes, gastrectomy, dumping syndrome.
- Vitamin D deficiency.
- Hepatobiliary and pancreatic disease: Loss of bile acids or pancreatic lipase reduce absorption of fat-soluble vitamins.
- Extremely low-fat diets.

- Renal osteodystrophy: Decreased renal hydroxylation of vitamin D.
- Decreased serum PO_4^-.
- Renal tubular acidosis, Fanconi's syndrome, hypophosphatasia.

SIGNS AND SYMPTOMS

- Bone pain.
- Weakness.
- Difficulty walking: Broad-based waddling gait with short strides.
- Thoracic kyphosis.

DIAGNOSIS

- **Radiographs:**
  - Show diffuse, nonspecific osteopenia.
  - Vertebrae may be biconcave from compression by intervertebral disks.
  - Pseudofractures (radiolucent lines perpendicular to bone cortex).
- **Labs:**
  - Ca^{2+} and PO_4^- low to normal.
  - High alkaline phosphatase.
  - PTH may be elevated in response to low Ca^{2+}.

TREATMENT

- Address underlying disorder.
- Calcium, vitamin D supplements.

Osteoporosis

Systemic disorder resulting in a reduction of bone mass that leads to increased risk of fracture.

EPIDEMIOLOGY

Risk factors for osteoporosis include:

- Female and elderly.
- Postmenopause.
- Family history of osteoporosis.
- Cigarette smoking.
- Thin body habitus.
- Sedentary lifestyle.

PATHOPHYSIOLOGY

- Reduction in bone mass occurs due to an imbalance between bone acquisition and bone reabsorption.
- There is no change in the ratio of mineral to organic bone.
- Histology: Decreased cortical thickness and decreased number and size of cancellous bone trabeculae (especially horizontal).
- **Clinical findings:**
- Osteoporosis is asymptomatic until fracture occurs.
- Vertebral body fractures:
  - Pain in the lumbar region.
  - Acute in onset.
  - Radiating to the flank.

Prior to surgery for tumor resection, patient must be properly alpha blocked with phenoxybenzamine or other alpha blockers to prevent intraoperative hypertensive crisis. Also, prior to starting beta-blocker therapy, alpha blockers must be on board to prevent unopposed alpha receptor stimulation.

Abnormalities of vitamin D synthesis and metabolism are common in osteomalacia.

Oncogenic osteomalacia can be cured with removal of the tumor.

Bone Mineral Density Scoring

T score > −1 = normal bone mass

T score −2.5 to −1 = osteopenia

T score ≤ −2.5 = osteoporosis

ENDOCRINOLOGY

- Usually occur after sudden bending or lifting.
- Radiation of the pain down one leg is common.
- Spinal cord compression is rare.
- Hip fractures:
  - Most serious complication.
  - Most resulting from a fall from a standing position.
  - Incidence of fracture increases with age in both men and women.
- **Laboratory findings:**
  - Serum calcium and phosphorus usually *normal.*
  - Alkaline phosphatase is increased after fractures but is usually normal if fractures aren't present.
  - Bone-specific alkaline phosphatase assays are useful for monitoring response to therapy.
  - Twenty percent of postmenopausal women have hypercalciuria.

DIAGNOSIS

- Since bone loss is a universal process of aging, 2° osteoporosis should be diagnosed definitively and other causes should be ruled out.
- Biconcavity of vertebral bodies with pathologic fractures is highly suggestive of osteoporosis.
- Bone densitometry establishes the diagnosis.
- Measure bone mineral density using dual x-ray absorptiometry (DEXA) scan (not a bone scan).
- **Indications for measurement of bone mass:**
  - Women age $\geq$ 65 years.
  - Postmenopausal women age < 65 years who have at lease one risk factor for osteoporosis other than menopause.
  - Postmenopausal women who present with fractures.
  - Women who are considering therapy for osteoporosis and for whom bone mineral densitometry tests results would influence this decision.
  - Women who have been receiving hormone replacement therapy for a prolonged period.
  - Radiographic findings suggestive of osteoporosis or vertebral deformity.
  - Corticosteroid therapy for > 3 months.
  - Primary hyperparathyroidism.
  - Treatment for osteoporosis (to monitor therapeutic response).

PREVENTION AND THERAPY

- Prevention of low bone mass by adequate dietary calcium and weight-bearing exercise. These measures increase peak bone mass earlier in life and prevent accelerated bone loss later in life.
- Estrogen replacement therapy prevents rapid bone loss and subsequently decreases rate of fractures.
- Calcitonin decreases bone reabsorption.
- Bisphosphonates (alendronate) increase density of spinal bone and decreases incidence of fractures when used in conjunction with vitamin D and calcium supplementation.

Paget's Disease of Bone

Chronic disease of adult bone in which localized areas of bone become hyperactive and the normal bone matrix is replaced by softened and enlarged bone.

Bone mineral densitometry is the only reliable method for measuring bone mass; osteoporosis is present when the T score is < – 2.5.

Differential in osteoporosis:
- Malignancy: Multiple myeloma, lymphoma, leukemia, and metastatic carcinoma
- Hyperparathyroidism
- Osteomalacia
- Paget's disease of bone

Treatment of osteoporosis is determined by bone mass and risk factors for osteoporosis.

Bisphosphonates and teriparatide are the agents that decrease nonvertebral fractures in osteoporosis.

ETIOLOGY

Cause is unknown, but it is suspected that a viral infection plays a role.

EPIDEMIOLOGY

- Rare for age > 40 years.
- 3:2 male predominance.

PATHOPHYSIOLOGY

- Hyperactive bone turnover.
- Increased bone formation.
- Pelvis, femur, skull, tibiae, and vertebrae all affected.
- Enlarged multinucleated osteoclasts.

CLINICAL FINDINGS

- Most patients are asymptomatic; diagnosis is made at autopsy.
- Incidental radiographic findings: Area of hyperlucency surrounded by a hyperdense border.
- Elevated alkaline phosphatase.
- Symptomatic patients:
  - Increasing hat size due to skull involvement.
  - Swelling or lengthening of a long bone, causing gait disturbance.
  - Dull aching pain, usually in the back; may radiate to the buttocks or lower extremities.
  - Rarely hearing loss due to involvement of the ossicles or auditory canal impinging on CN VIII.
- Complications:
  - Pathologic fractures.
  - Rarely "high-output" cardiac failure due to high vascularity of lesions.
  - Urinary stones due to high calcium excretion.
  - Sarcoma occurs in 1% of patients; poor prognosis.

 A patient is found to have an elevated alkaline phosphatase during a routine blood test. No other abnormalities were found. Further workup revealed the enzyme to be heat labile. *Think: Paget's disease.*

TREATMENT

- Most patients require no treatment.
- Indications for therapy are excessive pain, neural compression, profound alteration in posture or gait, high-output heart failure, hypercalcemia, and excessive calciuria, with or without renal calculi.
- Indomethacin is usually satisfactory for pain relief.
- Osteotomy is useful in selected cases of anatomic deformity or impingement.
- Bisphosphonates decrease bone reabsorption and are usually well tolerated.
- Calcitonin may be instituted in cases with cardiac failure or neurologic deficits. Calcitonin also has an analgesic effect.

When alkaline phosphatase is elevated, send gamma-glutamyl transpeptidase (GGT) to determine if hepatic or bone (elevated in liver but not bone).

Paget's disease is associated with elevated serum alkaline phosphatase levels and typical radiographic abnormalities; most patients are asymptomatic.

The primary indication for treatment in Paget's disease is the presence of symptoms and lytic involvement of vertebrae, skull, weight-bearing bones, or areas adjacent to major joints.

The therapy of choice for uncomplicated Paget's disease is an oral bisphosphonate.

ENDOCRINOLOGY

Gastroenterology

- **Visceral pain:**
  - Dull, and poorly localized pain.
  - Midline location due to bilateral innervation of organs.
  - Associated with stretching, inflammation, or ischemia, involving bowel walls or organ capsules.
- **Parietal pain:**
  - Sharp, well-localized pain; peritonitis associated with rebound tenderness and involuntary guarding.
  - Pain location correlates with associated dermatomes.
  - Occurs commonly with inflammation, air, frank pus, blood, or bile in or adjacent to the peritoneum.
- **Referred pain:**
  - Pain stimuli generated at an afflicted location are perceived as originating from a site in which there is no current pathology.
  - These sites are usually related by a common embryological origin.
  - The pain can sometimes be perceived in both locations.

Visceral pain is **V**ague. **Example:** Early appendicitis; initially dull, periumbilical pain.

Parietal pain is **P**inpoint. **Example:** Late appendicitis; local inflammation of the peritoneum → tenderness in the right lower quadrant.

Causes of Abdominal Pain

There are no hard-and-fast rules for localizing different types of abdominal pain. The following are classic examples for the exam:

- **Epigastric, upper abdominal pain:**
  - Gastroduodenal: Gastritis, peptic ulcer/perforation.
  - Pancreatic: Acute/chronic pancreatitis.
  - Aorta: Ruptured abdominal aortic aneurysm, dissecting abdominal aortic aneurysm.
  - Cardiac: Angina, myocardial infarction, pericarditis.
- **Right upper quadrant (RUQ):**
  - Hepatobiliary: Cholelithiasis, cholecystitis, cholangitis, hepatitis, abscess.
  - Peptic ulcer.
- **Left upper quadrant (LUQ):**
  - Spleen: Trauma, infarction, abscess, rupture (mononucleosis).
  - Gastric ulcer.
- **Right lower quadrant (RLQ):**
  - Appendicitis
  - Small bowel obstruction
  - Crohn's disease
  - Mesenteric lymphadenitis
  - Meckel's diverticulum
- **Left lower quadrant (LLQ):**
  - Diverticulitis
  - Inflammatory bowel disease
- **Flank pain:**
  - Nephrolithiasis
  - Pyelonephritis
  - Testicular torsion
  - Prostatitis
  - Epididymitis
- **Adnexal (lower abdominal pain):**
  - Ectopic pregnancy
  - Tubo-ovarian abscess

Example of referred pain: Ureteral obstruction can produce pain in the ipsilateral testicle.

- Pelvic inflammatory disease
- Ovarian torsion
- Salpingitis
- Cystitis
- **Anywhere:**
  - Strangulated hernia
  - Large bowel obstruction
  - Sigmoid volvulus
  - Mesenteric ischemia

Note: All premenopausal women with abdominal pain must have a pregnancy test, even if they say they are not sexually active.

 A 45-year-old obese woman complains of fever, RUQ pain, and nausea that is worse when she eats fatty foods. *Think: Cholecystitis.* **Next step:** Check RUQ ultrasound and LFTs.

A 26-year-old woman complains of severe left lower quadrant pain, vaginal bleeding, and light-headedness. Last menstrual period was 6 weeks ago. *Think: Ectopic pregnancy.* **Next step:** Pelvic exam and abdominal ultrasound. Consider OB/GYN and surgical consultation.

Other Causes of Abdominal Pain

- **Abdominal wall:** Hernia, rectus sheath hematoma.
- **Metabolic:** Diabetic ketoacidosis, acute intermittent porphyria, hypercalcemia.
- **Infectious:** Herpes zoster, mononucleosis, HIV.
- **Drugs/toxins:** Heavy metal poisoning, black widow spider envenomation.
- **Other:** Sickle cell anemia, foreign body.

Abdominal Pain in the Elderly

Elderly patients who present with abdominal pain must be treated with particular caution. Common problems include:

- Difficulty communicating.
- Comorbid disease.
- Inability to tolerate intravascular volume loss.
- Unusual presentation of common disease.
- May not mount a white blood cell count or a fever.
- Complaint often incommensurate with severity of disease.

Note: Up to 2% of elderly patients with a myocardial infarction (MI) will present with abdominal pain.

In elderly patients with abdominal pain, always consider vascular causes, including:

- AAA
- Mesenteric ischemia
- Myocardial infarction

GASTROENTEROLOGY

Abdominal Aortic Aneurysm (AAA)

- Dilation of the abdominal aorta usually involves the infrarenal arteries.
- AAAs are the most common site of atherosclerotic aneurysms.
- Men are more frequently affected.
- Acute expansion or leak of an AAA causes pain and may precede rupture, a life-threatening emergency.

RISK FACTORS

- Familial.
- Smoking.
- Atherosclerosis.
- Trauma/infection.
- Aneurysms > 5 cm associated with 20–40% 5-year risk of rupture.

SIGNS AND SYMPTOMS

- Abdominal or back pain.
- Pulsatile mass in abdomen.
- Hypotension (or symptoms of).
- History of vascular disease or atherosclerosis.

DIAGNOSIS

- **Screening:** U.S. Preventive Services Task Force recommends one-time screening with ultrasound (US) in men > 65–75 years of age who ever smoked. Screening of first-degree relatives usually begins at 50 years of age.
- **Ultrasonography, magnetic resonance imaging (MRI) or computed tomography (CT) scan with IV contrast:** Can demonstrate size of aneurysm and location of leak or rupture. May replace angiogram as gold standard.
- **Angiogram:** Usually done when treatment is planned to visualize renal and peripheral arteries. Can underestimate size of aneurysm with mural thrombus. Gold standard.

TREATMENT

- **Medical management:** Control hypertension, smoking cessation, treat coronary artery disease (CAD) and carotid artery disease and serial non-invasive assessment.
- **Surgical management:** Usually when diameter is > 5.0–5.5 cm, rapidly progressive (> 0.5cm/yr), symptomatic, or traumatic/infectious.
- **Dissection/rupture:** Requires emergent surgical repair/consult. All patients should have good IV access along with type and crossmatch of blood for transfusions if necessary.

 A 63-year-old man complains of pain in his "kidney" for 3 days. He is a smoker and has a history of MI × 2. He has no back tenderness but you feel a large pulsatile mass in his abdomen. *Think: Abdominal aortic aneurysm.* **Next step:** CT with IV contrast, blood pressure control, consider vascular surgery consult depending on results of CT.

Acute Mesenteric Ischemia vs. Chronic Mesenteric Ischemia

Acute mesenteric ischemia: Sudden onset of abdominal pain due to acute occlusion of mesenteric vessel by emboli or thrombosis; emergency.

Chronic mesenteric ischemia: Episodic, postprandial pain, due to slow narrowing of vessels due to atherosclerosis; weight loss associated; not emergency.

Mesenteric Ischemia

Interruption of intestinal blood flow resulting in abdominal pain and potentially catastrophic intestinal pathology depending on the severity of vascular compromise.

- Ischemia of celiac trunk affects stomach, duodenum and liver.
- Ischemia of superior mesenteric artery (SMA) affects jejunum, ileum, and right colon.
- Inferior mesenteric artery (IMA) affects left colon and rectum.

CAUSES

- **Atherosclerosis** causing obstruction of SMA, IMA, or celiac artery (chronic).
- Atrial fibrillation causing **embolus** (acute presentation).
- **Hypertension**, diabetes.
- Low-flow state (hypotension, poor cardiac output).
- **Hypercoagulability** (acute thrombus).

SIGNS AND SYMPTOMS

- Severe abdominal **pain out of proportion to exam**, nausea, vomiting and may have rectal bleed.
- History of **gnawing abdominal pain after eating**.
- Labs may show ↑ lactate, metabolic acidosis.

DIAGNOSIS

- Gold standard is **angiography**.
- Spiral CT scan with contrast and magnetic resonance angiography (MRA) of the abdomen also can diagnose.

TREATMENT

- Maintain tissue perfusion with fluids.
- Surgery revascularization (bypass).

 A 72-year-old man with a history of atrial fibrillation, on digoxin, complains of severe abdominal pain out of proportion to the exam. *Think: Acute mesenteric ischemia.* **Next step:** Abdominal angiogram, hydration, check serum lactate level, surgical consult.

 A 75-year-old woman with a history of myocardial infarction complains of gnawing abdominal pain after eating. She has lost 15 pounds in the past month. *Think: Chronic mesenteric ischemia.* **Next step:** Check abdominal CT angiogram or abdominal angiogram and refer patient for revascularization if positive.

Dysphagia

- May be distinguished as mechanical, functional or oropharyngeal.
- Intermittent dysphagia is usually caused by a ring, a web, or a functional cause (motility disorder).
- **Mechanical:** Progressive, associated with weight loss, solid more than liquid. Causes include lyomyoma, squamous cell carcinoma, adenocarcinoma, Barrett's esophagus.
- **Functional:** Intermittent with both solids and liquids. Common causes include achalasia, diffuse esophageal spasms, and scleroderma.
- **Oropharyngeal:** Choking, coughing, or regurgitations result of faulty transfer of bolus from oropharynx to esophagus. Usually structural or neuromuscular causes.

Esophagitis

Inflammation of the esophagus causing pain and discomfort.

ETIOLOGY

- Infectious:
  - **Viral:** herpes simplex virus (HSV), varicella-zoster virus (VZV), cytomegalovirus (CMV).
  - **Bacterial:** *Lactobacillus, Streptococcus, Cryptosporidium, Pneumocystis jiroveci* pneumonia (PCP), *Mycobacterium tuberculosis, Candida.*
- Other causes: Radiation, corrosives.

SIGNS AND SYMPTOMS

- Odynophagia.
- Dysphagia.
- Esophageal bleeding.
- Nausea/vomiting.
- Chest pain.
- May be asymptomatic.

A patient with HIV and odynophagia (pain on swallowing) has esophagitis most likely due to:
- Candida
- CMV
- Herpes

DIAGNOSIS

- Either barium esophogram or upper endoscopy.
- Remember some classic findings: HSV, VZV have vesicles; CMV has intranuclear inclusions. Candida will have white plaques.

TREATMENT

Treat the cause: Gancyclovir for CMV; acyclovir for HSV/VZV; fluconazole for candida.

Esophageal Rupture or Perforation

Iatrogenic or pathologic trauma to the esophagus, which may result in leakage of air and esophageal contents into the mediastinum. Carries a 50% mortality.

ETIOLOGY/TYPES

- **Iatrogenic:** This often occurs in an already diseased esophagus. Comprises 50–75% of cases of esophageal rupture: endoscopy, dilation, Blakemore tubes, intubation of the esophagus, nasogastric tube placement.
- **Boerhaave's syndrome:** A *full-thickness* tear. Generally occurs in the relatively weak left posterolateral wall of distal esophagus. **Due to** forceful vomiting, cough, trauma.
- **Mallory-Weiss syndrome:** A *partial-thickness* tear. Usually occurs in the right posterolateral wall of the distal esophagus and results in bleeding that generally resolves spontaneously. **Due to** forceful vomiting/retching.
- **Foreign body ingestion:** Objects usually lodge near anatomic narrowings—distal to the upper esophageal sphincter, near the aortic arch or at lower esophageal sphincter.

 An alcoholic man presents after severe retching, complaining of retrosternal and upper abdominal pain. *Think: Boerhaave's syndrome.* **Next step:** Immediate chest x-ray looking for subcutaneous and/or mediastinal air. Immediate cardiothoracic surgical evaluation if positive.

SIGNS AND SYMPTOMS

- Severe, constant pain in chest, abdomen, and back.
- Dysphagia.
- Dyspnea.
- **Subcutaneous emphysema.**
- Mediastinal emphysema heard as a "crunching sound" with heartbeat (Hammon's crunch).

DIAGNOSIS

- **Chest x-ray:** Left-sided pleural effusion, mediastinal or subcutaneous emphysema.
- **Esophagogram with water-soluble contrast:** Shows extravasation of contrast.
- **Other studies:** Endoscopy, CT, and pleurocentesis (check fluid for low pH and high salivary amylase).

TREATMENT

Surgical repair of full-thickness tears. Partial-thickness tears may resolve spontaneously.

A 56-year-old man complains of food feeling "stuck" on its way down and vomiting food he ate days ago. His breath is terrible. *Think: Zenker's diverticulum.* **Next step:** Check barium swallow looking for outpouching of esophagus.

Zenker's Diverticulum

Pharyngeal or esophageal pouch due to a defect in the muscular wall of the posterior hypopharynx.

SIGNS AND SYMPTOMS

- Halitosis.
- Regurgitation of food days after eating it ("spit-ups").
- Frequent aspiration.
- Esophageal obstruction.

DIAGNOSIS

Barium swallow or endoscopy.

TREATMENT

Surgical removal or cricopharyngeal myotomy.

Esophageal Spasm and Achalasia

- **Achalasia:** A neurogenic disorder of esophageal motility with absence of normal peristalsis and impaired relaxation of lower esophageal sphincter (food doesn't get pushed down normally). Thought to arise from scarring in Auerbach's plexus (nerve damage).
- **Diffuse esophageal spasm (DES):** Motility disorder with frequent non-peristaltic contractions. Believed to come from hypoactive inhibitory neurons within Auerbach's plexus. See Table 2.3-1.

DIAGNOSIS

- **Barium swallow** (see Figures 2.3-1 and 2.3-2).
- **Manometry** (measures esophageal pressures): Achalasia will show normal to ↑ pressure at LES with no relaxation upon swallowing; DES will show high-amplitude contractions, possibly including proximal esophagus.

TABLE 2.3-1. Comparison of Achalasia and Diffuse Esophageal Spasm

	ACHALASIA	DIFFUSE ESOPHAGEAL SPASM
Signs and symptoms	Weight loss, cough, diffuse chest pain.	Dysphagia, diffuse chest pain.
Pattern of contraction	Failure of LES to relax on swallowing. ■ Classic: Simultaneous small wave. ■ Vigorous: Simultaneous large wave.	Swallow-induced large wave.
Relieved by	Nitroglycerin.	Nitroglycerin.
Barium swallow	"Bird's beak" narrowing of terminal esophagus.	Corkscrew appearance.
Treatment	Nitroglycerin, local botulinum toxin, balloon dilatation, sphincter myotomy.	Nitroglycerin, anticholinergics.

FIGURE 2.3-1. Achalasia.

Barium esophagogram in a patient with achalasia demonstrates a dilated esophagus with a sharply tapered "bird's beak" narrowing. (Reproduced, with permission, from Waters PF, DeMeester TR. Foregut motor disorders and their surgical management. *Med Clin North Am* 65: 1244, 1981.)

FIGURE 2.3-2. Diffuse esophageal spasm.

Barium esophagogram in a patient with diffuse esophageal spasm demonstrates the characteristic "corkscrew" pattern. (Reproduced, with permission, from Schwartz SI, Fischer JE, Spencer FC, Shires GT, Daly JM. *Schwartz's Principles of Surgery*, 7th ed. New York: McGraw-Hill, 1998: 1129.)

GI Webs and Rings

The following conditions are anatomical obstructions, usually presenting with dysphagia to solids:

- **Plummer-Vinson syndrome:** Hypopharyngeal webs (thin mucosal structures protruding into lumen) associated with iron deficiency anemia.
- **Schatzki's ring:** A narrow lower esophageal ringlike outgrowth associated with dysphagia (see Figure 2.3-3).

Dysphagia to solids *and* liquids often indicates a motility problem (ie, achalasia and esophageal spasm). Dysphagia to *only* solids indicates mechanical obstruction (ie, tumor or Schatzki's ring).

Gastroesophageal Reflux Disease (GERD)

Reflux of acidic gastric contents into the esophagus.

CAUSES OF GERD

- Relaxed or incompetent lower esophageal sphincter (LES).
- Hiatal hernia.
- Delayed gastric emptying.
- ↓ esophageal motility.

CAUSES OF DELAYED GASTRIC EMPTYING

- Diabetes mellitus.
- Gastroparesis.

FIGURE 2.3-3. Schatzki's ring.

Barium esophagogram in a patient with Schatzki's ring demonstrates a distal esophageal ring at the gastroesophageal junction. (Reproduced, with permission, from Schwartz SI, Fischer JE, Spencer FC, Shires GT, Daly JM. *Schwartz's Principles of Surgery,* 7th ed. New York: McGraw-Hill, 1998: 1168.)

- Gastric outlet obstruction.
- Anticholinergic use.
- Fatty foods.

CAUSES OF LOWERED LES TONE

- Foods (coffee, chocolate).
- Alcohol.
- Cigarettes.
- Drugs (nitrates, calcium channel blockers).
- Hormones (estrogen, progesterone).

SIGNS AND SYMPTOMS

- Substernal burning pain.
- Dysphagia (secondary to stricture formation).
- Hypersalivation, with *sour* taste in mouth (water brash).
- Cough (particularly nocturnal), hoarseness.
- Wheezing.

DIAGNOSIS

Often, a trial of proton pump inhibitor (PPI) will be given to relieve symptoms without further workup. However, if "alarm signals" are present (long duration, weight loss, advanced age, nausea, refractory symptoms, guaiac positive), an endoscopy to rule out cancer is *required*.

TREATMENT

- **Lifestyle modification:** Elevate head of bed, discontinue foods that ↓ LES tone, avoid food < 3 hours before bed.
- **Pharmacologic:** H_2 blocker, PPI (continued indefinitely if severe).
- **Surgical:** Surgical correction such as Nissen fundoplication if all else fails.

COMPLICATIONS OF GERD

- **Esophagitis:** Esophageal damage, bleeding, and friability due to prolonged exposure to gastric contents.
- **Peptic stricture:** Occurs in about 10% of patients with GERD.
- **Barrett's esophagus:** Transformation of normal squamous epithelium to columnar epithelium, sometimes accompanied by an ulcer or stricture. This carries a significant risk of cancerous transformation. High-grade Barrett's requires resection. Other grades of Barrett's require surveillance endoscopy regularly for **life**; Barrett's does **not** regress, even if GERD is successfully treated.
- **Esophageal cancer:** Upper two-thirds of esophagus is usually squamous; lower one-third is usually adenocarcinoma.

Differential of chronic cough:
- **Asthma**
- **GERD**
- **Postnasal drip**

Barrett's esophagus carries an ↑ risk of development of esophageal adenocarcinoma; numbers vary but about 0.5% chance per year.

DISORDERS OF THE STOMACH

Peptic Ulcer Disease (PUD)

PUD consists of duodenal ulcers (DU) and gastric ulcers (GU).

GASTROENTEROLOGY

COMMON CAUSES

- *Helicobacter pylori.*
- Nonsteroidal anti-inflammatory drugs (NSAIDs).
- Miscellaneous causes including Zollinger-Ellison syndrome and idiopathic hypersecretion.

CLINICAL FEATURES

- Burning, gnawing, epigastric pain that occurs with an empty stomach. Pain is relieved within 30 minutes by food. Nighttime awakening with pain (when stomach empties); nausea/vomiting.
- When bleeding, melana or hematochezia is present.
- Associated with blood type O.

EPIDEMIOLOGY

- Two times more common in men.
- Incidence ↑ with age.
- Smoking ↑ risk.

A patient with known PUD presents with sudden onset of severe epigastric pain. Physical exam reveals guarding and rebound tenderness. *Think: Perforation.* **Next step:** Order a supine and upright abdominal x-ray, looking for free air under the diaphragm.

Causes of Peptic Ulcer Disease

NSAIDs and steroids inhibit production of PGE, which helps produce the gastric mucosal barrier.

H pylori produces urease, which breaks down the gastric mucosal barrier.

Gastric ulcers can even occur with achlorhydria.

PHYSIOLOGY KEY CONCEPTS

- **Gastrin is made by G cells** in the antrum of stomach and in the duodenum.
- Gastrin release is stimulated by gastrin-releasing peptide.
- Gastrin release is **inhibited by somatostatin.**
- **Gastrin stimulates parietal cells to secrete HCl into the gastric lumen.**
- Parietal cells are stimulated by gastrin, acetyl choline (from vagus nerve) and **histamine.**
- When stimulated, **parietal cells secrete acid into the lumen via a proton pump** that exchanges potassium for protons.
- **Gastrin also stimulates secretion of bicarbonate into the gastric venous circulation** (alkaline tide) and **into the protective gastric mucous gel**.
- Gastric bicarbonate secretion into the mucous gel **is inhibited by nonsteroidal anti-inflammatory drugs (NSAIDs), acetazolamide, alpha blockers, and alcohol.**
- Gel thickness is ↑ **by prostaglandin E (PGE)** and reduced by steroids and NSAIDs.
- **Zollinger-Ellison syndrome (ZE):**
  - A gastrin-secreting tumor in or near the pancreas. ZE can be part of multiple endocrine neoplasia type I (MEN I). Diarrhea is common.

Smoking is a risk factor for gastric ulcer.

- ZE has a triad of PUD, gastric acid hypersecretion, and an elevated gastrin level.

 A 52-year-old woman presents due to 3 months of early satiety, weight loss, and vomiting. *Think: Gastric outlet obstruction.*

Over 90% of patients with ZE have peptic ulcer disease.

DIAGNOSIS

- **Duodenal ulcer (DU):** Diagnose via endoscopy; however, most symptomatic cases of DU are easily diagnosed clinically. If patient responds to DU therapy, there is no need to do the biopsy.
- ***H pylori:*** Endoscopy with biopsy—allows culture and sensitivity for *H pylori* (organism is notoriously hard to culture—multiple specimens required during biopsy).
  - Serology: Anti–*H pylori* IgG indicates current or prior infection.
  - Urease breath test: $C^{13/14}$ labeled urea is ingested. If gastric urease is present, the carbon isotope can be detected as CO_2 isotopes in the breath.
- **ZE:** Secretin stimulation test—secretin, a gastrin inhibitor, is delivered parenterally (usually with Ca^{2+}), and its effect on gastrin secretion is measured. In ZE syndrome, there is a paradoxical astronomic rise in serum gastrin.
  - Gastrin level (must be taken when off antacid meds): If elevated, test for hyperacidity with gastric pH monitor.

H pylori may colonize 90% of the population — infection does not necessitate disease.

TREATMENT

Mainly depends on the cause:

- **Discontinue** NSAIDs, steroids, and smoking.
- **Triple therapy for *H pylori*** (eg, PPI, amoxicillin, and clarithromycin).
- **Antacid agents:** H_2 blockers and PPIs.
- **If bleeding, endoscopy** is done and sucralfate (enhances mucosal barrier) or misoprostol (prostaglandin analog) is used.
- **Surgery is indicated when ulcer is refractory** to 12 weeks of medical treatment or if hemorrhage, obstruction, or perforation is present.

 A 33-year-old female smoker presents with burning epigastric pain that is improved after eating a meal. *Think: Duodenal ulcer.* **Next step:** Trial of PPI. If not resolved in 4–6 weeks, then esophagogastroduodenoscopy (EGD).

Gastric ulcer pain is typically exacerbated by food. Duodenal ulcer pain is typically relieved by food.

COMPLICATIONS

- **Bleeding:** 20% incidence.
- **Perforation:** 7% incidence.
  - Posterior perforation of a duodenal ulcer will cause pain that radiates to the back and can cause pancreatitis. A chest or abdominal film will not show free air because the posterior duodenum is retroperitoneal.
  - Anterior perforation will show free air under the diaphragm in 70% of cases (see Figure 2.3-4).

FIGURE 2.3-4. Free air.

Upright chest film in a patient with perforated duodenal ulcer demonstrates free air underneath both right and left hemidiaphragms. (Reproduced, with permission, from Schwartz SI, Fischer JE, Spencer FC, Shires GT, Daly JM. *Schwartz's Principles of Surgery*, 7th ed. New York: McGraw-Hill, 1998: 1195.)

- **Gastric outlet obstruction**, due to scarring and edema (can also be a complication of neoplasm).

 A 45-year-old Japanese male smoker presents with epigastric pain, exacerbated by eating, and weight loss. *Think: Gastric ulcer.* **Next step:** Must get EGD, as patient has weight loss.

Gastritis

Acute or chronic inflammation of the stomach lining.

ETIOLOGY

- ↑ **acid:** Smoking, alcohol, stress.
- ↓ **mucosal barrier:** NSAIDs, steroids, *H pylori*.
- **Direct irritant:** Pancreatic and biliary reflux, infection.
- **Autoimmune.**

SIGNS AND SYMPTOMS

- Burning or gnawing pain usually **worsened with food** and relieved by antacids.
- Vomiting may relieve the pain after eating.

Cimetidine is a p450 inhibitor and, therefore, prolongs the action of drugs cleared in the liver by this system.

DIAGNOSIS

Endoscopy.

TREATMENT

Similar to PUD:

- Discontinue NSAIDs.
- Triple therapy to eradicate *H pylori* if present (PPI, amoxicillin, clarithromycin).
- Abstain from cigarettes and alcohol.
- H_2 blockers (eg, cimetidine, ranitidine), sucralfate, or misoprostol and PPI.
- Over-the-counter antacids.

COMPLICATIONS OF CHRONIC GASTRITIS

- Gastric atrophy.
- Gastric metaplasia.
- Pernicious anemia ($\downarrow$ production of intrinsic factor from gastric parietal cells due to **idiopathic** atrophy of the gastric mucosa and subsequent malabsorption of vitamin B_{12}).
- Gastric carcinoma, gastric lymphoma.

Etiologies of gastritis—

GNASHING

Gastric reflux (bile or pancreatic secretions)
Nicotine
Alcohol
Stress
*H*elicobacter pylori and other infections
Ischemia
NSAIDs
Glucocorticoids (long-term use)

DISORDERS OF THE PANCREAS

Normal Secretions from the Pancreas

- **Exocrine:** Bicarbonate, amylase, lipase, tyrosine, and other digestive enzymes.
- **Endocrine:** Insulin, glucagon, somatostatin.

Acute Pancreatitis

- Inflammation of the pancreas due to parenchymal autodigestion by proteolytic enzymes.
- Two varieties: Interstitial and necrotizing.
- In severe cases, it can be associated with a *systemic inflammatory response syndrome* (SIRS), which can progress to multiorgan system failure and acute respiratory distress syndrome (ARDS).

Hypercalcemia can cause pancreatitis, and pancreatitis can cause *hypocalcemia.*

ETIOLOGIES

- Gallstones.
- Alcohol.
- Hypertriglyceridemia.
- Complication of endoscopic retrograde cholangiopancreatography (ERCP).
- Drugs: Thiazides, furosemide, estrogen, antiretrovirals.
- Other rare problems: Neoplasm, hypercalcemia, idiopathic.

Most common causes of pancreatitis: Gallstones and alcohol.

SIGNS AND SYMPTOMS

- Severe, constant midepigastric or LUQ pain, *radiates to the back.*
- Pain sometimes improved when patient sits up and leans forward.

- Nausea, vomiting.
- Low-grade fever.
- Abdomen is usually tender with guarding, but no rebound.
- **The Grey-Turner sign** (flank discoloration) and Cullen sign (peri-umbilical discoloration) suggests **retroperitoneal hemorrhage.**

DIAGNOSIS

- Diagnostic markers in blood:
  - **Amylase:** Normally secreted by pancreas to break down carbohydrates. Elevation in pancreatitis, but not specific—can be found in small bowel inflammation, among other settings (in salivary glands, ovaries, testes, muscle).
  - **Lipase:** Normally secreted by the pancreas to break down triglycerides. Elevation in pancreatitis is fairly specific, though also found in gastric and intestinal mucosa. Level two times the upper limit of normal is 90% specific and 80–90% sensitive.
- Diagnostic imaging:
  - **Contrast-enhanced dynamic CT (CECT):** May show degree of pancreatic necrosis.
  - **Abdominal film:** May see calcification of pancreas, which is indicative of chronic pancreatitis, the "sentinel loop" of a localized small bowel ileus, and colon cutoff sign.
  - **Ultrasound:** May identify gallstones as the cause.
  - **ERCP:** Should be avoided in acute cases, but may be useful in endoscopic when associated with jaundice and cholangitis.

Ranson's criteria on admission—

GA LAW

Glucose
Age
LDH
AST
WBC

A 50-year-old male alcoholic presents with midepigastric pain radiating to the back. He is leaning forward on his stretcher and vomiting. *Think: Pancreatitis.* **Next step:** Establish IV access and start large-volume resuscitation with crystalloid.

Elevated lipase is more specific than amylase for diagnosing pancreatitis.

TREATMENT

- **IV hydration.**
- **Bowel rest.**
- NG tube for severe nausea, vomiting, or associated ileus.
- Analgesics and antiemetics as needed.
- **Antibiotics** (eg, imipenem) if infection is suspected, or necrosis identified on CT abdomen.

A "sentinel loop" on x-ray is distention and/or air-fluid levels near a site of abdominal distention. In pancreatitis, it is secondary to pancreatitis-associated ileus.

SEQUELAE

- **< 48 hours:** Usually isolated left pleural effusion containing high-amylase peripancreatic fluid.
- **1–4 weeks: Pseudocyst** (diagnosed by CT); if it persists, it can rupture or create a fistula, so surgical drainage is required. Ascites may result from pancreatic duct disruption or leaking pseudocyst.
- **4–6 weeks: Abscess;** requires surgical drainage.

PROGNOSIS

Ranson's criteria (see Table 2.3-2).

Gastric varices (without esopohageal varices) indicates splenic vein thrombosis, which is a complication of pancreatitis.

TABLE 2.3-2. Ranson's Criteria (Predicts Risk of Mortality in Pancreatitis)

ON ADMISSION	AFTER 48 HOURS
Glucose (serum) > 200	Drop in hematocrit > 10%
Age > 55	↑ in BUN > 5
LDH > 700	Calcium < 8
AST > 250	PO_2 < 60 mm Hg
WBC > 16,000	Base deficit > 4
	Fluid deficit > 6 L

NUMBER OF RISK FACTORS	MORTALITY
< 3	1%
3 or 4	16%
5 or 6	40%
> 6	Approaches 100%

Chronic Pancreatitis

Recurrent episodes of acute pancreatitis, usually from alcohol abuse (70–80%), which → inflammation, scarring, and duct obstruction.

OTHER CAUSES

- Hereditary pancreatitis.
- Protein energy malnutrition may cause chronic pancreatitis.

SIGNS AND SYMPTOMS

- Pain similar to acute pancreatitis.
- Malabsorption.
- Steatorrhea.
- Elevated blood sugars.
- Polyuria.
- Associated with chronic liver disease.

DIAGNOSIS

Pancreatic calcifications on x-ray or CT abdomen, diabetes, steatorrhea.

WORKUP

Abdominal x-ray (may show calcifications), trypsin level (low indicates poorly functioning pancreas). If these are inconclusive, do CT and/or ERCP (looking for abnormal duct anatomy). Finally, if all is still inconclusive, do secretin stimulation test.

Chole = of or pertaining to bile
Cyst = bladder
Cholecyst = gallbladder
Lith(o) = stones, calculus
Cholang = bile duct
Choledocholithiasis = stones in the bile duct

GASTROENTEROLOGY

TREATMENT

Same as for acute pancreatitis, with emphasis on pain control and abstinence from alcohol and fatty foods. May need pancreatic enzyme supplements. Surgical treatment when conservative measures fail.

 A patient with a history of alcohol abuse presents with severe abdominal pain exacerbated by food. Imaging shows calcifications of pancreas. *Think: Chronic pancreatitis.*

ERCP (endoscopic retrograde cholangiopancreatography): Endoscope inserted through mouth into the duodenum. A smaller scope is then inserted through the ampulla of Vater of the common bile duct allowing visualization (by injecting dye) of the pancreatic duct, hepatic duct, common bile duct, duodenal papilla, and gallbladder. ERCP can be interventional, as well as diagnostic. Stones can be removed, obstructed ducts can be stented, and biopsies can be performed.

DISORDERS OF THE BILIARY TREE

Bile is produced in the liver and stored in the gallbladder where it is acidified and concentrated. The presence of fat and amino acids in the proximal duodenum causes release of cholecystokinin, which stimulates gallbladder contraction.

Cholelithiasis

Gallstones.

MECHANISMS OF GALLSTONE FORMATION

- ↑ secretion of cholesterol in bile.
- ↑ formation of solid cholesterol nuclei.
- ↓ gallbladder emptying.

SIGNS AND SYMPTOMS

- RUQ pain that lasts between 2 and 6 hours.
- About two-thirds of patients will have pain after meals—often worse with fatty foods.
- Nausea and vomiting are common.
- On exam, the patient will be mildly tender in the RUQ *without* guarding or rebound.

DIAGNOSIS

RUQ ultrasound to detect gallstones.

ADDITIONAL WORKUP

- Aspartate transaminase (AST)/alanine transaminase (ALT) to evaluate for hepatitis.
- Alkaline phosphatase and bilirubin (direct fraction more elevated than indirect) to evaluate for common duct stones.
- Amylase/lipase for concomitant pancreatitis.

- Cholecystectomy is definitive; if asymptomatic, do nothing, as only 20% develop symptoms.
- Also can do lithotripsy (extracorporeal shock wave treatment; breaks up stones).
- Low-fat diet for prevention.
- Chenodeoxycholate to dissolve stones (not very effective).

Cholecystitis

- Gallbladder inflammation, ischemia, or infection usually due to an obstructing stone.
- *Note*: Infection *is not necessary* to make the diagnosis of acute cholecystitis but may complicate up to 75% of the cases.

ETIOLOGY

- Obstruction with gallstones.
- Infection (*E coli*, *Klebsiella*, *Enterococcus*, *Bacteroides*).
- Abscess.
- Tumor.

SIGNS AND SYMPTOMS

- RUQ pain often longer than the 6 hours' duration.
- Guarding and rebound may occur.
- Fever.
- Tachycardia.
- Murphy's sign (see box).

DIAGNOSIS

- **HIDA** (the study of choice): For this test, technetium 99m–labeled iminodiacetic acid is injected IV and is taken up by hepatocytes. In normals, the gallbladder is outlined within 1 hour; absence of visible gallbladder on HIDA = cholecystitis.
- **Ultrasound findings:** Presence of gallstones, **thickened gallbladder wall,** pericholecystic fluid (presence of all three has a positive predictive value of > 90%).
- **Other findings:**
  - Elevated white blood cell count with ↑ polymorphonuclear neutrophils (PMNs).
  - Elevated alkaline phosphatase, total bilirubin, gamma-glutamyl transpeptidase (GGT). May see mild elevation of AST/ALT.

TREATMENT

- **Cholecystectomy.**
- **Antibiotics** (usually second- or third-generation cephalosporin).
- Pain control.
- Fluids.

COMPLICATIONS

Fistula, gallstone ileus, perforation, pancreatitis, sepsis, gangrenous gallbladder.

Risk factors for cholelithiasis: 8 Fs
Female
Fat
Fertile
Forty
Fibrosis, cystic
Familial
Fasting
F-Hgb (sickle cell disease)
Also:
Diabetes
Oral contraceptives

Gallstone composition:
- Cholesterol (70%): Radiolucent (seen in rapid weight loss, oral contraception, ileal disease)
- Pigment (20%): Radiodense (seen in hemolysis)
- Mixed (10%)

Meperidine (Demerol) is thought to produce less spasm of the sphincter of Oddi than morphine, *although clinical evidence is lacking.*

GASTROENTEROLOGY

Acalculous Cholecystitis

Cholecystitis without stones.

- Makes up 5–10% of cases of cholecystitis.
- Usually occurs in seriously ill patients (eg, trauma, burns).
- Associated with more rapid clinical deterioration and ↑ morbidity and mortality.

Risk Factors

- ↑ age
- Diabetes mellitus (DM)
- Multiple trauma
- HIV
- Extensive burns
- Major surgery
- Prolonged labor
- Systemic vasculitides
- Gallbladder torsion
- Infections of the biliary tract

Murphy's sign: The arrest of inspiration while palpating the RUQ. This test is > 95% sensitive for acute cholecystitis, but less sensitive in the elderly.

Gold standard test for cholecystitis is HIDA scan.

Ascending Cholangitis

Inflammation/infection of the biliary outflow tract usually due to a stone (choledocholelithiasis), a stricture, or tumor.

- The biliary system becomes superinfected (usually with gram-negative bacteria), and without drainage, the patient becomes septic, and may die without immediate intervention.
- Another cause for this is ERCP (iatrogenic), though it is also the treatment (see below).
- Ascending cholangitis is an **emergency.**

Signs and Symptoms

- **Charcot's triad** (RUQ pain, jaundice, fever) occurs in only about 25% of patients and lacks specificity.
- **Reynolds' pentad** (Charcot's triad + shock and altered mental status) carries a worse prognosis.

Diagnosis

- **Ultrasound** may show stones in the common bile duct.
- Also, intrahepatic **biliary ductal dilatation** is an important finding, as well as **peri-cholecystic fluid.**
- If ultrasound does not give a diagnosis, magnetic resonance cholangiopancreatography (MRCP) is the next diagnostic study.

Charcot's triad:
- RUQ pain
- Jaundice
- Fever

For Reynolds' pentad; add:
- Shock (hypotension)
- Altered mental status

Treatment

Biliary drainage, which can be achieved in several ways:

- ERCP with stone extraction.
- Endoscopic sphincterotomy.
- Percutaneous drain.
- Surgery.
- Also:
  - Fluid resuscitation, vasopressors as needed for hemodynamic support.
  - Broad-spectrum antibiotics to cover *E coli, Klebsiella, Enterococcus,* and *Bacteroides* (gram negative).

Primary Sclerosing Cholangitis

A chronic progressive disorder of unknown etiology characterized by inflammation, fibrosis, and strictures of the medium- and large-diameter intrahepatic and extrahepatic biliary tree.

- Many develop cholangiocarcinoma.
- There is a strong association with **ulcerative colitis.**

TREATMENT

Balloon dilatation of obstructed biliary tree. The only cure is a liver transplant.

> A 34-year-old man with a history of ulcerative colitis presents with jaundice and elevated GGT and alkaline phosphatase. *Think: Primary sclerosing cholangitis.* **Next step:** ERCP showing "string-of-beads" appearance of biliary tree is diagnostic.

DISORDERS OF THE LIVER

Normal Function of the Liver

General rule: When **indirect bilirubin is much higher than direct** bilirubin, it usually means there is an ↑ bilirubin production by **hemolysis.** The other common cause is **Gilbert's syndrome** (harmless, common defect in bilirubin conjugation).

- Carbohydrate metabolism (glucose homeostasis).
- Plasma protein synthesis (albumin).
- Bile acid synthesis.
- Coagulation factor synthesis.
- Lipid synthesis.
- Vitamin storage.
- Detoxification of many endogenous and exogenous substances.
- Hormone metabolism.
- Nitrogenous waste processing (urea cycle).
- See Table 2.3-3 for explanation of liver function tests.

Cirrhosis

Chronic hepatic injury associated with hepatocellular necrosis, fibrosis, and nodular regeneration. There are many causes of cirrhosis (alcohol, hepatitis, etc.) listed below. They all share common clinical picture.

DIAGNOSIS

Can be made by liver biopsy; CT scan can suggest cirrhosis.

If the transaminases (AST/ALT) stand out as the most abnormal, the defect is usually parenchymal liver damage. If the alkaline phosphatase stands out as most abnormal, it is usually obstructive.

SIGNS AND SYMPTOMS

These can be seen with cirrhosis from any cause:

- Loss of appetite, nausea, vomiting.
- Jaundice (from high bilirubin) and pruritis.
- Signs of portal hypertension (varices, spider telangiectasia, ascites, edema, caput madusae).
- Bleeding (from ↓ clotting factors made in liver).

TABLE 2.3-3. A Comparison of Lab Findings in Obstructive and Parenchymal Liver Disease

TEST	OBSTRUCTIVE	PARENCHYMAL
AST/ALT	Slight elevation	Very high
Alkaline phosphatase	Very high	Slight elevation
Albumin	Normal	$\downarrow$
PT	Normal–slight elevation	Very high
Bilirubin: Direct (conjugated)	Normal–very high	Normal–very high
Bilirubin: Indirect (unconjugated)	Normal–slight elevation	Normal–very high
GGT	Very high	Normal–very high

ALT: alanine transaminase; AST: aspartate transaminase; GGT: gamma-glutamyl transpeptidase; PT: prothrombin time.

- Encephalopathy (mental status change possibly due to ↑ NH_3 and ↑ gamma-aminobutyric acid [GABA]).
- Palmar erythema (redness of palms).
- Dupuytren's contractures (contractures of palmar fascia resulting in flexion of fourth digit).
- Gynecomastia and hypogonadism.
- Early in cirrhosis, LFTs are high and there is hepatomegaly; as cirrhosis advances, LFTs begin to normalize (liver is burned out) and liver atrophies (nonpalpable).

TREATMENT

- Cease alcohol consumption.
- High-protein diet (1 g/kg body weight) and multivitamins.
- Avoid hepatotoxins (eg, acetaminophen, isoniazid).
- Spironolactone (potassium-sparing diuretic) for ascites.
- Lactulose for hepatic encephalopathy (broken down by colonic bacteria and causes NH_3 to convert to NH_4, which cannot cross the blood-brain barrier).

ALCOHOLIC CIRRHOSIS

Most common cause of cirrhosis in North America.

ETIOLOGY

- Caused by chronic alcoholism.
- *Alcoholic fatty liver*, a mostly asymptomatic, reversible form of liver injury, often precedes cirrhosis.
- *Alcoholic hepatitis* initiates the necrosis.

FINDINGS SPECIFIC TO ALCOHOLIC CIRRHOSIS/LIVER DAMAGE

- AST/ALT ratio > 2.
- GGT is most sensitive serum marker for alcohol bingeing.

NONALCOHOLIC CAUSES OF CIRRHOSIS

- Viral hepatitis.
- Primary biliary cirrhosis.
- Hemochromatosis.
- Cardiac cirrhosis (CHF causing congestive hepatopathy).
- Wilson's disease.
- Alpha-1-antitrypsin deficiency.

Primary Biliary Cirrhosis

Autoimmune disease causing destruction of *intrahepatic* bile ducts.

ETIOLOGY

Unknown, but *antimitochondrial antibodies* are the serologic hallmark, and the pathology results from an autoimmune response to the biliary epithelium.

EPIDEMIOLOGY

More common in middle-aged women, often associated with autoimmune disease (scleroderma, Sjögren's).

SIGNS AND SYMPTOMS

- Pruritus.
- Jaundice.
- Xanthomas (deposits of cholesterol in skin). Presence of an additional (extrahepatic) autoimmune disorder (eg, rheumatoid arthritis or Sjögren's).

Primary biliary cirrhosis: Women, autoimmune diseases
vs.
Primary sclerosing cholangitis: Men, ulcerative colitis

DIAGNOSIS

Presence of antimitochondrial antibodies (90% sensitive).

TREATMENT

- Liver transplant is the only cure.
- Ursodiol (ursodeoxycholate [synthetic bile acid]) may slow progression.

Portal Hypertension

↑ portal vascular resistance caused by cirrhosis, portal vein obstruction, or hepatic vein thrombosis.

Schistosomiasis is the most common cause of portal hypertension worldwide.

COMPLICATIONS

- Esophageal varices.
- Splenomegaly.
- Ascites.
- Hemorrhoids.
- Caput medusae (periumbilical collateral vessels visible on abdomen).

TREATMENT

- Creation of shunts to ↓ pressure: Portosystemic shunt surgery.
- Transjugular intrahepatic portocaval shunt (TIPS) between hepatic and portal veins.
- Propranolol reduces portal pressure and reduces chance of variceal bleeds.
- Liver transplant.

Acute variceal bleeds have a 50% mortality.

GASTROENTEROLOGY

Esophageal Variceal Bleeding

- Bleeding from esophageal vessels that have ↑ pressure 2° to portal hypertension.
- **Variceal bleeding** presents as hematemesis or hypotension from blood loss.
- This is a **high-pressure bleed and is an emergency.**

TREATMENT

- **Immediate:** Aggressive hydration (place large-bore catheters and give fluid!) and endoscopic sclerotherapy or banding.
- Balloon tamponade is a last resort.
- **Other therapy:** Somatostatin (**octreotide**).
- Beta blockade.
- Replace clotting factors with fresh frozen plasma if there is a coagulopathy from liver dysfunction.

 A patient presents with bleeding esophageal varices. After stabilizing with IV fluid, what is the next step? *Octreotide* followed by EGD for banding of varices.

Somatostatin (octreotide)
Inhibits visceral blood flow and that's why it works for upper GI and variceal bleeds.
Inhibits GI motility and that's why it can be used for refractory diarrhea.

Hepatic Encephalopathy

- A reversible (usually) mental status change associated with hepatocellular dysfunction.
- It can happen at any time in a cirrhotic patient, but can be precipitated by infection, GI bleed, or ↑ dietary protein.
- Its cause is unclear, but theorized to be related to ↑ NH_3 and ↑ GABA in the central nervous system (CNS).

SIGNS AND SYMPTOMS

- **Mental status changes,** ranging from mild to marked obtundation/coma.
- **Asterixis** (flapping of hands when arms extended).
- **Fetor hepaticus** (peculiar breath smell) may be present.

DIAGNOSIS

- Mainly clinical grounds, but exclude other causes (acute alcohol intoxication, delirium tremens, metabolic disorders, etc).
- Elevated NH_3 can also help.

TREATMENT

- **Protein restriction.**
- **Lactulose** (involving gut bacteria, it converts ammonia to ammonium ion, which is excreted in stool).
- **Neomycin** (kills urease-producing bacteria in the gut).

In early liver disease, patients are placed on a high-protein diet because the general state of protein malnutrition puts the body at a disadvantage to fight other stresses such as infection. In end-stage liver disease, the liver cannot break down protein, and the excess accumulation can cause encephalopathy. At this stage, the patient is protein restricted.

Spontaneous Bacterial Peritonitis

- An acute bacterial infection of the peritoneal fluid in patients with ascites.
- Presents with **ascites, fever, and abdominal pain.**

Most common organism in spontaneous bacterial peritonitis: *E coli.*

Miscellaneous scoring systems of liver failure (don't memorize, just know about):

MELD scoring: Predicts the survival of a patient with end-stage hepatic disease taking account of International Normalized Ratio (INR), bilirubin, and serum creatinine level.

Child-Turcotte-Pugh score: Used to assess the prognosis of chronic liver disease, mainly cirrhosis, and the necessity of liver transplantation. This scoring system employs bilirubin, presence of ascites, INR, serum albumin, and hepatic encephalopathy.

Hepatotoxicity due to acetaminophen (APAP) poisoning can be *prevented* by early determination of APAP levels and administration of *N*-acetylcysteine (NAC).

DIAGNOSIS

Perform **abdominal paracentesis.** Positive results are any of the following: **> 250 polymorphonuclear cells/µL** considered diagnostic (or >100 PMN/µL when patient is receiving peritoneal dialysis) + Gram stain or culture of ascetic fluid.

TREATMENT

Antibiotics with enteric gram negative coverage (eg, cefuroxime).

Hepatorenal Syndrome

- The development of acute renal failure in patients with advanced hepatic disease, characterized by azotemia, renal sodium sparing, and oliguria.
- It is usually seen as worsening renal failure/oliguria and hypotension (from low albumin).
- It can be precipitated by any large fluid shift in a liver-failure patient (eg, diuresis or paracentesis).

DIAGNOSIS

- Urine sodium < 10 mEq/L
- Hyponatremia

TREATMENT

- None proven effective.
- Infusion of albumin has never proven definitively effective (but it's commonly done).

Hepatitis

Infection or inflammation of the liver due to:

- Viral hepatitis A, B, C, D ("delta"), E, or G; CMV; Epstein-Barr virus (EBV), or herpes virus.
- Alcohol.
- Toxins: Acetaminophen, aflatoxin (found in peanuts).

SIGNS AND SYMPTOMS

- Right upper quadrant pain.
- Nausea, vomiting, malaise, fever.
- Jaundice.

HEPATITIS A VIRUS

- RNA virus.
- Spread by fecal-oral route.
- Incubation period: 15–50 days.
- No chronic carrier or infection state.

DIAGNOSIS

- Anti-HAV IgM: Acute infection.
- Anti-HAV IgG: Immunity from prior infection.

TREATMENT

- Symptomatic.
- **Self-limited, no progression to chronic liver disease.**

PREVENTION

- Safe dietary practices.
- If exposed: Anti-HAV immunoglobulin.
- HAV vaccine is given to all with chronic liver disease (especially hepatitis C), travel to high-risk countries, high-risk behavior, high-risk communities.

HEPATITIS B VIRUS

- DNA virus.
- Spread by percutaneous or mucous membrane exposure to blood, semen, and saliva.
- Incubation period: 45–160 days.

DIAGNOSIS

See Table 2.3-4 for more complete, but quick rules:

- HbsAg positive: Infection is present.
- Anti-HBc IgM: Acute infection (window period).
- Anti-HBs IgG: Past infection or vaccine (indicates immunity).

Etiology of viral hepatitis:
Vowels from the bowels (A and E, fecal-oral route)
Consonants from "consumance" (B, C, D, G from sex and blood)

HBV is the *only* DNA hepatic virus.

TABLE 2.3-4. Hepatitis B Markers

DISEASE STATE	MARKER	APPROXIMATE TIME FROM EXPOSURE TO DETECTION IN SERUM	EXPLANATION
Early infection	HBcAg (hepatitis B core antigen)	Never detectable	Intracellular antigen expressed in infected hepatocytes; not detectable in the serum.
Acute infection	Anti-HBc IgM	1.5–6 months	Window period (there can be a several-week gap between the disappearance of HBsAg and the appearance of anti-HBs in the serum, during this time infection can be detected with anti-HBc IgM).
Active hepatitis or carrier	HBsAg	1–6 months	Viral protein coat.
High infectivity, chronic hepatitis	HBeAg	1–4 months	Indicates ongoing viral replication.
Low infectivity	Anti-HBe	4 months–years	Present in acute phase.
Immunity (past infection or vaccine)	Anti-HBs IgG	6 months–years	In serum after disappearance of HBsAg.
Remote infection	Anti-HBc IgG	6 months–years	Remains detectable longest.

- Vaccine.
- Hepatitis B immune globulin (HBIG) (if < 7 days of exposure).
- HbsAg positive pregnancy: Infant should receive HBIG and hepatitis B vaccine.

TREATMENT

Lamivudine.

COMPLICATIONS

- One percent will develop fulminant hepatic necrosis.
- Ten percent of adults (90% neonates) will develop chronic carrier state or chronic hepatitis with an ↑ risk of hepatocellular carcinoma (HCC).

Hepatitis B exposure scenarios:

- Exposed newborn: Give HBIG vaccine.
- Infected blood exposure: Test for hepatitis B and if negative, give HBIG alone.
- Vaccine is okay in pregnancy.

HEPATITIS C VIRUS

- RNA virus.
- Spread by blood and body fluid contact (common from past blood transfusions and tattoos, IV drugs).
- Incubation 15–160 days.
- Most common form of hepatitis in the United States.
- Hepatitis G is similar to hepatitis C.

DIAGNOSIS

- Anti-HCV IgG presents 1–6 months after infectivity and indicates chronic or past infection.
- Polymerase chain reaction (PCR) for hepatitis C RNA measures viral load.

TREATMENT

- Interferon and ribavirin (reduce risk of hepatoma).
- Hepatitis C genotype can predict response to therapy.

COMPLICATIONS

Seventy to eighty percent develop chronic hepatitis, and 25% of these develop cirrhosis and/or hepatocellular carcinoma.

HEPATITIS D VIRUS OR "DELTA" AGENT

- Hepatitis D/"delta": "Defective" RNA virus that **requires coinfection with HBV** for replication and expression.
- Spread by blood or body fluid exposure as a *coinfection* (simultaneously with HBV) or a *superinfection* (patient already infected with HBV).
- **Makes hepatitis B more severe.**

DIAGNOSIS

Anti-HDV IgM.

HEPATITIS E VIRUS

- RNA virus.
- Incubation period: 15–60 days.
- Fecal-oral transmission.
- Occurs in India, Asia, Africa, and Central America.

- High rate of fulminant liver failure, especially if pregnant.
- No chronic carrier or infection state.
- Only supportive treatment.

 A medical resident develops severe symptoms of fever, jaundice, and *signs of severe liver failure* after returning from a trip to India. *Think: Hepatitis E.* **Next step:** Supportive management.

Liver Transplantation

- Liver transplant is used in selected cases of severe, irreversible liver disease.
- If successful, has a 5-year survival rate of better than 80%.
- Factors to determine eligibility reflect severity of disease: Bilirubin, INR, creatinine.
- Immunosuppression is often required to prevent rejection (cyclophosphamide, tacrolimus, OKT3 (anti–T cell).
- **Acute rejection** is suspected in a patient with RUQ pain, fever, ↑ LFTs. Treat with immunosuppression.
- Donor liver needs to be ABO and size matched, but not HLA matched.
- **Indications for liver transplant** can include select cases of sclerosing cholangitis, primary biliary sclerosis, or specific cases in any cause of liver failure.

DISORDERS OF THE COLON

Carcinoid Tumor

- A neuroendocrine tumor arising from ectodermal stem cells in the gut, usually in the ileum (often in appendix), making up about 30% of gut neoplasms.
- It is generally slow growing and causes symptoms by the aberrant secretion of various neurotransmitters/hormones (most often **serotonin [5-HT]**, **bradykinin**, and **histamine**).
- Though slow growing, it can metastasize to lymph nodes, lung, or liver.
- Most are idiopathic, but can be part of **MEN type I.**

SIGNS AND SYMPTOMS

- One or several of the following: flushing (bradykinin); diarrhea (serotonin); wheezing (histamine). Can also get bowel obstruction or appendicitis.
- **Carcinoid syndrome** occurs in 5–10% and consists of severe symptoms of the following triad: cutaneous flushing, diarrhea, and right-sided valvular heart disease (from serotonin).

DIAGNOSIS

Testing for enzyme and hormone levels: Urine levels of 5-hydroxyindoleacetic acid (5-HIAA) and 5-HT (serotonin) + abdominal CT to look for mass.

- **Surgical excision** or radioablation for local treatment.
- **Somatostatin** (octreotide) has been found to ↓ symptoms (unlikely that it slows progression, but this is controversial).
- Prognosis depends on size of tumor and whether or not there is metastasis.
- The occurrence of carcinoid syndrome usually is associated with worse prognosis.

PROGNOSIS

- Multifactorial. Typically, prognosis can be determined by the size of the primary tumor, the presence or absence of metastases, as well as the anatomic location of the primary tumor.
- Patients with a carcinoid tumor found in the appendix tend to have superior prognoses (probably due to its being found early on, before mets).

Diverticulosis

- An *acquired* condition of the colon in which saclike protrusions of colonic mucosa herniate through a defect in the muscle layer (where nutrient arteries insert) (see Figure 2.3-5).
- Diverticulae are most common in the sigmoid colon, probably because this is the narrowest area of the colon and therefore subject to the highest pressures.
- **Risk factors** are **low-fiber diet** and advanced age.
- Can cause **severe painless bleeding** when there is erosion through a vessel.

TREATMENT

Bleeding scan to localize the vessel and **embolize,** or **colectomy** if refractory.

Diverticulitis

Diverticulitis is inflammation and/or infection of a diverticulum due to impaction of fecal material in the diverticular neck.

SIGNS AND SYMPTOMS

LLQ pain, fever, and may have sigmoid mass on exam.

DIAGNOSIS

Typically done with CT (show inflamed diverticula and pericolic fat).

TREATMENT

- NPO, IV fluids, pain control.
- Antibiotics to cover gram-negative anaerobes, particularly *E coli, Klebsiella, Enterobacter, Bacteroides*, and *Enterococcus* (typically ciprofloxacin and metronidazole [Flagyl] or clindamycin and gentamicin).
- **Never do colonoscopy in a patient with diverticulitis (risk of perforation).**

Types of GI cancer differ based on region:

- Esophagus: Squamous or adenocarcinoma
- Stomach, duodenum and jejunum, and colon: Adenocarcinoma
- Ileum: Carcinoid, lipoma, and lymphoma

Diverticulosis is the most common cause of massive lower GI bleeding in patients over age 60.

GASTROENTEROLOGY

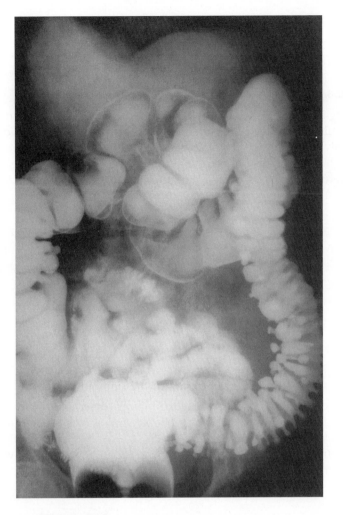

FIGURE 2.3-5. Diverticulosis.

Barium study in a patient with diverticulosis demonstrates many small contrast-filled outpouch-ings in the sigmoid colon. (Reproduced, with permission, from *Schwartz's Principles of Surgery*, 7th ed. New York: McGraw-Hill, 2000: 1277.)

Pseudomembranous Colitis

- A colonic infection caused by *Clostridium difficile*, a spore-forming an-aerobe sometimes found normally in the GI tract. When *C difficile* overgrows, due to eradication of competing gut flora by antibiotics, it may release exotoxins A and B, which damage colonic mucosa.
- Classically associated with **clindamycin**, *but any antibiotic can do it.*

SIGNS AND SYMPTOMS

- Crampy, diffuse abdominal pain and *foul-smelling diarrhea* with his-tory of antibiotic use.
- Can have fever.

DIAGNOSIS

- *C difficile* toxin in stool (insensitive).
- Sigmoidoscopy/colonoscopy shows pathognomonic yellowish membra-nous plaques (pseudomembranes) adherent to colonic mucosa.

C difficile is the most common cause of nosocomial enteric infection.

TREATMENT

- Stop the offending antibiotic if possible.
- **Metronidazole PO** or **vancomycin PO** (if Flagyl fails).

COMPLICATIONS

Toxic megacolon is a dreaded complication that can occur when inflammation and infection spread through all layers of the colon wall. Severe diarrhea and toxicity develop. Plain radiography may show a long colon loop with diameter > 8 cm and "thumbprinting" (bowel-wall edema)—these patients require careful monitoring, serial abdominal exams, and imaging, as well as a surgical evaluation for possible colectomy.

 A 68-year-old man in the hospital for 3 weeks for pneumonia returns with new-onset diarrhea. *Think: C difficile.* **Next step:** Send stool for C. diff Toxin A and B from three different samples.

Irritable Bowel Syndrome (IBS)

- Irritable bowel syndrome is an alteration of intestinal motility that → changes in bowel habits. Symptoms in patients with IBS may **fluctuate between spasm (constipation) and laxity (diarrhea)**.
- It typically presents in young people and is twice as common in females.
- It usually has no systemic symptoms and can be **associated with stress**.
- Diagnosis requires that other causes of diarrhea are ruled out.

Giardia infection and lactose intolerance may present similarly to IBS, so they must be ruled out.

TREATMENT

- Reassurance.
- High-fiber and low-fat diet.
- Anxiolytic, antispasmodic, or antidiarrheal in severe cases.

Inflammatory Bowel Disease

- A chronic inflammation affecting the GI tract.
- Two types: Crohn's disease (CD) and ulcerative colitis (UC).

SIGNS AND SYMPTOMS

UC	CD
- Bloody diarrhea (more prominent than in CD)	- Tender RLQ mass
- Rectal pain	- More indolent, chronic
- More acute flares	

See Table 2.3-5 for extraintestinal manifestations.

Crohn's: Lower incidence, lower risk of cancer, but more common in men than ulcerative colitis.

EPIDEMIOLOGY

- More common in people of Caucasian and Jewish background.
- Peak incidence in ages 15–35.
- Occurs with familial clustering.

Eye involvement	■ Uveitis	CD > UC
	■ Episcleritis	Uveitis, erythema nodosum, and colitic arthritis are commonly seen together.
Dermatologic	■ Erythema nodosum	CD, especially in children > UC
		Parallels disease course (gets better as IBD improves)
	■ Pyoderma gangrenosum	UC > CD
		May or may not follow disease course
	■ Aphthous ulcers	CD
Arthritis	■ Colitic arthritis	CD > UC
		Parallels disease course
	■ Ankylosing spondylitis	30 times more common in UC
		Unrelated to disease course
Hematologic	■ Anemia	UC = CD
	■ Thromboembolism	UC = CD
Hepatobiliary	■ Fatty liver	UC = CD
	■ Hepatitis	UC = CD
	■ Cholelithiasis	UC = CD
	■ Primary sclerosing cholangitis	
Renal	■ Secondary amyloidosis → renal failure	UC > CD
		CD
		Unrelated to disease course

- UC more common in women; CD more common in men.
- Associated **risk of colon cancer is 10–30 times for UC** and 3 times for CD.

PATHOLOGY

UC

- Inflammation of the **mucosa only** (exudate of pus, blood, and mucous from the *crypt abscess*).
- Always **starts in rectum** (up to one-third don't progress).
- Primary pathology limited to colon.

CD

- Inflammation involves **all bowel-wall layers**, which is what may → fistulas and abscess.
- Rectal sparing in 50%.
- Granulomas.
- Mouth to anus involvement.

INDICATIONS FOR COLONOSCOPY

- Primary diagnosis.
- Biopsy of the stricture or filling defects.
- **Surveillance for cancer** if had for > 8 years.

DIAGNOSIS (COLONOSCOPY FINDINGS)

UC
- **Continuous lesions** (always includes rectum).
- **Aphthous ulcers rare.**
- **Lead pipe colon** appearance due to chronic scarring and subsequent retraction and loss of haustra.

CD
- **Skip lesions:** Interspersed normal and diseased bowel.
- **Aphthous ulcers common.**
- **Cobblestone** appearance (from submucosal thickening interspersed with mucosal ulceration).

TREATMENT
- **Sulfasalazine:**
  - Consists of 5-ASA (active component) and sulfapyridine (toxic effects are due to this moiety).
  - How it works in IBD is unknown (because other NSAIDs do not work). It is activated in the colon by colonic bacteria, so it is ineffective for small bowel.
- **Mesalamine/olsalazine:**
  - Given topically (enema) or orally.
  - Similar to sulfasalazine but active in small bowel if taken orally; active in colon only if given by enema.
- **Corticosteroids:** Given in severe cases; works better in UC than CD.
- **Antibiotics (used for CD):** Metronidazole can be effective.
- **Immunomodulators:**
  - Used in refractory cases, especially in CD on chronic steroids.
  - Include azathioprine and 6-mercaptopurine (both purine analogs) and methotrexate.
  - Infliximab (Remicade) (antibody to TNF-α) is used in refractory CD and in fistulizing forms. It is also used as a steroid-sparing agent for maintenance of remission in the treatment of CD.
- **Surgical treatment:**
  - Surgery in UC can be curative, and is done in intractable disease or complications such as perforation, hemorrhage, or cancer.
  - Surgery in CD is typically not curative (recurrence often seen at anastomosis site) but still done in certain of the above situations.

COMPLICATIONS

UC
- Perforation.
- Stricture (presence may suggest cancer).
- Megacolon.

CD
- Abscess.
- Fistulas.
- Perianal disease (abscess, fistula).

Colorectal Cancer
- The second most common cause of cancer death in the United States.
- Most cases are thought to arise from adenomatous polyps, usually sessile, **villous polyps** ("villains" that cause cancer).
- **Diagnosed with colonoscopy.**

Inflammatory bowel disease symptoms **improve with nicotine (smoking).** Patients can wear dermal patches.

RISK FACTORS

- Age > 40 years.
- Personal history of adenoma or colon cancer.
- Inflammatory bowel disease.
- Family history.

SIGNS AND SYMPTOMS

- Can be consequence of blood loss (weakness, pallor), constipation (obstructing lesion), frank bleeding, pencil-thin stools, pain, or weight loss.
- **Left colon lesions** usually cause thin stools, rectal bleeding, obstruction.
- **Right colon lesions** usually cause more insidious blood loss (not frank bleeding) and can present with severe anemia.
- **Labs** can demonstrate **Fe-deficient anemia,** elevated carcinoembryonic antigen (CEA)—not recommended for screen or diagnosis, but can be useful to follow disease. Preoperative levels useful in assessing prognosis and follow-up, but otherwise of no diagnostic value. Elevated LFTs may indicate liver metastasis.

SCREENING (AMERICAN CANCER SOCIETY RECOMMENDATIONS)

- Annual digital rectal exam beginning at age 40.
- Annual fecal occult blood test (FOBT) screening beginning at age 50.
- Flexible sigmoidoscopy—every 3–5 years beginning at age 50, if asymptomatic with no risk factors.
- Colonoscopy is recommended for positive FOBT or positive sigmoidoscopy and for patients with inflammatory bowel disease or hereditary colorectal cancer syndromes.
- Colonoscopy generally has been used with ↑ frequency over flexible sigmoidoscopy and may be a better alternative (it views entire colon rather than just sigmoid).
- Diagnosis requires biopsy (see Figure 2.3-6).

COLON CANCER STAGING AND TREATMENT

- Dukes and TNM are both staging systems for colon cancer. TNM is preferred (see Table 2.3-6).
- Radiation is typically used only in rectal cancer.
- Chemotherapy typically consists of 5-fluorouracil (FU) and levimasole with the addition (sometimes) of oxaliplatinum or irinotecan.
- Colonoscopy is needed within 6–12 months postoperatively to exclude synchronous lesions; if negative, then every 3 years.
- Most early-stage cancers are cured.
- TNM staging and treatment made simple:
  - Stage I and II are local lesions confined to colon with no nodes. Usually treat with resection only (5-year survival > 70%).
  - Stage III is node positive. Usually treat with resection + adjuvant chemotherapy (5-year survival 40–60%).
  - Stage IV is metastatic disease. Usually chemotherapy only (can resect lesion if bleeding or obstructed for palliation; 5-year survival < 10%).
- **Duke's staging system for colorectal cancer:**
  - **A:** Mucosal involvement only, above muscularis propria, no lymph node involvement.
  - **B1:** Into muscularis propria but above pericolic fat, no lymph node involvement.
  - **B2:** Into pericolic or perirectal fat, no lymph node involvement.

Many colorectal cancers are within reach of the examiner's finger on rectal exam. Many patients with colon cancer have negative FOBT (insensitive).

Polyps:
- Tubular—benign.
- Villous or tubulovillous—have malignant potential.
- The larger the polyp, the more malignant potential (> 1 cm).

If a polyp is found on colonoscopy, perform polypectomy/biopsy and repeat colonoscopy in 3 years.

Endocarditis with *Streptococcus bovis* or *Clostridium septicum* is associated with colon cancer.

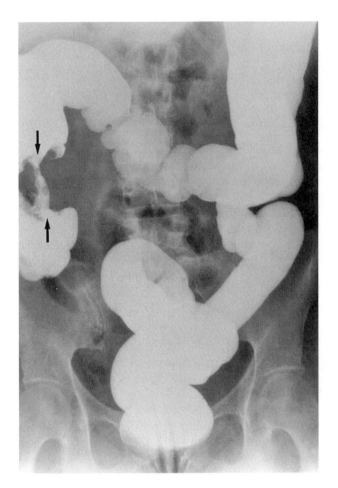

FIGURE 2.3-6.   Colon cancer.

Barium study in a patient with colon cancer demonstrates an "apple core"–shaped filling defect at the site of a circumferential neoplasm. (Reproduced, with permission, from Schwartz SI, Fischer JE, Spencer FC, Shires GT, Daly JM. *Schwartz's Principles of Surgery*, 7th ed. New York: McGraw-Hill, 1998: 1347.)

- ◾ **C1:** Same penetration as B1 with nodal metastases.
- ◾ **C2:** Same penetration as B2 with nodal metastases.
- ◾ **D:** Distant metastases.

 A 70-year-old woman presents with microcytic anemia, weight loss, and a vague abdominal pain that is not related to food or time of day. *Think: Colorectal cancer.* **Next step:** Colonoscopy.

Hereditary Colon Cancer Syndromes

- ◾ **Familial polyposis coli** (high risk for colorectal cancer):
  - ◾ Autosomal dominant condition in which thousands of adenomatous polyps appear throughout the colon by age 25.
  - ◾ Most untreated patients develop colon cancer by age 40.
  - ◾ Treatment: Prophylactic *total colectomy.*

TABLE 2.3-6. TNM Staging (Preferred)

Tis	Carcinoma in situ.
T1	Tumor invades submucosa.
T2	Tumor invades muscularis propria.
T3	Tumor invades through the muscularis propria into the subserosa, pericolic or perirectal tissues.
T4	Tumor directly invades other organs or structures.
NX	Regional nodes cannot be assessed.
N0	No positive nodes.
N1	Metastasis in 1–3 regional lymph nodes.
N2	Metastasis in 4 or more regional lymph nodes.
MX	Distant metastasis cannot be assessed.
M0	No distant metastasis.
M1	Distant metastasis.

Stage 0	Tis	N0	M0
Stage I	T1–2	N0	M0
Stage IIA	T3	N0	M0
Stage IIB	T4	N0	M0
Stage IIIA	T1–2	N1	M0
Stage IIIB	T3–4	N1	M0
Stage IIIC	Any T	N2	M0
Stage IV	Any T	Any N	M1

- **Hereditary nonpolyposis colon cancer (HNPCC)** (high risk):
  - Autosomal dominant condition in which three or more relatives of a patient, and at least one first-degree relative, develop colon cancer at an early age.
  - Often multiple other primary cancers in family.
- **Gardner's syndrome** (high risk): Autosomal-dominant disorder characterized by polyposis coli, supernumerary teeth, osteomas, and fibrous dysplasia of the skull.
- **Peutz-Jeghers syndrome** (low to moderate risk):

- Multiple polyposis of small intestine with multiple pigmented melanin macules in oral mucosa.
- Associated with gynecological cancers.

General Approach to Bleeding

- **Resuscitation:**
  - Establish IV access with two large-bore IV catheters and transfuse fluids and blood.
  - Evaluate patient for hemodynamic instability (hypotension, tachycardia, orthostasis).
  - Type and crossmatch, complete blood count (CBC), coagulation studies.
- **Determining the source of bleed** (upper GI [UGI] vs. lower GI [LGI] bleed [UGI bleed anatomically defined as bleeding above the ligament of Treitz]):
  - **History and physical:** Evaluate for localization of abdominal pain or tenderness; significant past medical history of peptic ulcer disease, chronic NSAID use, liver disease, recent vomiting or retching.
  - **Rectal exam** for hemorrhoids, mass, or tenderness.
  - **Stool exam for melana/guaiac.**
  - **Nasogastric lavage** looking for bright red blood or coffee grounds (UGI bleed).
    - **UGI bleed may present as hematemesis** (bloody vomitus), **coffee ground emesis** (dark-colored material representing a mixture of blood and gastric acid), **melena, hematochezia** (bright red blood per rectum), or maroon-colored stools with rapid GI bleeds.
    - **LGI bleeds may present as hematochezia** or **melena** (less common) associated with cecal or right colonic bleeds with slow transit of blood.

Etiology of UGI bleeds:
Mallory's **V**ices **G**ave (her) **A**n **U**lcer.

Coffee grounds is the term used to describe old, brown, digested blood found on gastric lavage. It usually indicates a source of bleeding proximal to the ligament of Treitz.

UPPER GI BLEEDS

ETIOLOGY

- Mallory-Weiss tear.
- Varices.
- Gastritis/esophagitis.
- Arteriovenous malformation.
- Ulcer: Peptic/duodenal.

SIGNS AND SYMPTOMS

- Hematemesis (bright red or coffee grounds).
- Hypotension.
- Tachycardia.
- Black, tarry stool.
- Very brisk UGI bleeds can be associated with bright red blood per rectum.

GASTROENTEROLOGY

DIAGNOSIS

- Gastric lavage severity of bleeding (old vs. new blood).
- Rectal exam with FOBT.
- Endoscopy (also therapeutic): Bleeding scan or arteriography can be done if can not localized bleed.

TREATMENT

Depends on etiology and severity:

- IV fluids and blood.
- Endoscopy with epinephrine injection, cautery or ligation if bleeding ulcers or varices.
- IV proton pump inhibitor.
- Most Mallory–Weiss tears resolve spontaneously.
- For bleeding varices:
  - Somatostatin inhibits gastric, intestinal, and biliary motility, ↓ visceral blood flow.
  - Consider balloon tamponade (rarely used at present).

LOWER GI BLEEDS

ETIOLOGY

- Cancer or polyps.
- Upper GI bleed (need to rule it out).
- Colitis (infectious, inflammatory bowel disease, ischemic, etc.).
- Angiodysplasia.
- Diverticulosis.
- Hemorrhoids.

SIGNS AND SYMPTOMS

- Hematochezia.
- Melena.
- Signs of blood loss (tachycardia, hypotension).
- Diarrhea (as seen with colitis).

DIAGNOSIS

- Gastric lavage to rule out upper GI source.
- Rectal exam.
- CBC.
- Colonoscopy.
- Bleeding scan or arteriography can be done if colonoscopy cannot be done, or if undiagnostic.

TREATMENT

- IV fluids.
- Blood (RBCs).
- Embolization or surgery.

A bleeding scan detects *active* bleeding by infusing a radioactive colloid or radiolabeled autologous RBCs and watching for their collection in the GI tract.

A patient comes in vomiting blood. What do you do?
1. Two large-bore IVs and fluid.
2. Type and crossmatch blood.
3. Endoscopy (for diagnosis and treatment).

Etiology of LGI bleeds: **C**an **U** **C**ure **A**unt **Di**'s **H**emorrhoids?

CBC in acute hemorrhage will not reflect the true severity of the bleed for 4–6 hours, as it takes time for the concentrations to change.

GASTROENTEROLOGY

The passage of fluid or semisolid stool with ↑ frequency. Initially, you need to differentiate between infectious versus noninfectious.

HISTORY

- **Quantity of diarrhea**: Large-volume (usually small bowel cause) vs. small volume (usually large bowel cause).
- **Quality of stool**: Color, foul odor, blood, mucus, fatty consistency.
- **Length of symptoms**: Acute (< 2 weeks) vs. **persistent** (> 2 weeks) vs. **chronic** (> 4 weeks).
- **Associated symptoms**: Fever, chills, abdominal pain, nausea, vomiting, weight loss.
- **Other questions**: Food intake prior to onset of diarrhea, travel history, presence of predisposing conditions (IBD, small bowel resection, pancreatic disease, immunodeficiency, etc.), medications, recent antibiotic use or hospitalization ↑ risk for *Clostridium difficile* colitis, lactose intolerance, sick contacts.

EXAM

General appearance: Does the patient look acutely ill? The presence of one or more of the following will dictate your immediate management of the patient:

- **Vital signs**: Fever, tachycardia, hypotension, orthostatic hypotension.
- **Abdominal exam**: Tenderness, distention, hepatomegaly, ascites.
- **Rectal exam**: Tenderness, mass, stool appearance, occult blood.
- **Skin**: Turgor, rash.

Acute Diarrhea

- Less than 2–4 weeks in duration; usually due to infectious etiology.
- **Workup:**
  - Fecal **leukocytes** (may be suggestive of infectious or inflammatory causes).
  - Stool **culture** for enteric pathogens.
  - Stool test for **C difficile** toxins (for pseudomembranous colitis).
  - Stool examination for **ova** and **parasites** (insensitive—must do with three different bowel movements over 3 days).

COMMON INFECTIOUS PATHOGENS

- **Bacterial:**
  - Noninvasive, all foodborne:
    - Enterotoxigenic *Escherichia coli*: Most common cause of traveler's diarrhea.
    - *Staphylococcus aureus*: Quick onset (3–4 hrs), mostly vomiting, toxin mediated, associated with mayonnaise consumption; patients commonly report having been to a picnic or other such event.
    - *Bacillus cereus*: Associated with reheated rice, commonly from day-old Chinese food.
    - *Clostridium perfringens*.
    - *Vibrio cholerae*: Contaminated water in third-world countries.

GASTROENTEROLOGY

- ▪ Invasive (bloody):
  - ▪ *Campylobacter*: Associated with Guillain-Barré syndrome.
  - ▪ *Yersinia*.
  - ▪ *Shigella*.
  - ▪ *Salmonella*: Raw eggs, uncooked chicken.
  - ▪ Enterohemorrhagic *E coli*: Shiga toxin producing *E coli* O157:H7; hemolytic uremic syndrome (HUS).
  - ▪ *C difficile*: Pseudomembranous colitis.
- ▪ **Viral:** Rotavirus, Norwalk virus, cytomegalovirus (CMV, in the immunocompromised patient).
- ▪ **Protozoa** (can also cause chronic diarrhea): *Giardia lamblia* (after hiking trip), *Entamoeba histolytica*, *Cryptosporidium* (common in AIDS).

> **Bloody diarrhea—**
>
> **CASES**
>
> **C**ampylobacter
> **A**moeba (*E. histolytica*)
> **S**higella
> **E** coli
> **S**almonella

 A patient vomits within 6 hours of eating something with mayonnaise (eg, potato salad) at a picnic on a hot day. *Think:* Staphylococcus.

 A patient has vomiting/diarrhea after eating reheated rice from leftover Chinese food. *Think:* Bacillus cereus.

 A patient has vomiting and severe watery diarrhea after eating spoiled shellfish. *Think:* Vibrio cholerae.

 A patient has flatulence and foul-smelling diarrhea after a camping trip. *Think:* Giardia lamblia. **Next step:** Treat with metronidazole.

MANAGEMENT

- ▪ Oral or intravenous rehydration and electrolyte replacement.
- ▪ Antibiotic therapy when infectious etiology is suspected and patient is moderately to severely ill:
  - ▪ If bacterial infections suspected: Empiric treatment with ciprofloxacin or trimethoprim-sulfamethoxazole (TMP-SMX) plus metronidazole for anaerobic coverage. Can also use piperacillin-tazobactam (Zosyn) as monotherapy.
  - ▪ If *C difficile* is suspected: PO metronidazole.
  - ▪ Treat the underlying disorder (eg, IBD, bacterial overgrowth).
  - ▪ Antimotility agents in noninfectious diarrhea (loperamide).

Chronic Diarrhea

GENERAL CLASSIFICATIONS AND COMMON TESTS

- **Osmotic diarrhea:** Ingestion of nonabsorbable solutes → osmotic water loss in the stool.
  - **Examples:** Magnesium-containing antacids, sodium phosphates, carbohydrates (lactose intolerance).
  - **Test: Fecal electrolytes and calculation of osmotic gap:** Osmotic gap = 290 − 2(Na + K) > 50 mOsm suggestive of an unmeasured solute indicating osmotic component to diarrhea.
- **Secretory diarrhea:** Oversecretion of water by the small and large bowel, which may be caused by bacteria, bacterial toxins, medications, GI hormones (eg, vasoactive intestinal peptide [VIP]), unabsorbed dietary fat.
  - **Examples:** Enteroinvasive bacteria, laxatives, hyperthyroidism, neuroendocrine tumors (eg, carcinoid, VIPoma), irritable bowel syndrome.
- **Inflammatory diarrhea:** Gastrointestinal mucosal irritation and inflammation → an exudative diarrhea.
  - **Examples:** Inflammatory bowel disease (Crohn's, ulcerative colitis).
  - **Tests: Sigmoidoscopy/colonoscopy** in certain cases of colitis will show pseudomembranes or inflammation.
- **Malabsorption diarrhea:** A problem with **either digestion** (ie, lack of digestive enzymes or bile acids) **or transport** (ie, problem with the small bowel mucosa).
  - **Examples:** *Digestive enzyme problems*—chronic pancreatitis, bile acid malabsorption; *transport problems*—celiac sprue, tropical sprue, Whipple's disease.
  - **Tests:**
    - **D-xylose test:** Distinguishes **digestion problem vs. transport problem.** A set amount of D-xylose given PO followed by measuring blood and urine levels to assess for adequate absorption. Xylose requires transport but not digestive enzymes to be absorbed; therefore, adequate amounts in blood/urine demonstrate intact absorption. Low levels of xylose indicate a problem with the small bowel mucosal transport.
    - **Small bowel biopsy:** If a transport problem is suspected in the small bowel, a biopsy will diagnose the cause (eg, Whipple's disease, celiac sprue).
    - **72-hour fecal fat analysis:** Steatorrhea (↑ fecal fat) may be seen in malabsorption due to pancreatic exocrine insufficiency.
- **↓ transit time:** May → diarrhea by an osmotic mechanism.
  - **Examples:** Dumping syndrome, short gut syndrome.

> Opiate antidiarrheal agents such as loperamide are generally *contraindicated* in diarrhea due to infectious agents; they promote longer contact time between bacteria and intestinal mucosa.

MAJOR TYPES OF MALABSORPTION

Celiac Sprue

- An **autoimmune condition** affecting the small bowel, triggered by gluten (high-molecular-weight proteins found in wheat, rye, and barley), resulting in malabsorption and diarrhea.
- It is associated with HLA-DR3 and HLA-DQw2.
- Manifestations include vitamin deficiencies, iron deficiency anemia, and malnutrition.

GASTROENTEROLOGY

- Diagnosis is made with a small bowel biopsy showing flattened (atrophic) intestinal villi.
- Other tests findings can be the presence of anti-gliadin IgG/IgA, anti-endomysial antibody.
- Treatment is the avoidance of gluten-containing foods (all grains except rice and corn).
- Steroids can be given if severe.

Tropical Sprue

- **A** malabsorption disease with flattened villi in the **jejunum** similar to celiac sprue—but likely from an infectious etiology.
- It typically occurs to people living in (or visiting) the tropics.
- Symptoms and findings are similar to celiac sprue, but often have megaloblastic anemia due to B_{12} deficiency.
- **Diagnosed by small bowel biopsy demonstrating flattened intestinal villi.**
- Treatment is vitamin B_{12} and folate supplementation in addition to tetracycline.

Lactase Deficiency

- Lactase is required to digest lactose, a carbohydrate found in dairy products. Deficiency of lactase results in cramping and diarrhea after ingestion of dairy products.
- Congenital deficiency is rare; a milder late-onset form is commonly found in adults at any time.
- Treat with lactase supplementation and/or the avoidance of dairy products.

Whipple's Disease vs. Sprue
They can have similar symptoms, but Whipple's is far more severe and has more *constitutional symptoms*, particularly with CNS involvement.

Whipple's Disease

- **Whipple's disease** is a severe illness beginning in the GI tract, but spreading systemically, often manifesting with fevers, arthralgias, and CNS symptoms (cranial nerve palsies, memory loss, nystagmus).
- Patients have profound malabsorption syndrome due to destruction of intestinal lamina propria.
- The causative organism is *Tropheryma whippelii*.
- More common in white males.
- **Diagnosis** is made by **PCR testing for *T whippelii*** of the saliva, stool or blood.
- Biopsy demonstrates the replacement of intestinal lamina propria by PAS-positive macrophages.
- **Treatment** is antibiotic therapy with ceftriaxone + TMP-SMX, or tetracycline. Fatal if untreated, curable if treated—a favorite on exams!

A 54-year-old farmer who has been suffering with diarrhea, weight loss, and arthralgias for the past few months is brought in by his wife for memory deficits that have been occurring for the past 3 weeks. *Think: Whipple's disease.* **Next step:** Small bowel biopsy and PCR of fluid from affected organs.

Protein-Losing Enteropathy

- A condition in which plasma proteins (principally albumin and gamma globulin) fail to be reabsorbed by the gut lumen and are lost in the GI tract; normally they are absorbed by the gut and sent into the portal circulation.
- This occurs due to mucosal injury (inflammatory bowel disease or celiac disease) or ↑ lymphatic pressure (where the proteins are normally absorbed) in gut wall (occurs with neoplasm, CHF).
- Patients get diarrhea and anasarca from protein loss.
- **Diagnose** with alpha-1-antitrypsin levels measured simultaneously in stool and serum.
- **Treatment** is to address underlying cause.

Hematology-Oncology

BENIGN RED CELL DISORDERS

Iron Deficiency Anemia

Anemia from ↓ iron stores, resulting in ↓ hemoglobin synthesis. Most common cause of anemia.

 A 47-year-old-man presents with iron deficiency anemia. *Think: Colon cancer unless proven otherwise (up to 20%).* **Next step:** Colonoscopy and endoscopy.

ETIOLOGY

- Blood loss.
- Premenopausal women from menorrhagia.
- Gastrointestinal (GI) blood loss in postmenopausal women and adult men.
- Hookworm in tropical areas.
- Malnutrition/malabsorption (think celiac, etc.).
- Pregnancy.

SIGNS AND SYMPTOMS

- Multigravid woman in her 40s, with tiredness, fatigue, and exertional dyspnea from menorrhagia.
- Pica (ingestion of clay or ice).
- Glossitis and cheilosis (also seen in folate deficiency).
- Spoon nails (koilonychia).

DIAGNOSIS

- Microcytic anemia (mean corpuscular volume [MCV] < 80) with ↑ red cell distribution width (RDW; > 15).
- Differential:
  - Thalassemia.
  - Anemia of chronic disease.
  - Sideroblastic anemia (lead poisoning).
- Low iron, ferritin, and high total iron-binding capacity (TIBC) or transferrin.

TREATMENT

Look for the cause, and supplement with oral ferrous sulfate (side effect is lots of constipation—iron is difficult to pass out).

Macrocytic Anemia

 A 38-year-old with HIV on HAART presents with macrocytosis. *Think:* AZT.

Glossitis means red, beefy (glossy) swollen tongue without papillae, and cheilosis is crusting of angle of mouth.

Features of iron deficiency anemia—

Fe KAP

Fe (iron)/**F**atigue
Exercise tolerance ↓
Koilonychia
Angular cheilosis
Pica/**P**allor

Causes of macrocytosis—

FEeD THeM

Folate and vitamin B_{12} deficiency
Ethanol and liver disease
Drugs (AZT, Methotrexate)
Thyroid (hypo)
Hemolysis (Reticulocytosis)
Myelodysplastic syndrome

There are a variety of causes of macrocytic anemia, including but not limited to folate and vitamin B_{12} deficiency. Other causes include alcohol abuse, certain drugs, metabolic disorders such as hypothyroidism, hemolysis, and bone marrow disorders including myelodysplastic syndrome.

Folate Deficiency Anemia

Anemia from folate deficiency resulting in impaired DNA synthesis.

ETIOLOGY

Most common causes of folate deficiency include pregnancy, malabsorption, alcoholism, and malnutrition. Green vegetables are an excellent source of folate and overcooking or lack of adequate intake can lead to deficiencies. In addition, folic acid is absorbed in the upper third of the small intestine, so any disease affecting absorption such as sprue or short gut syndromes will lead to folate deficiency. A thorough history usually reveals the etiology in most cases.

SIGNS AND SYMPTOMS

A typical patient is an elderly, depressed female, living alone and consuming a "tea and toast" diet, presenting with macrocytic anemia, diarrhea, glossitis, and cheilosis. Further questioning reveals that she abuses alcohol daily.

DIAGNOSIS

- High MCV.
- Hypersegmented neutrophils (right shift).
- High homocystiene (also seen in B_{12} deficiency).
- Low red blood cells (RBCs) and serum folate.

TREATMENT

Treat with oral folate.

Vitamin B_{12} Deficiency

Anemia from B_{12} (cobalamin) deficiency resulting in impaired DNA synthesis.

ETIOLOGY

- Lack of intrinsic factor (pernicious anemia).
- Vegan diet (no dairy).
- Fish tapeworm (*Diphyllobothrium latum*).
- Malabsorption (celiac, Crohn's, bacterial overgrowth, and ileal resection).

SIGNS AND SYMPTOMS

- Anemia (before neurological symptoms).
- Dementia.
- Neurological "megaloblastic madness" symptoms (**not seen in folate deficiency**):
  - Subacute combined degeneration of the dorsal (sensory) and lateral (upper motor neuron) spinal cord columns from myelin deficiency.
  - Symmetrical, affecting the legs and beginning with paresthesias and ataxia (loss of vibration and position sense) and progressing to weakness, spasticity, clonus, and hyperreflexia (upper motor neuron symptoms).

Causes of folate deficiency anemia—

Pregnant MAN!

Pregnancy and lactation
Malabsorption (celiac and Crohn's)
Alcoholism
Nutritional (toast and tea elderly diet)

All nutritional anemias (iron, B_{12}, and folate) will have low reticulocytes. Subsequently, reticulocytosis should occur in 3–4 days after replacement.

Folate deficiency can be differentiated from vitamin B_{12} deficiency by the lack of neurologic abnormalities.

Anemia precedes neurologic symptoms in vitamin B_{12} deficiency.

DIAGNOSIS

- High MCV.
- Hypersegmented neutrophils (right shift).
- High homocystiene (also seen in folate deficiency).
- **High methylmalonate in urine.**
- Low serum B_{12} level.

TREATMENT

Treat with intramuscular (IM) vitamin B_{12} injections.

Pernicious Anemia

PATHOPHYSIOLOGY

- Vitamin B_{12} needs hydrogen ions (gastric acid from parietal cells) to bind to intrinsic factor (IF), which carries it to the terminal ileum where it is absorbed.
- In pernicious anemia, antibodies are made against intrinsic factor and parietal cells, thus impairing the absorption of vitamin B_{12}.
- As parietal cells are destroyed, chronic gastritis and eventually gastric cancer can ensue.
- Other autoimmune processes such as vitiligo are also seen with pernicious anemia.

SIGNS AND SYMPTOMS

- Same as B_{12} deficiency; insidious onset.
- Associated with chronic gastritis, vitiligo, and gastric cancer.

DIAGNOSIS

- Anti-intrinsic factor antibody is the diagnosis of choice (IF-Ab).
- Anti-parietal cell antibody is less sensitive.
- Schilling test (now obsolete): First give IM radioactive vitamin B_{12}. Then give *oral* radioactive iodide. If there is no pernicious anemia, B_{12} will be absorbed and will "spill" in a 24-hour urine specimen (> 10%) as tissue receptors are already saturated.

TREATMENT

Give IM B_{12} shots for life. Newer studies show oral B_{12} in high doses (300–1000 μg/day) is also equally effective.

Glucose-6-Phosphate Dehydrogenase (G6PD) Deficiency

NORMOCYTIC ANEMIA

There are a myriad of causes of normocytc anemia. Listed below are a few of the more common etiologies encountered in clinical practice.

PATHOPHYSIOLOGY

- An X-linked disease that results from ↓ glutathione in the RBCs.
- G6PD is an enzyme needed to make nicotinamide adenine dinucleotide phosphate (NADPH), which is needed to make glutathione. It helps protect RBCs from the oxidative stress of free radicals.
- In the setting of infections, diabetic ketoacidosis, and medications such as sulfa drugs (trimethoprim-sulfamethoxazole, primaquine), quino-

Potassium can drop dramatically during B_{12} replenishment!

Causes of vitamin B_{12} deficiency—

VITAMIN B

Vegan diet
Ileal resection
Tapeworm
Autoimmune (pernicious anemia)
Megaloblastic anemia
Inflammation of terminal ileum
Nitrous oxide
Bacterial overgrowth

Causes of normocytic normochromic (normal size, normal shape) anemia include:

- Bone marrow problems (aplastic bone marrow, leukemia, myelodysplastic syndromes, etc.)
- ↑ destruction (hemolytic anemias)
- Early nutritional anemias (iron, B_{12}, folate)

lones, and also fava beans, hemoglobin (Hb) may precipitate within cells and cause hemolysis. Cells with precipitated Hb have **Heinz bodies,** which are removed by the spleen, resulting in **bite cells.**

- More common in Mediterraneans (Italians, Greeks, Arabs) and African-Americans.

SIGNS AND SYMPTOMS

- Acute hemolysis causing anemia.
- Sudden onset of jaundice (high indirect bilirubin).
- Dark urine (hemoglobinuria).
- Abdominal and back pain.
- Acute tubular necrosis.
- Important cause of neonatal jaundice.

A 31-year-old Italian male with back pain, dark urine, jaundice, and anemia after 2 days of ciprofloxacin. *Think: G6PD deficiency.* **Next step:** Check peripheral smear looking for "bite cells," transfuse if severe anemia, and check renal function.

DIAGNOSIS

- Evidence of intravascular hemolysis:
  - Indirect bilirubin elevated.
  - ↓ haptoglobin.
  - Hemoglobinuria.
- Smear will show reticulocytes, **bite cells,** and **Heinz bodies.**
- Negative Coombs' tests (nonautoimmune).
- G6PD assay.

Aplastic Anemia

PATHOPHYSIOLOGY

Marrow failure resulting in **pancytopenia** from stem cell defect, which is usually from immune-mediated injury (idiopathic or after exposure to radiation, drugs, infections, or certain chemicals).

ETIOLOGY

- Viral infections (viral hepatitis, **parvovirus B19**).
- Drugs (**chloramphenicol,** benzene, DDT, etc.).

SIGNS AND SYMPTOMS

- Anemia: Weakness, fatigue, and pallor.
- Thrombocytopenia: Mucosal bleeding.
- Neutropenia: Fever and infections.

DIAGNOSIS

- Low reticulocyte count.
- Bone marrow biopsy (hypocellular marrow with lots of white fat cells).
- Normal MCV

ABCs of G6PD deficiency—

ABCDEFG

Antimalarials
Bactrim/**B**ite cells
Ciprofloxacin
DKA
Inf**E**ction
Fava beans (can be **F**atal without transfusion)
G6PD deficiency

The genetic defect causes a ↓ half-life of enzyme, so older RBCs without G6PD die. Testing after acute attack will show younger RBCs that still have the enzyme, revealing a false-negative test. *Check G6PD assay 3 weeks after acute episode.*

Pure red cell aplasia (anemia only) can be seen in sickle cell patients after parvovirus B19 infection (erythema infectiosum).

TREATMENT

- Immunosuppression (antithymocyte globulin (ATG), cyclosporine, and steroids).
- Young patients: Bone marrow transplant if immunosuppression fails.

Anemia of Chronic Disease

PATHOPHYSIOLOGY

Anemia from chronic diseases (infectious, malignant, and rheumatologic) from impairment in iron mobilization (likely from inflammatory cytokines and an acute phase reactant called hepcidin). These patients have features similar to iron deficiency anemia despite adequate iron stores on lab evaluation.

ETIOLOGY

- Infections (tuberculosis, etc.).
- Malignancies.
- Rheumatologic diseases (systemic lupus erythematosus [SLE], rheumatoid arthritis).

DIAGNOSIS

- ↑ ferritin (acute phase reactant).
- ↓ **TIBC and transferrin** (unlike iron deficiency anemia).
- ↓ serum iron.
- Normocytic to microcytic anemia.
- Normal erythropoietin.

TREATMENT

Treat the underlying cause.

Hemoglobinopathies

Normal electrophoresis pattern in adult:

- Hemoglobin A (96%): α_2/β_2 (normal hemoglobin).
- Hemoglobin F (3%): α_2/γ_2 (fetal hemoglobin, normal till 6 months of age).
- Hemoglobin A_2 (1%): α_2/δ_2.
- There are two α genes and one β gene on each chromosome, making a total of four α genes and two β genes.

α-THALASSEMIA

Genetic defect causing gene deletions of α chains (normal: $\alpha\alpha/\alpha\alpha$).

EPIDEMIOLOGY

- $\alpha\alpha/$— thalassemia trait is most common in Asians (hydrops fetalis may result if heterozygotes mate and their offspring lack any alpha genes).
- α–/α– thalassemia trait is most common in Africans.

PATHOPHYSIOLOGY

Ineffective production of α globin chains causes overproduction of β chains that results in unstable soluble tetramers which can precipitate within the

153

cell. Because of this instability, α-thalassemia can cause chronic hemolysis. Severity depends on how many of the four foci get deleted or mutated.

SIGNS AND SYMPTOMS

- 1/4 foci involved = silent thalassemia: Asymptomatic.
- 2/4 foci involved = thalassemia trait: Mild anemia (very low MCV).
- 3/4 foci involved = hemoglobin H (HbH) disease: A significant amount of HbH, consisting of β_4 tetramers in circulation resulting in moderate to severe microcytic, hypochromic, hemolytic anemia with marked splenomegally.
- 4/4 foci involved = hemoglobin Barts, hydrops fetalis (**Bart drops a (α) fetus**): Incompatible with life. Fetal death.
- HbH has extremely high oxygen affinity, and failure to release oxygen in peripheral tissues results in severe CHF and anasarca, termed *hydrops fetalis.*

DIAGNOSIS

- Blood smear: Microcytic anemia, hypochromia, target cells, Heinz bodies.
- HbH precipitates on staining with brilliant **cresyl blue.**

β-THALASSEMIA

Gene defects including deletions, abnormalities of transcription and translation, and instability of mRNA in β globin hemoglobin.

PATHOPHYSIOLOGY

- Ineffective production of β globin chains causes α globin chains to accumulate in the cell.
- The accumulation of α chains form insoluble aggregates that damage cell membranes.
- A partial compensatory ↑ of the δ and γ chains yields elevated levels of HbA_2 ($\alpha_2\delta_2$) or HbF ($\alpha_2\gamma_2$).

SIGNS AND SYMPTOMS

- β-*Thalassemia major* (Cooley's anemia): Associated with jaundice, hepatosplenomegaly, and jaundice.
- β-*Thalassemia minor*: Mild or no anemia.

DIAGNOSIS

Elevated HbF and HbA_2 measurements on hemoglobin electrophoresis.

TREATMENT

- β-*Thalassemia major*: Aggressive transfusions, splenectomy to enhance survival of RBCs, bone marrow transplant.
- β-*Thalassemia minor*: No treatment indicated.

Sickle Cell Anemia (SCA)

- Autosomal recessive genetic disease characterized by the presence of hemoglobin S in RBCs.
- Hemoglobin S is formed by substitution of valine for glutamic acid in the sixth position of the β-hemoglobin chain.

Yersinia enterocolitica is a significant cause of morbidity in patients with thalassemia and other iron overload syndromes (cirrhosis and hereditary hemochromatosis).

Sickle cell patients should always be on folate! Chronic hemolysis causes folate loss and deficiency.

- This change causes Hb S to polymerize in hypoxic conditions, distorting the red cell into the classic crescent or sickle shape. The ↓ deformability can cause hemolysis and vascular occlusion, causing crisis.
- Sickle cell trait: Heterozygous for sickle gene.
- Sickle cell disease: Homozygous for sickle gene.

> A young African-American man with microcytic hypochromic anemia is found to have a high ferritin and iron with normal RDW. *Think: Sickle cell anemia.* **Next step:** Hemoglobin electrophoresis.

EPIDEMIOLOGY

↑ incidence in African-Americans, and in populations from Africa, the Mediterranean, Middle East, and India.

SIGNS AND SYMPTOMS

Acute Crisis
- Symptoms include arthralgias and pain (back, extremities, chest and abdomen, etc.).
- Caused by vascular sludging and thrombosis. These vaso-occlusive crises may cause organ failure (secondary to infarction), dehydration, fever, and leukocytosis.
- **Acute chest syndrome: Hypoxia, chest pain,** shortness of breath, infiltrates caused by occlusion of pulmonary vasculature by sickled cells and/or infection). It is the most common **cause of death** in sickle patients and is an emergency requiring exchange transfusion with normal red cells. **Treat with exchange transfusion.**
- **Priapism** can occur acutely or chronically. This is a medical emergency, as permanent damage can occur. Genitourinary evaluation is needed.

Chronic Disease Manifestations
- Skeletal: **Aseptic necrosis of femoral head** and *Salmonella* osteomyelitis.
- Biliary disease: Pigmented gallstones (↑ bilirubin).
- Renal: Chronic hematuria, renal papillary necrosis.
- Liver disease: Viral hepatitis (transfusions) and secondary hemochromatosis.
- Pulmonary: Local infection and vascular occlusions (acute chest syndrome), **pulmonary hypertension.**
- Heart: Enlarged, flow murmur, MI.
- Immune: ↑ susceptibility to infections, **functional asplenism** (due to repeated infarction). ↑ **sepsis with encapsulated organisms** (*Streptococcus pneumoniae*, *Salmonella* osteomyelitis, and *Haemophilus influenzae*).
- Eye: Ischemic retinopathy.
- Neuro: Cerebrovascular accident (CVA) and transient ischemic attacks (TIAs) (25% risk by age 45).

DIAGNOSIS

- **Hemoglobin electrophoresis will show HbS.**
- Blood smear: Howell-Jolly bodies (cytoplasmic remnants of nuclear chromatin that are normally removed by the spleen), sickled cells.

- Blood tests show anemia and evidence of hemolysis: ↑ reticulocyte count, ↑ indirect bilirubin and leukocytosis.

TREATMENT

- **Acute crisis:** Analgesia and hydration (and antibiotics if signs of infection).
- **Acute chest syndrome:** Respiratory support, exchange transfusion, and empiric antibiotics for pneumonia.
- **Long-term treatment:**
  - **Hydroxyurea** acts by increasing amount of fetal hemoglobin; may ↓ frequency of crisis.
  - *H. influenzae* and pneumococcal **vaccines** for prophylaxis.
  - Frequent follow-up.

Hemolytic Anemias

- **Immune-mediated hemolytic anemia:** Presence of autoantibodies to one's RBCs, resulting in hemolysis.
  - Features of hemolysis:
    - Reticulocytosis (bone marrow pushes out immature RBCs).
    - ↑ indirect bilirubin (by-product of lysed cells [globin]).
    - ↑ lactic dehydrogenase (LDH; by-product of lysed cells) and ↓ haptoglobin (binds free hemoglobin released from lysed cells).
    - ⊕ direct Coombs' test (presence of antibody on RBC surface).
    - Splenomegaly (site of clearance).
- **Warm hemolytic anemia:**
  - Most common form of immune-mediated hemolytic anemia.
  - **IgG** antibodies to different RBC antigens (eg, Rh).
  - Do not usually fix complement (IgG).
  - Active at body temperature.
  - **Treat with steroids.** Transfuse if severe anemia. Splenectomy for steroid resistant.
  - Seen with chronic lymphocytic leukemia (CLL), leukemias, SLE, and other autoimmune diseases, and drugs (penicillin, sulfas and antimalarials).
  - Sixty percent of cases are idiopathic.
- **Cold hemolytic anemia:**
  - **Immunoglobulin M (IgM)** antibodies.
  - Active at cool temperatures (dissociate at 30°C) such as in distal body parts (blue fingers and toes).
  - **Fixes complement (IgM).**
  - Presence of a high titer of cold agglutinins.
  - Seen acutely with ***Mycoplasma*** and **infectious mononucleosis** (resolve spontaneously) and chronically with **lymphomas** and **Waldenström's macroglobulinemia.**
  - Degree of hemolysis is variable.
  - **Treatment includes keeping warm;** corticosteroids don't work well.
- **Paroxysmal cold hemoglobinuria:**
  - Also called cold hemolysis (hemoglobinuria after exposure to cold).
  - **IgG** antibodies against P group antigen (Donath-Landsteiner Ab).
  - Active at cool temperatures, dissociate at 30°C to cause hemolysis.
  - **Fix complement.**
  - Clinically characterized by **acute intermittent massive hemolysis** and hemoglobinuria following exposure to cold.

Indications for exchange transfusion in sickle cell disease:
- Stroke/TIA
- Acute chest syndrome
- Priapism
- Third-term pregnancy
- Intractable vaso-occlusive crisis

Signs of SCA—

SICKLE

Splenomegaly/**S**ludging
Infection
Cholelithiasis/acute **C**hest syndrome
Kidney (hematuria, papillary necrosis)
Liver congestion/**L**eg ulcers
Eye changes

Renal papillary necrosis occurs in SCA because of the very high osmolalities in the renal medulla needed to pull the water from the collecting ducts, causing the RBCs to sickle.

A young woman feels weak. Labs show a normocytic, normochromic anemia, with an elevated LDH. Peripheral blood smear shows schistocytes. What is the diagnosis? Microangiopathic hemolytic anemia. When might you see this? TTP or DIC.

TRANSFUSION REACTIONS

Acute Hemolytic Transfusion Reactions

- Life threatening!
- Due to ABO incompatibility.
- These reactions involve naturally occurring host IgM anti-A and anti-B, which fix complement and cause rapid intravascular hemolysis.
- Direct Coombs' test is positive (antibodies on RBCs).
- **Usually due to human error** (improper identification or mislabeling of blood).

SIGNS AND SYMPTOMS

- Begins soon after starting the transfusion.
- **Usually sudden clinical deterioration.**
- Fever +/– chills.
- **Dyspnea** and tachycardia.
- **Back pain,** chest pain, abdominal pain.
- Hypotension.
- Sequelae:
  - Death (40%).
  - Acute renal failure (ATN).
  - Shock.
  - Disseminated intravascular coagulation (DIC).

TREATMENT

- Discontinue transfusion immediately!
- Hemodynamic support/supportive care/IV fluids.
- Recheck compatibility of blood with blood bank.

General anesthesia is a frequent setting for blood transfusion. In this setting, immediate hemolytic transfusion reaction should be suspected with:
- Severe hypotension
- Coagulopathic oozing
- Hemoglobinuria/pink serum
- Fevers

A young woman in the hospital was transfused 2 units of red cells after severe bleeding in childbirth. Several hours later, she developed acute shortness of breath, fever, and hypoxia. **Next step:** Chest x-ray. X-ray findings demonstrate diffuse bilateral infiltrates. What is likely diagnosis? Transfusion-related lung injury.

Delayed Hemolytic Transfusion Reactions

- **Mild** and occurs days to weeks after transfusion.
- Patient received a transfusion in the past and is now having immune response after being reexposed to antigen. Due to **anamnestic antibody response to a minor antigen** (Rh or Kidd, **not ABO**).

- Pretransfusion antibody level low → screening and crossmatch tests usually negative.
- Signs of mild hemolysis: Has high LDH, high total bilirubin, low haptoglobin.

SIGNS AND SYMPTOMS

Commonly: Fever, anemia, or asymptomatic. Rarely, there are serious manifestations that look more like acute transfusion reactions.

TREATMENT

Milder than acute reactions and usually no treatment or just supportive care is required.

Febrile Nonhemolytic Transfusion Reactions

- Common.
- Chills followed by fever within a few hours of transfusion; mild.
- Lasts only a few hours.
- Due to host immune response against transfused leukocytes/platelets or cytokines from donor leukocytes.

TREATMENT

- Discontinue transfusion (can occur after) to rule out acute hemolysis (see Acute Hemolytic Transfusion Reactions).
- Can give Tylenol and Benadryl as prophylaxis, although studies have shown no benefit.
- Not routinely recommended; however, the use of leukocyte-reduced blood products may reduce the incidence of febrile nonhemolytic transfusion reactions.

Allergic Reactions to Plasma

- **Rare.** Usually occurs in patients with congenital IgA deficiency; have anaphylactic reactions to the IgA in donor blood. Anti-IgA antibodies present.
- Can get hives, bronchospasm, anaphylaxis.
- Treatment: Maintain airway and give epinephrine.

Transfusion-Related Acute Lung Injury (TRALI)

- Sudden severe respiratory distress similar to adult respiratory distress syndrome (ARDS).
- Occurs within 6 hours of transfusion.
- Incidence ~ 1 in 5000 transfusions (all types of blood products).
- Caused by donor Ab against recipient granulocytes → agglutination of granulocytes and complement activation in the pulmonary vascular bed → capillary endothelial damage → fluid leak into the alveoli.

SIGNS AND SYMPTOMS

- Chills/fever.
- Chest pain.
- Hypotension.
- Cyanosis, dyspnea, crackles/rales.

- **Chest x-ray (CXR)** shows diffuse pulmonary edema (diffuse congestion).
- Resolves within 48–96 hours without residual effects (interim ventilatory support often required).
- Treatment is supportive.

COAGULATION

Coagulation Cascade

Common pathway factors: I, II, V, X (see Figure 2.4-1).

Heparin

- ↑ partial thromboplastin time (PTT).
- Affects intrinsic pathway.
- Acts as cofactor to antithrombin III (antithrombin III inhibits factor Xa and thrombin).
- Low-molecular-weight heparins have 10 times activity against factor Xa.
- Safe in pregnancy.
- Adverse effects include bleeding, heparin-induced thrombocytopenia (HIT). Less HIT with low-molecular-weight heparin.

FIGURE 2.4-1. Coagulation cascade.

The Three 3's of Heparin:
PTT (3 letters), in**TRI**nsic, AT**III**
Heparin prolongs **PTT**.
PTT measures in**TRI**nsic pathway.
Heparin activates antithrombin **III**.

Leafy green vegetables have high vitamin K content, and an ↑ consumption will ↓ the PT (and may go below the therapeutic level) for patients on warfarin.

Warfarin has an initial *procoagulant* effect. Due the shorter half-life of protein C, warfarin inhibits protein C earlier than factors II, VII, IX, and X. Due to the early inhibition of protein C (protein C is a vitamin K–dependent factor that acts with protein S to prevent clot formation). **Heparin** therapy is recommended as a *bridge* until warfarin takes full effect.

■ HIT can be a catastrophic complication of heparin therapy, causing a **paradoxical hypercoagulable state** and high risk of blood clots. Diagnosed with the finding of low platelets and a ⊕ HIT (heparin-platelet factor 4) antibodies. Treated by stopping heparin immediately and anticoagulating with argatroban (a direct thrombin inhibitor). **Suspect this with anyone on heparin and dropping platelets. Assume this diagnosis for anyone on heparin with low platelets and a blood clot.**

Warfarin

■ ↑ prothrombin time (PT).
■ Affects extrinsic pathway.
■ Inhibits vitamin K–dependent factors.
■ Primarily affects II, VII, IX, X.
■ Teratogenic.

Activated Partial Thromboplastin Time (aPTT)

■ Tests **intrinsic** and common pathways.
■ Isolated elevation of PTT (with normal PT) seen in:
  ■ Heparin therapy.
  ■ Deficiencies of factors VIII (hemophilia A and von Willebrand's disease), factor IX (hemophilia B), factor XI, and factor XII (asymptomatic).
  ■ Antiphospholipid antibody (prothrombotic state).

Prothrombin Time (PT)

■ Tests **extrinsic** and common pathways.
■ Isolated elevation of PT (with normal PTT) seen in:
  ■ Vitamin K deficiency.
  ■ Warfarin therapy.
  ■ Liver disease (↓ factor production).
  ■ Congenital (rare).

Thrombin Time (Tt)

Measures the time it takes to convert fibrinogen into a fibrin clot.

Bleeding Time

■ Measures time from start of skin incision to formation of clot (normal: 3–8 min). **Not very reliable.**
■ Independent of coagulation cascade.
■ Elevated in:
  ■ Thrombocytopenia.
  ■ Qualitative platelet disorders (eg, renal failure).
  ■ Antiplatelet therapy (clopidogrel, aspirin).
  ■ von Willebrand's disease.

Direct Coombs'

- Tests for antibodies on red blood cells.
- Elevated in:
    - Drug therapy (α-methyldopa, penicillin, tetracyclines, quinidine, insulin).
    - SLE.
    - Autoimmune hemolytic anemia.
    - Transfusion reactions.

Indirect Coombs'

- Tests for antibodies to red blood cells in the serum (not on the cells).
- Elevated in:
    - Acquired hemolytic anemia.
    - Incompatible crossmatched blood.
    - Rh: Women can develop anti-Rh antibodies during pregnancy/ delivery of an Rh-⊕ child.
    - Drug therapy (mefenamic acid, α-methyldopa).

Thrombocytopenia

Low platelets can be due to:

- ↓ production (bone marrow problem, as in leukemia).
- ↑ consumption (DIC, TTP, ITP).
- Hypersplenism (sequestration of platelets).
- Lab error: Platelet clumping.

Idiopathic Thrombocytopenic Purpura (ITP)

Immune-mediated thrombocytopenia of unknown etiology.

PATHOPHYSIOLOGY

Development of antibodies against a platelet surface antigen. The antibody-antigen complexes effectively ↓ platelet count by being removed from circulation.

SIGNS AND SYMPTOMS

- Petechiae and purpura over trunk and limbs.
- Mucosal bleeding.

DIAGNOSIS

- Thrombocytopenia on CBC.
- Absence of other factors to explain thrombocytopenia (diagnosis of exclusion).
- Antiplatelet antibodies **not useful.**

TREATMENT

- Corticosteroids acutely.
- Intravenous immunoglobulin (IVIG).
- **Platelet transfusion** if significant bleeding present.
- Splenectomy electively to ↓ recurrence.

Hypercoagulability and **skin necrosis** are feared complications of warfarin therapy and are easily avoided by using heparin-based therapy at the initiation of warfarin.

ITP vs. Aplastic Anemia vs. MDS
- **ITP** has **normal RBCs, normal WBCs, only low platelets** with giant (young) platelets on the peripheral smear. Usually don't give platelets—treat with steroids or IVIG.
- **Aplastic anemia** has low RBCs, low WBCs, and low platelets **(all cell lines low)**. No dysmorphic cells on smear.
- **Myelodysplastic syndrome (MDS)** can have **any one or all lineages low.** The smear can show dysplastic neutrophils (hypolobulated), and RBCs with ringed sideroblasts.

Causes of thrombocytopenia—

PLATELETS

Platelet disorders: TTP, ITP, DIC
Leukemia
Anemia
Trauma
Enlarged spleen
Liver disease
EtOH
Toxins (benzene, heparins, aspirin, chemotherapy agents, etc.)
Sepsis

Thrombocytopenia vs. Factor Deficiencies

Thrombocytopenia presents as oozing from mucosal sites (gums) and petechiae. Petechiae = Platelet Problem

Factor deficiencies (eg, hemophilia) present with large bleeds (typically hemarthrosis).

Typically, one transfuses platelets if they drop below 10,000 or if there are signs of bleeding. One unit ↑ platelets by 10,000.

Classic Pentad for TTP—

FAT RN

Fever
Anemia (hemolytic)
Thrombocytopenia
Renal dysfunction
Neurologic dysfunction

Thrombotic Thrombocytopenic Purpura (TTP)

- A microangiopathic hemolytic anemia that results from circulation and deposition of abnormal von Willebrand factor (vWF) multimers (large precursor proteins that are normally cleaved).
- **ADAMTS13** is the protease that normally cleaves these multimers, but is deficient in this condition.
- **This is a life-threatening emergency, with mortality approaching 90% if untreated!**
- Usually caused by an immune process that clears ADAMTS13 after an infection, but some cases are genetic.

 A 37-year-old female presents with fever, confusion, rash, and hematuria. CBC shows low platelets and ↑ creatinine. *Think: TTP.*
Next step: Plasma exchange, not platelets.

ETIOLOGY

- Infection (especially HIV and *E. coli* O157:H7).
- Malignancy.
- Drugs (antiplatelet agents, chemotherapy agents, contraceptives).
- Autoimmune disorders.
- Pregnancy.

SIGNS AND SYMPTOMS

Classic pentad—not all have to be present:

- Fever.
- Altered mental status (waxing and waning).
- Renal dysfunction (hematuria, oliguria).
- Thrombocytopenia—can be mild to severe.
- Microangiopathic hemolytic anemia.

DIAGNOSIS

- Low platelets.
- Evidence of hemolysis: **Schistocytes on peripheral smear,** ↓ haptoglobin, elevated LDH, elevated total bilirubin.
- Renal failure: Elevated blood urea nitrogen (BUN), creatinine.
- Fever.
- Altered mental status.
- **Do not need all;** based on clinical suspicion.

TREATMENT

- **Plasma exchange** (plasmapheresis) is the **mainstay** of treatment.
- **Do not transfuse platelets!**
- Fresh frozen plasma may help (contains missing ADAMTS13).

Disseminated Intravascular Coagulation (DIC)

CONSUMPTIVE COAGULOPATHY

- Acquired coagulation defect that results in consumption of coagulation factors, including **fibrinogen,** causing bleeding and thrombosis.

- Usually secondary to exposure of blood to procoagulants such as tissue factor (fetus, bacteria) and cancer procoagulant resulting in depletion of clotting factors and microangiopathic hemolytic anemia.
- Can be acute and life threatening or can be chronic, as seen with malignancies.

ETIOLOGY

- Obstetric problems (retained dead fetus, abruptio placentae, second-trimester abortion, amniotic fluid embolism, preeclampsia).
- Sepsis (particularly with gram-negatives, *Rickettsia*, HUS, malaria).
- Local tissue damage (snake bites, burns, frostbite).
- Extensive trauma.
- Chronic illness: Malignancy (acute myelocytic leukemia [AML]), liver disease.

SIGNS AND SYMPTOMS

- Diffuse, systemic bleeding (not from a single site).
- Usually have some other severe underlying condition also (eg, sepsis).

DIAGNOSIS

- ↓ fibrinogen.
- Elevated PT, aPTT, and thrombin time (TT).
- Thrombocytopenia.
- Presence of fibrin split products (elevated D-dimers).
- Evidence of microangiopathic hemolysis (schistocytes) on peripheral smear.

TREATMENT

- Treat underlying cause.
- Platelets, fresh frozen plasma (FFP), and cryoprecipitate to control bleeding can support until underlying cause is under control.

 A 50-year-old woman who is in the ICU for sepsis has purpura and gingival bleeding on day 2 of her hospital stay, and blood coming from her urinary catheter. PT and PTT are ↑, fibrinogen is ↓. *Think:* *DIC.* **Next step:** Transfuse FFP and cryoprecipitate.

E. coli O157:H7 is the causative organism in a bloody diarrhea syndrome, which has been associated with the subsequent development of HUS. HUS differs from TTP in severity and lack of neurologic symptoms.

Transfusing platelets in TTP is thought to "fuel the fire" and exacerbate consumption of platelets and clotting factors, resulting in more thrombi in the microvasculature.

Etiology of DIC—

How do you "SPELL" DIC?

Sepsis/**S**urgery/**S**nake bite
Pregnancy
Extensive trauma
Liver disease/**L**eukemia
Local tissue damage

MISCELLANEOUS BLEEDING DISORDERS

von Willebrand's Disease

Genetic disease, most commonly autosomal dominant, characterized by **lack, or functional defect** of von Willebrand factor (vWF)

PATHOPHYSIOLOGY

- Three functions of von Willebrand factor:
  - Forms an adhesive bridge between platelets and endothelium.
  - Also bridges adjacent platelets (aggregation).
  - Acts as a carrier protein for factor VIII.

- Three types of disease:
  - **Type 1** (by far the most common, and will likely be the one on exam): ↓ in amount (quantitative defect) autosomal dominant inheritance.
  - **Type 2: Qualitative defect** of vWF (several subtypes but all with functional defect).
  - **Type 3:** Severely ↓ (**essentially absent**) vWF.

AML type M3 (promyelocytic leukemia) often presents with DIC.

SIGNS AND SYMPTOMS

- Mostly asymptomatic.
- Often have history of very heavy menstruation, or bleeding with dental procedures, and then might have an episode of severe bleeding during a major surgery.

DIAGNOSIS

Test three parameters: the amount of vWF (vWF antigen); the function of vWF (ristocetin aggregation test, also called ristocetin cofactor assay); and size (multimers). **PTT can also be elevated because vWF carries factor 8.**

PT and PTT are normal in TTP, whereas they are elevated in DIC.

- **Type 1:** vWF antigen ↓; ristocetin aggregation test ↓ *in proportion to the ↓ antigen.* Multimers normal size.
- **Type 2:** vWF antigen normal or ↓; *ristocetin test low—out of proportion to any ↓ in the vWF antigen;* multimers usually small (these are abnormal proteins).
- **Type 3:** Both vWF antigen and ristocetin test **very low.**

TREATMENT

- Mild bleeding or minor surgery: DDAVP (desmopressin) ↑ vWF levels by releasing it from endothelium.
- Serious bleeding or major surgery: vWF and factor 8 concentrates.

 A young man presents with bleeding profusely after having his tooth pulled. Labs demonstrate normal platelets and normal PT, but a prolonged aPTT. What is the likely diagnosis? von Willebrand's disease. First-line treatment? Desmospressin.

Hemophilia

PATHOPHYSIOLOGY

von Willebrand's disease is the most common bleeding disorder.

Sex-linked recessive disease (only males affected) causing a deficiency of factor VIII or IX. Hemophilia A is factor VIII deficiency, and hemophilia B is factor IX deficiency (Christmas disease). They are both X-linked recessive.

SIGNS AND SYMPTOMS

Dependent on amount of active factor (usually measured as a % of normal):

- **5–25% factor VIII or IX activity (mild):** Abnormal bleeding when subjected to surgery or dental procedures, excessive bleeding following **circumcision** of newborns is a clue.
- **1–5% (moderate) and < 1% (severe) factor VIII or IX activity:** Deep tissue bleeding (muscles), typically **intra-articular hemorrhages** or **hemarthrosis** (usually knees).

DIAGNOSIS

- Prolonged aPTT, normal bleeding time.
- Clinical picture, family history, and the factor VIII and IX coagulant activity level.

TREATMENT

- Recombinant factor VIII or IX.
- DDAVP (desmopressin) for patients with mild hemophilia A but not hemophilia B.

Hemophilia vs. von Willebrand's Disease
Unlike in vWD, bleeding time in hemophilia A is unaffected because no abnormality with platelets is present. More importantly, hemophilia typically has bleeding into a joint (hemarthrosis), and vWF is usually mucosal bleeding or postsurgical procedure bleeding.

HEMATOLOGIC MALIGNANCIES

Hemolytic malignancies include any cancer of blood cells. In the context of malignancies, the term *clone* or *clonal* refers to a process in which the abnormal cells or process have **arisen from a single precursor.** This is the basic concept of cancer. When there is an abnormal growth of a specific cell, it is important to determine if they are clonal (cancer or precancer) or **polyclonal** (from multiple parent cells, and usually a **reaction** to another process). For example, if the lymphocytes in a patient with a lymphocytosis are clonal, then the patient has leukemia; if they are polyclonal, these cells are likely reacting to an infection.

Glanzmann's thrombasthenia is a *qualitative* disorder of platelets with a defect in GP IIb/IIIa. Normal number of platelets, but don't work. If bleeding, give platelets!

Acute Leukemias

- Acute leukemia is a disease in which patients present with a relatively sudden acute illness, which can be manifested by bleeding or extreme weakness or infection. This is in contrast to chronic leukemias, in which the patients can be asymptomatic for months or years, and are often picked up on routine blood tests. Any leukemia is a cancer of the blood.
- **Two basic types: lymphocytic and myeloid.** Each has subsets within: acute lymphocytic leukemia (ALL) and acute myelocytic leukemia (AML), discussed in detail below.

PATHOPHYSIOLOGY

- The clonal progenitor cells (*lymphoblast* or *myeloblast*) proliferate, eventually taking over the bone marrow and inhibiting the growth of normal cells.
- Clinical manifestations occur because of the loss of normal bone marrow elements and by infiltration of the body's tissues by malignant cells.

A 22-year-old woman recently received her first dose of chemotherapy for acute lymphocytic leukemia (or could be lymphoma). She has extreme fatigue and a fever. Labs reveal a high LDH with low calcium and high phosphate. What is likely diagnosis? Tumor lysis syndrome. Next step: Aggressive hydration. What are you worried about? Renal failure.

A patient presents to the ER feeling extremely weak. CBC shows Hgb 7.2 g, platelets of 9, and WBCs of 49,000. **Next step:** Check coags, correct coagulopathy emergently (platelets and blood products), then bone marrow biopsy.

SIGNS AND SYMPTOMS

- **Acutely ill!**
- Anemia: Weakness, fatigue, pallor, cardiopulmonary compromise.
- Neutropenia: Infections, fever.
- Thrombocytopenia: Petechiae, purpura, hemorrhages.
- Marrow infiltration: Bone pain.

A 25-year-old man presented to the clinic with ↑ night sweats, fever, and weight loss. On laboratory testing, leukemoid reaction was detected, with ↓ LAP score. Peripheral smear showed ↑ blast cells with intracytoplasmic rods. What would you do to confirm the diagnosis? Bone marrow aspiration and biopsy. (LAP score - Leukocyte Alkaline Phosphatase score, typically low in malignancy.)

Tumor lysis syndrome is seen in leukemias (especially after initiation of chemo) and other aggressive hematological malignancies. Rapid cell breakdown → high uric acid, hyperkalemia, hyperphosphatemia, hypocalcemia, acute renal failure, and ↑ LDH. **Treated with fluids, correcting electrolyte imbalance, and allopurinol.**

DIAGNOSIS

- **Initial finding:** Numerous and monotonous **blasts** found on the peripheral smear (large, immature cells with large nuclei, unclumped chromatin). Other cells are ↓.
- **Bone marrow biopsy** showing > 30% infiltration with blasts (usually almost entirely made of blasts).
- **Other tests** (used for leukemias and lymphomas):
  - **Flow cytometry:** Evaluates which proteins are expressed on the cell surface; expression of different proteins is associated with different stages of development (ie, blasts), and specific constellations of proteins are associated with different lymphomas.
  - **Fluorescent in situ hybridization (FISH):** A sensitive method to look for specific cytogenetic lesions associated with different leukemias and lymphomas.

TREATMENT

Please see Table 2.4-3 for complete list of the various chemotherapies available for selected malignancies.

- Three steps of chemotherapy:
  - *Induction:* High doses of chemotherapy are used to induce remission.
  - *Consolidation:* Chemotherapy is then administered to eradicate residual, undetectable malignant cells.
  - *Maintenance:* Ongoing chemotherapy to keep the number of malignant cells low.
- Complete remission is the goal in cancer patients. This is achieved if normal marrow elements are being produced and less than 5% residual blasts are present in the bone marrow.

ACUTE MYELOCYTIC LEUKEMIA (AML)

EPIDEMIOLOGY

- More common in **adults.**
- Association with history of benzene exposure.
- Eight subtypes: M0–M7:
  - M1–M3 have granulocytic differentiation.
  - M4 and M5 are monocytic precursors.

Signs of LEUKEMIA

Light skin (pallor)
Energy ↓
Underweight
Kidney failure
Excess heat (fever)
Mottled skin (hemorrhages)
Infections
Anemia

- M6 have predominance of erythroblasts.
- M7 is mainly megakaryocytic.

SIGNS AND SYMPTOMS

- Fatigue, hemorrhage, or bruising (30%).
- Infection of lung, skin (25%).
- Splenomegaly is rare (25%) compared to other types of leukemia.

DIAGNOSIS

Specific characteristics:

- M3—acute promyelocytic leukemia: Associated with DIC, Auer rods, t(15;17); in which there is a defect in the vitamin A receptor, treatment is different than others: all-trans retinoic acid (ATRA—vitamin A) + chemotherapy. Prognosis is better than other AMLs.
- **AML** related to **prior exposure to chemotherapy** (for a previous cancer) has a poor prognosis. Likewise, AML that evolves from **underlying myelodysplasia (MDS)** (often seen in elderly) has a **poor prognosis.**
- M5: Associated with gingival hyperplasia.
- M4, M5: Central nervous system (CNS) manifestations.
- t(8;21) seen in M2 and t(15;17) seen in M3 have better prognosis.

TREATMENT

- **Induction:** Cytarabine + an anthracycline (daunorubicin)—50–80% receive remission.
- **Consolidation:** Same chemotherapy as induction.
- **Maintenance:** Clinical trials determining best drugs.
- Stem cell transplantation is also potentially curative, usually for relapsing or high-risk patients.
- M3 treated with ATRA in addition to chemotherapy.

ACUTE LYMPHOCYTIC LEUKEMIA (ALL)

EPIDEMIOLOGY

- Primarily a disease of children, but accounts for 20% of adult leukemias.
- Generally, prognosis is inversely related to age. Younger patients (kids to young adults) have good prognosis, but older have a poor prognosis.
- Three subtypes:
  - **L1** occurs in 80% of ALL cases in **children.**
  - **L2** most **adult cases.**
  - **L3** cell is leukemic manifestation of Burkitt's lymphoma t(8;14) involving c-myk gene.

A 27-year-old woman presents to your office with night sweats, weakness, and weight loss. Laboratory work reveals anemia, thrombocytopenia, and a WBC of 47,000. Peripheral smear demonstrates blasts with intracytoplasmic rods. How do you confirm the diagnosis? Bone marrow aspiration and biopsy. What is likely diagnosis? Acute promyelocytic leukemia (M3). What translocation would you find on cytogenetic studies? t(15;17).

Signs and Symptoms

- Acute onset.
- Malaise, fever, lethargy, weight loss, bone pain, infection, and hemorrhage.
- **Lymphadenopathy**, can have mediastinal mass.
- CNS involvement.
- Testicular involvement.
- Splenomegaly and hepatomegaly can be seen.

Diagnosis

- Blasts in peripheral blood.
- Blasts taking over bone marrow on bone marrow biopsy; other cells ↓.
- 25–30%: Philadelphia chromosome (chromosome 22) arising from t(9;22)—poorer prognosis.

Treatment

- **Various regimens—you don't have to know details of chemo types.**
- General concept is that there is an induction, consolidation, and maintenance, as with AML (AML maintenance is only in specific patients).
- ALL treatment goes on for about 2 years, as opposed to AML treatment, which is shorter.
- The other difference is that ALL patients typically require CNS prophylaxis/treatment (intrathecal chemotherapy, usually given through lumbar puncture).
- *Induction:* Four or five drugs such as vincristine, prednisone, daunorubicin, L-asparaginase, and cyclophosphamide are used.
- *Consolidation:* Cell-cycle phase-specific antimetabolites.
- *Maintenance:* Low-dose chemotherapy is standard.
- Specific case: Patients with Philadelphia chromosome often need to go straight to bone marrow transplantation because their prognosis is so poor.

ATRA → maturation of immature cells in M3 and reduces the life-threatening DIC that can worsen with chemotherapy.

M3 = Acute promyelocytic anemia or APL: **DIC** (main cause of death), t(15;17) treated with ATRA, better prognosis. M5 = gingival hyperplasia.

Chronic Leukemias

Chronic leukemias—chronic myelogenous (or myelocytic leukemia and chronic lymphocytic leukemia)—differ from acute leukemias in that these patients are often **asymptomatic for years** before having clinical problems. Though ultimately life threatening, they are rarely an emergency on presentation. **Patients generally look clinically well—not acutely ill.**

Chronic Myelocytic Leukemia (CML)

- A clonal proliferation (cancer) of cells in the myeloid lineage.
- One of several myeloproliferative disorders (others are polycythemia vera, essential thrombocythemia and general myeloproliferative disease).
- It has 25% risk/year of transforming to acute leukemia (blastic transformation).

PATHOPHYSIOLOGY

- Philadelphia chromosome t(9;22) causes fusion of Bcr and Abl, forming a protein (a tyrosine kinase) that constantly sends cell proliferation signals.
- Phases:
  - **Chronic phase** (most common presentation): High peripheral white counts (can be several hundred thousand **myeloid cells of varying stages of maturation—most not blasts**), big spleen (can cause early satiety and abdominal fullness). **These patients are often asymptomatic!** (You will likely be tested on chronic phase, so focus on this!)
  - **Accelerated phase:** More than 15% blasts in peripheral blood. RBCs and platelets begin to ↓. Symptoms of bone pain and weakness start.
  - **Blastic phase:** Looks like an **acute leukemia** with many blasts (> 30% in the peripheral blood and marrow). Sick patient—severe **fatigue and weakness!**

Philadelphia chromosome t(9;22) represents a poor prognosis in ALL, but in the setting of a myeloid disorder, it is diagnostic for CML which has a good prognosis.

 A 60-year-old male presenting with fever, **petechiae, bleeding gums,** and fatigue for 2 weeks is found to have hemoglobin of 6, platelets of 30,000, WBC of 80,000 comprised of 80% blasts with Auer rods. *Think:* APL. **Next step:** Stabilize patient, treat infection, and give blood products as needed, then bone marrow biopsy (check cytogenetics for targeting therapy because t(15;17) will benefit from ATRA).

DIAGNOSIS

- Examining the peripheral blood smear shows leukocytosis with **immature myeloid cells of varying stages of maturation** (some totally mature neutrophils, too). This is in contrast with any acute leukemia in which there are monotonous immature cells (blasts).
- Bone marrow biopsy and cytogenetics showing Philadelphia chromosome t(9;22) are diagnostic.
- Leukocyte alkaline phosphatase is *low* in CML cells (*high* in infectious causes of leukocytosis).

TREATMENT

- **Imatinib** (Gleevec) is a tyrosine kinase inhibitor that inhibits Philadelphia chromosome and induces indefinite remission (a revolutionary breakthrough!). It is the treatment of choice. Side effects include bone marrow suppression and cardiac toxicity.
- **Allogenic bone marrow transplant** may still have a role for younger or refractory patients.

Better prognosis of CML is associated with:
- Young age (< 40)
- No thrombocytopenia
- Early stage
- Low percentage of blasts

CHRONIC LYMPHOCYTIC LEUKEMIA (CLL)

- Most common type of leukemia in the Western world and is **often asymptomatic.**
- Malignant clonal disorder of **mature B lymphocytes** (rarely T cells) that **can but does not always** progress to cause lymphadenopathy, splenomegaly, and bone marrow failure.
- Generally a chronic disorder that can last for years.
- Identical to small lymphocytic lymphoma (SLL)—which is the term when the disease is confined only to lymph nodes.

Ninety percent of patients with CML have the Philadelphia chromosome t(9;22).

- Some patients have immune dysfunction that → infection or autoimmune processes.
- **Richter's transformation** is the rare transformation to an aggressive large cell lymphoma. Typically very refractory to treatment.

SIGNS AND SYMPTOMS

- Many are asymptomatic, and a routine CBC shows a lymphocytosis.
- Lymphadenopathy, splenomegaly, and cytopenias in later stages.
- At later stages of disease, patient may have classic "B" symptoms of fever, night sweats, and weight loss.
- Can have infections, **hemolytic anemia (classic complication)**, or ITP from a dysfunctional immune system.

> A 32-year-old male presents to his doctor with fullness after only eating a small portion of food. Otherwise, he feels fine. His CBC is normal except for a WBC count of 120,000. Peripheral smear shows myeloid cells in varying stages of maturation. Likely diagnosis? CML. What would you likely find? t(9;22) on cytogenetics. What would you treat with? Imatinib.

DIAGNOSIS

- Often suspected or found incidentally on routine CBC (↑ lymphocytes, > 5000 needed to make diagnosis but often > 100,000). Diagnosis is made with flow cytometry of peripheral blood demonstrating CLL clone.
- Peripheral smear will reveal **numerous mature-appearing lymphocytes** (small cells with dense nuclei and scant cytoplasm).
- Lymph node biopsy can also be used for diagnosis.

STAGE/SURVIVAL

	RAI STAGE	SURVIVAL
0	Lymphocytosis only	> 10 yrs
I	Adenopathy	6–7 yrs
II	Splenomegaly	6–7 yrs
III	Hgb < 10	2–3 yrs
IV	Thrombocytopenia	2–3 yrs

TREATMENT

- **Observation only for early asymptomatic patients in early stages.**
- There is no cure, but many therapies and combinations are effective, including fludarabine (purine analog), rituximab (antibody to CD20), chlorambucil (alkylating agent).
- Autoimmune hemolytic anemia can be treated with steroids.

- Frequent infections with hypogammaglobulinemia can be treated with intravenous immunoglobulin.

> A 72-year-old man presents for a normal checkup. He feels great, and exam is entirely normal except for some palpable small axillary lymph nodes. Laboratory revealed a normal CBC except a WBC of 80,000 made up of primarlily lymphocytes. What is your most likely recommendation? *Observation.*

> A 75-year-old man has had CLL for 8 years and has never required treatment. Over the past 2 weeks he has had dramatic weakness, night sweats, and rapidly enlarging nodes, and he has lost 10 pounds. What do you suspect? Richter's tranformation.

Myeloproliferative Disorders

- Myeloproliferative diseases are a group of disorders originating from clones of different granulocyte cell lines: neutrophils (CML), RBC (polycythemia vera), or platelets (essential thrombocytosis).
- General myeloproliferative disease (neutrophils, RBCs, and platelets all elevated) and primary myelofibrosis are other types of myeloproliferative diseases.
- In any of these disorders, there may be a mixed picture, with more than just the primary cells being elevated (eg, patients with polycythemia vera may have elevated neutrophils as well as RBCs).
- Patients with any of these disorders are at risk for progression to AML or myelofibrosis (ultimately resulting from the cytokine secretion of myeloid cells). CML is discussed in the chronic leukemias section.

Polycythemia Vera (PV)

A myeloproliferative disease that results in ↑ red blood cells.

Etiology

- **Primary PV:** A primary bone marrow cause (*low* erythropoietin). This is a clonal process.
- **Secondary PV** (other causes that result in ↑ erythropoietin); nonclonal.
- Hypoxia (high altitudes, lung disease).
- Smoking (due to carboxyhemoglobin).
- Paraneoplastic (usually renal cell carcinoma and hepatoma aberrantly producing erythropoietin).

Epidemiology

- Males are more commonly affected.
- More common in people > 60.

Why is a lymphocyte count of 200,000 an emergency in a patient with acute leukemia, but not so in a patient with CLL? CLL cells are small and nonsticky mature cells that have little risk of hyperviscosity. Acute leukemic cells are large, sticky blasts that can cause sludging in the CNS or pulmonary vasculature.

CLL patients can commonly have either de novo hemolytic anemia, or treatement-associated hemolytic anemia after receiving a purine analog (fludarabine).

SIGNS AND SYMPTOMS

- Ruddy complexion.
- Pruritus after shower.
- Abdominal fullness (from splenomegaly).

RISKS

- Thrombosis (deep venous thrombosis [DVT], stroke, myocardial infarction [MI]).
- Bleeding.
- Transformation to AML or to myelofibrosis.

DIAGNOSIS

- Hemoglobin usually > 16.5 g/dL (females) and > 18.5 g/dL (males) and low erythropoietin in primary (must rule out secondary causes).
- Ninety percent of patients with PV have a JAK2 mutation.

TREATMENT

- Serial phlebotomy to keep Hct down and aspirin.
- Add hydroxyurea in elderly or history of thrombosis.

Why do patients with essential thrombocytosis bleed? The excess platelets consume von Willebrand factor and deplete it—thereby causing an acquired form of von Willebrand's disease.

ESSENTIAL THROMBOCYTOSIS

- Elevation of platelets—the most benign of the myeloproliferative diseases.
- Often, patients are **asymptomatic**. They are at **risk for thrombosis or bleeding.**
- One must rule out secondary causes of thrombocytosis to make the diagnosis. Examples of secondary: iron deficiency (classically associated with high platelets) and reactive (platelets can go up in response to any inflammatory process).
- **Treat with aspirin + either hydroxyurea or anagrelide** (used to suppress platelet production).

PRIMARY MYELOFIBROSIS

- Also called agnogenic myeloid metaplasia.
- Can occur either de novo or as a progressive manifestation of other myeloproliferative diseases.
- Other causes of bone marrow fibrosis are M7 AML and hairy cell leukemia, among other conditions.
- Often presents with weakness from severe anemia and symptoms from splenomegaly or hepatomegaly (both caused by extramedullary hematopoiesis).
- Peripheral smear shows teardrop cells and immature cells (cells forced out of the marrow).
- Treatment is steroids or thalidomide—and neither work well.

MYELODYSPLASTIC SYNDROME (MDS)

- A clonal myeloid disorder (not usually classified as a myeloproliferative disorder) in which abnormal myeloid precursors give rise to dysplastic and ineffective myeloid cells.
- Can manifest in multiple ways and levels of severity.

- Patients can have a single cell line affected (ie, **anemia**) or be pancytopenic.
- It is typically a disease of the **elderly**, but can also result from prior chemotherapy ("treatment-induced MDS").
- Peripheral smear often shows nucleated red blood cells (pushed out from bone marrow) or **dysmorphic neutrophils.**
- There are various treatments with moderate efficacy, though no cure.
- Demethylating agents (decitabine or 5-azacitadine) are recent advancements, but often transfusion support is the only treatment used.
- Complications include infection, transformation to AML or myelofibrosis.

Lymphomas and Multiple Myeloma

HODGKIN'S LYMPHOMA

PATHOPHYSIOLOGY

- Follicular B cells undergo a transformation to malignant cells.
- The malignant cell in Hodgkin's lymphoma is called the **Reed-Sternberg cell.**
- Often, biopsies reveal few Reed-Sternberg cells surrounded by numerous immune and inflammatory cells.
- Two major types of Hodgkin's lymphoma exist:
  - **Classical,** composed of subtypes nodular sclerosing (most common), mixed cellularity, lymphocyte depleted, and lymphocyte rich. Reed-Sternberg cells have very little similarity to their normal B-cell counterpart in this group.
  - **Nonclassical** has only one subgroup, which is the lymphocyte predominant.

EPIDEMIOLOGY

- Bimodal distribution having peaks in 30s and 70s.
- Some cases have an association with Epstein-Barr virus (EBV).

CLINICAL PRESENTATION

- Typically presents with cervical lymph node enlargement or a mediastinal mass.
- "B" symptoms: Fever, night sweats, weight loss without trying.
- Pruritus is another classic symptom of Hodgkin's lymphoma.

DIAGNOSIS

- Lymph node biopsy (excisional) demonstrating the presence of Reed-Sternberg cells.
- Staging:
  - **Stage I:** One lymph node enlarged.
  - **Stage II:** More than one node, on same side of the diaphragm.
  - **Stage III:** Nodes on both sides of diaphragm.
  - **Stage IV:** Extranodal involvement (eg, bone marrow).
  - If there are "B" symptoms, add a "B" to any stage (ie, one node + "B" symptoms = stage IB).

TREATMENT

- Usually a good prognosis, particularly in young patients.
- Numerous regimens exist but currently ABVD (**A**driamycin, **B**leomycin, **V**inblastine, and **D**acarbazine) is the treatment of choice.
- Occasionally, radiation has a role in bulky lymph nodes, or when there is only one site of disease.
- New biologic chemotherapy agents (see Table 2.4-1)

NON-HODGKIN'S LYMPHOMA

Non-Hodgkin's lymphoma can arise from B or T lymphocytes, but B-cell lymphomas are far more common. They can be divided into **aggressive or indolent types:**

- **Aggressive or high-grade lymphomas** (eg, large B-cell lymphoma, Burkitt's, lymphoblastic lymphoma) are often symptomatic with "B" symptoms. Untreated survival is short, but many cases are highly curable with treatment.
- **Indolent or low-grade lymphomas** (eg, follicular lymphoma, marginal zone lymphoma) are often asymptomatic and slow growing, but with time can cause symptoms and clinical deterioration. Untreated patients can survive for years, but even with treatment, these diseases are usually *not* curable. Typically treated only if symptomatic.

TABLE 2.4-1. **Biologic Chemotherapeutics**

DRUG	TARGET	USES
Biologics: all ending with **-Mab** are **M**onoclonal antibodies:		
Rituximab	Antibody to CD20 of B cells	B-cell non-Hodgkin's lymphomas
Infliximab	Antibody to TNF	Crohn's, rheumatoid arthritis
Bevacizumab	Antibody to VEGF	Lung, colon, kidney cancers
Abciximab	Gp IIb/IIIa of platelets	MI, angioplasty
Trastuzumab	Her2/neu	Breast cancer
Those ending with **-NIB** are small molecule tyrosine kinase i**N**(h)**IB**itors:		
Imatinib (Gleevec)	bcr/abl	CML, ALL
Erlotinib	EGF receptor	Lung/pancreas cancer
Sorafenib/Sunitinib	VEGF inhibitors	Kidney and liver cancer

ALL, acute lymphocytic leukemia; CML, chronic myelocytic leukemia; EGF, endothelial growth factor; MI, myocardial infarction; TNF, tumor necrosis factor; VEGF, vascular endothelial growth factor.

SIGNS AND SYMPTOMS

These symptoms can occur in any lymphoma, even in advanced stages of indolent lymphomas:

- "B" symptoms (fatigue, fever, night sweats, weight loss, infections).
- Lymphadenopathy.
- Cytopenias from bone marrow involvement.

DIAGNOSIS

- Lymph node biopsy: This is critical to evaluate the tissue architecture.
- Flow cytometry—this evaluates which proteins are expressed on the cell surface; specific constellations of proteins are associated with different lymphomas (this method is also important in any leukemia diagnosis).
- **FISH** is a sensitive method to look for specific cytogenetic lesions associated with different leukemias and lymphomas.
- Unlike Hodgkin's disease, histology of the nodes is a major predictor of prognosis.

TREATMENT

- Add rituximab to chemotherapy for all B-cell lymphomas.
- Do no treat asymptomatic indolent lymphomas.

SPECIFIC TYPES

- **Follicular lymphoma:**
  - Typically a low-grade lymphoma seen in middle aged or elderly.
- Commonly asymptomatic, painless, diffuse, long-standing lymphadenopathy in a middle-aged individual.
- Bone marrow involvement and disseminated disease is present in the majority of patients.
- Classic cytogenetic lesion is t(14;18) involving BCL-2 (anti-apoptosis protein).
- Divided into low, intermediate, and high grades; high-grade behaves like an aggressive lymphoma.
- **Treat only if symptomatic.** Among many acceptable treatments/combinations are alkylating agents (cyclophosphamide), monoclonal antibodies (rituximab), and corticosteroids.
- **Diffuse large cell lymphoma:**
  - Most common intermediate/high grade lymphoma.
  - May present in a variety of extranodal sites, particularly the gastrointestinal tract and the head and neck.
  - **Often curable.** Treat with chemotherapy—R-CHOP (**R**ituximab, **C**yclophosphamide, Doxorubicin [**H**ydroxydaunomycin], Vincristine [**O**ncovin], **P**rednisone).
- **Lymphoblastic lymphoma:**
  - Very high-grade lymphoma often seen in children; behaves like an acute leukemia.
  - Derived from thymic T-cells and often presents with large mediastinal mass.
  - Often seen in children.
  - Associated with testicular, CNS, and marrow involvement.

Why are there lytic lesions and hypercalcemia in multiple myeloma patients? Myeloma cells overproduce osteoclast activating factor that causes ↑ bone turnover.

- **Adult T-cell leukemia/lymphoma:**
  - **Associated with HLTV-1 virus,** seen in patients from Japan and the Caribbean.
  - Often presents with hypercalcemia.
  - Although high grade, not typically curable.
- **Burkitt's lymphoma:**
  - **High-grade lymphoma** more common in children than adults.
  - **Endemic type (African)** associated with EBV and jaw lesions.
  - **Nonendemic type:** Diffuse lymphadenopathy.
  - Classic cytogenetic lesion is t(8;14) involving the **c-myc gene.**
  - Bone marrow can have a "starry sky" appearance (from macrophages eating away the necrotic cells and leaving spaces between cells).
  - Treatment includes high-dose cyclophosphamide, methotrexate, and cytarabine and intensive CNS prophylaxis.
- **Mantle cell lymphoma:**
  - Has both high- and low-grade features.
  - Can be very aggressive (high-grade feature) but usually relapses after treatment (low-grade feature).

MULTIPLE MYELOMA

- Plasma cells normally produce antibodies to fight infections. Multiple myeloma is the clonal proliferation of plasma cells usually characterized by the **presence of monoclonal immunoglobulin** or **immunoglobulin fragments (light chains)** in the serum and urine.
- Other manifestations include bone destruction **(lytic lesions)** and **hypercalcemia.**
- Patients also can get renal failure, usually from protein damage.

EPIDEMIOLOGY

Typically elderly; twice as common in African-Americans than whites.

SIGNS AND SYMPTOMS

Patients can present with a pathologic fracture (where a lytic lesion was), hypercalcemia, renal failure, weakness, infection, hyperviscosity from high protein, anemia from bone marrow failure.

DIAGNOSIS

- **Serum and urine electrophoresis (SPEP/UPEP):** These will detect the presence of a monoclonal protein in the serum or urine. Light chains (without the rest of the immunoglobulin) are referred to as **Bence Jones proteins.**
- **Immunofixation** is another method to detect monoclonal proteins.
- **Bone marrow biopsy** shows elevated plasma cells (normal is < 5%).
- Other possible findings:
- Peripheral blood smear: **Rouleaux formation.**
- Radiography: **Lytic lesions** on x-ray (needs whole body skeletal survey or x-rays, *not* bone scan).
- **Elevated total protein** on chemistry.

TREATMENT

- There is no cure.
- Multiple effective therapies exist, including older chemotherapies (melphalan) and newer (bortezomib and lenalidomide). Steroids are effective.

- Autologous bone marrow transplant (use the person's own stem cells) is also used.
- Bisphosphonates may delay or prevent lytic lesions, and ↓ hypercalcemia.

 A 60-year-old man with punched out lytic lesions in the skull and mild anemia. *Think: Multiple myeloma.* **Next step:** Check serum and urine protein electrophoresis (SPEP and UPEP).

 A 68-year-old man presents with low back pain, hypercalcemia, anemia, and azotemia. *Think: Multiple myeloma* (common triad of back pain, anemia, and renal insufficiency).

Adverse effects of chemotherapy agents:
Cisplatin: Nephrotoxicity
Bleomycin and **Meth**otrexate: Pulmonary fibrosis (**bleo**mycin blasts the lungs with **METH**ane)
Vin**cristine** = neurotoxic, palsies (**Kristine** lost her **nerves**)
Doxo**rubi**cin = cardiotoxic (**Rubi** lost his heart)
Tamoxifen = uterine cancer (selective estrogen antagonist at breast is an agonist at uterus causing uterine hyperplasia/cancer)
Asparaginase = pancreatitis
CYclophosphamide = hemorrhagic **CY**stitis

SOLID TUMOR MALIGNANCIES

Breast Cancer

EPIDEMIOLOGY

- Second most common cause of **cancer death** in women in the United States (most common is lung cancer, as in men). One in eight lifetime risk.
- One percent of all breast cancer occurs in men.
- Ten percent caused by mutations in one or more of the following genes: p53 (tumor suppressor), BRCA-1, BRCA-2, erbB2 (HER-2/neu).

RISK FACTORS

- Age, prior breast cancer, family history, previous benign biopsy, ↑ estrogen exposure.
- **Causes of ↑ estrogen exposure:** Early menarche, late menopause, nulliparity/late pregnancy, no breast-feeding.
- Oral contraceptives **do not** ↑ risk; but hormone replacement therapy **does** ↑ risk.
- BRCA-1 and BRCA-2 have ↑ risk of breast (50–85%) and ovarian cancer (50%). Prophylactic bilateral mastectomy and oophorectomy should be considered.
- Ductal carcinoma in situ (DCIS) and lobular carcinoma in situ (LCIS).

SCREENING

- **Breast exams:**
  - Annually by physician (starting at age 20).
  - Monthly self-exam (best time is 3–5 days after onset of menses) does not ↓ mortality.
- **Mammograms:**
  - Not done if < **35 years** because of a dense breast.
  - **40–49 years:** q1–2y is controversial but recommended by most.
  - **50+:** Annually until age 70, then only if life expectancy is > 10 years.

- **Evaluation of breast masses:**
  - Cancer is usually painless.
  - Sonography—differentiate cystic from solid masses.
  - Fine-needle aspiration (FNA).
  - **Excisional/open biopsy**—definitive diagnosis.
  - **Diffusely inflamed and indurated breast (peau d'orange**—looks like the skin of an orange): Signifies inflammatory breast cancer in which the cancer has infiltrated the dermal lymphatics. Typically very aggressive with poor prognosis.

PROGNOSIS

Prognosis depends on staging, tumor grade, and hormone receptor status (estrogen/progesterone positive is better).

TREATMENT

- For **nonmetastatic disease:** Surgical resection.
  - Breast conservation (lumpectomy) is usually possible, but mastectomy is required for very large tumors (> 7 cm) and other specific situation.
  - If lumpectomy only, adding radiation reduces the risk of local recurrence (but not mortality).
  - Adjuvant systemic (chemo) treatment is needed if tumor > 2 cm or there are $\oplus$ axillary lymph nodes.
  - Special cases:
    - In estrogen/progestin receptor-$\oplus$ patients, tamoxifen (an estrogen/progesterone receptor blocker) is used in premenopausal women and an aromatase inhibitor should be used for postmenopausal women.
    - Trastuzumab (herceptin) is used for HER-2/neu-$\oplus$ patients.
    - Chemotherapy typically used includes adriamycin, cyclophosphamide, and taxanes, or a combination of two of the three.
- For **metastatic disease:** Chemotherapy, hormonal therapy, and/or trastuzumab can be used, depending on receptor status.

Ovarian Cancer

EPIDEMIOLOGY

- Ovarian cancer is the fourth most common cause of death from cancer among women of all ages in the United States.
- Most patients present in advanced stages.

SIGNS AND SYMPTOMS

Abdominal bloating, **enlarging pants size**, ascites.

RISK FACTORS

- ↑ **risk:** Older age at first pregnancy/nulliparous; family history/BRCA1 and 2.
- ↓ **risk** (by prolonging periods of anovulation): Childbearing and breastfeeding, oral contraceptives, tubal sterilization.

FIGO STAGING

- **Stage I:** Ovary only.
- **Stage II:** Ovary + pelvic extension.

Most cases of breast cancer are *not* associated with known gene mutations.

One in eight women who live to age 80 will develop breast cancer.

The breasts of young women contain a high proportion of fibrous tissue, rendering mammograms uninterpretable. As women age, the fiber is replaced by fat, which mammograms can evaluate effectively. At age 35 a woman is still at low risk for breast cancer, yet has undergone fatty replacement of a substantial amount of the fiber, making it a good time for the baseline mammogram.

- **Stage III:** Ovary + peritoneal carcinomatosis with ascites (70% of patients)—but confined to abdominal cavity.
- **Stage IV:** Metastasis outside of abdominal cavity.

SCREENING

Not recommended.

PROGNOSIS

Forty percent 5-year survival depending on stage and presentation.

TREATMENT

- Surgery alone for stages IA and IB.
- Surgery (debulking) followed by chemo (paclitaxel + platinum agent) for more advanced stages (**surgical debulking is done even when there are metastases**).

Cervical Cancer

Cervical cancer is a consequence of sexually transmitted infection of human papillomavirus (HPV) types 16 & 18 accounting for 70%.

RISK FACTORS

- HPV.
- Human immunodeficiency virus (HIV).
- Smoking.
- Early age at first intercourse.
- Large number of sexual partners.

SIGNS AND SYMPTOMS

- Foul-smelling vaginal discharge.
- **Postcoital** and irregular vaginal bleeding.
- Pelvic pain.
- Dyspareunia.

SCREENING

- Yearly Papanicolaou (Pap) smear test starting at age 21 in virgins or age at first sexual intercourse until age 65. Perform every 2–3 years if three consecutive negative Pap smears.
- Counsel patients about protective effect of barrier contraceptives.

FIGO STAGING

- **Stage I:** Confined to cervix.
- **Stage II:** Cervix + uterus but not to pelvic wall or lower third of vagina.
- **Stage III:** Invades pelvic wall or lower third of vagina.
- **Stage IV:** Invades other organs in pelvis (bladder) or distant mets.

TREATMENT

- Colposcopic-directed cervical or cone biopsy for carcinoma in situ (stage 0).
- Radical hysterectomy for disease invading cervix (**stage I**). Fertility preservation, if desired, may be possible in limited disease.

- Radiation therapy (usually with cisplatinum chemotherapy) for disease that invades beyond cervix (**stages II–IV**) but without distant metastasis.
- Recurrent or distant metastasis: Radiation for palliation and/or chemotherapy.

PROGNOSIS

Depends on nodal status and stage:

- **Stages I and II:** 5-year survival is 80%.
- **Stage III:** 5-year survival is 40%.

Prostate Cancer

- Prostate cancer is an adenocarcinoma that is the most common cancer in men and third most common cause of cancer death in men in the United States.
- Incidence ↑ with age, with most in men older than 50 years.
- There is a higher incidence in African-Americans.

SIGNS AND SYMPTOMS

- Usually asymptomatic, diagnosed by elevated prostate-specific antigen (PSA).
- Dysuria and urinary hesitancy (more common with benign prostatic hyperplasia [BPH] than prostate cancer) or hematuria.
- New-onset erectile dysfunction.
- Back pain—when presenting with bone mets to spine.

SCREENING

- Screening (PSA) begins at age 50 until age 75 (or when life expectancy < 10 years); start at age 40 for African-American men or those with BRCA-1 or family history.
- Yearly digital rectal exam to look for nodules.
- Yearly PSA (controversial).
- For PSA > 4.1, transrectal ultrasonography (TRUS) with biopsy of suspicious areas.

STAGING AND TREATMENT

- In addition to staging, factors that define high risk are high PSA score and high Gleason score.
- Generally, treatment is surgery or radiation for local disease.
- Prostate cancer typically grows in response to testosterone, so blocking testosterone is an important part of treatment in advanced stages.
- Those with high risk (as defined by a high Gleason score or high PSA) but local disease may benefit from adjuvant hormonal deprivation ("hormonal therapy").
- Metastatic disease can be treated with hormonal therapy alone.
- Commonly used hormonal therapies are anti-androgen agents (eg, flutamide), gonadotropin-releasing hormone (GnRH) agonists (paradoxically, this can ↓ testosterone production), and orchiectomy.
- **T1 (nonpalpable) and T2 (palpable) disease:**
  - Prostatectomy or radiotherapy.
  - Consider both or adding anti-androgen therapy if pathologically high Gleason score or high PSA.
- **T3 disease (extracapsular extension):**

- Radical prostatectomy or radiation.
- Consider hormonal therapy.
  - **Metastasis:**
    - Hormonal therapy.
    - Consider chemotherapy if refractory to hormonal therapy.

PROGNOSIS

Ten-year survival rates are 75% when the cancer is confined to the prostate, 55% for those with regional extension, and 15% for those with distant metastases.

Testicular Cancer

- A common cancer in men age 20–40, and is seen more frequently in whites.
- Though other types exist, 95% are germ cell tumors.

CLASSIFICATION

- Germ cell tumors are divided into **seminomas (50%)** and **nonseminomas (50%).**
- Nonseminomas have the following subtypes: choriocarcinoma (secretes human chorionic gonadotropin [hCG]); endodermal sinus tumor (yolk sac tumor; secretes alpha-fetoprotein [AFP]); embryonal carcinoma (secretes hCG and AFP); teratoma (cell types from more than one layer—ecto-, meso-, or endoderm).

FINDINGS

- Painless testicular mass or persistent swelling is cancer unless proven otherwise.
- Metastases may present as back pain (retroperitoneal), para-aortic/supraclavicular nodes, or dyspnea (lung mets).

DIAGNOSIS

- **Do not perform scrotal biopsy** (risk of seeding retroperitoneum by disruption of fascial planes).
- **Orchiectomy from inguinal approach.** Ultrasound should be done prior to surgery to rule out infections or benign conditions such as varicoceles.
- Tumor markers: **LDH for seminoma** (if β-hCG or AFP is elevated, it is automatically considered a nonseminoma regardless of LDH), **β-hCG for choriocarcinoma,** and **AFP for yolk sac tumor.**

TREATMENT

- Cure rates are high, even in advanced stages due to the chemosensitivity of nonseminomas and the radiation sensitivity of seminomas.
- **Nonseminoma:** Orchiectomy, retroperitoneal lymph node dissection (RPLND), and chemotherapy for lymph node involvement or metastasis. Patients without lymph node involvement or metastases have a 95% cure rate.
- **Seminoma:** Orchiectomy and retroperitoneal radiation has 98% cure rate for nonmetastasized seminomas; chemotherapy for metastases.

> A 23-year-old man presents with gynecomastia and substernal pain, and physical exam reveals painless testicular mass. *Think: Malignancy.* **Next step?** CXR. Finding? Mediastinal mass = germ cell tumor. Young men with mediastinal mass. *Think:* Lymphoma or germ cell tumor.

Renal Cell Carcinoma

PRESENTATION

- Triad of flank mass, hematuria, and abdominal pain. Diagnosed with abdominal CT scan.
- Paraneoplastic syndromes: Hypercalcemia, polycythemia.
- **Renal vein thrombosis** and **IVC thrombus** are classic findings (see Table 2.4-2).

TREATMENT

- Early stages (within kidney): Radical nephrectomy.
- Advanced stages (mets or invading the capsule): Interleukin-2 (IL-2) may → remission in 10% of patients who can tolerate it; vascular endothelial growth factor (VEGF) inhibitors (sunitinib or sorafenib).

Bladder Cancer

Usually, cell type is transitional cell carcinoma. Rarely can be "small cell" (neuroendocrine tumor).

RISK FACTORS

Smoking and occupational (dye) exposure.

TABLE 2.4-2. Paraneoplastic and Distant Effects of Tumors

EFFECT	MOLECULE	ASSOCIATED NEOPLASM
Cushing's syndrome	ACTH or ACTH-like peptide.	Small cell lung carcinoma.
SIADH	ADH or ANP.	Small cell lung carcinoma and intracranial neoplasms.
Hypercalcemia	PTH-related peptide, TGF-α, TNF-α, IL-2.	Squamous cell lung carcinoma, renal carcinoma, breast carcinoma, multiple myeloma, and bone metastasis (lysed bone).
Polycythemia	Erythropoietin.	Renal cell carcinoma (hypernephroma).
Lambert-Eaton syndrome	Antibodies against presynaptic Ca^{2+} channels at NMJ.	Thymoma, bronchogenic carcinoma.
Gout	Hyperuricemia due to excess nucleic acid turnover (ie, cytotoxic therapy).	

ACTH, adrenocorticotropic hormone; ADH, antidiuretic hormone; ANP, atrial natriuretic peptide; IL-2, interleukin-2; NMJ, neuromuscular junction; PTH, parathyroid hormone; TGF, transforming growth factor; TNF-α, tumor necrosis factor-α.

PRESENTATION

Painless hematuria.

DIAGNOSIS

CT urogram and cystoscopy. Urine for cytology (10% yield).

TREATMENT

- Localized (not invading bladder muscle): Surgery + intravesical chemo or bacillus Calmette-Guerin (BCG).
- Advanced: Chemotherapy.

Hepatocellular Carcinoma

EPIDEMIOLOGY

- More common in Asia.
- Seen in patients with cirrhosis, especially hepatitis B and hemochromatosis.

SCREENING

- Liver ultrasound +/– **AFP (tumor marker)** every 6 months in patients with cirrhosis or chronic hepatitis B.
- MRI for more definitive diagnosis.

TREATMENT

- Depends on the degree of cirrhosis and the size of the tumor.
- For local disease, options include surgery, radiofrequency ablation, and chemoembolization.
- For metastatic disease, VEGF inhibitors (sunitinib or sorafenib) can be given.

MISCELLANEOUS METASTATIC DISEASE

- **Liver metastasis:**
  - Liver and lung are the most common sites for metastatic disease.
  - Primary tumors that metastasize to the liver: **Colon > Stomach > Pancreas (all three GI from portal circulation) > Breast > Lung.**
- **Bone metastasis:**
  - Breast and prostate are the most common.
  - Kidney, thyroid, testes, lung, prostate, breast.
    - Lung = **L**ytic
    - Breast = **B**oth lytic and blastic
    - Prostate = blastic
- **Brain metastasis:**
  - Fifty percent of brain tumors are metastatic lesions.
  - Primary tumors metastasizing to the brain: **L**ung, **B**reast, **S**kin (melanoma), **K**idney (renal cell carcinoma), **G**I.

Lots of Bad Stuff Kills Glia
(Origin of brain mets:
Lung, Breast, Skin, Kidney,
GI)

Hypercalcemia

- The most common metabolic emergency of malignancy.
- Symptoms and signs include confusion, nausea, fatigue, ↓ PO intake, polyuria, depression, psychosis/confusion, nephrolithiasis (**BONES, STONES, GROANS, and PSYCHIATRIC OVERTONES**).
- Can progress to severe confusion and coma.
- Electrocardiogram (ECG) may show QT interval shortening.
- Usual cancers: Multiple myeloma, breast cancer, squamous cell (lung cancer, head and neck), renal cell cancer, lymphomas.
- Either from bone mets, PTH related peptide or 1-25 vitamin D (lymphomas).
- **Treatment: Aggressive rehydration with normal saline**, furosemide if patient is fluid overloaded, **bisphosphonates (takes 2–3 days)**. Calcitonin as a temporizing measure has limited role due to tachyphylaxis.

Febrile Neutropenia

Fever in the setting of clinically significant neutropenia (absolute neutrophil count < 500).

WORKUP

- Careful history and physical.
- Chest x-ray.
- Pan-culture.

TREATMENT

- Antibiotics should be started empirically (usually cefepime +/− aminoglycoside); add vancomycin if the person has hypotension, history of methicillin-resistant *Staphylococcus aureus* (MRSA), or an **infusaport** (access device for transfusions or chemotherapy) or a skin source).
- If vancomycin is not added initially, then add vanco at day 3 if patient continues to have fever and neutropenia. Add antifungals (voriconazole) on day 5 if no improvement.

Tumor Lysis Syndrome

- Cell breakdown causes release of intracellular ions (potassium and phosphorus) and DNA breakdown causing **hyperuricemia.**
- Seen in leukemias, lymphomas, and after chemotherapy in bulky tumors.
- Uric acid can cause acute renal failure and gout.
- Electrolyte disturbances: Hyperkalemia, hyperphosphatemia and hypocalcemia (from binding to phosphorus). **High LDH.**
- Treat with IV fluids, allopurinol.
- Severe cases require urine alkalinization and IV therapy with rasburicase (an enzyme that degrades uric acid).

Superior Vena Cava (SVC) Syndrome

Caused by obstruction of the superior vena cava by external compression, tumor invasion, or thrombus formation in the SVC lumen.

SIGNS/SYMPTOMS

Dyspnea, facial edema and plethora, cough, neck and arm edema.

DIAGNOSIS

CT chest, chest x-ray.

TREATMENT

- Chemotherapy, **radiation.**
- Intubation/tracheal stent if airway compromise.
- Steroids (controversial).

Spinal Cord Compression

- Compression of spinal cord secondary to vertebral collapse or extension of tumor from vertebra.
- Most commonly affects the thoracic spine.
- Back pain in cancer patient with neurological symptoms = cord compression.

SIGNS/SYMPTOMS

- Back pain.
- Loss of bowel or bladder function.
- Muscle weakness.
- Saddle anesthesia.

DIAGNOSIS

- Thorough neurologic exam, including rectal exam for evaluation of sphincter tone.
- MRI spine with gadolinium.

TREATMENT

High-dose steroids + radiation therapy or surgical decompression.

TABLE 2.4-3 Common Classes of Chemotherapies

SPECIFIC DRUGS (EXAMPLES)	INDICATIONS	SPECIFIC TOXICITY
Drug Class: Alkylating agents	**Mechanism:** Formation of DNA cross-links and hence inhibition of DNA function and synthesis.	**General Toxicities:** Myelosuppression, mucosal toxicity-mucosal ulceration, diarrhea, nausea and vomiting.
Cyclophosphamide/ Ifosfamide	HL, NHL, ALL/CLL, Multiple myeloma, breast/ lung/ovary/ testicular cancer.	Hemorrhagic cystitis.
Melphalan	Multiple myeloma, ovarian cancer.	Myelosuppression, hypersensitivity.
Chlorambucil	CLL, HL/NHL.	Myelosuppression, bone marrow failure.
Bendamustine	CLL, NHL.	Pancytopenia, hyperbilirubinemia.
Temozolomide	Brain cancer, malignant melanoma.	Myelosuppression, elevated LFTs.
Procarbazine	HL, NHL.	Myelosuppression, reproductive dysfunction, hemolysis (in G6PD deficiency).
Dacarbazine	HL, malignant melanoma.	Myelosuppression, metallic taste, rash.
Drug Class: Platinum compounds	**Mechanism:** Form intrastrand and interstrand DNA cross-links; bind to nuclear and cytoplasmic proteins.	
Cisplatin	NSCLC, breast cancer, bladder cancer, head and neck cancer, ovarian cancer.	**Nephrotoxicity,** peripheral **neuropathy,** myelosuppression, ototoxicity.
Carboplatin	NSCLC, breast cancer, bladder cancer, head and neck cancer, ovarian cancer.	Myelosuppression.
Oxaliplatin	Colorectal cancer, pancreatic cancer.	Myelosuppression, peripheral neuropathy.

DRUG	MECHANISM OF ACTION	INDICATIONS	TOXICITY
Drug Class: Antimetabolites			
Subclass: Folic acid analogs			
Methotrexate	Inhibits dihydrofolate reductase, inhibits thymidylate synthetase.	NHL, bladder cancer, head and neck cancer.	Mucositis, diarrhea, myelosuppression. **Don't give if any effusions (drug will stay there).**

TABLE 2.4-3   Common Classes of Chemotherapies *(continued)*

DRUG	MECHANISM OF ACTION	INDICATIONS	TOXICITY
Subclass: Pyrimidine analogs			
Cytarabine	Inhibits DNA synthesis and repair.	Acute leukemias (AML and ALL).	Myelosuppression, **cerebellar toxicity.**
5-Fluorouracil (5-FU)	Interferes with DNA synthesis, Inhibits thymidylate synthetase, incorporates into RNA.	Colorectal cancer, stomach cancer, head and neck cancer, breast cancer.	Mucositis, bone marrow suppression.
Capecitabine	Oral version of 5-FU. Interferes with DNA synthesis, inhibits thymidylate synthetase, incorporates into RNA.	Colorectal cancer, gastroesophageal cancer, pancreatic cancer, breast cancer.	Hand-foot syndrome, myelosuppression.
Gemcitabine	Inhibits DNA synthesis, inhibits ribonucleotide reductase.	Pancreatic cancer, NSCLC, breast cancer.	Myelosuppression, edema, hepatotoxicity.
Subclass: Purine analogs			
6-mercaptopurine (6-MP)	Inhibits purine nucleotide synthesis, inhibits DNA/RNA synthesis.	ALL, AML.	Myelosuppression, hepatotoxicity.
Cladribine	Incorporates into DNA, inhibits DNA synthesis and repair.	**Hairy cell leukemia.**	Myelosuppression.
Fludarabine	Incorporates into DNA, inhibits DNA synthesis and repair.	NHL, **CLL.**	Myelosuppression, myalgias, arthralgias.
Hydroxyurea	Interferes DNA synthesis (antimetabolite), ↑**Hb F level in sickle cell anemia.**	CML, polycythemia vera, essential thrombosis, **sickle cell disease.**	
Drug Class (sort of): Natural products			
Subtype: Vinca alkaloids (from plant)			
Vinblastine	Inhibits microtubule formation and mitosis.	**HL,** NHL, breast cancer, testicular cancer, Kaposi's sarcoma.	Myelosuppression, hypertension.
Vincristine	Inhibits microtubule formation and mitosis.	Leukemias, HL, NHL.	**Neuropathy,** myelosuppression.

(continued)

TABLE 2.4-3 Common Classes of Chemotherapies *(continued)*

DRUG	MECHANISM OF ACTION	INDICATIONS	TOXICITY
Subtype: Taxanes (from plant)			
Docetaxel	Interfere with microtubules, inhibit mitosis.	Breast cancer, metastatic prostate cancer, NSCLC.	**Fluid retention**, neurotoxicity, myelosuppression.
Paclitaxel	Interfere with microtubules, inhibit mitosis.	Breast cancer, NSCLS, ovarian cancer.	**Neuropathy,** myelosuppression.
Subtype: Camptothecins (topoisomerase I inhibitors) (from plant)			
Topotecan	Inhibits topoisomerase I.	Ovarian cancer, small cell lung cancer.	Myelosuppression.
Irinotecan	Inhibits topoisomerase I.	Lung cancer, colorectal cancer.	Diarrhea, nausea, myelosuppression.
Subtype: Epipodophyllotoxins (topoisomerase II inhibitors) (Podophyllotoxin derivative)			
Etoposide	Inhibits topoisomerase II.	NHL, NSCLC, gastric cancer.	Mucositis, myelosuppression, alopecia.
Teniposide	Inhibits topoisomerase II.	ALL.	Mucositis, myelosuppression.
Miscellaneous			
Arsenic	DNA fragmentation, induces apoptosis, degrades PML/RAR alpha protein.	Acute promyelocytic leukemia (M3).	
Asparaginase (enzyme)	Hydrolyzes asparagine and hence inhibits protein synthesis.	ALL.	**Pancreatitis**, coagulation abnormalities—bleeding and clotting
ATRA (tretinoin)	**Induces differentiation of promyelocytes, thereby reducing DIC when chemo starts.**	Acute promyelocytic leukemia **(M3).**	**ATRA syndrome:** Severe fluid retention that can cause respiratory failure. Treat with steroids.
Drug Class: Antibiotics			
Bleomycin	Binds to DNA, causing DNA breaking.	HL, NHL, germ cell cancer, squamous cell cancer.	**Pulmonary fibrosis,** mucositis, dermatotoxicity.
Daunorubicin/Doxorubicin (adriamycin)	Binds to DNA causing DNA breaking, inhibits toposiomerase II.	ALL, lymphomas, breast cancer.	**Cardiotoxicity,** myelosuppression.

TABLE 2.4-3 **Common Classes of Chemotherapies** *(continued)*

DRUG	MECHANISM OF ACTION	INDICATIONS	TOXICITY
Small molecules (usually inhibit a tyrosine kinase in the cell signaling)			
Erlotinib	Inhibits EGFR tyrosine kinase.	**NSCLC**, pancreatic cancer.	**Skin rash,** interstitial lung disease.
Imatinib	**Inhibits Bcr-Abl tyrosine kinase.**	**CML (revolutionary breakthrough with great results),** GIST.	Fluid retention and edema, myalgias.
Sorafenib and sunitinib	Inhibits multiple kinase receptors involved with VEGF.	Unresectable hepatocellular cancer, renal cell carcinoma.	Skin rash, fatigue, ↑ INR.

ALL, acute lymphocytic leukemia; ATRA: all-trans retinoic acid; CML, chronic myelocytic leukemia; CLL, chronic lymphocytic lymphoma; EGFR, endothelial growth factor; HL, Hodgkin's lymphoma; GIST, gastrointestinal stromal tumor; G6PD, glucose-6-phosphate dehydrogenase; INR, International Normalized Ratio; NHL, non-Hodgkin's lymphoma; NSCLC, non–small cell lung cancer; PML, promyelocytic leukemia; RAR, retinoic acid receptor; VEGF, vascular endothelial growth factor.

Infectious Disease

- **Infection:** Microbial process characterized by an inflammatory response.
- **Bacteremia:** Invasion of and presence of bacteria in the blood.
- **Systemic inflammatory response syndrome (SIRS):** Characterized by two or more of the following:
  - Temperature > 38°C or < 36°C
  - Heart rate > 90
  - Respiratory rate > 20 per minute or $PaCO_2$ < 32
  - White blood cell count > 12 or < 4 or greater than 10% immature neutrophils
- **Sepsis:** SIRS and a nidus of infection.
- **Severe sepsis:** Sepsis with evidence of organ hypoperfusion.
- **Septic shock:** Severe sepsis with hypotension despite adequate fluid resuscitation requiring vasopressors to maintain blood pressure.

GENITOURINARY INFECTIONS

Urinary Tract Infection (UTI), Cystitis, and Pyelonephritis

DEFINITIONS

- A **urinary tract infection (UTI)** is a general term encompassing infection anywhere from the urethral meatus to the kidneys. **An uncomplicated UTI** is one that occurs in healthy, nonpregnant females, all others are generally **complicated UTIs.**
- **Cystitis** is infection of the bladder.
- **Pyelonephritis** is infection involving the renal parenchyma.
- **Bacteriuria** is the presence of bacteria in the urine, which may or may not be symptomatic.
- **Pyuria** is the presence of WBCs in the urine, usually associated with bacteriuria.
- **Hematuria** is the presence of RBCs in the urine, often seen with cystitis.

EPIDEMIOLOGY

- More common in women by a ratio of 30:1 from age 1 through 50; beyond age 50 the ratio is 2:1.
- UTI is the most common infectious complication of pregnancy.
- In the elderly, UTI is the most frequently documented infection, the most common cause of sepsis, and the most common nosocomial infection.

RISK FACTORS

- **Men:**
  - Uncircumcised males.
  - Prostatic hypertrophy.
  - Phimosis.
  - Anal intercourse or vaginal intercourse with urinary tract infected partner.

Always treat a pregnant woman for a UTI, even if it's asymptomatic. First-line treatments are nitrofurantoin or a beta-lactam (penicillin or cephalosporin).

- Asymptomatic bacteremia should **not** be treated in the following populations: women (premenopausal, nonpregnant), diabetics, elderly, nursing home residents or patients with spinal cord injury or indwelling urethral catheters. These patients tend to have colonized or contaminated specimens.
- Asymptomatic bacteremia **always** should be treated in pregnant women.
- Asymptomatic pyuria (WBCs in urine) should **not** be treated in most cases.

INFECTIOUS DISEASE

Men with cystitis should be investigated for an underlying cause such as prostatitis or urinary retention.

An alkaline urine is suggestive of infection with *Proteus mirabilis* or *Ureaplasma urealyticum.*

- **Women:**
  - Recent sexual intercourse.
  - History of prior UTI.
  - Use of spermicide.
  - Postmenopausal state.
- **Both:**
  - Instrumentation/catheterization (see Table 2.5-1 for common procedures).
  - Immunocompromise.
  - Genitourinary tract abnormalities.

ETIOLOGY

- *Escherichia coli* is by far the most common pathogen, accounting for 80–85% of community-acquired UTIs and 50% of nosocomial ones.
- *Staphylococcus saprophyticus* contributes to 5–15% of uncomplicated cases, mostly in young women.
- *Klebsiella, Proteus, Pseudomonas,* and enterococci account for most of the remainder of cases.
- Group B strep accounts for only ~ 1% of cases but is a clinically important pathogen in the pregnant patient at term—**always test third-trimester pregnant patients for this.**

TABLE 2.5-1. Common Genitourinary Procedures

TEST	DESCRIPTION	USES
Intravenous pyelography	Contrast is injected into a peripheral vein, followed by radiographs, allowing visualization of the renal parenchyma and the ureters.	Basically anytime you want to visualize the ureters and kidneys. Examples: suspicion of infection, tumor, renal damage of any sort (e,g., pyelonephritis).
Voiding cystourethrogram	Contrast medium is placed into the bladder via catheter and visualized with x-ray during active micturition.	Investigation of abnormalities of bladder and ureters. Examples: **structural abnormality** (congenital, ectopic drainage, strictures, vesicoureteral reflux, ureteroceles) or **functional abnormality** (neurogenic bladder, stress incontinence) of ureters.
Cystometry	Bladder is filled with water via catheter. Bladder is emptied into a measuring device. The pressure is recorded during this process.	Investigation of bladder function in the setting of incontinence or urgency (eg, is benign prostatic hypertrophy obstructing bladder outflow? Is there outflow obstruction, or is bladder not contracting for other reasons?)
Cystoscopy	Introduction of either a flexible or rigid scope into the urethra.	Visualize inside of bladder. For example, investigate hematuria—is there tumor there (can biopsy also)? Bladder stone? Also therapeutic—can crush bladder stones.
Renal ultrasound	Advantage is that it is noninvasive.	Visualize kidneys. First step in investigating kidney failure. "Atrophic kidneys" suggest kidney damage. Also can see tumors, hydronephrosis, thrombus.

SIGNS AND SYMPTOMS

- **General UTI:** Dysuria, frequency, urgency, nocturia, suprapubic pain, cloudy, malodorous urine, or bloody urine.
- **Pyelonephritis:** Spiking fever, shaking chills, costovertebral angle tenderness, nausea, vomiting, anorexia.

DIAGNOSIS

- **Urine dipstick** can detect **leukocyte esterase** (correlates to pyuria—or leukocytes in the urine) and **nitrites** (made by certain common UTI bugs, eg, Enterobacteriaceae); the most widely available and cost-effective test; fairly sensitive and specific.
- The presence of leukocyte esterase and nitrites usually indicate a UTI.
- **Urine analysis** involves spinning down and directly visualizing the presence of WBCs (pyuria) (> 5 WBCs is ⊕).
- **Interpretation of all tests must take into account the presence or absence of symptoms.**
  - **Nitrites:** May have false ⊖ if bacteria that do not produce nitrite, or if already on antibiotics or if voided urine not in bladder long; may have **false** ⊕ due to meds altering dipstick color, or if not fresh urine.
  - **Leukocyte esterase:** False-⊕ leukocyte esterase results are seen with fecal contamination; false ⊖—patient already on antibiotics.
- **Pyuria** is present in nearly all UTIs; its absence suggests another diagnosis. Greater than 5 WBC per high power field is definitively ⊕ (2–5 is a gray area); this is around > 8 WBC/μL or 8000 WBC/mL.
- **Urine culture** is the definitive test. A ⊕ result is defined as > 10,000 colony-forming units (CFUs) per milliliter with a single organism in symptomatic patients, and > 100,000 CFU/mL in an asymptomatic patient. Urine cultures should always be obtained for complicated UTIs, due to high rate of bacterial resistance.
- **Imaging** is not indicated for uncomplicated UTI. CT scan or renal ultrasound can demonstrate perinephric/intrarenal abscesses, nephrolithiasis, or obstruction. If pyelonephritis does not improve after 48–72 hours, these causes should be sought.

TREATMENT

- Most uncomplicated UTIs are treated with a short course (3–5 days) of oral antibiotics on an outpatient basis. Complicated UTI requires a longer duration of antibiotics.
- Bacteriuria in pregnancy is *always* treated, regardless of the presence of symptoms, due to high rate of progression to pyelonephritis. Empiric category B antibiotics are nitrofurantoin and ampicillin.
- Consider hospitalization and intravenous antibiotics for high-risk patients: elderly, immunocompromised, those with indwelling catheters, sepsis, and patients who are unable to tolerate oral intake.

Vaginitis

The normal flora of the vagina creates an acidic environment (pH 3.5–4.5) in large part through the colonization of lactobacilli. This protects the vagina from pathogenic organisms. When this environment is disturbed, infections become possible.

> **Bugs that cause UTI—**
>
> **SEEKS PP**
>
> **S.** saprophyticus
> **E.** coli
> **E**nterobacter
> **K**lebsiella
> **S**erratia
> **P**roteus
> **P**seudomonas
>   (especially with GU instrumentation)

> Lactobacilli are used to make yogurt. A Yoplait a day keeps vaginitis away.

INFECTIOUS DISEASE

The "whiff" test: Application of KOH to the wet mount will enhance the odor of both *Gardnerella* and *Trichomonas*. **On wet mount:** "Clue cells" = bacterial vaginosis; motile flagellated organisms = trichomoniasis.

Metronidazole is contraindicated in first-trimester pregnancy. Use clotrimazole instead.

Warn patients against having any alcohol while on metronidazole. It can cause a disulfiram-like reaction when co-ingested with alcohol.

De Musset's sign (head bobbing seen in aortic insufficiency) was first described in prostitutes with syphilitic aortitis.

Argyll Robertson (syphilitic) pupil is like a prostitute: It accommodates but doesn't react.

CAUSES

- Bacterial vaginosis (BV)—*Gardnerella*.
- *Trichomonas vaginalis* (sexually transmitted).
- Yeast—*Candida albicans*.

SIGNS AND SYMPTOMS

- Vaginal itch and burning sensation.
- Abnormal odor.
- Discharge:
  - **BV:** Fishy odor of discharge.
  - ***Trichomonas:*** Fishy odor of discharge, strawberry cervix.
  - **Yeast:** Cottage cheese–like discharge.

DIAGNOSIS

Wet mount:

- BV: Clue cells (epithelial cells coated with bacteria).
- *Trichomonas:* Motile trichomonads.
- Yeast: Pseudohyphae.

TREATMENT

- Metronidazole for BV and *Trichomonas*.
- Treat sexual partners as well in *Trichomonas* (sexually transmitted).
- Azole antifungals or nystatin for yeast infection.

SEXUALLY TRANSMITTED DISEASES (STDS)

Syphilis

- A sexually transmitted or congenital disease with variable clinical manifestations, depending on stage of the disease.
- Transmitted primarily through sexual contact but can be spread through any mucosal or epithelial abrasion.
- The causative organism is *Treponema pallidum*, a spirochete.
- Once the spirochete has entered the body, it spreads throughout most organ systems and the disease then progresses through three active stages.

SIGNS AND SYMPTOMS

All patients develop a *painless* chancre at inoculation site. If untreated, some patients progress to a disseminated (2°) stage, during which the organism is spread throughout the entire body and is highly infectious.

- 1° syphilis:
  - A **painless "buttonlike" chancre** with indurated borders develops at inoculation site within 2–6 weeks after exposure.
  - Accompanied by regional lymphadenopathy (**"bubo"**) within 1 week.
  - Chancre can last up to 6 weeks if untreated.
- 2° syphilis:
  - Appears 4–6 weeks after 1° syphilis resolves, lasts for 6–8 weeks.
  - Maculopapular rash (multiple, discrete, firm, "ham-colored" papules scattered symmetrically over trunk, **palms and soles,** and genitals).

- **Condylomata lata:** Soft, flat-topped pink papules on anogenital region that are painless, wartlike lesions.
- Flulike symptoms: Fever, malaise, arthralgia, generalized lymphadenopathy, and splenomegaly.
- **Latent phase:**
  - This stage can last for several years.
  - Patients are asymptomatic but remain seropositive.
- **3° syphilis:**
  - Develops at any time during the latent phase and continues indefinitely if not treated.
  - **Gummas:** Rubbery granulomatous lesions in subcutaneous tissues of central nervous system (CNS), heart, aorta.
  - Cardiovascular: Vasa vasorum vasculitis, aortic insufficiency.
  - Neurosyphilis: Seizures, personality changes, psychosis, **tabes dorsalis** (posterior column degeneration).
  - The syphilitic pupil is also known as **Argyll Robertson pupil.**

LABORATORY

- **Venereal Disease Research Laboratory (VDRL) and rapid plasma reagin (RPR):** Good screening tests but nonspecific.
- **Fluorescent treponemal antibody-absorption test (FTA-ABS):** Done when VDRL or RPR is ⊕. Good sensitivity and specificity. Remains ⊕ for life, regardless of treatment.
- **Darkfield microscopy:** Smear of exudate from primary chancre or secondary papular lesions reveal a 5- to 20-μm-long spirochete, with kinking and contractile movements but without locomotion.
- *T. pallidum* does not grow in regular blood cultures.
- If neurosyphilis is suspected, cerebrospinal fluid (CSF) should be sent for WBC count, protein, glucose, and VDRL.

TREATMENT

Penicillin G; can consider tetracycline for nonpregnant patients with severe penicillin allergies; however, desensitization therapy is preferred in these cases whenever possible.

Balanitis

Inflammation of the glans penis.

CAUSES

- *Candida albicans*, other infectious agents.
- Allergic reaction (often to latex condoms).
- Reactive arthritis (formerly known as Reiter's syndrome).

TREATMENT

Treat underlying cause: Candidal infections are treated with nystatin/topical azoles. Reactive arthritis is treated with NSAIDs.

Genital Herpes

Infection with herpes simplex virus. Type 1 usually associated with oral lesions, and type 2 with genital lesions, but not always.

Rapid plasma reagin (RPR) syphilis screening is part of dementia workup.

VDRL/RPR false ⊕ are seen in:
- Systemic lupus erythematosus (SLE)
- Infectious mononucleosis
- Hepatitis C

Jarisch-Herxheimer reaction: Fever, fatigue, and transient worsening of mucocutaneous symptoms, typically seen in treatment of 2° syphilis with penicillin. *It is not a drug allergy!*

If maternal syphilis infection is untreated by 16 weeks' gestation, child may be born with congenital syphilis and is at risk of stillbirth.

Any patient who presents with balanitis should be screened for diabetes (candidal infections are common in diabetics and uncommon in normal men).

Reactive Arthritis: Can't See, Can't Pee, Can't Climb a Tree! Reactive arthritis is a condition described by Hans Reiter (**no longer called Reiter's syndrome** secondary to his involvement with the Nazis in WWII) with the classic triad of nongonococcal urethritis, conjuctivitis, and arthritis.

Infections can remain dormant for years, but the herpesvirus is continuously shed and can be transmitted during latent phases.

HSV meningitis presents with fever, confusion, and photophobia, and MRI usually shows a temporal lobe lesion. Give: IV acyclovir.

HPV types 16, 18, 31, 45, 51, 52, and 53 are associated with cervical cancer.

SIGNS AND SYMPTOMS

- **Painful** vesicular lesions on erythematous base.
- Local lymphadenopathy.
- Neuralgia often precedes an outbreak.

LABORATORY

- Tzanck smear test and culture.
- Herpes serology.

TREATMENT

Antiviral agents acyclovir, famciclovir, and valacyclovir are not curative but effective in reducing the severity and frequency of outbreaks, as well as the degree of viral shedding.

Human Papillomavirus (HPV)

STD caused by the human papillomavirus, of which there are many subtypes.

EPIDEMIOLOGY

- Most common sexually transmitted disease.
- Commonly asymptomatic in men.
- Certain serotypes have been implicated as causative agent in cervical cancer (16, 18, 31 most common).

SIGNS AND SYMPTOMS

- Bowenoid papules on penis.
- Condyloma acuminata (papillomatous growths with a soft, macerated surface).
- Warts grow on mucous membrane of penis, perineum, vulva, vagina, and vaginal canal.

DIAGNOSIS

Most HPV warts are flat and invisible to the unaided eye. Coating them with 1% acetic acid turns them white. All white lesions on colposcopy are biopsied for HPV.

TREATMENT

- Lesions are removed via cryosurgery, laser ablation, or chemical ablation (podophyllin).
- **Gardasil (HPV vaccine)** is used to prevent infection with cervical cancer-associated serotypes.

Urethritis

Neisseria gonorrhoeae and *Chlamydia trachomatis* are the two most common organisms:

- **N. gonorrhoeae** (gonococcus [GC]) can cause cervicitis, urethritis, epididymitis, conjunctivitis, PID, pneumonia, and lymphogranuloma venereum.
- *C. trachomatis* can cause cervicitis, urethritis, epididymitis, conjunctivitis, pelvic inflammatory disease (PID), pneumonia, and lymphogranuloma venereum.

DIAGNOSIS

Polymerase chain reaction (PCR) analysis of vaginal or penile swab, or urine culture.

HPV: Mother may infect newborn during delivery, causing **laryngeal papillomatosis.**

TREATMENT

- Single-dose therapy:
  - **For GC:** 125 mg ceftriaxone IM.
  - **For *Chlamydia:*** 1 g azithromycin PO.
- Above combination often given empirically, thereby avoiding compliance issues.
- Multiple 7-day combinations exist, if above regimen is not chosen.
- Sexual partners should be treated concurrently; if the partner is not present, the patient is often given an extra prescription to be taken by their partner.

Always treat *Chlamydia* and GC concurrently because coinfection is often present.

Pelvic Inflammatory Disease (PID)

- Infection of the upper genital structures in women (uterus, oviducts, ovaries), often with involvement of neighboring organs.
- Usually, this is GC or *Chlamydia* untreated and progressing (see urethritis).
- Both, particularly *Chlamydia*, can be chronic and cause scarring of the fallopian tubes and infertility.

RISK FACTORS

- Younger age at first sexual contact.
- Multiple sexual partners.
- Use of intrauterine device (IUD).
- Prior history of PID.
- Recent intrauterine instrumentation.

The discharge of GC is purulent, whereas that of *Chlamydia* is nonpurulent.

SIGNS AND SYMPTOMS

- Lower abdominal pain.
- Tenderness to pelvic exam.

DIAGNOSTIC CRITERIA

Cervical motion and adnexal tenderness *plus* one or more of the following:

- Fever > 101°F.
- Abnormal vaginal/cervical discharge.
- Lab evidence of GC or *C. trachomatis*.
- Elevated erythrocyte sedimentation rate (ESR) or C-reactive protein.

Chlamydia is the leading infectious cause of blindness worldwide (trachoma).

TREATMENT

- **Outpatient:**
  - Treat for GC and *C. trachomatis*, major causative organisms.
  - Offer HIV testing.
  - Remove any infected foreign body.
  - Treat all sexual partners.
- **Inpatient:** Hospital admission and IV antibiotics (ceftriaxone and azithromycin) is warranted if any of the following: high fever, uncertain diagnosis, pregnancy, can't take PO, immunosuppression, first episode in nulligravida, can't follow up in 48 hours, failure of outpatient therapy.

C. trachomatis is a major cause of PID and infertility (fallopian tube scarring causes infertility).

INFECTIOUS DISEASE

Prostatitis

Two types—bacterial and nonbacterial.

> A 19-year-old sexually active female presents with left lower quadrant crampy pelvic pain for 1 week. Physical exam reveals a temperature of 101°F, cervical motion tenderness, and a mucopurulent vaginal discharge. Laboratory results reveal ESR 65 and WBC 16. *Think: Pelvic inflammatory disease.* Check for GC and chlamydia. **Next step:** Give IV antibiotics (ceftriaxone and azithromycin).

BACTERIAL PROSTATITIS

Inflammation of the prostate due to bacteria ascending the urethra and then passing into the prostate through the prostatic ducts.

CAUSES

- *E. coli.*
- *Pseudomonas*

SIGNS AND SYMPTOMS

- Perineal and suprapubic pain.
- Dysuria and urinary frequency.
- Fever.
- Tender, boggy prostate on physical exam.
- Chronic bacterial prostatitis is uncommon and presents as recurrent UTI.

LABORATORY FINDINGS

- Leukocytosis with neutrophil predominance.
- Urinalysis (U/A) shows bacteriuria and pyuria.

TREATMENT

- Outpatient therapy consists of TMP-SMZ or ciprofloxacin (flouroquinolone is preferred) for 21 days.
- Indications for hospitalization include severe comorbidities, poor patient compliance, or sepsis.

NONBACTERIAL PROSTATITIS

- An inflammatory process in the prostate from an unknown etiology.
- Viral agents or an autoimmune reaction are possible causes.
- This is the most common cause of chronic prostatitis.

SIGNS AND SYMPTOMS

- Urinary frequency and dysuria.
- Nontender, enlarged prostate on physical exam.

LABORATORY

- U/A and urine culture are $\ominus$.
- Leukocytes can be seen in prostatic secretions.

Care must be taken during the rectal exam on a prostatis patient. Vigorously massaging the prostate can → bacteremia.

INFECTIOUS DISEASE

TREATMENT

- A trial of antibiotics is often given.
- Anti-inflammatories for symptomatic relief.

Community-Acquired Pneumonias (CAPs)

Top five bacterial etiologies of CAP:

1. *Streptococcus pneumoniae* (most common).
2. *Staphylococcus aureus* (methicillin-resistant [MRSA] becoming more common in the community).
3. *Legionella*.
4. *Haemophilus influenzae*.
5. Atypicals: *Chlamydia pneumoniae* and *Mycoplasma pneumoniae*.

TREATMENT

Treatment is almost always initiated with an empirically selected antibiotic: macrolide in simple cases; respiratory flouroquinolone (levofloxacin, moxifloxacin) or beta-lactam plus a macrolide for patients with significant comorbidities.

Typical Pneumonias

- *S. pneumoniae*:
  - Most common CAP; typically has lobar consolidation with "rusty-colored" sputum.
  - Gram-⊕ cocci, grows in chains.
  - Causes multiple infections, including acute sinusitis, otitis media, meningitis, septic arthritis, pneumonia, cellulitis, erysipelas, bacteremia, and others.
  - People with defective complement/antibody function, prior hospitalization, splenectomy, renal insufficiency, diabetes, and other conditions are predisposed to community-acquired S. *pneumoniae*.
  - Treat with beta-lactam antibiotics; most also susceptible to flouroquinolones, macrolides.
  - Prophylaxis against common serotypes is available with polysaccharide vaccine (especially adults age 65 and over) or conjugate vaccine (infants and small children).
- *Staphylococcus aureus* pneumonia:
  - Consider this in a patient with viral infection ~ 2 weeks before. "Salmon pink" sputum and cavitary lesions.
  - Gram-⊕ cocci in clusters.
  - Treat with beta-lactams or vancomycin if MRSA is suspected.
- *Klebsiella pneumoniae*:
  - "Currant jelly" sputum, "bulging fissure" on chest x-ray (CXR).
  - "Friedlander's bacillus."
  - May cause biliary or urinary tract infections in hospitalized patients.
  - Treat with cephalosporin +/– aminoglycoside.
- *Haemophilus influenzae*:
  - Gram-⊖ coccobacilli.

Austrian syndrome is the triad of pneumococcal endocarditis, pneumonia, and meningitis. Rare, but seen in alcoholics and IV drug users.

INFECTIOUS DISEASE

- Has many types; the most commonly known is *H. influenzae* type B (Hib).
- Nontypable *H. influenzae* is responsible for sinusitis, otitis media, and CAP, especially in chronic obstructive pulmonary disease (COPD) patients.
- Infection with Hib causes meningitis, especially in children < 3 years of age; currently, there is an Hib vaccine to protect against this.
- Treat with third-generation cephalosporin, quinolone, doxycycline.
- *Moraxella catarrhalis:*
  - Gram-$\ominus$ coccus.
  - Mostly in COPD and immunocompromised patients; causes upper respiratory infections and pneumonia.
  - Susceptible to penicillin/clavulanic acid, macrolides, and trimethoprim-sulfamethoxazole (TMP-SMZ).

All HIV-$\oplus$ patients should receive the pneumococcal and *H. flu* vaccines.

Atypical Pneumonias

- *Mycoplasma pneumoniae:*
  - One of the most common community-acquired pathogens causing pneumonia in healthy persons under age 40; most common in ages 5–20.
  - Causes atypical pneumonia ("walking" pneumonia).
  - Insidious onset with an incubation period of up to 3 weeks.
  - Patients present with fever, pharyngitis, headaches, chills, tonsillitis, arthritis, hemolytic anemia, change in mental status, or erythema multiforme.
- *Chlamydia pneumoniae:*
  - Common cause of CAP in children and young adults.
  - Transmission is person to person.
  - Patients often present with fever, nonproductive cough.
  - CXR shows segmental infiltrates.
  - Treat with quinolone or cephalosporin and macrolide.
- *Chlamydia psittaci:*
  - Obligate intracellular parasite.
  - Host is avian species (**think prior exposure to bird**).
  - Transmitted via the respiratory route.
  - Patient presents with fever, headache, chills, cough, myalgias, abdominal pain, nausea, vomiting.
  - On physical exam ~ 70% of patients will have splenomegaly.
  - Can be treated with tetracyclines.
- *Legionella pneumophila:*
  - Gram-$\ominus$ rod, anaerobic.
  - Source is typically bodies of water; can be spread through air conditioning systems.
  - Causes Legionnaire's disease, which consists of **pneumonia**, change in mental status, headaches, **diarrhea**, abdominal pain, nausea, vomiting, high fever, hyponatremia (**think Legionnaire's anytime you hear pneumonia + GI symptoms**).
  - Elderly and those with chronic lung diseases are at greatest risk.
  - Diagnose with direct immunofluorescent antigen or urinary antigen.
  - Treat with macrolides, quinolones, doxycycline.

A patient who works in a pet store presents with diffuse, bilateral infiltrate. *Think*: Chlamydia psittaci.

A 21-year-old woman who complains of dry cough, malaise, and low-grade fevers for 2 weeks has a CXR with hazy infiltrates. *Think:* Mycoplasma pneumoniae. **Next step:** Treat with macrolide if no comorbidities.

A patient presents with confusion and diarrhea and is found to have a large infiltrate on CXR with a pleural effusion. *Think:* Legionella pneumophila. **Next step:** Check *Legionella* antigen in the urine and serum PCR for *Legionella* antigen; start macrolide therapy and third-generation cephalosporin empirically until results become available.

Hospital-Acquired Pneumonias

- **HAP:** Fever, leukocytosis, and infiltrate on CXR in any patient receiving care within the hospital for 48 hours or more.
- *Pseudomonas, Enterobacter, Klebsiella pneumoniae, E coli, H influenzae, S aureus.*
- **Must always cover for *Pseudomonas*;** use fourth-generation cephalosporin, carbapenem, or piperacillin/tazobactam.
- Cover for MRSA with vancomycin in high-risk cases.
- *Pseudomonas aeruginosa:*
  - Gram-⊖ bacillus.
  - Usually acquired in the hospital.
  - Most common organism in ventilator-associated pneumonia.
  - Cystic fibrosis patients can be colonized by *P. aeruginosa*, which correlates with severity of airway disease.
  - Common infectious agent associated with exacerbations of bronchiectasis.
- *Acinetobacter baumanii:*
  - Small gram-⊖ coccobacilli.
  - Often colonize respiratory secretions and endotracheal tubes but also causes nosocomial infections, **particularly ventilator-associated pneumonia.**
  - Often multidrug resistant.
  - Treat with a third-generation cephalosporin and an aminoglycoside.

An elderly patient hospitalized for 3 weeks following an episode of decompensated heart failure now has fever, elevated WBC, and infiltrate on CXR. *Think: Hospital-acquired pneumonia.* **Next step:** Start pipercillin-tazobactam + vancomycin to cover *Pseudomonas aeruginosa*, resistant *S. pneumoniae*, and MRSA.

Health Care–Associated Pneumonias

- Patients from the community who received acute hospital care for more than 48 hours within the past 90 days, reside in a long-term care or other health care facility, or frequent facilities such as dialysis centers.
- Microbiology and management are similar to **hospital-acquired pneumonia.**

Aspiration Pneumonias

- Patients with a history of losing consciousness (eg, alcoholic binge, seizures, etc.) or with neurologic impairment (cerebrovascular accident [CVA], multiple sclerosis, etc.) presenting with a right middle lobe or right lower lobe infiltrate.
- Typical organisms include **anaerobes** such as *Bacteroides, Fusobacterium nucleatum, Peptostreptococcus,* along with gram negatives like *E coli, Pseudomonas,* and *Klebsiella.*
- Must provide broad-spectrum coverage for gram-⊖ and anaerobic organisms, with agents such as piperacillin-tazobactam or carbapenems.

 One week following a CVA, a 78-year-old patient develops fever and a right lower lobe infiltrate. *Think: Aspiration pneumonia.* **Next step:** Start imipenem empirically and obtain induced sputum cultures.

Other Respiratory Infections

- Adenovirus:
  - DNA virus.
  - Infections occur primarily during the fall and spring seasons.
  - Causes upper respiratory tract infection.
  - Supportive treatment.
- Epstein-Barr virus (EBV):
  - DNA virus.
  - Causes **infectious mononucleosis,** which is characterized by pharyngitis, fever, tender cervical **lymphadenopathy, +/– splenomegaly.**
  - Patients with mononucleosis should not engage in contact sports due to the risk of splenic rupture.
  - Laboratory studies will show abnormal liver function tests (LFTs) and lymphocytosis.
  - **Diagnose with heterophile antibody titers or, serum IgG/IgM for EBV.**
  - May be associated with hairy leukoplakia.
  - Supportive treatment.
- Influenza virus:
  - RNA virus.
  - Three types: A and B constitute one genus, and C makes up the other.
  - Influenza A periodically undergoes major antigenic changes, known as **antigenic shifts,** causing epidemics.
  - Transmission is via areosolized particles.
  - Patients present with fever, headache, malaise, myalgias, cough, pharyngitis, arthralgias, or lymphadenopathy.

- Influenza may be complicated by a primary viral pneumonia or a 2° bacterial pneumonia caused by *S aureus*, *S. pneumoniae*, or *H. influenzae*.
- Prophylaxis is with yearly flu vaccinations.
- May treat with amantadine/rimantadine or oseltamavir; however, treatment is largely supportive.
- **Parvovirus B19:**
  - DNA virus.
  - Causes **erythema infectiosum, also known as "fifth disease,"** in children.
  - Spread through respiratory secretions in people who appear to have the common cold.
  - In adults, parvovirus B19 presents as acute, symmetric **arthritis of the hands,** wrists, and knees.
  - Can also cause an aplastic anemia syndrome, particularly in sickle cell patients.
  - Treat supportively; may treat arthritis with nonsteroidals.

 A day care worker presents with fever and arthritis of the hands. *Think: Parvovirus B19.* **Next step:** Check serum parvovirus B19 antigen, IgG, and IgM.

- **Rhinovirus:**
  - RNA virus.
  - Causes the common cold, which presents as nasal congestion, rhinorrhea, sneezing, headache, and malaise.
  - Self-limited.
  - Treatment is supportive.
- ***Corynebacterium diphtheriae:***
  - Gram-⊕ bacillus.
  - Diphtheria presents as upper respiratory infection (not pneumonia) with low-grade fevers, sore throat, nausea, vomiting.
  - On exam, may find **grayish exudates in oropharynx that can coalesce to become a pseudomembrane.**
  - Treat with macrolide or penicillin, diphtheria antitoxin (IV infusion).
  - Prevent with TDaP (tetanus, diphtheria, pertussis) vaccine for kids and boosters for adults.

COMMON SKIN INFECTIONS

Staphylococcus aureus

- Gram ⊕, coagulase ⊕.
- Commonly causes infections of skin, septic arthritis, catheter infections, and endocarditis. **See *S aureus* syndromes below.**

Toxic Shock Syndrome

- Seen in menstruating women using "super-absorbent" tampons.
- Exotoxin mediated, produced by strains of *Staph A* and some group A strep species.

- Consists of fever, rash, desquamation of skin, nausea, along with evidence of organ failure (kidney, liver, respiratory, cardiovascular).
- Treat by removing foreign body and supportive care (antibiotics are controversial, but clindamycin may ↓ toxin; beta-lactams and vancomycin are also sometimes used in conjunction with clindamycin).

Scalded Skin Syndrome

- The most severe form is toxic epidermal necrolysis (TEN).
- Starts as periorbital or perioral erythematous rash and progresses to limbs.
- In days, the skin sloughs off.
- Must treat as burn, with careful monitoring and aggressive fluid administration depending on the extent of skin involvement.
- Also, meticulous skin care must be provided to prevent super-infection.

Streptococcus pyogenes

- Gram-⊕ cocci, group A beta-hemolytic.
- Causes soft tissue infections such as cellulitis, impetigo, and necrotizing fasciitis.
- Also causes pharyngitis, pneumonia, toxic shock–like syndrome.
- Treat with penicillin.
- **Postinfection sequelae:**
  - **Scarlet fever:** Presents as pharyngitis, strawberry tongue, and a rash that begins on the trunk and spreads to the extremities. Palms and soles have no rash but undergo desquamation.
  - **Poststreptococcal glomerulonephritis:** Glomerulonephritis ~ 2 weeks after strep infection.
  - **Streptococcal toxic shock syndrome:** Similar to staphylococcal type.

IMMUNITY

Humoral Immunity

- Branch of immune system composed of circulating or cell-bound proteins.
- Facilitates and directs cell destruction.
- Inactivates toxins.
- Two main components:
  1. **Immunoglobulins:** Produced by B lymphocytes and plasma cells (see Table 2.5-2).
  2. **Complement:** Produced by the liver.

Cellular Immunity

- Branch of immune system composed of *cells* (as opposed to immunoglobulins/proteins).
- T lymphocytes:
  - Cytotoxic T cells: Kill cells expressing foreign antigens, CD8+.
  - Helper T cells: Enhance activity of other T cells, B cells, and macrophages, CD4+.
  - Suppressor T cells: Inhibit cellular immune response, CD8+.

TABLE 2.5-2. Immunoglobulins and Their Functions

IgG	■ ~ 70% of total immunoglobulins.
	■ Predominant antibody in secondary immune response.
	■ Fixes complement (sometimes).
	■ Crosses placenta.
	■ Four subtypes.
	■ **Long lasting, evidence of previous exposure to antigen.**
IgA	■ ~ 20% of total immunoglobulins.
	■ Present in serum, colostrum, saliva, tears, and respiratory and intestinal mucosa **(think of it as the first line of defense in mucosa—defects result in lots of mucosal infections).**
IgM	■ ~ 10% of total immunoglobulins.
	■ **Fixes complement strongly!**
	■ Predominant antibody in primary immune response **(it is the first responder to infection before IgG is made).**
	■ Is a pentamer (huge protein).
	■ **Indicates acute infections.**
IgD	■ ~ 1% of total immunoglobulins.
	■ B cell surface receptor.
IgE	■ 0.01% of total immunoglobulins.
	■ Triggers histamine release from mast cells: Immediate hypersensitivity reactions (allergy, anaphylaxis, asthma).
	■ Also rises in parasitic infections.
	■ **When elevated think: allergy/hypersensitivity or parasite!**

- Neutrophils.
- Eosinophils.
- Mast cells.
- Reticuloendothelial system (monocytes, macrophages, histiocytes, Langerhans' cells, Kupffer cells, etc.).
- Natural killer cells.

IMMUNODEFICIENCY

Cell-Mediated Immunodeficiency (CMI)

- Major diseases causing cell-mediated immunodeficiency (CMI):
  - AIDS.
  - Leukemias and lymphomas.
  - Diabetes mellitus (**test questions: diabetics are prone to** *Mucor* **and** *Rhizopus* **infections.**).
  - Sarcoidosis.
  - Iatrogenic CMI:
    - High-dose corticosteroids.
    - Chemotherapy.
    - Radiation therapy.

Mucor—who gets it? Diabetics and immunosuppressed. How do you treat it? Surgery (actual resection of the fungus) and amphotericin.

207

- **CMI-associated infections** (think about classic infections AIDS patients get):
  - **Viruses:** Herpesviruses, cytomegalovirus (CMV), human papillomavirus (HPV), human herpes virus (HHV)-6.
  - **Fungi:** *Cryptococcus, Candida, Histoplasma, Coccidioides, Aspergillus, Pneumocystis jiroveci* (PCP).
  - **Protozoa:** *Toxoplasma, Cryptosporidium, Giardia lamblia.*
  - **Helminths:** *Strongyloides stercoralis.*
  - **Bacteria:** *Listeria, Nocardia, **Mycobacterium tuberculosis** reactivation,* nontuberculous mycobacteria, *Legionella, Salmonella.*

Humoral Immune Deficiency Disorders

- Patients with humoral immune deficiency disorders are commonly infected with encapsulated bacteria (similar to asplenic patients).
- **Common variable hypogammaglobulinemia:**
  - Can be acquired at any age.
  - Low levels of IgG, IgA, and IgM.
  - Normal numbers of B cells, but are defective.
  - Patients usually well until 15–30 years of age.
  - Classically get sinopulmonary infections with ***Streptococcus pneumoniae, Haemophilus influenzae, Klebsiella pneumoniae,* and *Mycoplasma;*** also autoimmune diseases.
- **Selective IgA deficiency:**
  - Most common of the selective immunoglobulin deficiencies.
  - Present with mucous membrane infections (URI, UTI, GI).
  - Low-molecular-weight IgM ↑ in partial compensation.
  - Serum may contain anti-IgA, IgE.
  - IgA replacement may cause **anaphylaxis** (don't do it).
  - Patients who are transfused with blood products and get anaphylaxis—think: **IgA deficiency responding to the IgA in donor's blood.**
- **Other:** CLL, multiple myeloma (these conditions leave people with abnormal antibody production). They also get sinopulmonary infections similar to common variable hypogammaglobulinemia (above).

Major Causes of Fever in the Immunocompromised

- **Cancer patients:** Certain types of cancer can create an immune abnormality. Leukemias, lymphomas, and multiple myeloma are examples. Although leukocytosis may be present, these white cells are dysfunctional and immunity is impaired.
  - Fever of unknown origin; often tumor related.
  - Bacteria: Gram-positive or gram-negative aerobes, anaerobes at site of mixed infection.
  - Viruses: Respiratory syncytial virus (RSV), parainfluenza, adenoviruses, herpes simplex virus (HSV), CMV.
  - Fungi: *Candida, Aspergillus, Cryptococcus, Trichosporon, Mucor, Pneumocystis jirovecii* and *Toxoplasma* also seen.
  - **Classic test examples** are **shingles in a multiple myeloma** patient, ***Listeria* meningitis in a CLL** patient.
  - Any cancer that is **treated with chemotherapy** is at risk for both cellular and humoral deficiencies.

- Neutropenia typically occurs 7–10 days after the last chemotherapy, when the "nadir" of all cell lines occurs. If a patient presents with fever any time during chemotherapy, neutropenia must be suspected and counts must be checked.
- If the patient is neutropenic, they must be treated empirically with IV antibiotics covering for bacterial (especially gram-⊖/*Pseudomonas*) infections (see below).
- Fevers of unknown causes in cancer patients are often due to the tumor itself.

- **Transplant patients:** These patients are extremely immunosuppressed around the transplant procedure (whichever type) itself, and less so later on, due to the use of ongoing immunosuppressive agents (usually steroids or a T-cell suppressive agent such as temsirolimus or cyclosporine) that prevent rejection of the transplanted organ or bone marrow.
- **Bone marrow transplant:**
  - There are basically two types: allogeneic (utilizes donor marrow from someone else) and autologous (uses stem cells harvested from the patient's own bone marrow).
  - Whereas both these types of patients are severely immunosuppressed soon after the transplant, this is far greater in allogeneic transplant patients.
  - Allogeneic patients also have longer suppression due to the common ongoing requirement of immunosuppressive agents to prevent host-versus-graft rejection.
  - **Classic infections** include the following:
    - **Early (1–4 weeks) infections:** HSV, bacteria, *Candida, Aspergillus.*
    - **Mid (4–26 weeks):** HSV, CMV, varicella-zoster, *Aspergillus,* PCP.
    - **Late:** Encapsulated bacteria (*S. pneumoniae, Neisseria meningitidis,* and *H. influenzae*), aspergillosis, HSV, CMV.
- **Solid organ transplant:** Influenced by time since transplant, and type of transplant.
- **Organisms include:**
  - **Bacteria:** Includes gram positive and negative.
  - **Viruses:** CMV, EBV, HBV, hepatitis C virus (HCV), adenovirus.
  - **Fungi:** *Aspergillus, Pneumocystis jiroveci.*
- **Splenectomy patients:** Encapsulated organisms (*S. pneumoniae, N. meningitidis,* and *H. influenzae*); **parasites:** malaria, *Babesia.*

Functionally asplenic patients (sickle cell disease) or postsplenectomy patients are at ↑ risk for infection with encapsulated organisms even if they are not neutropenic. Asplenic patients require vaccinations against *S. pneumoniae, N. meningitidis,* and *H. influenzae.*

Sickle cell patients can commonly get osteomyelitis caused by *Staphylococcus.*

General Principles of Evaluation and Management of Fever in Immunocompromised Patients

Diagnostic Studies

- Complete blood count (CBC) with manual differential and coagulation studies.
- Culture urine and blood.
- CXR regardless of physical exam findings.
- Culture sputum with cough or if CXR warrants.
- Culture stool and CSF in AIDS patients, look for cryptococcal antigen.
- In AIDS and transplant patients, obtain CMV antigen.
- **If neutropenic:**
  - Immediately start broad-spectrum therapy (eg, piperacillin/tazobactam, third-/fourth-generation cephalosporin, or carbapenem).
  - If patient has an indwelling catheter (eg, central line or chemotherapy port), add vancomycin to cover MRSA.

Neutropenic patients are vulnerable to more than one infection at a time. More than one organism may emerge during a single febrile episode. Be aggressive with broad-spectrum antibiotics.

- Adjust therapy based on culture results.
- If still febrile in 3 days, add antifungal (eg, voriconizole, amphotericin).
- **If pulmonary infiltrate on CXR:** Immediately begin with broad-spectrum therapy (eg, piperacillin/tazobactam, third-/fourth-generation cephalosporin, or carbapenem) and adjust according to culture (similar to neutropenic patients).

HUMAN IMMUNODEFICIENCY VIRUS (HIV) AND ACQUIRED IMMUNODEFICIENCY SYNDROME (AIDS)

AIDS Definition

Any HIV-infected individual with:

- A CD4 count of < 200/µL, regardless of the presence of symptoms or opportunistic diseases.
- An AIDS-defining clinical condition, regardless of CD4 count.

A CD4 count of < 100 requires prophylaxis against toxoplasmosis.

Major AIDS-Defining Conditions

- Candidiasis (pulmonary or esophageal).
- Cervical cancer (invasive).
- *Cryptococcus* (extrapulmonary).
- CMV retinitis with vision loss.
- Encephalopathy, HIV-related.
- Herpes simplex (chronic ulcers, pulmonary, or esophageal).
- Kaposi's sarcoma.
- Lymphoma (Burkitt's or 1° brain).
- *Mycobacterium avium* complex.
- *Mycobacterium tuberculosis.*
- Atypical mycobacteriosis.
- PCP.
- Recurrent pneumonias.
- CNS toxoplasmosis.
- Wasting syndrome due to HIV.

Life Cycle of HIV

Antiretroviral medications work against reverse transcriptase and proteases that cleave the newly formed viral proteins after translation. Newer targets are cell-entry mechanisms and integrase.

- HIV is an **RNA virus** that binds CD4 molecule on a CD4+ human leukocytes.
- HIV RNA internalized into host cell.
- **HIV reverse transcriptase transcribes HIV RNA into dsDNA** (step inhibited by therapy).
- DNA translocates to nucleus and integrates into host genome.
- Translated into long HIV polypeptides.
- **Virally encoded protease** cleaves polypeptides at specific sites to generate functional proteins (step inhibited by therapy).
- New infective virus particle (proteins plus genomic viral RNA) assembles at host cell membrane.
- Budding of new virus particle.

Transmission of HIV

- **Sexual contact:**
  - Worldwide, HIV is predominantly transmitted by heterosexual sex.
  - One-half of U.S. cases are still among homosexual men.
  - Incidence of heterosexual transmission in the United States is increasing, mainly among women and minorities.
  - HIV is present in infective quantities in seminal fluid and vaginal and cervical secretions.
  - Strong association of HIV transmission with receptive anal intercourse.
  - Vaginal intercourse: 20-fold greater chance of transmission from man to a woman than woman to a man.
  - Oral sex: Much less efficient mode of transmission.
  - Genital ulceration ↑ chances of transmission (both infectivity and susceptibility to infection).
  - Lack of circumcision is associated with higher risk of infection.
- **Blood products:**
  - Sharing contaminated injection drug syringes.
  - Transfusion of contaminated blood products.
  - An estimated 10,000 individuals in the United States were infected by contaminated blood products (many hemophilia patients, for example) before spring 1985; currently minimal risk of HIV from transfusions due to sensitive screen procedures.
  - **Occupational transmission:**
    - Transmission risk after skin puncture from blood contaminated sharp object from person with documented HIV infection is 0.3%.
    - Transmission for hepatitis B following similar exposure is 20–30%.
    - The higher the viral load of the infected patient, the greater the chances of transmission.
    - Postexposure prophylaxis and wound cleansing after exposure ↓ rate of HIV seroconversion by 79% (to 0.06% for HIV).
- **HIV-⊕ mothers to infants intrapartum, perinatally, or via breast milk:**
  - HIV can be transmitted from mother to fetus during pregnancy, delivery, or through infected breast milk.
  - Transmission rate from untreated mother to newborn is approximately 25% in the United States.
  - Zidovudine treatment of HIV-infected pregnant women from the beginning of the third trimester through delivery, with treatment of the infant for 6 weeks after birth, ↓ transmission rate to 8%.
  - Breast milk transmission (7–22%) is most important in developing countries where other means of infant nutrition are not readily available.
- **Transmission by other body fluids:** HIV can be identified in almost any body fluid but transmission risk via saliva, sweat, tears, and urine is very small.
- There is **no evidence** that HIV can be transmitted by insects.

Centers for Disease Control and Prevention (CDC) recommendations for HIV post-exposure prophylaxis (ie, a needle stick): Zidovudine, lamivudine, and indinavir for 4 weeks.

AIDS Epidemiology

- **Worldwide:**
  - Approximately 33 million people were living with HIV infection worldwide as of December 2007.
  - Sixty-eight percent live in sub-Saharan African countries.

- **United States:**
  - AIDS was the sixth leading cause of death in Americans aged 25–44 years in 2006.
  - Among new infections diagnosed in 2006, 26% were women, 53% were men who have sex with men. Nearly half were African-American.
  - The overall incidence of AIDS has remained stable since the late 1990s.
  - African-Americans and Hispanic-Americans constitute a disproportionately high number of HIV cases.

HIV Disease Course (Without Therapy)

0–12 Weeks (Acute HIV syndrome; see below)
- Virus enters bloodstream and is cleared by lymphoid organs or spleen.
- Virus replicates to critical level in lymphoid organs (lymphadenopathy).
- Burst of viremia occurs, disseminating virus throughout body.
- Eventually partial immunologic control of virus replication occurs.
- **Acute HIV syndrome:**
  - Approximately 60% experience acute viral syndrome within 3–6 weeks of primary infection.
  - Symptoms (usually last ~ 1 week):
    - **General:** Fever, pharyngitis, lymphadenopathy, headache, lethargy, nausea, vomiting, diarrhea.
    - **Neuro:** Meningitis, encephalitis, peripheral neuropathy.
    - **Dermatologic:** Erythematous maculopapular rash and mucocutaneous ulceration.
  - Ten percent have fulminant course—clinical and immune deterioration immediately after the initial viral syndrome subsides.
  - Ninety percent become asymptomatic (clinically latent phase).

12 Weeks to 8–10 Years
- HIV evades immune system by:
  - Killing off most of the HIV-specific cytotoxic T cells with an overwhelming burst of HIV antigen.
  - Saturating the antigen presenting cells in lymphoid tissue with HIV antigen (these cells would otherwise help create more virus specific cytotoxic T cells).
- Clinical latency is the disease-free state when opportunistic infections do not occur, but continued decline of CD4 T cells occurs due to viral cytotoxicity.
- CD4 counts fall approximately 50 cells/μL/year.

> 10 Years
- CD4 count falls below critical level (usually about 200 cells/μL).
- Patient becomes highly susceptible to opportunistic diseases (see Table 2.5-3).
- CD4 counts may drop to < 10 cells/μL, yet patients can survive for months.
- Patient eventually succumbs to opportunistic infection or neoplasm.

Measures of AIDS progression (2 parameters looked at):
- Status of disease: CD4 count
- Rate of activity/progression: Viral load (measure of HIV RNA)

TABLE 2.5-3. Diseases Associated with CD4 Thresholds in AIDS

CD4 Counts			
350	**200**	**100**	**50**
▪ Pneumococcal pneumonia	▪ Kaposi's sarcoma	▪ Toxoplasmosis	▪ MAC
	▪ Tuberculosis	▪ Disseminated *Candida*	▪ Cytomegalovirus
	▪ Oral thrush	▪ Cryptococcosis	▪ PML
	▪ Oral hairy leukoplakia		
	▪ PCP		
	▪ Lymphoma		

MAC, *Mycobacterium avium* complex; PCP, *Pneumocystis jiroveci* pneumonia; PML, progressive multifocal leukoencephalopathy (JC virus)

Treatment of HIV Infection

GENERAL PATIENT MANAGEMENT

- ▪ Disease necessitates patient education about complications, transmission, and prognosis.
- ▪ All patients with HIV (especially those with CD4 counts < 200) should designate an individual with durable power of attorney.

INITIAL AND FOLLOW-UP STUDIES

- ▪ Routine chemistry, CBC, and CXR.
- ▪ CD4 counts.
- ▪ Two separate HIV RNA levels.
- ▪ VDRL.
- ▪ Anti-*Toxoplasma* Ab titer.
- ▪ Purified protein derivative (PPD) skin test.
- ▪ Mini mental status exam.

Generally you will not be required to know the specific drug names, however you should familiarize yourself with the classes of drugs available and their mechanisms of action.

ANTIRETROVIRAL THERAPY

Major drug classes for HIV therapy are reverse transcriptase inhibitors (nucleoside analogs and non-nucleoside), protease inhibitors, fusion inhibitors, and integrase inhibitors.

- ▪ **Nucleoside analog reverse transcriptase inhibitors (NRTIs):** Act as DNA chain terminator.
  - ▪ **Zidovudine (AZT):**
    - ▪ First drug approved for HIV treatment.
    - ▪ Most appropriately used as part of combination retroviral therapy.
    - ▪ Also used as monotherapy for prevention of maternal-fetal transmission of HIV.
    - ▪ **Side effects:** Headache, malaise, nausea, fatigue (often subside with extended therapy), macrocytic anemia secondary to low erythropoietin (can be managed with recombinant erythropoietin injections), proximal myopathy.

- **Lamivudine (3TC):**
  - Only for use in combination with AZT.
  - Strains of HIV that are resistant to lamivudine are sensitive to zidovudine.
  - **Toxicities: Pancreatitis, peripheral neuropathies.**
- Others include **didanosine, stavudine, abacavir, emtricitabine,** and **tenofovir** (nucleotide analog).
- **Non-nucleoside reverse transcriptase inhibitors (NNRTIs):**
  - **Nevirapine, delavirdine** (rarely used), **efavirenz,** and **etravirine.**
  - Bind to reverse transcriptase outside the active site and cause conformational changes that ↓ enzyme activity.
  - Monotherapy causes rapid resistance.
  - Main toxicity is maculopapular rash.
- **Protease inhibitors:**
  - **Saquinavir, ritonavir, indinavir, nelfinavir, lopinavir, atazanavir** inhibit the activity of HIV protease.
  - Less toxic than the reverse transcriptase inhibitors.
  - Monotherapy results in rapid emergence of drug-resistant strains.
  - Indinavir: Main side effects are nephrolithiasis and asymptomatic indirect hyperbilirubinemia. Potent and well tolerated compared to saquinavir and ritonavir.
  - Ritonavir: Mainly used in low doses to boost other protease inhibitors.
- **Fusion inhibitors:**
  - **Maraviroc** prevents HIV binding and entry into cells by binding CCR5.
  - **Enfuvirtide** prevents HIV virion fusion with cells by binding gp41; available only as injection.
  - Used in combination therapy regimens for patients with drug-resistant virus.
- **Integrase inhibitor:**
  - Single agent approved—raltegravir.
  - Prevents the insertion of viral genome into host DNA (integration).
  - Used in salvage therapy regimens.

TREATMENT RECOMMENDATIONS

- Initiate therapy with two nucleoside reverse transcriptase inhibitors (eg, AZT, 3TC) and a boosted protease inhibitor (eg, indinavir/ritonavir) or a non-nucleoside reverse transcriptase inhibitor (eg, efavirenz) in any one of these conditions:
  - Symptomatic/history of AIDS-defining illness.
  - CD4 count < 200–350.
  - HIV-associated nephropathy.
  - Pregnancy.
  - Co-infection with HBV requiring treatment.
- Recent studies have shown no benefit in treating asymptomatic individuals with CD4 counts > 500. In fact, due to emergence of resistant strains, deferring antiretroviral therapy until necessary is recommended.
- Newer regimens use combination pills which can be taken daily, making patient compliance less of a factor in disease control.

Opportunistic Infections in AIDS and Other Immunocompromised States

PNEUMOCYSTIS JIROVECI PNEUMONIA (PCP)

- Formerly known as *Pneumocystis carinii.*
- PCP is declining, but remains the most common initial AIDS-defining illness in the United States.
- Seen largely in patients who are not aware of their HIV status or are not receiving treatment.
- PCP is most common in those with a previous episode of PCP.

CLINICAL FINDINGS

- Patients often appear nontoxic and have clear lungs but low oxygen saturation.
- Often have dyspnea on exertion and weight loss.
- Spontaneous pneumothorax complicates PCP in 2% of cases.

DIAGNOSIS

- **Definitive:** Bronchoalveolar lavage/or transbronchial biopsy.
- **Other findings:**
  - ↓ oxygen saturation.
  - CXR usually normal or shows faint, bilateral interstitial infiltrate.
  - Lactate dehydrogenase (LDH) is often elevated.

 A 34-year-old patient with unknown HIV status presents with weight loss, dry cough, dyspnea, **hypoxemia,** and vague bilateral infiltrates on chest x-ray. *Think: PCP.* **Next step:** Provide supplemental oxygen and start TMP-SMZ.

TREATMENT

- **TMP-SMZ:**
  - Fifty to sixty percent have side effects including rash, fever, leukopenia, thrombocytopenia, and hepatitis.
  - Twenty-one-day course.
  - Patients get worse before they get better and will not improve until the end of the first week of treatment.
  - May give pentamidine for patients intolerant of TMP-SMZ.
- Glucocorticoids:
  - Initiate in any AIDS patient with PCP if $PaO_2 < 70$ mmHg or a-A gradient > 35 mmHg.
  - Start no later than 36–72 hours after starting TMP-SMZ.
  - Twenty-one-day course (with subsequent taper).
  - ↓ mortality by approximately 50%.
- **Prophylaxis in patients with CD4 < 200 or previous PCP:** Give TMP-SMZ (three times/week instead of daily), or dapsone in sulfa-allergic patients or aerosolized pentamidine for those unable to take systemic prophylaxis (see Table 2.5-4).

 An HIV patient presents with dry cough for 1 week. He denies fever, night sweats, and chills. His WBC is normal. *Likely diagnosis?* Mycoplasma pneumoniae (Lesson: community-acquired pneumonias are still most common, even in AIDS patients.) Always treat for CAP also until any suspected opportunistic organisms are confirmed.

TABLE 2.5-4. Prophylaxis in AIDS

INFECTION	PROPHYLAXIS	INDICATION
Pneumocystis jiroveci pneumonia	Bactrim or dapsone in patients with sulfa allergies	CD4 < 200
Toxoplasmosis	Bactrim or dapsone in patients with sulfa allergies	CD4 < 100
Tuberculosis	Isoniazid	PPD > 5-mm induration (not erythema)
Mycobacterium avium complex	Azithromycin or clarithromycin	CD4 < 100

TOXOPLASMOSIS

- Most common cause of secondary CNS infection in AIDS.
- Seroprevalence in United States is 15%; toxoplasmic encephalitis occurs in one-third of all seropositive AIDS patients without prophylaxis.
- Late complication.

CLINICAL PRESENTATION

- Fever, headache, and focal neurological deficits (90%).
- Seizure, hemiparesis, and aphasia also occur.
- **AIDS patient with meningitis:**
  - Sensation of smell and behavior changes: *Think HSV (temporal lobe involvement).*
  - India ink stain with round organisms: *Think Cryptococcus.*

DIAGNOSIS

- Magnetic resonance imaging (MRI) or head computed tomography (CT) with contrast shows **multiple ring-enhancing lesions** (see Figure 2.5-1).
- IgG antibodies to *Toxoplasma.*

TREATMENT

- Pyrimethamine and sulfadiazine: Leukopenia is the major side effect (treat leukopenia with folinic acid).
- Lifelong treatment for toxoplasmosis is necessary, due to relapse rate of 50% within 6 months.
- TMP-SMZ given for PCP prophylaxis is also effective as prophylaxis against toxoplasmic encephalitis. Patients with CD4 count < 100 should receive prophylaxis against *Toxoplasma.*
- **AIDS patient with brain lesion:**
  - Ring-enhancing lesion with mass effect: Toxo
  - Periventricular ring: CMV
  - Other: CNS lymphoma (associated with EBV)

PROTOZOAL DIARRHEA IN AIDS

ETIOLOGY

Cryptosporidia, microsporidia, and *Isospora belli* are the most common bugs.

FIGURE 2.5-1. **Toxoplasmosis in an AIDS patient.**

Note ring-enhancing lesions. (Reproduced, with permission, from Lee SH, Rao K, Zimmerman RA [eds]. *Cranial MRI and CT.* New York: McGraw-Hill, 1999: 505.)

TREATMENT

- Cryptosporidia and microsporidia: Paromomycin or erythromycin.
- *Isospora:* TMP-SMZ.

A 32-year-old HIV-⊕ patient with a low CD4 count presents with 3 months of watery diarrhea. *Think: Cryptosporidiosis.* **Next step:** Check stool for ova and parasites (O&P). Effective antiretroviral treatment is best therapy + Nitazoxanide.

> **AIDS patient with diarrhea:**
> - Cryptosporidia (round)
> - *Isospora* (oral)
> - Microsporidia

MYCOBACTERIUM AVIUM COMPLEX (MAC)

EPIDEMIOLOGY

- Disseminated *Mycobacterium avium* is a marker of advanced immune suppression; it typically occurs when CD4 count is < 50.
- Median survival after MAC diagnosis is 6–8 months.

SYMPTOMS

- Fever
- Cough
- Weight loss
- Night sweats
- Lymphadenopathy
- Abdominal pain
- Diarrhea

A 29-year-old HIV-⊕ patient presents with CD4 count of 100, unexplained fever, and elevated alkaline phosphatase. *Think: MAC.*

DIAGNOSIS

- Long, slender, acid-fast bacilli (AFB) seen in biopsy specimens or sputum.
- **Other findings:**
  - Eighty-five percent of MAC patients have mycobacteremia.
  - Alkaline phosphatase level often elevated.
  - CXR: 25% have bilateral lower lobe interstitial infiltrate.
  - Blood culture confirms diagnosis (turns ⊕ within 2 weeks).

TREATMENT

- Clarithromycin and ethambutol.
- Prophylaxis: Azithromycin or clarithromycin when CD4 drops below 50.

TUBERCULOSIS

See Pulmonary chapter for full discussion.

EPIDEMIOLOGY

- Estimated to be the cause of death in 13% of AIDS patients worldwide.
- HIV ↑ risk of developing active TB by 15–30 times.
- HIV disease progresses more rapidly in patients with active TB.

An AIDS patient being treated for TB has clinical worsening of his TB following initiation of highly active antiretroviral therapy (HAART). *Think: Immune reconstitution inflammatory syndrome (IRIS).* **Next step:** Supportive care.

FUNGAL INFECTIONS

- **Candidiasis:**
  - *Candida* infections are the most common fungal infections in HIV-⊕ patients, and virtually all patients experience some form of *Candida* infection during their illness.
  - Infections occur early: They are often the first sign of immunosuppression.
- **Thrush:**
  - Very early finding in immunocompromise.
  - White, cheesy exudates on posterior oropharynx.
  - Pseudohyphae detectable on wet-mount KOH preps.
- **AIDS-defining *Candida* infections:**
  - *Candida* infections of lungs, esophagus, trachea, and bronchi.
  - **Esophagitis** is most common; presents with retrosternal pain and odynophagia and diagnosed with upper GI endoscopy.

TREATMENT

- Oral and vaginal candida: Oral fluconazole; topical nystatin or clotrimazole troches are also effective.
- Severe cases including esophageal candidiasis must be treated with systemic therapy (oral itraconazole or oral/IV fluconazole).

CRYPTOCOCCOSIS

- *Cryptococcus neoformans* is the leading cause of **meningitis** in AIDS patients.
- Highest risk when CD4 count is < 50.
- Serious, life-threatening infection.

SIGNS AND SYMPTOMS

- **Subacute meningoencephalitis.**
- Fever (virtually all patients).
- Nausea and vomiting (40%).
- Altered mental status.
- Headache.
- Meningeal signs.

DIAGNOSIS

- Cryptococcomas.
- Variety of findings on **CT or MRI:** Can be normal or show atrophy, mass lesions, hydrocephalus, or ring-enhancing or cystic lesions.
- **Serology:** CSF or serum cryptococcal antigen or ⊕ culture from any site.
- **India ink stain of CSF** shows organism.

TREATMENT

- Amphotericin B for 6 weeks in combination with flucytosine for CSF disease.
- Since 50% of patients relapse after therapy is stopped, fluconazole should be given indefinitely.

ASPERGILLUS FUMIGATUS

- **Fungus ball (aspergilloma)** in preexisting lung cavity.
- Mold with septated hyphae.
- Acquired through inhalation of spores in soil and decay.
- Immunocompetent individuals can get an allergic hypersensitivity reaction; not invasive (wheezing); treat with steroids.
- **Invasive aspergillosis** is seen in immunocompromised patients and can present as rapidly progressive necrotizing pulmonary infiltrates, tracheobronchitis. Can cause **life-threatening hemoptysis.**
- Lung biopsy is needed for definitive diagnosis.
- Extrapulmonary sites: Sinusitis, CNS, skin, osteomyelitis.
- Treat with amphotericin B; some patients may benefit from surgery (removing the fungus ball). Voriconazole is usual drug of choice but interacts with antiretroviral drugs.

Fluconazole prophylaxis can be given to all AIDS patients once CD4 < 100/ μL to prevent both cryptococcosis and candidal infections.

Invasive aspergillosis: Infection in immunocompromised people sometimes causing a fungus ball.

Allergic aspergillosis: A hypersensitivity reaction in immunocompetent people, causing severe obstructive lung disease, wheezing, bronchiectasis. Treat with steroids. Not an infection!

Viral Infections and AIDS/Immunocompromise

CYTOMEGALOVIRUS (CMV)

- Ninety-five percent of HIV-⊕ patients are CMV ⊕, and clinical syndromes most often represent reactivation of latent infection (see Figure 2.5-2).
- **CMV retinitis** is a dreaded HIV complications; presents with painless, progressive vision loss; may complain of "floaters."
- CMV can also cause many other systemic infections (pneumonia, hepatitis, colitis).

DIAGNOSIS

Retinitis: Fundoscopy shows perivascular hemorrhage and exudates; diagnose any systemic CMV reactivation by testing blood for CMV viral copies by PCR.

CLINICAL COURSE

Vision loss is irreversible; may be complicated by retinal detachment. Many other manifestations may reverse with therapy.

FIGURE 2.5-2.   Cytomegalovirus infection in an AIDS patient.

Note diffuse periventricular enhancement. (Reproduced, with permission, from Lee SH, Rao K, Zimmerman RA [eds]. *Cranial MRI and CT.* New York: McGraw-Hill, 1999.)

TREATMENT

- Ganciclovir (ocular implants can be used) or foscarnet.
- Recurrence is common; maintenance therapy with foscarnet.
- CMV Ab–⊖ patients should receive blood products from CMV-⊖ donors if at all possible.

Ganciclovir causes bone marrow suppression and cannot be given with TMP-SMZ or AZT.

HERPES SIMPLEX VIRUS (HSV)

- HSV in HIV manifests as recurrent orolabial, genital, and perianal lesions.
- Can cause herpetic esophagitis (beefy red and painful esophagus).
- Can cause recurrent **herpetic whitlow** (painful nodular lesions usually found on fingers).
- Treat with acyclovir, famciclovir, or valacyclovir.

 An HIV-⊕ patient presents with a painful, poorly healing, perirectal lesion. *Think: HSV.*

VARICELLA-ZOSTER VIRUS (VZV) AND HIV

- **Shingles:** The reactivation of chickenpox (or varicella-zoster) can happen in any person but is very common in AIDS patients.
  - Reactivation of latent infection.
  - Usually an early complication of HIV.
  - Painful, vesicular skin eruptions.
  - Can have extensive involvement of several dermatomes, but also may just follow one dermatome, which would classically be seen wrapping around the flank but not crossing midline.
  - Treatment with acyclovir may shorten course of disease.
- **Primary VZV infection** (chickenpox) may be *lethal* in the HIV patient. Treat aggressively with acyclovir and hyperimmune globulin.
- **Acute retinal necrosis syndrome:**
  - From zoster in the eye/orbital area (trigeminal nerve varicella-zoster or orolabial HSV).
  - Presents with pain, keratitis, and iritis.
  - Fundus exam shows widespread pale gray peripheral lesions.
  - Often complicated by retinal detachment.

Pain from zoster may precede the rash by a couple of days. Watch for zoster in any patient presenting with pain in a dermatomal distribution!

HEPATITIS

- Ninety-five percent of HIV-⊕ patients have serologic evidence of HBV or HCV infection.
- Patients with HBV and HIV have less severe inflammatory liver disease because of immunosuppression.

Shingles in any patient under 50 years of age mandates workup for underlying immunodeficiency.

INFECTIOUS DISEASE

Neoplastic Disease and HIV

Due to the immunosuppression, and particularly the absence of functional T cells (cellular immunity), which help find and kill abnormal cells, HIV patients are at high risk for developing neoplasms.

KAPOSI'S SARCOMA

EPIDEMIOLOGY

- Incidence has been ↓ since first recognized as an HIV-associated neoplasm.
- Mostly in homosexual men.
- Associated with human herpes virus type 8 (HHV-8).

CLINICAL FINDINGS

- Multiple vascular nodules appearing in the skin, mucous membranes, and viscera.
- Appearance is purplish macular or papular nodule on skin, or discoloration of the oral mucosa.
- Lesions often occur in sun-exposed areas.
- Pulmonary involvement can occur; presents as shortness of breath.
- May be seen with a normal CD4 count.

DIAGNOSIS

Biopsy of suspicious lesion.

TREATMENT

- Indicated when a single or multiple lesions are symptoms.
- Always give HAART.
- Can use topical all-trans retinoin or local radiation.
- Occasionally can use systemic chemotherapy.

LYMPHOMAS

EPIDEMIOLOGY

- Six percent of patients develop lymphoma at some point during their disease.
- Incidence is ↑ 120-fold in HIV compared with general population.
- **Three main types occur in HIV:**
  - Grade III or IV immunoblastic (60%).
  - Burkitt's lymphoma (20%).
  - Primary CNS lymphoma (20%).

CLINICAL PRESENTATION

- Dependent on the site of tumor.
- Persistent unexplained fever.
- Focal seizures if in CNS.
- Rapidly growing mass lesion in the oral mucosa.
- Eighty percent have extranodal disease.

TREATMENT

HAART + systemic chemotherapy.

HIV-associated malignancies:
- HHV-6,8: Kaposi's sarcoma
- HPV: Cervical cancer
- HBV: Hepatocellular cancer

- The following are agents with high potential for use in bioterrorism. The inhalational type is expected to be the most common form used in bioterrorism, due to ease of inoculation.
- Suspected or confirmed cases should be reported to local or state departments of health.
- Antibiotics are initially given parenterally and then switched to oral once patient improves clinically.
- In mass-casualty situations, parenteral therapy may not be possible; in this situation, oral antibiotics are administered.
- Antibiotics for treating patients infected in connection with a bioterrorist event are included in the national pharmaceutical stockpile maintained by the Centers for Disease Control and Prevention (CDC), as are ventilators and other emergency equipment.
- This information is compiled from the **CDC** Web site, where the latest surveillance information is available: *http://www.cdc.gov.*

Anthrax

INCUBATION PERIOD

Usually < 1 week.

TRANSMISSION

- **Skin:** Direct skin contact with spores; in nature, contact with infected animals or animal products (usually related to occupational exposure).
- **Respiratory tract:** Inhalation of aerosolized spores.
- **GI:** Consumption of undercooked or raw meat products or dairy products from infected animals.
- No person-to-person transmission of anthrax.

SIGNS AND SYMPTOMS OF INHALATIONAL ANTHRAX

- Initial phase consists of nonspecific symptoms such as low-grade fever, nonproductive cough, malaise, fatigue, myalgias, profound sweats, and chest discomfort.
- Upper respiratory tract symptoms are rare.
- Physical exam may reveal rhonchi, otherwise normal.
- One to five days after onset of initial symptoms, onset of high fever and severe respiratory distress (dyspnea, stridor, cyanosis) occur. Shock and death occur within 24–36 hours. An interim period of a few days of wellness can occur between the two stages, or they may occur in rapid succession.
- Hemorrhagic meningitis can also be seen.

DIAGNOSIS

- Gram-⊕ bacilli on unspun peripheral blood smear or CSF.
- **CXR** demonstrates **widened mediastinum with clear lung fields.**
- Aerobic blood culture growth of large, gram-⊕ bacilli provides preliminary identification of *Bacillus* species.

- Nasal swab for PCR available for epidemiological surveillance; not approved to make individual patient decisions.
- A blood test that detects antibodies to a component of the toxin of *Bacillus anthracis* is available, yielding results in 1 hour.

A group of previously healthy young people develop an acute respiratory illness. CXRs demonstrate a widened mediastinum with clear lung fields. *Think: Anthrax; keep bioterrorism in mind.*

TREATMENT

- Initiate antimicrobial therapy immediately upon suspicion with ciprofloxacin, doxycycline, and amoxicillin.
- Supportive care including controlling pleural effusions.
- Contact precautions.
- Vaccine available for military personnel and lab workers who handle organism directly.

Botulism

See the Neurology chapter.

Pneumonic Plague

- There are three types of plague: pneumonic, bubonic, and septicemic.
- The most common form is bubonic, which is not transmitted person to person.

ETIOLOGY

Yersinia pestis. Indications that plague had been artificially disseminated would be the occurrence of cases in locations not known to have enzootic infection, in persons without known risk factors, and in the absence of prior rodent deaths.

INCUBATION PERIOD

Two to four days.

TRANSMISSION

Via inhalation of respiratory droplets.

SIGNS AND SYMPTOMS

- Fever, headache, weakness.
- Rapidly developing pneumonia with shortness of breath, chest pain, cough, and sometimes bloody or watery sputum.
- Pneumonia progresses for 2–4 days and causes respiratory failure and shock.

A previously healthy 29-year-old banker living in a big city contracts a severe pneumonia characterized by the rapid development of respiratory failure, shock, bleeding, and other signs of the systemic inflammatory response syndrome. Sputum reveals gram-⊖ bacilli with bipolar staining. *Think:* Yersinia pestis.

DIAGNOSIS

- Gram stain of sputum or blood may reveal gram-⊖ bacilli or coccobacilli.
- Wright, Giemsa, Wayson stain will often show bipolar staining.
- Antigen detection, IgM enzyme immunoassay, immunostaining, and PCR.

TREATMENT

- Start streptomycin within 24 hours of start of symptoms.
- Other effective agents include gentamicin, tetracycline, doxycycline, and chloramphenicol.
- Isolation of patients using respiratory droplet precautions, but then are no longer contagious after 48 hours of antibiotic treatment.

A laboratory confirmation of *Y. pestis* is made on autopsy of a healthy 40-year-old living in a big city. There was no history of handling an animal carcass or any travel to an endemic area. *Think: This could be a sentinel event for a bioterrorist attack. Be on the lookout for cases of severe acute respiratory illness in others very shortly.*

PREVENTION

- Postexposure prophylaxis for people who have had direct, close contact with infected patients (7-day course).
- A plague vaccine is not currently available for use in the United States.

Smallpox

INCUBATION PERIOD

Seven to seventeen days.

TRANSMISSION

- Face-to-face contact is required.
- Can be spread through direct contact with infected bodily fluids or contaminated objects.
- Humans are the only natural hosts of variola.

SIGNS AND SYMPTOMS

- Prodrome: 2–4 days:
  - High fever, malaise, head and body aches, and sometimes vomiting.
  - Patients are acutely ill, in contrast to varicella infection.

The rash of smallpox consists of lesions that are all at the *same stage of development.* In contrast, the lesions of varicella are at all different stages.

- Rash:
  - First, small red spots on the tongue and in the mouth that become sores that break open and spread large amounts of the virus into the mouth and throat; person becomes most contagious at that time.
  - Next, rash appears on the skin, starting on the face and spreading to the arms and legs (**centrifugal**) and then to the palms and soles. Usually, the rash spreads to all parts of the body within 24 hours. Patient may start to feel better during rash appearing.
  - On the third day, the rash becomes raised bumps.
  - By the fourth day, bumps fill with a thick fluid and often pustules (characteristic feature of smallpox). Eventually scab, which fall off and form pitted scars.

DIAGNOSIS

Made by PCR or enzyme-linked immunosorbent assay (ELISA) of throat swab, or culture of fluid from pustules or CSF.

TREATMENT

- Patients are quarantined for 17 days or until scabs fall off.
- Treatment consists of fluid replacement and antibiotics for any 2° bacterial infections.
- No treatment against the virus itself.

PREVENTION

Smallpox vaccine contains live *vaccinia* virus, a weaker relative of the *variola* virus that causes smallpox. Some military and first responders vaccinated.

Tularemia

ETIOLOGY AND TRANSMISSION

- Bacterial zoonosis caused by *Francisella tularensis* (small nonmotile, aerobic, non-spore-forming, gram-$\ominus$ coccobacillus).
- Found in water, moist soil, hay, straw, and decaying animal carcasses.
- Very infectious.
- Mostly in south-central and western United States in summer.
- Humans infected through bite of an exposed tick, fly, or mosquito, or by direct contact with infectious animal (often carcasses) or environment (soil, water, food).
- No person-to-person transmission (no need for patient isolation).
- Rodents are reservoir.

Adverse effects of tetracyclines:
- Photosensitivity
- ↑ preexisting prerenal azotemia
- Brown/yellow deposits in teeth and brittle bones (children)

INCUBATION

Symptoms usually appear at 3–5 days, but may be as long as 14 days.

SIGNS AND SYMPTOMS

- Sudden onset of high fever, chills, diarrhea, headache, myalgia, cough.
- If inhaled, hemorrhagic inflammation, pneumonia, and pneumonitis.
- Airborne *F. tularensis* can also cause ocular involvement, ulcers in broken skin, and oropharyngeal disease.

DIAGNOSIS

Gram stain, direct fluorescent antibody, or immunohistochemical stains of respiratory secretions and blood.

TREATMENT

- **Streptomycin** is drug of choice.
- Gentamicin, tetracyclines, and chloramphenicol are also effective.

Lyme Disease

ETIOLOGY

- *Borrelia burgdorferi:* Microaerophilic spirochete.
- Transmitted by *Ixodes scapularis* tick.
- Found in the northeastern United States, in wooded areas.
- **Erythema chronicum migrans** is the pathognomonic skin rash that starts at bite and progresses until there is central clearing.

SIGNS AND SYMPTOMS

- **Initial stage:** Fevers, headaches, arthralgias, and myalgias.
- **Second stage** (weeks to months): Recurring rash, myocarditis with first-, second-, or third-degree heart block; meningitis; cranial nerve palsy; peripheral neuropathy.
- **Third stage:** Migratory or oligoarthritis.

DIAGNOSIS

- ELISA followed by Western blot. If clinical suspicion is high, then treat the patient before serologies come back.
- Treat with doxycycline or amoxicillin if there is no cardiac involvement.
- Treat with penicillin or cephalosporin if there is any cardiac or neurologic involvement.

 A 42-year-old woman who recently camped in the woods of Vermont presents to the ER with one-sided facial droop. *Think: Lyme disease (often presents with Bell's palsy).* **Next step:** Check Lyme serologies and EKG to rule out cardiac involvement.

Ehrlichiosis

Two types: Human monocytic ehrlichiosis (HME) and human granulocytic ehrlichiosis (HGE).

ETIOLOGY

- *Ehrlichia chaffeensis,* intracellular bacteria causing HME.
- *Ehrlichia phagocytophila,* intracellular bacteria causing HGE.

TRANSMISSION

- HME caused by the bite of the *lone star tick.*
- HGE caused by the bite of *Ixodes* tick.

SIGNS AND SYMPTOMS

Nonspecific flulike symptoms, high fever, headache, malaise, **leukopenia and thrombocytopenia** are most common presentations.

DIAGNOSIS

- Serum PCR.
- HME in southern United States and HGE in northern United States.

TREATMENT

Tetracycline or doxycycline.

Rocky Mountain Spotted Fever

ETIOLOGY

Rickettsia rickettsii, gram-⊖ coccobacillus, found in the southeastern United States.

TRANSMISSION

Bite of the wood tick *Dermacentor andersoni* or dog tick *Dermacentor variabilis*.

SIGNS AND SYMPTOMS

- Patients initially present with fever, nausea, severe headache, vomiting, and history of recent tick bite.
- After 3–4 days of symptoms, rash starts as a nonpruritic, maculopapular rash on the distal extremities starting on the wrists and ankles then involving the palms and soles, then progresses centrally to the trunk and face.
- Can be fatal if not treated aggressively.
- Disseminated intravascular coagulation (DIC) and pneumonia are serious complications of infection.

DIAGNOSIS

Indirect immunofluorescence assay or latex agglutination.

TREATMENT

Tetracyclines are the drug of choice.

Babesiosis

ETIOLOGY

Babesia microti, an intra-RBC parasite (like malaria) transmitted by the *Ixodes* tick in the Northeast and Midwest United States.

PRESENTATION

Fever, chills, myalgias, **hemolytic anemia.**

DIAGNOSIS

Thick and thin smears of whole blood reveal ring-shaped trophozoites and the characteristic cross-shaped tetrad of merozoites known as the **Maltese cross** within red blood cells.

TREATMENT

Quinine and clindamycin.

Tularemia

ETIOLOGY

Francisella tularensis, transmitted by tick or flea bites in Arkansas and Oklahoma.

TREATMENT

- Gentamicin or tetracycline.
- See tularemia discussion above.

EPIDURAL ABSCESS

- **Neurosurgical emergency!**
- **If suspected, get emergent MRI.**
- Spinal abscesses are most commonly found in the immunosuppressed, IV drug users, and the elderly.
- An abscess can form anywhere along the spinal cord and as it expands, it compresses against the spinal cord and occludes the vasculature.

ETIOLOGY

- The infection is generally spread from the skin or other tissue.
- *Staphylococcus aureus*, gram-⊖ bacilli, and *Mycobacterium tuberculosis* are most common causes.

SIGNS AND SYMPTOMS

Presents with a triad of pain, fever, and progressive weakness of legs (focal neuromuscular weakness). Can progress over a week.

DIAGNOSIS AND TREATMENT

- Magnetic resonance imaging (MRI) can localize the lesion.
- Lumbar puncture (LP) is not required unless meningitis is suspected.
- Emergent surgery + antibiotics is the definitive treatment, and must be initiated early.

 An IV drug user presents with fever of one week's duration and new-onset lower extremity weakness. *Think: Epidural abscess.* **Next step:** Order emergent MRI of spine, start empiric broad-spectrum antibiotics if ⊕.

PATHOPHYSIOLOGY

- **Vector:** *Anopheles* mosquito. Bites human to introduce sporozoites.
- Merozoites are then released from infected liver cells to infect RBCs.

EPIDEMIOLOGY

Three hundred million to five hundred million malaria cases, with three million deaths, occur annually worldwide.

- ***Plasmodium falciparum*** causes most deaths, endemic in Africa.
- ***Plasmodium vivax*** is endemic in India and central America.

SIGNS AND SYMPTOMS

- The organisms grow in the liver, then spread to the blood to reproduce in RBCs.
- When the RBC is full, it bursts, releasing the organism and exposing it to the host immune system; red cells burst at the same time, causing the characteristic intermittent fever.
- *P. falciparum* causes more severe disease because it infects erythrocytes of all ages. It can cause a microvascular blockade that → local anoxia affecting the brain (delirium, seizures), kidneys, lungs (pulmonary edema, acute respiratory distress syndrome [ARDS]), intestines (nausea, vomiting, diarrhea, abdominal pain), liver, and blood.
- *P. vivax* infects mostly younger erythrocytes.
- *P. vivax* and *P. ovale* cause persistent infection in the liver.
- Symptoms of fever and chills occur about 1–4 weeks after infection.
- Other symptoms include headache, ↑ sweating, back pain, myalgias, diarrhea, nausea, vomiting, and cough.
- Anemia, thrombocytopenia, and elevated liver enzymes may be present.

DIAGNOSIS

Thick and thin blood smears **show parasites in RBCs.**

TREATMENT

- Chloroquine for *P. falciparum* acquired in chloroquine-sensitive regions.
- Atovaquone when resistance is not known.
- If chloroquine resistant, use mefloquine or pyrimethamine/sulfadoxine.
- Quinidine for critically ill patients.
- Contact the CDC.

PREVENTION

- Prophylactic chloroquine or mefloquine for travelers to endemic areas.
- Check CDC recommendations.
- DEET-containing insect repellent and avoid mosquitos.

Patients from endemic areas with **fever that follows a cyclical pattern every 48 or 72 hours** should be considered for malaria.

(See Table 2.5-5.)

TABLE 2.5-5. Common Antibiotic Classes

ANTIMICROBIAL	MECHANISM OF ACTION	ANTIMICROBIAL SPECTRUM	SIDE EFFECTS	COMMON CLINICAL USE
Class: Beta Lactams	Inhibition of bacterial cell wall synthesis by inhibiting enzyme transpeptidases by binding to penicillin-binding proteins.			
Penicillins				
Penicillins (natural): ▪ PCN VK ▪ PCN G ▪ PCN benzathine		▪ **Gram ⊕:** *Listeria*, *Streptococcus* species, *Bacillus anthracis*. ▪ ***Treponema pallidum* (syphilis),** meningococci, dental infections.	Anaphylaxis, rash, pruritus, diarrhea.	**Syphilis.**
Aminopenicillins: ▪ Amoxicillin (PO) and (amoxicillin + clavulanic acid) ▪ Ampicillin (IV) and (ampicillin + sulbactam)		▪ Added gram-⊖ coverage *(H influenzae, E coli, Proteus, Salmonella)* and *Enterococcus faecalis* when compared to natural penicillins. ▪ Clavulanic acid and sulbactam add anaerobic coverage and some gram-⊖.	GI side effects.	Ampicillin is added in patients > 60 or immunocompromised in meningitis to cover *Listeria*.
Antistaphylococcal: ▪ Oxacillin (IV) ▪ Dicloxacillin (PO) ▪ Nafcillin (IV)		Added activity against beta-lactamase/ penicillinase producing *S aureus (but does not cover MRSA)*.	Interstitial nephritis.	▪ Oxacillin and nafcillin are first line for non-MRSA cellulitis if IV agent is required. ▪ Dicloxacillin (or cephalexin) is first-line oral agent for cellulitis.

INFECTIOUS DISEASE

TABLE 2.5-5. **Common Antibiotic Classes** *(continued)*

ANTIMICROBIAL	MECHANISM OF ACTION	ANTIMICROBIAL SPECTRUM	SIDE EFFECTS	COMMON CLINICAL USE
Antipseudomonal: ■ Piperacillin (piperacillin/ tazobactam) ■ Ticarcillin (ticarcillin / clavulanic acid)		Covers *Pseudomonas aeruginosa* and anaerobes (when in combination with beta-lactamase inhibitor like tazobactam and clavulanic acid).		Commonly used in hospital for broad pneumonia (particularly aspiration pneumonia) or gut coverage, including *Pseudomonas* and anaerobes. Also good for resistant bugs in UTIs.
Cephalosporins		Gram-⊖ coverage ↑ with increasing generations.		About 10% cross-reactivity with penicillin (less with higher generations).
First generation: ■ Cefazolin (IV) ■ Cephalexin, cefadroxil (PO)		MSSA and *Streptococcus,* plus some gram-⊖ (eg, *E. coli*).	■ Rash, hypersensitivity reaction. ■ GI upset.	Cephalexin is first-line oral agent for simple cellulitis.
Second generation: ■ Cefuroxime, cefoxitin, cefotetan (IV) ■ Cefaclor, cefprozil, cefuroxime axetil (PO)		■ *E coli, Klebsiella, Proteus, Haemophilus influenzae, Moraxella catarrhalis* ■ Cefotetan and cefoxitin cover some anaerobes also.		
Third generation: ■ Cefotaxime, ceftriaxone, ceftazidime (IV) ■ Ceftbuten, cefpodoxime, cefotaxime, cefdinir (PO)		■ Second-generation coverage plus: Enterobacteriaceae, *Serratia, Neisseria gonorrhoeae.* ■ Used for pneumonias and gonorrhea.		**Ceftriaxone:** (1) combined with azithromycin = first line for community-acquired pneumonia; (2) empiric treatment for meningitis (covers *Streptococcus pneumoniae + Neisseria*); (3) pyelonephritis.

INFECTIOUS DISEASE

TABLE 2.5-5. Common Antibiotic Classes (continued)

ANTIMICROBIAL	MECHANISM OF ACTION	ANTIMICROBIAL SPECTRUM	SIDE EFFECTS	COMMON CLINICAL USE
Fourth generation: Cefepime		▪ Ceftazidime, cefepime, have activity against *Pseudomonas aeruginosa*. ▪ Cefepime has MSSA and streptococcal coverage.		Cefipime is first line in neutropenic fever (with or without vancomycin).
Carbepenems			Cross-reactivity in penicillin allergic patients ~ 10%.	
▪ **D**oripenem ▪ **I**mipenem ▪ **M**eropenem ▪ **E**rtapenem		▪ **Very** broad coverage: gram ⊕ (but not MRSA), gram ⊖, and anaerobes (but ertapenem does not cover *Acinetobacter, Pseudomonas aeruginosa*). ▪ Cilastatitin is given with imipenem as it prevents its hydrolysis in the renal tubules, and maintains the drug for longer.	Lowers seizure threshold.	▪ Imipenem is used for very broad coverage for hospital infections/neutropenic fevers/immuno-compromised patients. ▪ Ertapenem very good for gut coverage.
Monobactam				
▪ Aztreonam	Same as other beta-lactams.	▪ Covers only aerobic gram-⊖. ▪ Effective in chromosomal produced beta-lactamases, but not ESBL gram ⊖.		▪ Safe in penicillin-allergic patients. ▪ Vancomycin + aztreonam is a common in-hospital regimen for gram-⊕ and -⊖ coverage in penicillin-allergic patients).

INFECTIOUS DISEASE

TABLE 2.5-5. **Common Antibiotic Classes** *(continued)*

ANTIMICROBIAL	MECHANISM OF ACTION	ANTIMICROBIAL SPECTRUM	SIDE EFFECTS	COMMON CLINICAL USE
Class: Fluoroquinolones				Gram-⊕ coverage ↑ with increasing generations (whereas cephalosporin generations ↑ gram-⊖ coverage).
First generation: Nalidixic acid **Second generation:** ▪ Ofloxacin ▪ Ciprofloxacin	Inhibit bacterial DNA synthesis by inhibiting DNA gyrase/ topoisomerase IV.	▪ *E coli, Salmonella, Shigella, Enterobacter, Campylobacter,* and *Neisseria.* ▪ Intracellular organisms such as *Chlamydia, Mycoplasma, Legionella, Brucella.*	▪ Tendonitis/tendon rupture. ▪ QTc prolongation. ▪ May damage growing cartilage and cause an arthropathy; not used in children.	▪ Ciprofloxacin's excellent gram-⊖ coverage good for UTIs, gut infections, infectious diarrhea. ▪ Moxifloxacin/ levofloxacin good for pneumonias (gram ⊕ and ⊖ and atypicals).
Third generation (respiratory): ▪ Levofloxacin ▪ Trovafloxacin **Fourth generation (respiratory):** ▪ Moxifloxacin ▪ Gemfloxacin		A respiratory quinolone covers the bugs listed above, plus more gram-⊕ coverage including penicillin-resistant *S. pneumoniae* and *S aureus.*		
Class: Aminoglycosides				
▪ **T**obramycin ▪ **A**mikacin ▪ **G**entamicin	Prevents bacterial protein synthesis by binding to the 30S ribosomal subunit.	▪ Aerobic gram-⊖ bacteria. ▪ Synergistic activity with beta-lactams, especially for endocarditis caused by streptococci, staphylococci, and enterococci.	▪ Nephrotoxicity, ototoxicity. ▪ Avoid in patients with myasthenia gravis (causes neuromuscular blockade).	▪ Often combined with cefipime for double coverage against *Pseudomonas* in neutropenic patients. ▪ Combined with beta-lactam for synergy in endocarditis.

TABLE 2.5-5. **Common Antibiotic Classes** *(continued)*

ANTIMICROBIAL	MECHANISM OF ACTION	ANTIMICROBIAL SPECTRUM	SIDE EFFECTS	COMMON CLINICAL USE
Class: Macrolides			Erythromycin and clarithromycin inhibit CYP3A4 enzymes.	
▪ Erythromycin ▪ Clarithromycin ▪ Azithromycin	Inhibits bacterial protein synthesis by binding reversibly to 50S ribosomal subunits.	▪ **Erythromycin:** Some gram ⊕ (including pneumococci, group *A streptococci,* some *Staphylococcus aureus*) and some gram ⊖ and treponemes, mycoplasmas, *Chlamydia,* and rickettsiae. ▪ **Clarithromycin:** More potent against streptococci and staphylococci + atypicals + *Helicobacter pylori.* ▪ **Azithromycin:** Good for atypical bugs (especially atypical pneumonias), plus some gram ⊕, some gram ⊖, and chlamydia and gonorrhea.	▪ **Erythromycin:** GI upset, cholestatic hepatitis. ▪ **Azithromycin:** GI upset (less common than erythromycin), LFT abnormalities. ▪ **Clarithromycin:** Metallic taste.	▪ Azithromycin is front line in uncomplicated community acquired pneumonias. ▪ For complicated pneumonias, combined with ceftriaxone.
Class: Tetracyclines ▪ Minocycline ▪ Doxycycline ▪ Tetracycline ▪ Demeclocycline	Blocks protein synthesis by binding to 30S ribosomes.	▪ More active against gram-⊕ than gram ⊖. ▪ Some microorganisms, such as *Rickettsia* and *Chlamydia.* ▪ Some atypical mycobacteria.	▪ Photosensitvity. ▪ Gray/yellow discoloration of teeth. ▪ Pseudotumor cerebri.	▪ Can be used for community-acquired MRSA infection. ▪ Treatment for chlamydia and gonorrhea and *Rickettsia* (Rocky Mountain spotted fever).

INFECTIOUS DISEASE

TABLE 2.5-5. **Common Antibiotic Classes** *(continued)*

INFECTIOUS DISEASE

ANTIMICROBIAL	MECHANISM OF ACTION	ANTIMICROBIAL SPECTRUM	SIDE EFFECTS	COMMON CLINICAL USE
Miscellaneous				
■ Vancomycin (a glycopeptide)	Inhibits bacterial cell wall synthesis by inhibiting elongation of peptidoglycan and cross-linking.	■ Covers only gram ⊕ including MSSA (second line), MRSA, but not some enterococci (VRE). ■ Used orally for treatment of *Clostridium difficile.*	■ **Red man syndrome:** Histamine-related reaction; avoid by giving slowly. ■ Nephrotoxicity.	MRSA.
■ Polymyxin B	Penetrates into and disrupts phospholipids in cell membranes.	Good for gram-⊖ aerobic bacilli except *Proteus, Serratia,* and *Providencia* species.	■ Nephrotoxicity, neurotoxicity. ■ Neuromuscular blockade. ■ Paresthesias around the lips, tongue, and extremities; peripheral neuropathy.	
■ Linezolid	Inhibits bacterial protein synthesis by binding to 23S ribosomal RNA of the 50S subunit.	■ Bacteriostatic against *Staphylococcus* and *Enterococcus* species. ■ Bactericidal against *Streptococcus* species.	■ Myelosuppression. ■ Linezolid is an MAOI and therefore can cause serotonin sydrome when used with SSRIs or TCAs.	■ Used primarily for VRE and MRSA infections.
■ Daptomycin	Binds to bacterial membranes resulting in depolarization, loss of membrane potential, and cell death.	Gram-⊕ coverage: *Staphylococcus, Streptococcus,* and *Enterococcus.*	■ Myopathy and rhabdomyalysis. ■ Produces false elevations in PT/INR. ■ Not for lung infections as it is denatured by pulmonary surfactant.	Covers MRSA and VRE.

ESBL: extended-spectrum beta-lactamase; INR: International Normalized Ratio; LFT: liver function test; MAOI: monoamine oxidase inhibitor; MRSA: methicillin-resistant *Staphylococcus aureus;* MSSA: methicillin-sensitive *S aureus;* PT: prothrombin time; SSRI: selective serotonin reuptake inhibitor; TCA: tricyclic antidepressant; UTI: urinary tract infection; VRE: vancomycin-resistant *Enterococcus.*

Nephrology and Acid-Base Disorders

Le Chatelier's principle is the key to understanding acid-base disorders.

General Principles

EQUATION

$$HCO_3^- + H+ \rightarrow\uparrow H_2CO_3^- \rightarrow\uparrow H_2O + CO_2$$

INITIAL DISTURBANCE

Understanding acid-base disorders requires only an understanding of very basic chemistry! Remember **Le Chatelier's principle:** If you change the concentration of one of the chemicals in an equilibrium, the equilibrium shifts to counteract the change.

- In a **respiratory acidosis,** hypoventilation $\rightarrow \uparrow CO_2$. This shifts the equilibrium to the left, causing a rise in H^+ (thus a fall in pH) and a rise in bicarbonate (HCO_3^-).
- In a **metabolic acidosis,** an overall gain of acid (H^+) causes the pH to fall. This shifts the equilibrium to the right causing a fall in HCO_3^-. Note that this is the case even with GI losses of bicarbonate because excess hydrochloride (HCl) in the gut $\rightarrow \uparrow$ acid reabsorption and $\uparrow$ blood acid concentration.
- In a **respiratory alkalosis,** hyperventilation $\rightarrow \downarrow CO_2$. This shifts the equilibrium to the right, causing a fall in H^+ (thus a rise in pH) and a drop in HCO_3^-.
- In a **metabolic alkalosis,** an overall loss of acid (H^+) causes the pH to rise. This shifts the equilibrium to the right, causing a rise in HCO_3^-.

Respiratory compensation is fast and may occur in a matter of minutes. Metabolic compensation is slow and will be seen only with a chronic respiratory disturbance.

COMPENSATION

In any acid-base disturbance, the body attempts to compensate for the disturbance (Table 2.6-1).

- In a respiratory acidosis, the kidneys attempt to generate more bicarbonate, leading to further $\uparrow$ in HCO_3^- and a compensatory $\uparrow$ in pH.
- In a metabolic acidosis, the body attempts respiratory compensation by hyperventilation. Hyperventilation $\downarrow PaCO_2$ and therefore helps shift the equilibrium to the right to $\downarrow H^+$ (and thus $\uparrow$ pH).
- In a respiratory alkalosis, the kidneys attempt to lose bicarbonate, leading to further $\downarrow$ in HCO_3^- and a compensatory $\downarrow$ in pH.
- In a metabolic alkalosis, the body attempts respiratory compensation by hypoventilation. Hypoventilation $\uparrow PaCO_2$ and therefore helps shift the equilibrium to the left to $\uparrow H^+$ and lower pH.

Remember, it is impossible to overcompensate for the primary disturbance. If it appears that a compensation "overcorrects" the pH, then look for a second primary acid-base disturbance.

TABLE 2.6-1. **Acid-Base Disturbances**

DISORDER	ABNORMALITY	COMPENSATION	pH	PaCO₂	HCO₃
Metabolic acidosis	Gain H⁺/lose bicarb	↑ ventilation	↓	↓	↓
Respiratory acidosis	*Hypo*ventilation	Generate bicarbonate	↓	↑	↑
Metabolic alkalosis	Lose H⁺/gain bicarb	↓ ventilation	↑	↑	↑
Respiratory alkalosis	*Hyper*ventilation	Bicarbonate consumption	↑	↓	↓

Bold arrows indicate compensatory response

Learn this ABG sequence as these values are frequently reported in this order without labels:
Normal ABG: 7.4/40/90/24/98

A high anion gap means there is another chemical in addition to the usual organic acids and albumin that is not measured by a basic metabolic panel. For example, a patient with diabetic ketoacidosis will have high ketones (acids), which will "consume" bicarbonate and generate an anion gap.

Use Winter's formula to determine if compensation is appropriate in the setting of metabolic acidosis: **1.5 × (HCO₃⁻) + 8 ± 2 = pCO₂**

ARTERIAL BLOOD GAS (ABG)

Normal Values

pH	7.4 (7.35–7.45)
PaCO₂	40 (35–45)
PaO₂	90 (80–100)
HCO₃	24 (21–27)
O₂ sat	98 (95–100)

- **Look for hypoxia** using PaO_2; correlate with the clinical scenario.
- **Determine the type of disturbance** using pH, $PaCO_2$, and HCO_3 (see Table 2.6-1).
- **Calculate the degree of compensation:**
  - A change in $PaCO_2$ of 10 mmHg, up or down, causes pH to ↑ or ↓ by 0.08 units (pH ↓ as $PaCO_2$ rises).
  - A pH change of 0.15 is the result of a bicarbonate change of 10 mEq/L.
- If compensation is not within the expected range, look for a second acid-base disturbance.

ANION GAP (FIGURE 2.6-1)

The concentration of serum anions not measured in routine electrolyte profiles, mostly organic acids (eg, lactic and keto acids) and albumin.

$$Anion\ Gap = Na - (Cl + HCO_3^-)$$

$$Normal = 8{-}12\ mEq/L$$

Though chiefly used to determine the etiology of a metabolic acidosis, it should be calculated on every patient with an acid-base disturbance to evaluate for an underlying anion gap metabolic acidosis.

Metabolic Acidosis

- ↓ in pH with ↓ in HCO_3.
- Etiology depends on presence or absence of an anion gap.

NEPHROLOGY AND ACID-BASE DISORDERS

FIGURE 2.6-1. Anion Gap

The sum of the positive and negative charges within the box (including AG) must be neutral. If negative, the there are unmeasured anions resulting in an anion gap metabolic acidosis.

NORMAL ANION GAP METABOLIC ACIDOSIS

ETIOLOGY

- **Renal losses:**
  - Renal tubular acidosis (RTA).
  - Medications (acetazolamide, spironolactone, beta blockers).
- **GI losses:**
  - Diarrhea
  - Ileostomy

ANION GAP METABOLIC ACIDOSIS

See Table. 2.6-2.

Always check the anion gap. It is the easiest way to pick up a secondary metabolic acidosis.

TABLE 2.6-2. Causes of Anion Gap Metabolic Acidosis: MUDPILES

CAUSE	FINDINGS/DIAGNOSTIC TOOL
Methanol	Tox screen, vision changes, ↑ osmolal gap
Uremia	History of renal failure, ↑ creatinine
Diabetic ketoacidosis	Diabetes, ↑ serum glucose
Paraldehyde	Tox screen
Isoniazid, **I**ron	Medication history
Lactic acidosis	Serum lactate
Ethanol, **E**thylene glycol	Tox screen, history of alcohol abuse
Salicylates	Respiratory alkalosis and metabolic acidosis, tox screen

DELTA GAP OR DELTA-DELTA

Used to calculate tertiary acid-base disorders. Use only to diagnose anion gap metabolic acidosis or metabolic alkalosis. Calculates whether the body is excreting bicarbonate properly to compensate for the presence of unmeasurable anions.

- Anion gap – 12 (nl gap) = excess anion gap.
- Excess anion gap + HCO_3 = delta gap.
- If delta gap is > 30, then underlying metabolic alkalosis is present.
- If delta gap is < 23, then underlying acidosis is present.
- If between 23 and 30, then no tertiary disorder is present.

TREATMENT

- Correct underlying cause.
- Often, HCO_3^- is given in IV solution (bicarb drip) when pH < 7.0, but this practice has **not** been proven to improve mortality.

 A 34-year-old diabetic man with renal insufficiency has normal anion gap. K is high; bicarbonate level is low. *Think: Type IV RTA (hyporeninemic hypoaldosteronism).*

Respiratory Acidosis

- Hypoventilation from any cause ↑ the $PaCO_2$ and ↓ the serum pH.
- There is a compensatory ↑ in bicarbonate. Remember the equation.
- With an ↑ in CO_2, the equation shifts to the left, creating more H^+ and HCO_3^-.
- More H^+ means the pH ↓.

ETIOLOGY

- Pulmonary (chronic obstructive pulmonary disease [COPD], severe alveolar infiltrates, pulmonary edema, interstitial restrictive lung disease).
- Airway obstruction (foreign body, severe bronchospasm, laryngospasm).
- Thoracic disorders (pneumothorax, flail chest).
- Alveolar hypoventilation (myasthenia gravis, severe hypokalemia causing weak muscles of respiration, muscular dystrophy).
- Peripheral nervous system disorders (Guillain-Barré syndrome, botulism, tetanus, organophosphate poisoning).
- Depression of central respiratory drive (narcotic overdose, general anesthesia, ↑ intracranial pressure [ICP]).

SIGNS AND SYMPTOMS

Confusion, encephalopathy, coma.

TREATMENT

- Treat underlying cause.
- Mechanical hyperventilation will ↓ the amount of CO_2 retention in severely hypoxic patients.

NEPHROLOGY AND ACID-BASE DISORDERS

Respiratory Alkalosis

- Elevated arterial pH and hyperventilation, resulting in $\downarrow$ PCO_2 and compensatory $\downarrow$ in serum bicarbonate. Remember the equation.
- With a $\downarrow$ in CO_2, the equation shifts to the right, H^+ $\downarrow$, so the pH $\downarrow$ and the HCO_3^- $\downarrow$ (though often the bicarb change is minimal).

ETIOLOGY

- Most commonly caused by anxiety, which provokes hyperventilation.
- Other causes include shock, sepsis, pulmonary disease, cerebrovascular accident (CVA), normal pregnancy, liver disease, hyperthyroidism, salicylates.

SIGNS AND SYMPTOMS

- Rapid, deep breathing.
- Chest tightness, chest pain, and anxiety.
- Circumoral paresthesias, tetany in severe cases.

TREATMENT

- Reassurance, if anxiety.
- If patient can be calmed enough, have him or her breathe into a paper bag. This $\uparrow$ PCO_2 and helps restore pH.
- $\downarrow$ the minute volume in the mechanically ventilated patient.

Metabolic Alkalosis

- Elevated pH, $\uparrow$ plasma bicarbonate, and a compensatory $\uparrow$ in $PaCO_2$.
- Usually seen in cases of volume contraction.
- Remember, an $\uparrow$ in HCO_3^- pushes the equation to the right and uses up H^+, therefore $\uparrow$ pH and $\uparrow$ CO_2.
- Also, in metabolic alkalosis, the respiratory compensation is hypoventilation, $\rightarrow$ a further $\uparrow$ in PCO_2.

ETIOLOGY

Divided into chloride-responsive and chloride-resistant forms:
- **Chloride-responsive:** Urine chloride < 20 mEq/L:
  - Vomiting or prolonged NG tube drainage.
  - Pyloric stenosis.
  - Laxative abuse.
  - Diuretics (urine chloride is high during active diuretic use and low after discontinuation of diuretic therapy).
  - Post-hypercapnic states.
- **Chloride-resistant:** Urine chloride > 20 mEq/L:
  - Severe Mg or K deficiency.
  - Diuretics (thiazides or loops).
  - $\uparrow$ mineralocorticoids (Cushing's syndrome, primary aldosteronism, renal artery stenosis).
  - Licorice, chewing tobacco.
  - Inherited disorders (Bartter's syndrome, Gitelman's syndrome, and Liddle's syndrome).

SIGNS AND SYMPTOMS

- Irritability and neuromuscular hyperexcitability.
- Concomitant signs of hypokalemia (muscular weakness, cramping, ileus).
- Suspect metabolic alkalosis when the physical exam suggests hypovolemia and chronic GI volume loss.

TREATMENT

- Mild metabolic alkalosis requires no specific treatment.
- Hydration if cause is volume contraction.
- In severe hypokalemia and hypermineralocorticoid states the alkalosis is chloride resistant and cannot be corrected until potassium is replaced. Specific therapy must address hypermineralocorticoid state.

COMPENSATION FORMULAS

You will not need to calculate the appropriateness of the compensation for an exam, but it may help you during your rotation when trying to decide if there is more than one acid-base disturbance. If you find that the measured change differs significantly from the expected, look for a second acid-base disturbance.

Important Rules

1. There can be only three acid-base disorders at the same time.
2. The body can **never** overcompensate for the primary acid-base disorder.

RESPIRATORY ACIDOSIS

- **Acute:** ↑ in HCO_3 by 1 for every 10 ↑ in CO_2.
- **Chronic:** ↑ in HCO_3 by 3 for every 10 ↑ in CO_2.

pH ↓ by 0.08 for every ↑ in CO_2 by 10 in acute, and pH ↓ by 0.04 for every ↑ CO_2 by 10 in chronic.

RESPIRATORY ALKALOSIS

- **Acute:** ↓ in HCO_3 by 2 for every ↓ in CO_2 by 10.
- **Chronic:** ↓ in HCO_3 by 4 for every ↓ in CO_2 by 10.

METABOLIC ACIDOSIS

Calculate Winter's formula to determine what the CO_2 should be in a primary metabolic acidosis.

$$1.5 \times (HCO_3^-) + 8 \pm 2 = pCO_2$$

A quick way to estimate the expected CO_2 should be is to look at the last two digits of the pH (ie, if the pH is 7.28, the CO_2 in a metabolic acidosis should be 28).

METABOLIC ALKALOSIS

CO_2 ↑ by .06 for every ↑ in HCO_3 by 1.

Putting It All Together

The primary distubance is always the factor that changes in the same directions as the pH. For example, in acidosis, the primary disturbance will be identified by either a low HCO_3 or a low CO_2.

1. Look at pH: If < 7.40, acidosis is present; if > 7.40, alkalosis is present.
2. Next, look at the CO_2. If acidosis is present and the CO_2 is < 40, the primary disorder is metabolic acidosis; if the CO_2 is > 40, the primary disorder is respiratory acidosis. If alkalosis is present and the CO_2 is < 40, the primary disorder is respiratory alkalosis. If the CO_2 is > 40, the primary disorder is metabolic alkalosis.
3. Calculate compensation for the primary disorder using the calculations above to diagnose secondary acid-base disorder.
4. Calculate the anion gap if an acidosis is present.
5. Calculate delta gap to diagnose tertiary acid-base disorder.

ELECTROLYTE DISORDERS

Body Fluids

- Total body water (TBW) is approximately 60% of lean body mass.
- Intracellular fluid (ICF) is two-thirds of TBW:
  - The major cations in ICF are K^+ and Mg^{2+}.
  - The major ICF anions are proteins and organic phosphates (adenosine triphosphate [ATP], adenosine diphosphate [ADP], adenosine monophosphate [AMP]).
- Extracellular fluid (ECF) is one-third of TBW:
  - Consists of interstitial fluid (third space) and plasma.
  - The major ECF cation is Na^+.
  - The major ECF anions are Cl^- and HCO_3^-.
  - Plasma comprises one-fourth of the ECF (one-twelfth of TBW). The major plasma proteins are albumin and globulins.
  - Interstitial fluid is three-fourths of the ECF (one-fourth of TBW). The electrolyte composition of interstitial fluid is the same as plasma. However, interstitial fluid contains little protein (ultrafiltrate).

Fluid Shifts Between Compartments

- Water shifts between ECF and ICF so the osmolarities of the two compartments remain equal.
- Solutes that do not cross the cell membranes freely contribute to ECF osmolarity (glucose, sodium, mannitol, IV contrast materials).
- **Serum osmolarity:**
  - Normal range: 280–300 mOsm/kg.
  - Serum osmolarity can be estimated with the following formula:

  $$\text{Serum Osmolarity} = 2(Na + K) + \text{Glucose}/18 + BUN/2.8$$

  - Elevated in dehydration, hypernatremia, diabetes insipidus, uremia, hyperglycemia, mannitol therapy, toxin ingestion, hypercalcemia, diuretic therapy.
  - $\downarrow$ in syndrome of inappropriate antidiuretic hormone (SIADH), hyponatremia, overhydration with 5% dextrose solution, Addison's disease, hypothyroidism.
  - Major toxins that $\uparrow$ the serum osmolarity: EtOH, methanol, ethylene glycol.

Hyponatremia

Plasma sodium < 134 mEq/L.

ETIOLOGY AND CLASSIFICATION

Calculate serum osmolarity and determine fluid status of a patient to determine classification of hyponatremia. Hyponatremia is subdivided into three categories based on the serum osmolarity and fluid status (Table 2.6-3):

- **Hypotonic hyponatremia** is further subdivided into three categories:
    1. *Hypervolemic:* CHF ($\uparrow$ free H_2O), nephrotic syndrome ($\downarrow$ albumin), cirrhosis ($\downarrow$ albumin).
    2. *Isovolemic:* Renal failure, SIADH, glucocorticoid deficiency (hypopituitarism or Addison's disease), hypothyroidism with myxedema, primary polydypsia, and medications.
    3. *Hypovolemic:*
        - Loss of both sodium and water.
        - Renal losses (diuretics, partial urinary tract obstruction, salt-wasting nephropathies).
        - Extrarenal losses (vomiting, diarrhea, extensive burns, third-spacing (pancreatitis, peritonitis).
- **Isotonic hyponatremia** (normal serum osmolarity):
    - SIADH.
    - Isotonic infusions (glucose, mannitol).
- **Hypertonic hyponatremia** ($\uparrow$ serum osmolarity):
    - *Hyperglycemia:* Each 100 mg/dL $\uparrow$ in serum glucose above normal (100 mg/dL) $\downarrow$ plasma sodium concentration by 1.6 mEq/L. To avoid missing a potentially severe *hypernatremia*, you must calculate the corrected serum sodium: Corrected Na = [(serum glucose -100)/100] $\times$ 1.6.
    - *Hypertonic infusions:* Mannitol, glucose.

SIGNS AND SYMPTOMS

- Moderate hyponatremia or gradual onset: Confusion, muscle cramps, lethargy, anorexia, nausea.
- Severe hyponatremia or rapid onset: Seizures or coma (no exact number, but Na^+ < 115 is always severe).

TABLE 2.6-3. Causes of Hyponatremia

		URINE OSM	URINE SODIUM
Hypovolemic	Extrarenal: GI losses, skin losses, lung losses, third-spacing (fistula, burns, vomiting, diarrhea, GI suction, edema, pancreatitis).	$\uparrow$	$\downarrow$ < 10 mEq/L
	Renal: Diuretics, intrinsic renal damage (including acute tubular necrosis), partial urinary tract obstruction, salt-wasting nephropathies.	$\uparrow$	$\uparrow$ > 20 mEq/ L
	Adrenal insufficiency (Addison's).	$\uparrow$	$\uparrow$
Isovolemic	Water intoxication.	$\downarrow$	$\downarrow$
	SIADH.	$\uparrow$	$\uparrow$
Hypervolemic	CHF, liver cirrhosis, and the nephrotic syndrome.	$\uparrow$	$\downarrow$

CHF, congestive heart failure; SIADH, syndrome of inappropriate antidiuretic hormone.

- **Normal osmolarity:** Consider pseudohyponatremia and overinfusion of non-sodium-containing isotonic solutions such as glucose and mannitol.
- **Low osmolarity:** Clinically assess the extracellular fluid volume. Look for tachycardia, hypotension, poor skin turgor (indicative of **hypovolemia**). Also look for peripheral edema (indicative of **hypervolemia**). Normal vital signs and no edema usually indicate **isovolemia**.
- **High osmolarity:** Measure serum glucose concentration to consider hyperglycemia. Also consider overinfusion of hypertonic, non-sodium-containing solutions (mannitol, glucose, glycine).

Pseudohyponatremia

- Simply an error in measurement of sodium due to an ↑ in other plasma components.
- Since plasma is 93% water and 7% plasma protein and lipid, and sodium ions are only dissolved in the plasma water, increasing the non-aqueous phase artificially lowers the Na^+ concentration.
- This occurs in multiple myeloma (due to ↑ plasma protein) or hyperlipidemia.

A patient presents with multiple myeloma and hyponatremia, but calculated serum tonicity is normal. *Think: Pseudohyponatremia/paraproteinemia.*

If kidneys are still functional in a hypovolemic patient, urine Na^+ should be < 10 mEq/L as the kidneys will be trying to conserve Na^+ to maintain intravascular volume.

Urine Na^+ can distinguish between renal and extrarenal causes of hypovolemic hyponatremia. Renal cause: UNa^+ > 20 $\mu Eq/L$ since kidneys cannot conserve Na^+ or H_2O. Nonrenal cause: UNa < 10 $\mu Eq/L$.

General Rules
- Treatment approach is twofold: Correction of the serum sodium and treatment of the underlying disorder.
- Serum sodium should be corrected only halfway to the lower range of normal within the first 24 hours.
- Unless patient has acute hyponatremia with seizure, do not correct sodium faster than 1 mEq/L/hr with a maximum correction of 10 mEq/L/24 hrs. Central pontine myelinolysis (CPM), seizures, coma, and death can result.

Type-Specific Treatment
- **Hypovolemic hyponatremia:** 0.9% NaCl (**normal saline**) infusion to correct volume deficit. Monitor the serum sodium to prevent complications of rapid correction. Hypertonic saline is rarely indicated.
- **Hypervolemic hyponatremia:** Sodium and **water restriction.** In congestive heart failure (CHF), the combination of captopril and furosemide is effective.

Pseudohyponatremia is suspected if the measured and calculated serum osmolarities are different.

Central pontine myelinolysis (CPM):

- Sometimes termed osmotic demyelination syndrome, occurs as a treatment complication of severe or chronic hyponatremia (< 110 mEq/L).

NEPHROLOGY AND ACID-BASE DISORDERS

- A symmetric zone of demyelination occurs in the basis pontis (and extrapontine areas), leading to stupor, lethargy, quiet and confused delirium, and quadriparesis.
- CPM can be avoided by increasing the serum sodium no faster than 1 mEq/L/hr. Some patients treated symptomatically will recover in 3–4 weeks; however, in some, the damage is irreversible.

Hypernatremia

Serum Na > 145 mEq/L.

ETIOLOGY AND CLASSIFICATION

See Table 2.6-4.

- **Hypovolemic** (most common):
  - Loss of water and sodium (water loss >> than sodium loss).
  - Renal losses (diuretics, glycosuria); GI, respiratory, or skin losses; adrenal deficiencies.
- **Isovolemic:**
  - ↓ TBW, normal total body sodium, and ↓ ECF.
  - Diabetes insipidus (neurogenic and nephrogenic), skin losses (hyperthermia), iatrogenic causes, reset osmostat.
- **Hypervolemic:**
  - ↑ TBW, markedly ↑ total body sodium, and ↑ ECF.
  - Iatrogenic (hypertonic fluid administration).
  - Mineralocorticoid excess (Conn's tumor, Cushing's syndrome).
  - Excess salt ingestion.

SIGNS AND SYMPTOMS

- Fatigue
- Confusion (can progress to coma and seizures)
- Lethargy
- Edema

Formula: Water deficit (WD) in hypernatremic patients:

WD (in liters) = 0.6 × body weight (kg) × (Measured Na/Normal Na) − 1)

Giving DDAVP (desmopressin) to a patient with hypernatremia will result in increased urine osmolarity and improvement in hypermatremia in central diabetes insipidus.

TABLE 2.6-4. Causes of Hypernatremia

		URINE OSM	URINE SODIUM
Hypovolemic	Renal loss: Osmotic diuresis (glycosuria, urea), acute/chronic renal failure, partial obstruction.	N/↓	↑
	Extrarenal loss: Hyperpnea, excessive sweating.	↑	↑
	Extrarenal loss: Diarrhea, burns, moderate sweating.	↑	↓
	Iatrogenic (bicarbonate, dialysis, salt tablets).	↑	↑
Isovolemic	Diabetes insipidus (from any cause).	↓	↓
Hypervolemic	Mineralocorticoid excess (eg, Conn's syndrome).	N/↓	N/↓

- **Hypovolemic hypernatremia:** Fluid replacement with normal saline. Correct plasma sodium no faster than 0.5mEq/L/hr.
- **Isovolemic hypernatremia:**
  - Fluid replacement with half normal (0.45%) saline. Correct only half of the estimated water deficit in the first 24 hours.
  - The correction rate should not exceed 1 mEq/L/hr in acute hypernatremia and 0.5 mEq/L/hr in chronic hypernatremia.
  - Vasopressin for central diabetes insipidus.
- **Hypervolemic hypernatremia:**
  - Fluid replacement with half normal (0.45%) saline (to correct hypertonicity).
  - Loop diuretic therapy (eg, furosemide) to ↑ sodium excretion.

In hypovolemic hypernatremia, always correct fluid deficit with normal saline before anything else.

Hypokalemia

Plasma potassium < 3.3 mEq/L.

ETIOLOGY AND CLASSIFICATION

Patients taking digitalis must have their potassium checked regularly because hypokalemia ↑ the risk and severity of digitalis toxicity.

- Extra- to intracellular potassium shifting (redistribution) and undetermined mechanisms:
  - Alkalosis (each 0.1 ↑ in pH ↓ serum K^+ by 0.4–0.6 mEq/L).
  - Insulin (drives K^+ into cells).
  - Vitamin B_{12}.
  - Beta-adrenergics.
  - Correction of digoxin toxicity with digitalis antibody fragments (Digibind).
- ↑ **renal potassium excretion:**
  - Medications (diuretics, amphotericin B, cisplatin, aminoglycosides, corticosteroids).
  - Renal tubular acidosis type I (distal) or type II (proximal).
  - Hypomagnesemia.
  - Osmotic diuresis (mannitol).
  - Bartter's syndrome: JG-cell hyperplasia causing ↑ renin/aldosterone, metabolic alkalosis, hypokalemia, hypercalciuria, muscle weakness, and tetany (seen in young adults).
  - Gitelman's syndrome: Defective distal tubule thiazide-sensitive Na^+ Cl^- transporter → metabolic alkalosis, hypokalemia, hypomagnesemia, and hypocalciuria. Presents similar to Bartter's syndrome, but less severe in presentation.
  - ↑ mineralocorticoid activity (primary hyperaldosteronism [tumor] or secondary hyperaldosteronism [CHF, cirrhosis, dehydration]), Cushing's syndrome.
- **GI losses:**
  - Vomiting, nasogastric suctioning.
  - Diarrhea, laxative abuse.
  - Inadequate dietary intake (anorexia nervosa).
  - Cutaneous losses from excessive sweating.

SIGNS AND SYMPTOMS

- Impaired gastric motility, nausea, and vomiting.
- Mild muscle weakness to overt paralysis depending on severity.
- Rhabdomyolysis.
- Atrial and ventricular dysrhythmias.

A 10-mEq infusion will raise the serum K by 1.0 mEq/L.

Chronic, slowly developing hyperkalemia is better tolerated than acute changes (ie, less likely to have cardiac changes).

Perform a STAT ECG on patients with moderate to severe hyperkalemia.

Treatments for hyperkalemia—

Controlling K Immediately Diverts Bad Arrhythmias

Calcium
Kayexalate, Diuretics
Insulin and glucose
Dialysis
Bicarbonate
Albuterol

Kayexalate and diuretics are the only treatments of hyperkalemia (other than dialysis) that remove potassium from the body.

TREATMENT

Replace potassium (PO or IV, depending on severity). IV infusion of K+ should not exceed 20 mEq/L/hr, but may be combined with simultaneous oral administration.

Hyperkalemia

Serum K > 5.5 mEq/L.

ETIOLOGY

- Always consider pseudohyperkalemia (falsely elevated measurement due to hemolysis of specimen and leakage of potassium from lysed cells in the tube). This is the most common cause of elevated potassium based on lab results. Repeat test.
- **Intra- to extracellular potassium shifting** occurs in acidosis, heavy exercise, insulin deficiency, and digitalis toxicity.
- ↑ **potassium load** occurs with IV potassium supplementation, potassium-containing medications, and ↑ cellular breakdown.
- ↓ **potassium excretion** occurs with oliguric renal failure, potassium sparing diuretics, beta blockers, angiotensin-converting enzyme (ACE) inhibitors, aldosterone deficiency, and obstructive uropathies.

SIGNS AND SYMPTOMS

- GI: Nausea, vomiting, diarrhea.
- Neuro: Muscle cramps, weakness, paresthesias, paralysis, areflexia, tetany, focal neurologic deficits, confusion.
- Respiratory insufficiency.
- Cardiac: Arrhythmias, arrest.

DIAGNOSIS

Electrocardiogram (ECG) changes:

- 6.5–7.5 mEq/L: **Tall peaked T-waves in ALL ECG leads** (see Figure 2.6-2), short QT interval, prolonged PR.
- 7.5–8.0 mEq/L: QRS widening, flattened P-wave.
- 10–12 mEq/L: QRS may degrade into a "sine-wave" pattern.
- V-fib, complete heart block, or asystole may occur.

TREATMENT

- **Immediate:** The following therapies are only **temporizing measures** of lowering potassium until definitive therapy is initiated. *Remember:* Your job is not done until definitive potassium lowering therapy is given.
  - IV calcium gluconate: **Goal is immediate cardiac membrane stabilization;** acts in minutes.
  - Insulin has the most potent effect on driving potassium into cells. Also can use albuterol (beta-adrenergic agonist), and lastly bicarbonate. Goal is shifting K+ from ECF to ICF; acts in minutes.
  - If giving insulin, must make sure to give the patient glucose, usually in the form of D50 IV push, to prevent hypoglycemia.
- **Definitive therapy:** The following therapies provide removal of total body potassium.
  - Cation exchange resin such as Kayexalate, diuretics, and hemodialysis are used with goal removal of potassium from the body; takes hours to work.

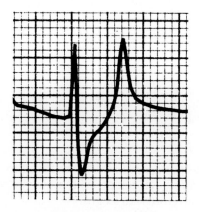

FIGURE 2.6-2. Peaked T-wave due to hyperkalemia.

- Diuretics (eg, furosemide) $\uparrow$ K$^+$ excretion and may be given with IV fluids if patient is euvolemic.
- Refractory hyperkalemia, or hyperkalemia with life-threatening arrhythmias, requires hemodialysis as the most effective therapy to lower total body potassium.

Hypocalcemia

- Serum Ca < 8.5 mg/dL.
- Calcium can be found bound to plasma proteins, complexed with anions (eg, phospate), or free (ionized). The free (ionized) fraction is biologically active.

ETIOLOGY

- Always consider hypoalbuminemia. Since a large amount of calcium is bound to albumin, patients with hypoalbuminemia (eg, liver failure, nephrotic syndrome) have low total calcium levels but normal ionized calcium levels.
- You can calculate a corrected calcium as follows for an estimate of effective calcium level, or you can check an ionized calcium level to be sure:

$$\text{Corrected Calcium} = \text{Measured Calcium} + [(4 - \text{Measured Albumin})] \times 0.8$$

- Parathyroid hormone (PTH) insufficiency. PTH secretion is stimulated by low free calcium and inhibited by increasing free calcium. Three major actions:
  1. In bone, PTH causes resorption of both calcium and phosphate.
  2. In the kidney, PTH facilitates resorption of calcium and excretion of phosphate.
  3. Also in the kidney, PTH stimulates conversion of 25-OH vitamin D to 1,25 dihydroxyvitamin D$_3$ (active vitamin D). Renal failure results in vitamin D deficiency $\rightarrow$ low Ca$^+$ $\rightarrow$ $\uparrow$ PTH. Vitamin D causes retention of both calcium and phosphate.

  Therefore, the net effect of PTH is to $\uparrow$ serum calcium and $\downarrow$ serum phosphate.
- Vitamin D deficiency (intestinal malabsorption, cholestyramine, primidone, renal disease).

Correcting for hypoalbuminemia: The measured Ca should be adjusted upward by 0.8 mg/dL for each 1.0 g/dL of albumin below normal.

- Pseudohypoparathyroidism (Albrights' hereditary osteodystropy) = end-organ resistance to PTH due to a defective PTH receptor.
- Toxins: Fluoride, cimetidine, ethanol, citrate, phenytoin.
- Sepsis.
- Pancreatitis.
- Rhabdomyolysis, tumor lysis syndrome ($\uparrow$ serum phosphate).
- Severe magnesium deficiency.

SIGNS AND SYMPTOMS

- Circumoral paresthesia is usually the first symptom.
- The next sign is muscular tetany, which may be observed by examining for Chvostek's and Trousseau's signs.
    - **Chvostek's sign:** Facial muscle spasm with tapping of the facial nerve.
    - **Trousseau's sign:** Carpal spasm after occluding blood flow in forearm with blood pressure cuff.
- Acute severe hypocalcemia may cause laryngospasm, seizures, confusion, or cardiovascular collapse with bradycardia and decompensated heart failure.

DIAGNOSIS

- Clues to diagnosis can be provided by careful bedside evaluation, looking for evidence of prior neck surgery, a thorough evaluation of medications, as well as detailed family history looking for cases of hypocalcemia, hypoparathyroidism, or pseudohypoparathyroidism.
- ECG findings: Prolonged QT and ST intervals (peaked T-waves are also possible, as in hyperkalemia).

TREATMENT

- For PTH deficiency: Replacement therapy with vitamin D or calcitriol combined with high oral calcium intake. Thiazide diuretics are used to lower urinary calcium and prevent calcium urolithiasis.
- Repletion of magnesium for hypomagnesemia.
- Oral calcium supplementation, dietary phosphate restriction, and calcitriol for chronic renal failure.
- Vitamin D and calcium supplementation for pseudohypoparathyroidism.
- IV calcium for severe, life-threatening hypocalcemia.

Hypercalcemia

Serum Ca > 10.2 mg/dL.

ETIOLOGY

- Drugs:
    - Calcium supplementation (IV).
    - Excess vitamin D $\uparrow$ intestinal calcium absorption.
    - Antacid abuse.
    - Thiazides (inhibit renal calcium excretion).
    - Lithium.

Neck surgery, even long after the procedure, can be associated with postoperative hypoparathyroidism, usually due to ischemia of the parathyroid glands.

Primary hyperparathyroidism is the most common cause of hypercalcemia in the outpatient. Malignancy is the most common cause in the inpatient.

NEPHROLOGY AND ACID-BASE DISORDERS

- **Malignancies:**
  - Colon, lung, breast, prostate (all cause metastasis to bone).
  - Multiple myeloma.
  - Zollinger-Ellison syndrome (as part of multiple endocrine neoplasia type I (MEN I).
- **Endocrinopathies:**
  - Hyperparathyroidism
  - Hyperthyroidism
  - Acromegaly
  - Addison's disease
  - Paget's disease (of bone)
- **Other:**
  - Immobility ($\rightarrow \uparrow$ bone turnover with $\uparrow$ bone resorption).
  - Granulomatous diseases such as sarcoidosis, tuberculosis (1,25-[OH]$_2$-vitamin D$_3$ production by macrophages within granulomatous tissue).

SIGNS AND SYMPTOMS

- Malaise, fatigue, headaches, diffuse aches and pains.
- Patients are often dehydrated and a vicious cycle ensues. Dehydration $\downarrow$ renal calcium excretion, while at the same time patients are losing fluids from vomiting and nausea induced by the hypercalcemia.
- Lethargy and psychosis occur when hypercalcemia is severe.
- Metastatic calcifications may occur in skin, cornea, conjunctiva, and kidneys.
- Severe hypercalcemia may cause QT interval shortening and variable degrees of AV block.

TREATMENT

- IV fluids +/– Lasix.
- Calcitonin.
- Bisphosphonate derivatives ($\downarrow$ osteoclastic activity).
- Dialysis for severe or symptomatic hypercalcemia.
- Parathyroidectomy if hyperparathyroid is cause.

MALIGNANCY AND HYPERCALCEMIA

- **Humoral hypercalcemia of malignancy:** Tumor production of PTH-related peptide (PTH-rp). Stimulates bone resorption and renal calcium reabsorption. PTH-related peptide is not detected by the usual PTH immunoassay. Specific immunoassay exists for PTH-related peptide.
- **Local osteolytic hypercalcemia:** Malignant cells in multiple myeloma or solid tumors with bone metastases may cause osteoclast stimulation. Osteoclast-activating factors (OAFs) are interleukins, transforming growth factors, and other cytokines.

MANAGEMENT OF SEVERE HYPERCALCEMIA

- Rehydration with normal saline to initiate calciuresis.
- IV infusion of **pamidronate** (bisphosphonate) should be initiated simultaneously.
- May also use calcitonin.
- May also use furosemide to $\uparrow$ diuresis once patient is hydrated.
- Dialysis if severe or refractory to medical treatment.

Causes of hypercalcemia—

CHIMPANZEES

Calcium supplementation
Hyperparathyroidism/**H**yperthyroidism
Immobility/**I**atrogenic
Metastasis/**M**ilk alkali syndrome
Paget's disease
Addison's disease/**A**cromegaly
Neoplasm
Zollinger-Ellison syndrome
Excessive vitamin A
Excessive vitamin D
Sarcoidosis

Acute pancreatitis can be precipitated by hypercalcemia.

Transient hypoparathyroidism can occur after removal of a parathyroid adenoma because the remaining glands take a few days to begin secreting PTH again.

Hypercalcemia: "Stones, bones, groans, and psychiatric overtones."

Hypercalcemic crisis is an uncommon manifestation of primary hyperparathyroidism. It presents with severe hypercalcemia, volume depletion, and altered mental status.

Hungry bone syndrome is the rapid transfer of calcium and phosphate into bones following removal of a hyperactive parathyroid nodule.

Hyperparathyroidism

PRIMARY

- Elevated parathyroid hormone and elevated serum calcium.
- May occur in conjunction with MEN I or MEN IIa (all glands are hyperplastic).
- Usually, only one parathyroid gland is enlarged, and hypercalcemia suppresses the function of the remaining glands.

EPIDEMIOLOGY

More common in middle-aged to elderly women.

SIGNS AND SYMPTOMS

- Usual presentation is asymptomatic hypercalcemia noted on routine laboratory examination.
- Patients may also have nonspecific complaints like fatigue, weight loss, depression, abdominal pain, or arthralgias.
- Hypercalciuria from the kidneys' inability to reabsorb the large calcium load may → nephrocalcinosis or renal calculi.
- Elevated PTH levels → bone remodeling and ↓ bone mass.

DIAGNOSIS

- Hypercalcemia.
- PTH level in the high-normal range.
- Hypophosphatemia.
- Hypercalciuria.

SECONDARY/RENAL OSTEODYSTROPHY

PATHOPHYSIOLOGY

- In chronic kidney disease, (CKD), nephron loss reduces phosphate excretion, causing hyperphosphatemia.
- This lowers serum calcium (thereby increasing PTH secretion) and impairs calcitriol formation.
- ↓ calcitriol formation (also due to nephron loss) reduces intestinal calcium absorption.
- This provides further stimulation for PTH secretion.
- The ↑ PTH → excessive bone resorption/turnover.

ETIOLOGY AND CLASSIFICATION

Three types of bone lesions are associated with secondary hyperparathyroidism:

1. **Osteitis fibrosa cystica:** Normal bone is replaced by fibrous tissue, primitive woven bone, and cysts due to high bone turnover.
2. **Osteomalacia:** Associated with vitamin D deficiency, characterized by defective osteoid mineralization.
3. **Adynamic bone disease:** Cause is unknown, but the disease is due to excessively low bone turnover.

- Bone pain.
- Proximal muscle weakness.
- Pruritus.
- Soft-tissue ulcerations.
- Diffuse soft-tissue calcifications.

TREATMENT

Goal is to normalize the calcium–phosphate balance:

- Dietary phosphate restriction.
- Reduce intestinal absorption of phosphate with aluminum-containing antacids and/or phosphate binders (PhosLo, Renagel, etc.).
- Vitamin D with calcitriol to ↑ serum calcium and reverse some of the bone changes.
- Cinacalcet (Sensipar), which mimics the action of calcium on the parathyroid gland reducing PTH levels.
- Subtotal parathyroidectomy may benefit patients who do not respond to medical therapy.
- Frequent dialysis.
- Renal transplant in selected patients.

Hypophosphatemia

- Serum phosphate < 2.5 mg/dL.
- Usually, alcoholism or malnutrition is the cause. Also seen with diabetic ketoacidosis (DKA) and hyperparathyroidism.
- Symptoms are neuro (mental status change, agitation) and muscle weakness.
- Severe hypophosphatemia (< 1 mg/dL) can result in rhabdomyolysis or seizures.
- Treat with phosphate supplementation orally, or if phosphate < 1 mg/dL intravenously.

Phosphate is especially important for weaning patients off ventilators since the diaphragm requires a lot of ATP (adenosine triPHOSPHATE) for energy.

Hyperphosphatemia

Plasma phosphate > 5 mg/dL.

ETIOLOGY

Renal failure, tumor lysis syndrome (rapid necrosis of tumor after chemotherapy), iatrogenic (excessive amounts given IV or PO).

TREATMENT

Oral calcium carbonate (binds phosphate in gut and ↓ absorption), low-phosphate diet, aluminum-containing antacids, phosphate binders (PhosLo, Renagel, etc.) depending on the level and cause of hyperphosphatemia.

Hypomagnesemia

Serum magnesium < 1.8 mg/dL.

A common cause of high phosphate serum values is *in vitro* hemolysis. Most labs will report that the specimen was hemolyzed, however.

When supplementing calcium or potassium, always check for hypomagnesemia. The calcium and potassium levels will not elevate if magnesium is low.

ETIOLOGY

- Drugs (loop diuretics, amphotericin, gentamicin), insulin, hungry bone syndrome.
- Low magnesium causes hypokalemia and hypocalcemia *refractory* to replacement.
- **You will be unable to correct the potassium or calcium deficit until magnesium is corrected.**
- ECG changes similar to hypokalemia.
- Treat with oral or IV supplementation.

Hypermagnesemia

Serum magnesium > 2.3 mg/dL.

ETIOLOGY

Iatrogenic (during treatment of eclampsia/preeclampsia), magnesium-containing drugs (some laxatives, antacids) if given to a patient with renal failure.

TREATMENT

IV fluids, calcium if there are ECG changes; dialysis if refractory.

General Principles of Electrolyte Disorder Management

- Always check the other electrolytes—isolated electrolyte abnormalities are uncommon.
- Abnormal calcium level is meaningless without an albumin level in an asymptomatic patient.
- Redraw labs if *in vitro* hemolysis is a possibility.
- If severe, place patient on continuous ECG monitoring.
- Neurological exam soon after treatment begun—focus on level of consciousness, presence of confusion, and deep tendon reflexes. Serial neuro exams during treatment can guide therapy while labs are pending.

IV magnesium infusion requires:

- Cardiac monitor
- Vitals q 10 min
- Monitor deep tendon reflexes
- Monitor urine output

ARF with oliguria has a worse prognosis. In addition, interventions to change renal failure from oliguric to nonoliguric (using high-dose diuretics) do not change the prognosis.

Oliguria: Urine output < 400 mL/day. Minimum volume needed to excrete daily production of metabolites and waste products.

ACUTE RENAL FAILURE (ARF)

- Also called **acute kidney injury (AKI).**
- Clear-cut definition does not exist.
- Usually rapid onset of increasing blood urea nitrogen (BUN) and creatinine.
- Often occurs in the hospitalized patient.
- May be heralded by ↓ urine production (oliguria).

CLASSIFICATION

Prerenal, postrenal, or intrinsic renal failure.

GENERAL APPROACH

- **Prerenal** (due to ↓ kidney perfusion):
  - BUN rising out of proportion to creatinine (> 20:1).
  - Volume depletion from hemorrhage, dehydration, surgery.
  - CHF causing ↓ cardiac output and secondary renal hypoperfusion.

- Third-spacing from cirrhosis, nephrotic syndrome, sepsis, burns.
- Most common cause of inpatient renal insufficiency is due to ↓ renal perfusion.
- Exacerbated by nonsteroidal anti-inflammatory drugs (NSAIDs), angiotensin-converting enzyme (ACE) inhibitors, and diuretics.
- **Postrenal** (due to obstruction of urinary excretion):
  - Bilateral ureteral obstruction: Urothelial tumor, benign prostatic hypertrophy (BPH), cervical cancer.
  - Unilateral ureteral obstruction from renal stones, stricture, or tumor may cause significant ↓ in glomerular filtration rate (GFR) and unilateral kidney failure.
  - Urethral obstruction: Bladder cancer.
  - Retroperitoneal fibrosis.
  - Renal sonogram: May show bilateral hydronephrosis; retrograde ureterogram is more sensitive for obstruction.
  - Reversible if obstruction removed in time.
  - If lower obstruction cannot be removed, nephrostomy tubes relieve the obstruction and prevent further kidney injury.
  - Postobstructive diuresis: Frequent temporary sequela of obstruction removal. Presents with overdiuresis by kidneys, resulting in dehydration and electrolyte disturbance. If present, hydrate and follow electrolytes.
- **Intrinsic:**
  - Acute tubular necrosis (ATN) due to ischemia (after prerenal insult/hypoperfusion), toxins such as medications (aminoglycosides, cisplatin, pentamidine, lithium, amphotericin), myoglobin from rhabdomyolysis, IV contrast.
  - Acute allergic interstitial nephritis (AIN).
  - Vascular disorders and atheromatous emboli.
  - Glomerular disorders (nephrotic and nephritic syndromes).
- **Urinary sodium:**
  - Prerenal failure has low urine sodium (< 15 mEq/L) and high urine osmolarity (> 500 mOsm/L). The urine specific gravity is usually around 1.020. This is a result of the kidney's trying to concentrate the urine and conserve volume when perfusion is ↓.
  - Intrinsic renal failure has high urine sodium (> 15 mEq/L) and low urine osmolarity (< 400 mOsm/L) because the kidneys are unable to concentrate the urine.
- **Urinary sediment:** Intrinsic renal disease shows large amounts of protein and an "active" sediment (blood, protein, and red and white cell casts) that often will point toward the underlying cause of the renal disease:
  - **Acute glomerulonephritis:** Red blood cell (RBC) casts with hematuria and proteinuria and low urine specific gravity.
  - **ATN:** Many renal epithelial cells and muddy brown granular casts.

Tubulointerstitial Diseases

- Most common cause of intrinsic ARF.
- Includes ATN and interstitial nephritis.
- Tubulointerstitial causes of renal failure are the most common etiologies of ARF in hospitalized patients, and are associated with the best outcomes if recognized early.

The fractional sodium excretion (FeNa+) is the best discriminator between prerenal and intrinsic renal failure:
FeNa <1% is pre-renal, FeNa >2% is intrinsic renal failure. A value between 1% – 2% is indeterminant.

Dopamine, diuretics, mannitol, and saline confound use of fractional sodium excretion in finding etiology of renal failure.

Acute Tubular Necrosis (ATN)

Acute necrosis of renal tubules due to ischemic or toxic insult.

ETIOLOGY

- **Ischemic:** Shock, trauma, sepsis, hypoxia.
- **Toxic:** IV contrast media, aminoglycosides, rhabdomyolysis (heme pigments), and tumor lysis.

COURSE

- Patients present with dramatic renal failure.
- Most survive and recover normal renal function.
- Severity correlates with survival.
- Failure lasts 1–2 weeks, during which intensive care and sometimes hemodialysis are required while kidneys recover.
- Approximately 50% have normal urine output (less severe).

DIAGNOSIS

- Muddy brown granular casts.
- High urine sodium.
- Rising creatinine.
- FeNa is > 1%.

PREVENTION

- Monitor creatinine in patients receiving nephrotoxic substances.
- Maintain adequate intravascular volume for patients pre and post surgical procedures.
- Provide hydration to patients that will receive iodinated contrast media as tolerated (typically use normal saline IV).
- Maintain good cardiac output.

TREATMENT

- Normal saline for volume replacement.
- Match fluid and salt intake to daily urine output.
- Discontinue precipitating cause/offending or exacerbating agents (eg, medications).
- Manage electrolyte disturbances.

Acute Interstitial Nephritis (AIN)

Inflammation of the renal parenchyma.

ETIOLOGY

- **Systemic diseases:** Sarcoidosis, Sjögren's syndrome, lymphoma.
- **Systemic infections:** Syphilis, toxoplasmosis, cytomegalovirus, Epstein-Barr virus, HIV.
- **Medications:** Beta-lactam antibiotics, diuretics, and NSAIDs, proton pump inhibitors, allopurinol.

NSAIDs usually do not cause AIN, but by inhibiting prostaglandin synthesis they ↓ the GFR, which can precipitate renal failure in a patient with underlying renal problems.

NEPHROLOGY AND ACID-BASE DISORDERS

TABLE 2.6-5.   ATN vs. AIN

	ATN	AIN
Classic clinical setting (but not limited to)	Hypotension/post-hypotension (shock)	▪ Drugs (beta-lactam antibiotics) ▪ Infections (*Legionella, Streptococcus*)
Findings	Muddy brown granular and epithelial casts	▪ Rash, fever ▪ Eosinophilia ▪ Eosinophils in urine ▪ White and red cell casts
Treatment	Fluids and treat hypotension	▪ Stop drug ▪ Give steroids (if severe)

A patient was treated with penicillin for streptococcal pharyngitis. Now he has a diffuse rash and renal failure. Urinalysis shows white and red cell casts. Complete blood count shows elevated eosinophils. *Think: Acute interstitial nephritis.* **Next step:** Stop antibiotic, give steroid.

CLINICAL AND LAB FINDINGS

- Clinical and lab findings similar to ATN (see Table 2.6-5).
- Drug-induced interstitial nephritis is associated with eosinophilia and eosinophiluria and may be accompanied by other signs of systemic hypersensitivity reaction (eg, rash).

TREATMENT

- Address underlying cause/discontinue offending agent.
- Manage renal failure as for ATN.
- Renal function recovers in most cases following discontinuation of offending agent.
- High-dose prednisone may improve recovery if infection is not a concern.

GLOMERULAR DISORDERS

Nephrotic Syndrome

- Glomerular lesion causing proteinuria > 3 g/day.
- Indicates a defect in the glomerular filtration barrier.
- Defined by the triad of proteinuria, hyperlipidemia, and peripheral edema.

- Onset of glomerular permeability to plasma proteins, resulting in proteinuria and loss of albumin (hypoalbuminemia).
- Hypoalbuminemia → a ↓ in oncotic pressure, resulting in edema and serosal effusions.
- Hyperlipidemia, particularly hypercholesterolemia, is also common.
- Hypercoagulability due to loss of proteins C and S and antithrombin III.

COMMON CAUSES

Rule of Thirds for membranous nephropathy:
One-third progress to CRF; one-third have spontaneous remission; one-third remain nephrotic but do not progress.

- **Minimal change disease** (nil disease, lipoid nephrosis):
  - Usually idiopathic, usually found in children.
  - Electron microscopy shows podocyte (epithelial) foot process fusion, but light microscopy shows no change.
  - Usually responds to steroid therapy, though sometimes cytotoxic therapy is required, especially in recurrent cases.
  - Recurs frequently.
  - Rarely progresses to chronic renal failure (unlike the other causes of nephrotic syndrome).
- **Focal segmental glomerulosclerosis (FSGS):**
  - Glomerular scarring involving limited number of glomeruli (segmental involvement).
  - May be primary (idiopathic) or secondary to a known disease.
  - Causes of secondary FSGS include HIV, hepatitis B virus (HBV), heroin abuse, vesicoureteric reflux, morbid obesity causing glomerular hyperfiltration.
  - Immunoglobulin and complement deposition may be detected by immunofluorescence.
  - → hypertension and chronic renal failure.
  - Treatment may include corticosteroids or cytotoxic therapy, as well as ACE inhibitors or angiotensin receptor blockers (ARBs) if non-nephrotic. If secondary FSGS, treatment must also be directed against the primary disease.
- **Membranous nephropathy:**
  - Common cause of adult nephrotic syndrome.
  - Caused by subepithelial immune complex deposition.
  - Idiopathic, or associated with systemic lupus erythematosus (SLE), HBV, or solid tumors.
  - Treat with steroids and cytotoxic agents (chlorambucil or cyclophosphamide).
  - Rule of thirds.
- **Systemic causes:**
  - Sickle cell anemia (papillary damage due to sickling in hyperosmotic medullary interstitium).
  - Diabetic glomerulopathies (diffuse glomerulosclerosis, nodular glomerulosclerosis). Most common secondary cause of nephrotic syndrome.
  - Multiple myeloma (Bence Jones proteinuria from immunoglobulin light chains or their breakdown products).

NEPHROLOGY AND ACID-BASE DISORDERS

Nephritic Syndrome (Glomerulonephritis)

- Indicates inflammation and glomerular damage.
- Involves abrupt-onset hematuria with RBC casts, mild proteinuria; often includes hypertension, edema, and azotemia.
- Acute glomerulonephritis (AGN): Nephritic syndrome (synonym).

POSTSTREPTOCOCCAL GLOMERULONEPHRITIS (PSGN)

- Also called **postinfectious glomerulonephritis.**
- Associated with group A, beta-hemolytic *Streptococcus* (usually associated with preceding pharyngitis or impetigo).
- On immunofluorescence, immune complex deposition with complement (IgG, C3) in a "lumpy-bumpy" pattern between the glomerular epithelial cell and the GBM → glomerular damage.
- Presents ~ 2 weeks after infection with dark urine and edema (periorbital or generalized).
- Usually reversible but occasionally progresses (children often have complete recovery).

LABS

Nephritic sediment (RBC casts), low complement, antistreptolysin O (ASO) antibody titers are helpful in diagnosis.

TREATMENT

- Treat underlying infection.
- Immunosuppressive drugs are ineffective.

IgA NEPHROPATHY (BERGER'S DISEASE)

- Most common glomerulonephritis.
- Presents as hematuria during a viral infection or after exercise.
- On immunofluorescence, immune complex deposition of IgA and C3 in mesangial matrix ("mesangial hypercellularity"). Mesangial proliferation on light microscopy.
- Conservative management with ACE inhibitors or ARBs in patients with normal renal function and minimal proteinuria.
- Pulse corticosteroids in severe cases may be beneficial.

MEMBRANOPROLIFERATIVE GLOMERULONEPHRITIS (MPGN)

- Idiopathic, associated with hepatitis C and cryoglobulinemia, bacterial endocarditis, and autoimmune diseases such as lupus and Sjögren's syndrome.
- On immunofluorescence, subendothelial immune deposits are seen. Basement membrane proliferation causes basement membrane to look double layered ("tram-track"); also mesangial proliferation.
- **Labs:** Nephritic sediment and low complement levels (C3 and C4).
- Frequently progresses to renal failure.
- **Treatment:** Depends on underlying disease, for example, successful treatment of hepatitis C, or plasmapheresis for patients with cryoglobulinemia.

RBC casts are pathognomonic of any glomerulonephritis.

If a patient presents with hematuria immediately after an infection, think *IgA nephropathy.* If a patient presents 2 weeks after infection, think *postinfectious glomerulonephritis.*

Antimicrobial therapy of the initial streptococcal infection does **not** prevent the onset of PSGN (as opposed to rheumatic fever).

NEPHROLOGY AND ACID-BASE DISORDERS

Rapidly Progressive Glomerulonephritis (RPGN)

- Any glomerulonephritis that progresses can subsequently become RPGN.
- Also called *crescentic* GN because biopsy shows epithelial cell proliferation (crescents) in glomeruli.
- Characterized by fulminant renal failure with proteinuria, hematuria, and RBC casts.
- Uncommon.

Classification

Three categories:

1. **Pauci-immune RPGN** (antineutrophil cytoplasmic antibody [ANCA]-associated vasculitis):
   - 50% of RPGN.
   - No immune complex or complement deposition.
   - ANCA is serologic marker for pauci-immune RPGN associated with systemic vasculitis.
   - **Examples:** Churg-Strauss, Wegener's (c-ANCA ⊕), polyarteritis nodosa (p-ANCA ⊕), microscopic polyangiitis (c- or p-ANCA ⊕).
2. **Immune complex RPGN** (granular immunoflourescence):
   - 40% of RPGN.
   - Can be associated with certain medications, syphilis, some malignancies.
   - **Examples:** Postinfectious glomerulonephritis, lupus nephritis, IgA nephropathy, membranoproliferative glomerulonephritis, idiopathic RPGN.
3. **Anti–glomerular basement membrane Ab disease** (linear immunofluorescence):
   - 10% of RPGN.
   - Anti-GBM Ab present in blood—can be seen on GBM with immunofluorescent microscopy.
   - Cytotoxic T-cells contribute to the pathogenesis.
   - **Example:** Goodpasture's syndrome.

> **Anti–glomerular basement membrane Ab disease:**
> In 60–90% of patients, the anti-GBM Ab cross-react with pulmonary alveolar basement membranes—you get both lung and renal manifestations.

Prognosis and Treatment

- Eighty percent of untreated patients progress to end-stage renal disease in 6 months.
- Treat with steroids and cyclophosphamide.

Other Diseases Associated with Acute Nephritic Syndrome

Secondary (multisystem-associated) glomerular diseases:

- **Collagen vascular disorders:**
  - Polyarteritis nodosa
  - SLE
  - Wegener's granulomatosis
  - Henoch-Schönlein purpura (HSP)
- **Hematologic disorders:**
  - Thrombotic thrombocytopenic purpura (TTP)
  - Hemolytic-uremic syndrome
  - Serum sickness

NEPHROLOGY AND ACID-BASE DISORDERS

- **Glomerular basement membrane diseases:**
  - Alport's syndrome
  - Goodpasture's syndrome
  - Thin basement membrane disease

CHRONIC KIDNEY DISEASE (CKD)

↓ renal function (GFR < 60 mL/min per 1.73m²) or evidence of kidney injury for > 3 months.

ETIOLOGY

- **Diabetes mellitus:** Diffuse glomerulosclerosis, nodular glomerulosclerosis (Kimmelstiel-Wilson lesions).
- **Hypertension:** Nephrosclerosis.
- Idiopathic failure.
- **Chronic glomerulonephritis:** RBC casts.
- **Chronic tubulointerstitial diseases:** Sodium wasting, no proteinuria, prolonged obstructive uropathies.
- **Polycystic kidney disease.**

PATHOPHYSIOLOGY

- Nephrons are lost and remaining healthy nephrons compensate by increasing their GFR. This process damages the healthy nephrons causing disease progression.
- Loss of renal endocrine function: ↓ synthesis of activated vitamin D, ammonia, and erythropoietin.

RENAL FUNCTION IN CKD

- Usually asymptomatic until GFR < 30 mL/min per 1.73m².
- **Water and sodium balance:**
  - Initially: ↓ urine concentrating ability, easy dehydration, sodium wasting.
  - Later: Volume overload once the kidneys are no longer able to excrete dietary sodium.
- **Potassium:** Once GFR becomes markedly diminished, the ability to excrete dietary potassium is lost. The distal tubule compensates for the loss of excretory function until there is oliguria.
- **Acid-base balance:** With decreasing GFR, the tubular excretion of H⁺ is impaired secondary to the impaired renal production of ammonia, resulting in anion gap metabolic acidosis.
- **Calcium and phosphate:**
  - Hypocalcemia, hyperphosphatemia.
  - ↓ activation of vitamin D due to loss of 1-hydroxylase activity.
  - Secondary hyperparathyroidism.
  - Renal osteodystrophy: Severe bone resorption.
  - Ectopic calcifications.
- Serum **creatinine** ↑ (creatinine clearance ↓ with ↓ GFR).
- BUN ↑, but to a lesser extent than the creatinine.

Renal biopsy should be performed **prior** (ie, don't wait) to development of end-stage renal disease (ESRD) to provide any hope of identifying the etiology and providing treatment. Once ESRD is established, biopsy will likely only show chronic scarring.

Anemia is common in CKD and is associated with ↑ cardiovascular disease risk as well as accelerated CKD progression. It is due, primarily, to erythropoietin deficiency and is treated to a target hemoglobin of 11 g/dL with erythropoiesis-stimulating agents.

Why creatinine is a measure of kidney function:
Creatinine is neither secreted nor reabsorbed by the nephron, it is only filtered. Therefore, the creatinine clearance is directly proportional to the GFR.

GFR and creatinine clearance:
For each doubling of the serum creatinine, the GFR has ↓ by 50%.

Large kidneys can be seen on sonogram in diabetes, amyloidosis, polycystic kidney disease, and HIV nephropathy, though in diabetes and HIV, they can ultimately become atrophic and small.

SIGNS AND SYMPTOMS

- Uremic syndrome, nephrotic syndrome.
- Ultrasound often reveals shrunken kidneys with cortical thinning.
- Rule out urinary tract infection (UTI) with urine culture.

TREATMENT

- ACE inhibitors may slow progression.
- Treat reversible causes.
- Diet: Modest protein restriction with near normal caloric intake ↓ nitrogen intake and avoids catabolism.
- Dialysis (see below).

Dialysis

- Chronic hemodialysis (HD) is the mainstay of therapy for chronic renal failure, but chronic ambulatory peritoneal dialysis (CAPD) is also an alternative.
- There is no absolute lab value that requires dialysis.
- **The decision is clinical** and based on a constellation of factors.

ABSOLUTE INDICATIONS FOR DIALYSIS

- Uremic pericarditis with or without cardiac tamponade.
- Progressive motor neuropathy.
- Intractable volume overload.
- Life-threatening and intractable hyperkalemia or acidosis.
- Toxins (eg, ethylene glycol).

Indications for Emergent Hemodialysis

A E I O U

Acidosis
Electrolytes (K⁺, Ca²⁺, PO₄⁻)
Ingestions (drugs, toxins)
Overload (volume)
Uremia

CLINICAL FINDINGS RESPONDING TO DIALYSIS (RELATIVE INDICATIONS)

- Fluid and electrolyte imbalances.
- Volume-dependent hypertension.
- Central nervous system (CNS) abnormalities.
- Anemia and bleeding diatheses.
- Anorexia, nausea, and vomiting.
- Weight loss.
- Pruritus and ecchymoses.

HEMODIALYSIS

- The two most commonly used vascular access sites are arteriovenous fistulae (AVF), (usually in the forearm) and artificial grafts inserted between an artery and a vein. Dialysis needles are placed directly into the graft.
- A tunneled dialysis catheter (TDC) is usually placed in the right internal jugular vein and serves as a bridge that allows hemodialysis to take place until AVF or graft is placed.
- Dialysis patients are frequently instrumented, and combined with the dialysis patient's impaired immunity, infection is common. Infective endocarditis may occur if the infections are not recognized early and treated correctly.
- Viral hepatitis is also a risk of hemodialysis, possibly from other patients using the same dialysis machine. For that reason, patients with hepatitis are dialyzed with separate machines.

Patients on chronic medications (cardiac meds, warfarin, chemotherapy, etc.) dramatically drop their serum drug levels during dialysis. The timing and dosing of medication must be decided with the dialysis schedule in mind.

CHRONIC AMBULATORY PERITONEAL DIALYSIS

- A permanent catheter is inserted into the peritoneum, allowing dialysis to be provided to the patient outside the hospital.
- Approximately 2 L of dialysis fluid is infused rapidly and allowed to remain in the peritoneal cavity for 4–6 hours. The fluid is then drained, and new fluid is immediately infused.
- Peritoneum acts as a dialysis membrane.
- Infusion of hypertonic glucose solution allows for concurrent volume reduction.
- Spontaneous bacterial peritonitis (SBP) is a common problem.
- Hypoalbuminemia, hypertriglyceridemia, hypokalemia, and anemia are common.

Uremic Syndrome

Uremia is a syndrome associated with chronic renal failure that affects multiple organ systems.

SIGNS AND SYMPTOMS

- Appearance: Pale complexion, wasting, purpura, excoriation.
- Complaints: Pruritus, polydipsia, nausea, anorexia, vomiting.
- Urinalysis: Isosthenuria, proteinuria, abnormal sediment with tubular casts.

> **Isosthenuria:** Inability of kidney to concentrate urine; fixes specific gravity at 1.010.

SYSTEMIC EFFECTS

- **CNS:** Foot drop, carpal tunnel syndrome, clonus, asterixis, seizures.
- **Cardiac and pulmonary:**
  - Hypertension → left ventricular hypertrophy (LVH) and diastolic dysfunction.
  - Accelerated atherosclerosis, development of ischemic heart disease.
  - Pleuropericardial inflammation (pericarditis with effusion and tamponade).
  - Calcification of mitral and aortic valves.
  - Pulmonary edema and pleural effusions.
- **Hematologic:**
  - Normochromic, normocytic anemia due to ↓ erythropoietin synthesis, among other reasons.
  - Defective platelet function—prolonged bleeding time.
  - White cell function and absolute counts are reduced, resulting in ↑ likelihood of infection.
- **GI:** Mild GI bleeding, nausea/vomiting, anorexia.
- **Metabolic:** Elevated triglycerides, ↓ insulin clearance may → hypoglycemia and perceived improvement in diabetes mellitus.

Polycystic Kidney Disease

- Autosomal dominant.
- Kidneys are enlarged and have multiple cysts.
- Patients typically present in their 30s or 40s with flank pain or hematuria.
- Approximately 50% of patients will develop end-stage renal disease by the age of 60.
- Associated extrarenal manifestations are berry aneurysms (subarachnoid hemorrhage), hepatic cysts, pancreatic cysts. and diverticula.

NEPHROLOGY AND ACID-BASE DISORDERS

- Complications of polycystic kidneys are hypertension, recurrent UTIs, and kidney stones (calcium oxalate and uric acid stones).
- Diagnose via ultrasound or computed tomography (CT) scan.

Renal Tubular Acidosis

Defect in renal tubular ability to excrete daily acid load created by the metabolism of protein or to reabsorb filtered bicarbonate, which results in a metabolic acidosis with a normal anion gap.

ETIOLOGY

- There are three types (see Table 2.6-6): 1, 2, and 4 (there is no type 3).
- May be inherited or acquired via medications or disease states.
- Types 1 and 4 occur in the distal tubules.
- Type 2 occurs in the proximal tubule.

PATHOPHYSIOLOGY

- **Type 1** is caused by a distal tubule defect in hydrogen secretion causing acidosis and hypokalemia.
  - Can be caused by autoimmune diseases (SLE, rheumatoid arthritis, Sjögren's syndrome), medication (lithium, amphotericin B).
  - Patients may also get renal stones due to hypercalcemia.
- **Type 2** is caused by a defect in proximal bicarbonate reabsorption (bicarbonate wasting), usually in the setting of Fanconi's syndrome (generalized proximal tubule dysfunction).
  - The bicarbonate loss is self-limiting as the distal tubules can absorb some bicarbonate and bicarbonate levels reach a new, lower set point.
  - Can be caused by multiple myeloma, heavy metals, carbonic anyhydrase inhibitors (acetazolamide).
  - Potassium can be low to normal.
- **Type 4 = hypoaldosteronism** and is caused by a defect in aldosterone secretion or aldosterone sensitivity by the renal tubules and ammonium excretion. The effect is similar to that of a potassium-sparing diuretic.
  - Patients usually have low renin and aldosterone levels.
  - The hallmark of type 4 RTA is **hyperkalemia,** and patients are usually managed with potassium-wasting diuretics or fludrocortisone.
  - May be a primary defect or caused by diabetic nephropathy, obstructive uropathy, or other kidney diseases.

Urolithiasis

Calculi in the urogenital system.

TABLE 2.6-6. RTA Types

	DEFECT	**PLASMA BICARBONATE LEVEL**	**URINE pH**	**PLASMA K+**
Type 1 RTA	Impaired acidification of urine	Low	> 5.3	Low
Type 2 RTA	↓ bicarbonate resorption	12–20	< 5.3	Low to normal
Type 4 RTA	↓ aldosterone	Typically > 17	< 5.3	**High**

- One of the most common diseases of the urinary tract.
- Two to five percent of the population will form a urinary stone at some point in their lives.
- Majority of stones form between the ages of 20 and 50.
- Male-to-female ratio of 3:1.
- Familial tendency in stone formation.
- Tendency for recurrence—36% of patients with a first stone will have another stone within 1 year.

TYPES OF STONES

- **Calcium oxalate stones** (75%):
  - Strongly radiopaque.
  - Treat with thiazides to ↓ calciuria.
  - ↑ incidence in inflammatory bowel disease (↑ oxalate), hypercalcemia (hyperparathyroidism), ↓ citrate (forms stable soluble complex with calcium), uricosuria (small urate crystals serve as nidus for larger calcium stones).
- **Struvite (Mg NH4 PO4) stones** (15%):
  - Moderately radiopaque.
  - Common in *Proteus* UTIs due to high urinary pH (*Proteus* makes urease, which cleaves urinary urea, yielding two molecules of ammonia—the conjugate base of ammonium ion).
  - Treat by lowering urine pH.
- **Uric acid stones** (< 1%):
  - Radiolucent.
  - ↑ incidence in myeloproliferative diseases and gout (due to ↑ purine turnover).
  - Treat by raising urine pH.
- **Cystine stones** (< 1%):
  - Moderately radiopaque.
  - Seen in congenital cystinuria (*not* homocystinuria).
  - Hexagonal crystals, positively birefringent.
  - Treat by raising urine pH.

PREDISPOSING FACTORS

- Dietary history—large calcium and alkali intake.
- Prolonged immobilization.
- Residence in hot climate.
- History of UTIs.
- History of calculus in the past and in family members.
- Drug ingestion (analgesics, alkalis, uricosuric agents, protease inhibitors).
- Prior history of gout.
- Underlying gastrointestinal disease (Crohn's, ulcerative colitis, peptic ulcer disease).

A 39-year-old man presents with severe back pain and hematuria. He is writhing in the bed, unable to find a comfortable position, and is nauseous. *Think: Renal colic due to urolithiasis.* **Next step:** Order noncontrast CT abdomen and pelvis to determine size and location of stone.

TABLE 2.6-7. Interpretation of the Urinalysis

FINDING	SIGNIFICANCE
Color	■ Red or brown indicates presence of hemoglobin, myoglobin (as with rhabdomyolysis), or red food (beets).
Clarity	■ Normal urine should be clear. ■ Turbidity or cloudiness can be caused by excessive cellular material (often as WBCs in pyuria or casts), protein, or precipitation of salts.

pH	Normal pH ranges from 4.5 to 7.5.
	  ■ Alkaline urine indicates type 1 RTA or UTI with *Proteus* or *Ureaplasma*.
	  ■ Acidic urine can be seen with aspirin overdose or type 2 RTA.

Specific gravity	■ Normal specific gravity is 1.002–1.035. ■ High (> 1.010) indicates dehydration. ■ Inability to concentrate urine in the setting of dehydration indicates renal disease.
Protein	■ Proteinuria indicates glomerular dysfunction. ■ Microalbuminuria is a marker for early diabetic nephropathy. ■ Protein loss in urine of > 3 g/day is nephritic syndrome.
Glucose	■ Glucose in urine can indicate hyperglycemia.
Ketones	Seen in diabetic ketoacidosis, isopropyl alcohol intoxication, and starvation ketosis.
Nitrite	■ Normal is $\ominus$. ■ $\oplus$ nitrite indicates bacteria present in the urine, usually gram-$\ominus$ rods.
Leukocyte esterase	■ $\oplus$ findings indicate the presence of white cells and infection.
RBCs	Present in glomerulonephritis, tumor, trauma, renal stones, renal infarct, malignant hypertension (also often erroneously $\oplus$ in menstruating females).
WBCs	■ Also called pyuria; seen in UTIs, prostatitis, vaginitis.
Eosinophils	■ Seen in acute interstitial nephritis (AIN).
Squamous epithelial cells	■ From the skin surface or outer urethra; a measure of contamination.

Casts	■ Urinary casts are formed in the distal convoluted tubule and the collecting duct.
	  ■ RBC casts: Glomerulonephritis.
	  ■ WBC casts: Pyelonephritis or glomerulonephritis.
	  ■ Muddy brown granular casts: ATN.
	  ■ Hyaline casts: Prerenal azotemia.

Crystals	■ Renal stones, ethylene glycol intoxication.
Bilirubin	■ Extravascular hemolysis.
Hemoglobin	■ Intravascular hemolysis.

- Severe, abrupt onset of colicky pain that begins in the flank and may radiate toward the groin. In males, the pain may radiate toward the testicle. In females, it may radiate toward the labia majoris.
- Nausea and vomiting are almost universal with acute renal colic.
- Abdominal distention from secondary ileus.
- Gross hematuria.

DIAGNOSIS

- **Urinalysis** (Table 2.6-7).
  - Vast majority of patients (about 85%) will have RBCs in the urine. However, a lack of RBCs on urinalysis does not rule out renal stones.
  - Urinary pH can aid in differentiating the type of stone present. Normal urinary pH is about 5.85. If the pH is > 6, one should suspect the presence of urea-splitting organisms (*Proteus*). A low urine pH (≤ 5) suggests uric acid stones.
  - WBCs or bacteria may suggest underlying urinary tract infection and should be aggressively treated.
- **Radiographic studies:**
  - See Infectious Disease chapter for table on common genitourinary procedures.
  - Plain abdominal film (KUB) will reveal only radiopaque stones (60–70%).
  - Renal ultrasound is useful to detect hydronephrosis and is easy, cheap, and doesn't require subjecting the patient to IV contrast. It misses small stones.
  - Noncontrast renal CT is most useful to diagnose small stones. It can accurately locate stones in the renal collecting system and detect the presence of hydronephrosis. Overall sensitivity is about 95%.
  - Intravenous pyelogram (IVP) has been the gold standard for the diagnosis of renal and ureteral calculi. It can clearly outline the entire urinary system making it easy to see hydronephrosis and the presence of any type of stones. In addition, an IVP can demonstrate renal function and allow for verification that the opposite kidney is functioning properly.

TREATMENT

- Analgesia.
- Hydration.
- **Passage of stones:**
  - Ninety percent of stones < 5 mm will pass spontaneously.
  - Fifteen percent of stones 5–8 mm will pass.
  - Five percent of stones > 8 mm will pass.
- **For stones unlikely to pass spontaneously:**
  - Extracorporeal shock wave lithotripsy (ESWL) has been effective for stones located in the kidney with 85% success rate.
  - Percutaneous nephrolithotomy, which establishes a tract from the skin to the collecting system, is used when stones are too large or too hard for lithotripsy.
  - New laser techniques are becoming mainstays of therapy for extracting large stones.

Pulmonology

↓ delivery/utilization of oxygen at tissue level. A variety of cardiorespiratory diseases can cause hypoxia by some basic mechanisms:

A married couple comes to the hospital complaining of "flulike" symptoms, including headache, nausea, vomiting, and disorientation. The wife thinks they caught the virus from a neighbor when they borrowed his home generator. *Think: Carbon monoxide poisoning.* **Next step:** Check carboxyhemoglobin levels.

> The most important determinant of the amount of oxygen delivery to tissues is *hemoglobin.*

- **V/Q mismatch:** When perfusion and ventilation to different areas of lungs are not proportionately matched, causing some of the ventilation or perfusion to go to waste. *Responds to supplemental oxygen.*
  - **Examples:** Chronic obstructive pulmonary disease (COPD), congestive heart failure (CHF), pulmonary fibrosis, and asthma.
  - **Dead space ventilation:** When a part of the lungs receives ventilation, but the blood supply is interrupted as in pulmonary embolism (PE).
- **Right-to-left shunt:** Intrapulmonary shunting of blood, due to perfusion of the nonventilated lung (as in lung consolidation), or extrapulmonary, such as congenital heart disease.
- **Diffusion defect:** Gas exchange compromised due to a defect in the alveolar interface, as seen in interstitial lung disease.
- In the *absence* of cardiorespiratory disease, hypoxia may be the result of:
  - **Anemia:** ↓ hemoglobin ↓ oxygen carrying capacity, has a normal PaO_2, ↓ PvO_2 (due to ↑ extraction from the tissues).

  Arterial oxygen content = $PaO_2 \times 0.0031 + 1.36 \times Hb \times SaO_2$

  - **Improper utilization of delivered oxygen in the tissues:** Cytochrome impairment due to cyanide poisoning, diphtheria toxin, etc.
  - **Low inspired oxygen:** At high altitude or other low-oxygen environment.
  - **Carbon monoxide (CO) poisoning:** CO has much higher affinity for hemoglogin than oxygen; carboxyhemoglobin is unavailable for oxygen transport; O_2 unloaded at much lower oxygen tensions, resulting in impaired delivery to tissues. CO poisoning does not cause cyanosis. At highly toxic levels, it can cause a "cherry red" discoloration of lips and nails.
  - **Hypoventilation:** Occurs with obesity-hypoventilation syndrome, neuromuscular disorders (Guillain-Barré, myasthenia gravis, amyotrophic lateral sclerosis [ALS]).

LUNG PHYSICAL EXAM

- **Inspection:** Best done with the patient standing.
  - Look for evidence of respiratory distress such as nasal flaring, accessory muscle use, pursed-lip breathing (common in COPD), and intercostal retractions.

PULMONOLOGY

- Also look for chest wall deformities such as kyphoscoliosis or pectus excavatum.
- Look for evidence of recent trauma such as bruising, bleeding, or "flail chest."

- **Auscultation:** See Table 2.7-1.
- **Breath sounds:**
  - **Normal** (vesicular): Breath sounds are low pitched and are heard throughout inspiration and most of early expiration.
  - **Bronchial:** Breath sounds are high pitched and heard equally well during both inspiration and expiration.
  - **Crackles (rales):** Short, discontinuous nonmusical sounds heard mostly during inspiration ("crunchy").
  - **Wheezes/rhonchi:** Continuous, musical, high-pitched sounds heard mostly during expiration. Both terms are usually used interchangeably.
  - **Pleural rub:** Grating sound produced by motion of pleura, heard best at end of inspiration/beginning of expiration.
  - **Stridor:** Discontinuous sound usually best heard during inspiration. Signifies upper airway narrowing or obstruction by foreign body, tumor, or laryngospasm.
  - **Egophony:** Spoken words by the patient are ↑ in intensity and take on different quality during auscultation. Patient says "eeee" and will be heard as "aaaa." Signifies "solid" lung tissue in communication with a patent bronchus, as in areas of consolidation and in areas of compressed lung above the upper level of a pleural effusion.
- **Palpation:**
  - **Tactile fremitus:** Performed by placing ulnar side of hand or palm against the patient's chest wall and having the patient say "ninety-nine." Vibrations are felt through the chest wall and can be compared from one side to the other. A local or unilateral difference in tactile fremitus is of clinical importance.
    - ↑ tactile fremitus = ↑ density of the lung parenchyma (consolidation).
    - ↓ tactile fremitus = excess subcutaneous tissue on the chest, air or fluid in pleural cavity (pneumothorax, pleural effusion) or overexpansion of lung.

Clinical Pearl: Sound travels better through *solid* (lung consolidation) than *liquid* (pleural effusion). For example, if you put your ear to the ground, you can hear the train coming, but if you are under water, you won't be able to hear your friend shout your name.

TABLE 2.7-1. Lung Auscultation

TERM	MECHANISM	CAUSES
Crackle (rale)	Excessive airway secretions.	Bronchitis, pneumonia, pulmonary edema, atelectasis, fibrosis.
Wheeze	Rapid airflow through obstructed airway.	Asthma, pulmonary edema, bronchitis.
Rhonchus	Transient airway plugging.	Bronchitis.
Pleural rub	Inflammation of the pleura.	Pneumonia, pulmonary infarction.

- **Percussion:** Tapping the chest wall to evaluate underlying structures. The sound produced depends on the air-tissue ratio of the structure involved.
  - **Dull:** Dullness over the chest implies ↑ density, as when the air in the lungs is replaced by fluid or solid tissue. Examples include consolidation, a lung mass, or fluid surrounding the lung as in pleural effusion. (Percussion over the liver will reveal *dull* sounds.)
  - **Flat:** Large muscle mass (thigh).
  - **Tympanic:** Hollow, air-containing structure (percussion over the stomach will yield *tympanic* sounds).
  - **Resonant:** Structure composed of air within tissue (normal lung).
  - **Hyperresonant:** Structure with ↓ density and ↑ amount of air, such as in emphysema, or a large pneumothorax.

PLEURAL EFFUSION

Abnormal accumulation of fluid within the space between the parietal and visceral pleural membranes of the lungs. Pleural effusion is classified as a transudative or exudative.
- **Transudative** pleural effusions are due to:
  - ↑ hydrostatic pressure as in heart failure.
  - ↓ oncotic pressure, as in nephrotic syndrome.
- **Exudative** pleural effusions are due to ↑ capillary permeability, usually secondary to an inflammatory process.

DIAGNOSIS

- Any pleural effusion of unclear etiology should be tapped for diagnostic pleural fluid analysis.
- Any pleural fluid should be analyzed for total and differential cell count, protein, glucose, lactate dehydrogenase (LDH), and pH (if there is suspicion of empyema).
- **Light's criteria** *(learn this for exam):* The effusion is an **exudate** if **one** or more of the following is present:
  - Ratio of pleural to serum protein > 0.5.
  - Ratio of pleural to serum lactic dehydrogenase (LDH) > 0.6.
  - Pleural fluid LDH > ⅔ upper normal limit of serum LDH.
- An effusion is a **transudate** if **none** of the above criteria is fulfilled.

Transudates	Exudates
■ **CHF**	■ **Infection**
■ Cirrhosis	■ Tumor
■ Nephrosis	■ Trauma

COMMON ASSOCIATIONS

- **Parapneumonic effusion:** As the name suggests, it should be suspected if an effusion develops in the setting of a pneumonia. Any parapneumonic effusion is an exudate, with a high neutrophil count.
  - A "simple" parapneumonic effusion can become "complex" and "complicated" if any of the following is present:
    - pH < 7.2
    - Glucose < 40 mg/dL
    - LDH > 1000
    - ⊕ Gram stain or culture

- When frank pus can be aspirated, the term *empyema* is used. Complicated parapneumonic effusions and empyemas can also become loculated.
- **Gross blood:**
  - Tumor (breast cancer, lung cancer, lymphoma).
  - Pulmonary infarction.
  - Hemothorax: Defined as pleural fluid hematocrit > 50% of serum hematocrit; this is a **surgical emergency!** Causes include trauma and aortic dissection.
- **Low glucose:**
  - Complicated parapneumonic effusion and empyema.
  - Rheumatoid arthritis (glucose extremely low, usually < 15 mg/dL).
  - Tumor: Indicator of poor prognosis.
  - Tuberculosis.
- **High amylase:**
  - Pancreatitis.
  - Renal failure.
  - Tumor.
  - Esophageal rupture: High *salivary* amylase is useful in diagnosis. **Surgical emergency** with high mortality if not treated immediately!

Empyema (pus in pleural space), ⊕ cultures, or loculated effusions always require chest tube.

PULMONARY FUNCTION TESTS (PFTs)

- **Spirometry:** Measures the rate at which the lung volume *changes* during forced breathing.
- **Forced vital capacity (FVC):** Patient inhales maximally, then exhales as rapidly and completely as possible for > 6 sec. The exhalation and subsequent inhalation are recorded as a flow volume curve.
- **FEV_1:** The volume of air exhaled in the first second of the FVC maneuver.
- FEV_1, FVC, and the ratio between them (FEV_1/FVC) are important parameters to determine the nature of lung disease and severity (see Table 2.7-2). The values obtained in a patient are compared with the expected normal values for that age, sex, height, and ethnic background.
  - Normal FEV_1 = > 80% of predicted.
  - Normal FVC = > 80% of predicted.
  - Normal FEV_1/FVC ratio = > 0.7.
- **Obstructive lung disease:** FEV_1 is disproportionately reduced compared to FVC; therefore FEV_1/FVC ratio is low. FEV_1/FVC ratio of < 70% is a key parameter to diagnose obstruction. Seen with airway diseases like chronic bronchitis, emphysema, and asthma.

TABLE 2.7-2. Pulmonary Function Tests

NORMAL SPIROMETRY	OBSTRUCTIVE LUNG DISEASE	RESTRICTIVE LUNG DISEASE
▪ FVC normal	▪ FVC normal or ↓	▪ FVC ↓
▪ FEV_1 normal	▪ FEV_1 ↓	▪ FEV_1 normal or ↓
▪ FEV_1/FVC > 0.7	▪ FEV_1/FVC < 0.7	▪ FEV_1/FVC > 0.7
	▪ Lung volume normal or ↑	▪ Lung volume *always* ↓

PULMONOLOGY

- **Restrictive lung disease:** Seen with interstitial lung diseases, neuromuscular diseases (ALS, myasthenia gravis, Guillain–Barré), chest wall disorders (obesity, kyphoscoliosis). Both FEV_1 and FVC are low, but their ratio is usually normal or elevated.
- **Lung volume measurements:** Lung volumes such as total lung capacity (TLC), functional residual capacity (FRC), and residual volume (RV) can be measured by using body plethysmography or helium dilution techniques.
- **Diffusion capacity of carbon monoxide (DL_{CO}):** Using trace amounts of CO in the inhaled gas mixture, diffusion of alveolar air across pulmonary capillaries can be assessed. DL_{CO} is a very useful test for diagnosis and follow up for patients with interstitial lung diseases, in which this value is usually ↓.

LUNG INFECTIONS

Pneumonia

Infection of the lung parenchyma by any microorganism.

- **Community-acquired pneumonia (CAP):** Pneumonia diagnosed in patients within 48 hours of hospital admission who do not meet criteria for health care–associated pneumonia.
- **Health care–associated pneumonia (HCAP):** Pneumonia diagnosed within 48 hours of hospital admission in patients who have ≥ 1 of the following risk factors for being infected with organisms resistant to multiple antibiotics:
  - Hospitalization for ≥ 2 days in an acute-care facility within previous 90 days (most common and also most likely to cause infection with resistant organisms).
  - Residence in a nursing home or long-term care facility.
  - Antibiotic therapy, chemotherapy, or wound care within 30 days of current infection (lower risk).
  - Hemodialysis treatment at a hospital or clinic (lower risk).
  - Home infusion therapy or home wound care (low risk).
- **Hospital acquired pneumonia (HAP):** Pneumonia developing at least 48 hours after hospital admission. HAP may be due to multidrug-resistant (MDR) organisms if any of the following are present:
  - Antibiotic therapy within 90 days of infection.
  - Current hospitalization of > 5 days.
  - High frequency of antibiotic resistance in the specific hospital unit.
  - Immunosuppressive disease or therapy.
  - Presence of HCAP risk factors for MDR.

 A 27-year-old patient has pneumonia, bullous myringitis, and a chest film that looks worse than expected. *Think:* Mycoplasma pneumoniae.

A patient with HIV who has a CD4 count of 52 does not take antiretroviral medications or trimethoprim-sulfamethoxazole, is hypoxic on room air, and has a diffuse bilateral infiltrates on chest film. *Think:* Pneumocystis jiroveci *pneumonia (PCP).*

An elderly man presents with pneumonia, GI symptoms, bradycardia, and hyponatremia. *Think: Legionella.*

ETIOLOGY

See Table 2.7-3 for organisms affecting immunocompetent host and Table 2.7-4 for those affecting immunocompromised hosts.

PATHOPHYSIOLOGY

Pathogenic bacteria reach alveoli in one of the following ways:

- **Inhalation:** Aspiration of (colonized) nasopharyngeal, oral, or gastric contents.
- **Hematogenous spread:** Direct inoculation (stab wounds, endotracheal tube).

SIGNS AND SYMPTOMS

Patients with pneumonia may have few signs or symptoms, or may be extremely ill.

- **Typical symptoms:**
  - Fever
  - Cough with sputum production
  - Pleuritic chest pain

Pneumonias causing relative bradycardia (slower-than-expected heart rate for temperature or disease, but above 60 bpm):
- *Legionella*
- *Salmonella*
- *Chlamydia psittaci*

TABLE 2.7-3. Likely Organisms Causing Pneumonia in Immunocompetent Host

Community acquired, typical
1. *Streptococcus pneumoniae*
2. *Haemophilus influenzae*
Community acquired, atypical
1. *Chlamydia pneumoniae*
2. *Legionella pneumophila*
3. *Mycoplasma pneumoniae*
Hospital acquired
1. *Pseudomonas aeruginosa*
2. *Staphylococcus aureus*
3. Enteric organisms

TABLE 2.7-4. Causes of Pneumonia in Immunocompromised Host

HIV INFECTION	CD4 COUNT/DL
Mycobacterium tuberculosis	< 500
Pneumocystis jiroveci (PCP)	< 200
Histoplasma capsulatum	< 200
Cryptococcus neoformans	< 200
Mycobacterium avium-intracellulare	< 50
Cytomegalovirus	< 50

Neutropenia:
1. *Pseudomonas aeruginosa*
2. Enterobacteriaceae
3. *Staphylococcus aureus*
4. *Aspergillus*

Splenectomy, sickle cell anemia:
Encapsulated organisms

Chronic steroid use:
1. *M tuberculosis*
2. *Nocardia*

Alcoholics:
1. *Streptococcus pneumoniae*
2. *Haemophilus influenzae*
3. *Klebsiella pneumoniae*
4. *M tuberculosis*

- Atypical symptoms:
  - Dry cough
  - Headache
  - Malaise
  - Gastrointestinal (GI) symptoms

PHYSICAL EXAM

- Dullness to percussion.
- Rales.
- Tactile fremitus in consolidated lobe or segment.
- Egophony (E to A changes) with stethoscope.
- Respiratory distress depending on severity.

DIAGNOSIS

- **Chest x-ray (CXR):** Most patients with pneumonia will have an infiltrate on x-ray corresponding to a lobe or segment. Sometimes they can have bilateral infiltrates. In some cases, the localization and/or nature of infiltrates can give clues to the etiologic agents:
  - Upper lobe (*Mycobacterium tuberculosis, Klebsiella*).
  - Small cavities without air-fluid levels (*M tuberculosis*).
  - Large cavities with air-fluid levels (*Staphylococcus* spp, anaerobes, gram-⊖, coccidiomycosis, nocardiosis).
  - Diffuse bilateral infiltrate (PCP, *Mycoplasma*).
- **Gram stain:** An adequate sputum sample should contain:
  - < 10 epithelial cells per low-power field (the fewer the better).
  - > 25 leukocytes per low-power field.
- **Culture:** Once an organism is identified on sputum culture, antibiotics should be tailored to cover this organism if possible.

SEVERITY ASSESSMENT

- Mainly used for CAP to determine need for admission and strategy for management.
- There are many scoring systems available. One of the simpler ways to assess severity of pneumonia is the **CURB-65 score** (see Table 2.7-5):
  - **0–1 point:** Low risk. Consider outpatient treatment.
  - **2 points:** Higher severity. Consider short hospitalization or closely observed outpatient therapy.
  - **3–5 points:** Severe pneumonia. Hospitalization strongly recommended, consider ICU care if higher score.
- Remember, there are many scoring systems out there, but they serve only as *guides*. The most important tool you have is your clinical judgment. If you feel a patient is very ill and requires more aggressive care, you should always provide it.

If a patient develops a postinfluenza pneumonia, think *Pneumococcus.*

If there are no bacteria on Gram stain, consider *Legionella* and *Mycoplasma.*

If you see **currant jelly sputum**, think *Klebsiella.*

If you see **rusty sputum**, think *Pneumococcus.*

Loeffler's pneumonia is idiopathic eosinophilic pneumonia.

TABLE 2.7-5. Pneumonia Severity Assessment

CURB-65	POINTS
Confusion	1
Blood **U**rea nitrogen > 19 mg per dL	1
Respiratory rate ≥ 30 breaths per minute	1
Systolic **B**lood pressure < 90 mmHg or Diastolic blood pressure ≤ 60 mmHg	1
Age ≥ **65** years	1
Total points:	

Steroid administration in PCP prevents respiratory failure and improves survival. Give for:
- A-a gradient > 35
- PaO$_2$ < 75

TREATMENT

The best choices for empiric coverage until cultures are completed depend on the type of pneumonia as defined above.

- **Community-acquired** (cover for both typicals and atypicals):
  - No risk factors: Macrolide (azithromycin).
  - Risk factors present (CHF, diabetes, etc.): Macrolide and second-/third-generation cephalosporin.
  - Alternatively, respiratory flouroquinolone such as moxifloxacin or levofloxacin.
- **Hospital-acquired:** Need *Pseudomonas* coverage with imipenem or piperacillin-tazobactam), if severe add coverage for methicillin-resistant *Staphylococcus aureus* (MRSA) with vancomycin.
- **Immunocompromised:** Add PCP coverage (trimethoprim-sulfamethoxazole ([TMP-SMZ]).

Tuberculosis

Tuberculosis (TB) is a leading cause of death worldwide. In the United States, the incidence of TB ↓ every year until 1984, with a resurgence during the HIV epidemic.

PATHOPHYSIOLOGY

Transmission occurs by inhalation of droplet nuclei produced by the cough or sneeze of a patient with pulmonary TB disease. Particles may remain suspended in air for several hours:

- Five percent of those infected will develop TB disease in 2 years.
- Five percent more will develop TB disease in their lifetime.
- Ninety percent will remain infected but disease free.

EPIDEMIOLOGY

Sites of TB disease:
- Lungs (85% of all cases)
- Central nervous system (TB meningitis)
- Lymphatics
- Genitourinary system
- Bones (Pott's disease)
- Disseminated TB (miliary)

- **High-prevalence groups:**
  - HIV-infected persons.
  - Close contacts of persons with TB disease.
  - IV drug users.
  - Immunocompromised persons (non-HIV).
  - Foreign-born persons.
  - Residents of medically underserved communities.
  - Prisoners.
  - Homeless.
- **High risk for active tuberculosis once infected:**
  - HIV-infected persons.
  - IV drug users.
  - Immunocompromised persons (non-HIV).
  - Abnormal CXR.

SYMPTOMS

- Productive cough
- **Night sweats**
- **Hemoptysis**
- Anorexia
- Weight loss
- Fever, chills, fatigue
- Chest pain

PULMONOLOGY

DIAGNOSIS

- **Findings:**
  - ⊕ purified protein derivative (PPD): Indicative of infection, *not* active disease.
  - Infiltrate or granuloma in upper lobes of lungs.
  - Acid-fast bacilli (AFB) on sputum microscopy.
- **How to use the TB skin test:**
  1. Screen patients in high-prevalence groups.
  2. Gives a ⊕ reaction 2–10 weeks after infection.
  3. Plant 0.1 mL of PPD intradermally on volar aspect of the forearm.
  4. Read 48–72 hours after placement.
  5. Measure induration, not erythema (see Table 2.7-6).
- **False ⊕:**
  - *Bacillus Calmette–Guérin (BCG)* vaccination will result in false ⊕ for a period of 10–15 years. Immigrants receiving BCG vaccine as children should not be ⊕ as adults over 25–30 years old.
  - Nontuberculous mycobacterial infection.
- **False ⊖:**
  - Ten to twenty-five percent of patients with TB infection have ⊖ skin tests.
  - The two-step TB skin test is used in high-prevalence patients who have a ⊖ first test: The first test boosts the immune response to a second skin test, which will turn ⊕ in infected patients.

Anergy (does not mount response) can be screened for, by planting the common antigens *mumps* and *Candida* intradermally. If no response, PPD testing is useless.

TREATMENT

- **Latent TB:**
  - Isoniazid (INH) daily for 9 months (may be given twice weekly if directly observed therapy [DOT] is used).
  - Rifampin daily for 4 months if in contact with people with INH-resistant TB.
  - Close contacts of active tuberculosis patients with ⊖ PPD should be retested in 10 weeks.
  - Pregnant women should wait until after delivery for treatment unless high risk (eg, HIV).

T A B L E 2 . 7 - 6 . Interpretation of PPD Skin Test

MEASURED INDURATION		
≥ 15 MM	≥ 10 MM	≥ 5 MM
All patients are considered infected	Considered infected if:	Considered infected if:
	■ IV drug user	■ HIV
	■ Foreign born	■ Close contact
	■ Medically underserved	■ Abnormal CXR
	■ Nursing home resident	■ Immunocompromised
	■ Prisoner	
	■ Child under age 4	
	■ Health care worker (you)	
	■ Other medical problems	

PULMONOLOGY

- **Active TB:**
  - Standard regimen for pulmonary TB: 2 months of INH, rifampin, pyrazinamide, and ethambutol followed by 4 months of INH/rifampin.
  - Pregnant with TB: 2 months of INH, rifampin, and ethambutol followed by INH and rifampin (no ethambutol) for 7 more months.
  - Meningeal, skeletal, and sometimes lymph node TB are treated with longer duration of antituberculous antibiotics.
- **Infectivity:** People are considered no longer infectious when they are undergoing appropriate therapy, improving clinically, and have had three consecutive sputum smears on different days ⊖ for TB.

TOXICITY OF TB MEDICATION

Pink puffers (emphysema):
- Barrel-shaped chest
- Thin and emaciated
- High PCO_2, normal to low PO_2

- **INH:**
  - Peripheral neuropathy (can be prevented with administration of pyridoxine).
  - Seizures in overdose: These can be very difficult to break with standard measures—remember to give pyridoxine!
  - Hepatitis (check liver function tests each month).
- **Rifampin:**
  - Induces hepatic microsomal enzymes; also hepatotoxic.
  - Is excreted as a **red-orange compound in urine,** stool, sweat, and tears; will discolor contact lenses.
- **Ethambutol:** Optic neuritis and impaired color vision are related to cumulative dose.

Blue bloaters (chronic bronchitis):
- Right heart failure
- Polycythemia
- High PCO_2, low PO_2

 A patient is brought in by ambulance in status epilepticus. The patient's family member says he has no medical history except TB. *Think:* INH toxicity. **Next step:** Treat with pyridoxine.

OBSTRUCTIVE AIRWAY DISORDERS

Chronic Obstructive Pulmonary Disease (COPD)

Chronic bronchitis and emphysema are forms of chronic obstructive pulmonary disease. COPD is defined by a chronic obstruction to expiratory airflow, largely irreversible, as evidenced by a ↓ in FEV_1. The term *COPD* is preferred to describe both chronic bronchitis and emphysema, as many patients have elements of each disease.

Patients with severe emphysema will lose weight for a variety of reasons. For example, the work of breathing is highly taxing metabolically; in addition, stopping to chew food and swallow prevents adequate oxygenation, so patients avoid eating in severe cases.

- **Chronic bronchitis:** Defined as chronic productive cough on most days for ≥ 3 months in each of 2 successive years; may or may not be accompanied by chronic expiratory airflow obstruction.
- **Emphysema:** Permanent enlargement of the air space distal to the terminal bronchioles due to destruction of alveolar septa. A pathological entity whose clinical correlate is chronic expiratory airflow obstruction with evidence of hyperinflation.

PULMONOLOGY

PATHOPHYSIOLOGY OF EMPHYSEMA

- **Centrilobular** emphysema affects the respiratory bronchioles and surrounding alveoli. Usually in smokers, predominantly in the *upper lobes*.
- **Panlobular or panacinar emphysema** occurs in patients with α_1-antitrypsin deficiency. α_1-antitrypsin protects against the degradation of lung elastin. The whole of pulmonary lobules are destroyed. Seen predominantly in *lower lobes*.

EPIDEMIOLOGY

- Higher prevalence in men.
- Mortality rates are higher in whites.
- Only 15% of smokers develop COPD.

RISK FACTORS

- Smoking.
- α_1-antitrypsin deficiency (autosomal recessive inheritance, more common in Mediterraneans).

DIAGNOSIS/FINDINGS

- **Clinical presentation:** Usually with slowly progressive shortness of breath on exertion.
- **Physical exam:** Barrel chest, ↓ air entry with prolonged expiration, wheezes.
- **CXR:** Hyperinflated lungs, low and flattened diaphragm.
- **PFTs:** Irreversible obstructive pattern (low FEV_1 low FEV_1/FVC. The severity of COPD is defined by the extent of loss of FEV_1.
- **Electrocardiogram (ECG):** May show right-sided strain pattern. Also, multifocal atrial tachycardia is a common supraventricular tachycardia seen in these patients.
- **Computed tomography (CT):** Shows loss of alveolar walls in emphysema.

TREATMENT

- **Smoking cessation:** The only intervention proven to slow down the loss of pulmonary function.
- **Oxygen:** Has also been shown to **improve** COPD patients' IQ, exercise tolerance, and **mortality!** Oxygen should be given to:
  - Patients with a resting PaO_2 of < 55 mmHg.
  - Patients with PaO_2 of 55–59 who have cor pulmonale, erythrocytosis, or who desaturate during exercise.
- Maintain vaccination against influenza and *Streptococcus pneumoniae*.
- Beta agonists and anticholinergics (ipratropium bromide, tiotropium) improve FEV_1 modestly.
- Inhaled corticosteroids (eg, fluticasone, budesonide) are helpful in patients with severe COPD (FEV_1 < 50% predicted and frequent infective exacerbations).
- Antibiotics for acute infective exacerbations of COPD reduce the duration of COPD exacerbation symptoms by 20% and ↓ hospital admissions by 50%. A course of steroids can also help in resolution of COPD exacerbations.

Supplemental oxygen is the only therapy for COPD proven to extend life.

NSAIDs can precipitate an asthma attack. Watch for this in a patient with a history of asthma who takes ibuprofen for a headache.

Cough-variant asthma: Cough is the patient's only symptom. The diagnosis of asthma is demonstrated by response to asthma-specific treatment.

MDIs deliver smaller particles than nebulizers and therefore reach the smallest airways better. Nebulizers are favored for hospital treatment because of ease of use.

Asthma

A chronic condition characterized by airway inflammation, bronchoconstriction, and hypersecretion. It is reversible (typically with bronchodilators).

PATHOPHYSIOLOGY

- Airway inflammation occurs in response to allergen exposure. The early phase of asthma is immunoglobulin E (IgE) mediated, associated with histamine release from mast cells.
- The late phase is associated with cytokine release and eosinophil infiltration, and is improved by steroids.

TRIGGERS

- Exposure to various allergens from pets, dust, pollen, etc., → inflammation and airway hyperreactivity.
- Once airway hyperreactivity is established, an asthma attack may be induced by nonspecific triggers like exercise, cold air, strong smells, etc.

SIGNS AND SYMPTOMS

The hallmark of airflow obstruction associated with asthma is its variability from day to day, at different times of the day and from season to season. Predominant symptoms include:

- Chest tightness
- Wheezing
- Shortness of breath
- Cough, usually dry (especially at night)

PHYSICAL EXAM

- Wheezing on exhalation.
- ↓ air entry, ↑ expiratory phase.
- ↓ peak flow and FEV_1.
- **Clinical features of acute severe asthma:**
  - Patient too breathless to complete a full sentence.
  - Respiratory rate > 30/min.
  - Use of accessory muscles.
  - ↓ air entry on auscultation.
  - Heart rate > 120/min, and presence of pulsus paradoxus > 20 mmHg.
  - Patient is drowsy or tells you that they're "tiring out."
  - Arterial blood gas analysis showing normal or ↑ CO_2 level (see below).

TREATMENT (TABLE 2.7-7)

- **Short-acting β_2 agonists** (eg, albuterol, terbutaline) (rapid onset):
  - Delivered by metered-dose inhaler (MDI) or nebulizer.
  - Promote bronchodilation.
- **Ipratropium bromide** (rapid onset):
  - Delivered by nebulizer or MDI.
  - Dries up bronchial secretions.
  - Effects of beta agonists and ipratropium bromide are additive.

PULMONOLOGY

TABLE 2.7-7. Asthma Classification and Treatment

CLASSIFICATION	FREQUENCY OF SYMPTOMS	TREATMENT
Mild intermittent	1–2 episodes per month	**PRN:** Short-acting β_2 agonists as needed.
Mild persistent	> 2 per week but < 1 per day	**PRN:** Short-acting β_2 agonists as needed.
		Maintenance: May add oral or inhaled steroids or cromolyn or leukotriene modifier.
Moderate persistent	Daily	**Maintenance:** Oral or inhaled steroids and long-acting β_2 agonist; may also use cromolyn or leukotriene modifier.
		PRN: Short-acting β_2 agonist as needed.
Severe persistent	Continuous	**Maintenance:** Oral or inhaled steroid + long-acting β_2 agonist.
		PRN: Short-acting β_2 agonist.

- **Steroids** (take 6 hours to work):
  - Reduce inflammation.
  - Inhaled corticosteroids, often used in combination with long acting β_2 agonists (eg, salmeterol, fomoterol) are the cornerstone of preventive and maintenance therapy for bronchial asthma.
  - Oral or IV use for acute exacerbations.
- Other preventative medications:
  - Leukotriene modifiers such as montelukast.
  - Mast cell stabilizers such as cromolyn.
- **Methylxanthines** such as theophylline are no longer regularly used for asthma due to the narrow therapeutic window and the frequency of adverse effects, including nausea, vomiting, headache, and, in severe toxicity, seizures and arrhythmias.
- **Allergen removal:** Common environmental triggers should be addressed, including smoking, dust, pets, carpets, cockroaches, and seasonal allergens.

INTERPRETATION OF ARTERIAL BLOOD GASES IN ASTHMA

The notation for arterial blood gases is: pH/P_{CO_2}/P_{O_2}/calculated HCO_3/calculated SaO_2.

Sample ABGs
- **Normal:** 7.4/40/98.
- Mild asthma: 7.48/30/60 (acute respiratory alkalosis).
- Severe asthma: 7.40/40/55 (the "normalization" of the pH and P_{CO_2} in the presence of continued symptoms and hypoxia indicate that the patient is getting fatigued and is no longer able to maintain CO_2 balance).

If an asthmatic in respiratory distress has a normal pH and normal P_{CO_2}, beware of *impending respiratory failure:* intubate (he is tiring out).

Obstructive Sleep Apnea (OSA)

Brief periods of breathing cessation (apnea) or marked reduction in tidal volume (hypopnea) occurring during sleep due to occlusion of upper airways.

Why does an obese patient known to snore have daytime sleepiness?
Obstructive sleep apnea/obesity hypoventilation syndrome.

SIGNS AND SYMPTOMS

- Snoring.
- Persistent daytime sleepiness.
- Morning headache.
- Obesity.
- Hypertension.
- Large neck circumference.
- OSA ↑ the risk of morbidity and mortality from hypertension and other cardiovascular disorders.

DIFFERENTIAL DIAGNOSIS

- Simple snoring.
- Central sleep apnea.
- Other disorders causing daytime sleepiness (insufficient sleep, circadian rhythm disturbances, narcolepsy, periodic limb movement disorder).

DIAGNOSIS

- Made with polysomnography (sleep study).
- OSA is defined by ≥ 5 episodes of apnea and hypopnea per hour of sleep (apnea-hypopnea index).

TREATMENT

- Lateral sleeping position, avoidance of alcohol or sedative medications, weight loss.
- Continuous positive airway pressure (CPAP) during sleep: Very effective, if consistently used by the patient.
- Surgery (tonsillectomy, uvulopalatopharyngoplasty, tracheostomy).

UPPER RESPIRATORY TRACT DISEASES

Acute Cough

- Cough is a common presenting complaint of patients.
- Acute cough, or cough of < 3 weeks' duration, is most commonly caused by the postnasal drip associated with the common cold.
- See Table 2.7-8 for causes of acute cough.

Chronic Cough

Cough of > 3 weeks' duration.

ETIOLOGY

- Postnasal drip.
- Asthma.
- Gastroesophageal reflux disease (GERD).
- See Table 2.7-9 for a complete list of causes.

TABLE 2.7-8. **Causes of Acute Cough**

PREVALENCE	CAUSE
Very common	Postnasal drip (due to common cold, acute bacterial sinusitis, allergic rhinitis, environmental irritant rhinitis)
Common	Pertussis
	COPD exacerbation
Less common	Asthma
	Congestive heart failure
	Pneumonia
	Aspiration syndromes
	Pulmonary embolism

Postnasal Drip Syndrome (PNDS)

PNDS is thought to be the single most common cause of both acute and chronic cough. It is now called upper airway cough syndrome.

ETIOLOGY

All causes of rhinosinusitis can cause postnasal drip and cough.

PATHOPHYSIOLOGY

PNDS may be caused by a mucus hypersecretory phenotype that develops following chronic exposure of the respiratory tract to particulate matter, allergens, irritants, and pathogens. The mechanical action of secretions dripping into the hypopharynx triggers the cough reflex.

PNDS, asthma, and GERD account for nearly 100% of causes of chronic cough in nonsmokers with normal CXR, who are not on angiotensin-converting enzyme (ACE) inhibitors.

TABLE 2.7-9. **Causes of Chronic Cough**

PREVALENCE	CAUSES
Common	PNDS
	Asthma
	GERD
Less common	Chronic bronchitis
	Bronchiectasis
	Postinfectious cough (pertussis)
Uncommon	Bronchogenic carcinoma
	ACE inhibitors
Rare in adults	Psychogenic cough

ACE, angiotensin-converting enzyme; GERD, gastroesophageal reflux disease; PNDS, postnasal drip syndrome.

- Cough, more on lying down and more at night when the patient sleeps.
- Nasal discharge or nasal obstruction.
- Dripping sensation or tickle in the throat; drainage may be present on the posterior pharyngeal wall.

- **PNDS** is treated with a first-generation antihistamine and a decongestant. Nonsedating antihistamines have been shown to be less effective in this case.
- Intranasal corticosteroids are used in cases where PNDS is secondary to allergic rhinitis or symptoms are more persistent.
- Treatment of PNDS due to sinusitis is addressed below.

Sinusitis

- Sinusitis is a common cause of PNDS and cough.
- Acute sinusitis is a bacterial infection that usually involves an obstructed maxillary sinus.
- Chronic sinusitis is the persistence of sinus inflammation for ≥ 3 months.
- Also associated with allergic rhinitis, dental infections, foreign body or tumor, cystic fibrosis, and asthma.

- Purulent nasal discharge.
- Sinus pain worse on bending forward.
- Fever.
- Tenderness to percussion over sinuses.

- Transillumination findings are inconsistent.
- CT scan is extremely sensitive but is not specific to sinusitis, and many false ⊕ occur. CT scan should be reserved for hospitalized patients, or for the diagnosis of chronic sinusitis.

- **Acute sinusitis:** Routine treatment with antibiotics is *not* indicated. If initial symptomatic treatment with antihistamines and anti-inflammatory medications is not effective, nasal corticosteroids are to be tried.
- If severe symptoms persist or there are indications of spreading infections, antibiotics are started and should be directed against the most likely bacterial organisms: *S. pneumoniae, Haemophilus influenzae,* and *Moraxella catarrhalis.* Amoxicillin or TMP-SMZ or amoxicillin–clavulanic acid for 1–2 weeks.
- **Persistent chronic sinusitis:** May require subspecialist involvement.

- Preseptal or periorbital cellulitis.
- Orbital cellulitis.
- Epidural, subdural, or cerebral abscess.
- Meningitis.
- Dural sinus venous thrombosis.

Pertussis (Whooping Cough)

Caused by *Bordetella pertussis*, a gram-⊖ coccobacillus.

EPIDEMIOLOGY

- Thought to be a common cause of cough in adults.
- The classic "whoop" caused by rapid air inspiration against a closed glottis is rarely seen in adults.

IMMUNIZATION

- Before routine immunization, whooping cough was a common cause of infant death.
- DTP (killed whole-cell) or DTaP (acellular) at 2, 4, 6, 18 months, and 4–6 years.

SIGNS AND SYMPTOMS

- **Catarrhal stage:**
  - Lasts 1–2 weeks.
  - Characterized by mild upper respiratory infection (URI) symptoms.
- **Paroxysmal stage:**
  - Lasts 2–4 weeks.
  - Characterized by prolonged paroxysmal cough.
  - Often worse at night.
- **Convalescent stage:** Characterized by gradual improvement of symptoms.

DIAGNOSIS

Nasopharyngeal swab and culture.

TREATMENT

- Macrolide antibiotics, such as erythromycin, will reduce the severity of the disease if started within 8 days.
- Identification and treatment of adult patients is important to help prevent transmission to unimmunized or incompletely immunized children.

MISCELLANEOUS LUNG DISORDERS

Acute Respiratory Distress Syndrome (ARDS)

- A condition that results from ↑ permeability of alveolar capillaries causing fluid to fill alveoli.
- Also known as noncardiogenic pulmonary edema.

ETIOLOGY

- Shock
- Septicemia
- Aspiration
- Severe pancreatitis
- Blood transfusion

- Ratio of $PaO_2/FiO_2 \leq 200$.
- Bilateral fluffy infiltrates.
- Pulmonary artery capillary pressure, which reflects pressures in the left side of the heart, < 18 mmHg (thereby ruling out cardiogenic pulmonary edema).

TREATMENT

- O_2 treatment does not improve hypoxia in ARDS. Fluid-filled, consolidated, or collapsed alveoli lead to effective arteriovenous shunting.
- Treatment usually involves hemodynamic support and treatment of the underlying disease.

Bronchiectasis

- A chronic condition characterized by pathological dilatation of the medium-sized airways.
- Usually caused by an abnormal inflammatory response to an initial infectious or toxic insult.

ETIOLOGY

- **Localized:** Usually the result of previous pneumonia.
- If **severe or bilateral,** the following causes should be considered:
  - Cystic fibrosis.
  - Immotile cilia syndromes (Kartagener's).
  - Immunodeficiency: Hypogammaglobulinemia, HIV.

PATHOPHYSIOLOGY

- The resulting airway damage allows bacterial colonization, buildup of secretions, and continued bronchial destruction.
- Bronchiectasis is the cause of chronic cough in about 4% of cases.

SIGNS AND SYMPTOMS

- Chronic cough often with large amount of expectoration.
- Hemoptysis is often the major or only presenting symptom.
- Wheezing.
- Failure to thrive.

DIAGNOSIS

- High-resolution CT scan will detect bronchial dilatation and destruction in 60–100% of cases.
- Patients with cystic fibrosis will have abnormal pancreatic function and an abnormal sweat test.

TREATMENT

- Chest physiotherapy and postural drainage.
- Antibiotics.
- Bronchodilators, mucolytics.

Clinical Pearl: ARDS is a diagnosis of exclusion. You must be certain that there is no other explanation for the acute onset of bilateral "fluffy" infiltrates.

A 54-year-old male with pancreatitis goes into respiratory failure. CXR shows bilateral infiltrates. Diagnosis? ARDS (sepsis is the most common cause of ARDS).

A patient with cystic fibrosis has chronic hypoxia that causes pulmonary hypertension and then cor pulmonale and right heart failure.

Most common organisms to colonize bronchiectatic lung:
- *H influenzae*
- *S aureus*
- *Pseudomonas aeruginosa*

PULMONOLOGY

Hemoptysis

- Coughing up of blood due to bleeding from the lower respiratory tract.
- See Table 2.7-10 for a list of causes.
- **Massive hemoptysis** is defined as bleeding > 600 mL in 48 hours (200–600 mL/24 hr), or any amount of bleeding causing clinical impairment of respiratory function.

 A patient presents with hemoptysis, sinusitis, and glomerulonephritis. On physical exam, you notice a "saddle-nose" deformity. *Think: Wegener's granulomatosis.* **Next step:** Send for circulating antineutrophil cytoplasmic antibody (c-ANCA).

A patient presents with dyspnea, hemoptysis, and acute renal failure. *Think: Goodpasture's syndrome.* **Next step:** Send for anti–glomerular basement membrane antibodies.

DIAGNOSIS

CXR, high-resolution CT, bronchoscopy.

TABLE 2.7-10. Causes of Hemoptysis

INCIDENCE	CAUSE
Common	Bronchitis
	TB
	Pneumonia
	Lung cancer
	Bronchiectasis
	Unknown
Uncommon	Coagulopathy
	Congestive heart failure
	Pulmonary embolism
	Wegener's granulomatosis
	Goodpasture's syndrome
Rare	Pulmonary hypertension
	Trauma
	Vasculitis
	Foreign body
	Collagen vascular disease
	Pulmonary arteriovenous malformation

TREATMENT

- Supplemental oxygen.
- Position patient with bleeding side down.
- Suppress cough reflex (ie, codeine).
- Patients with massive hemoptysis usually require surgical involvement. Initial therapy includes:
  - Protection of the good lung often by intubation with a double-lumen tube (selective intubation).
  - Endobronchial cold saline or epinephrine.
  - Bronchial artery embolization.

Pulmonary Embolism (PE)

- Usually results from the dislodging and migration of a deep venous thrombus, causing blockage of pulmonary blood flow beyond the embolus.
- Very large PEs that impede blood flow in both the right and left pulmonary arteries are called **saddle emboli.**

 A patient with a known history of antiphospholipid syndrome has acute shortness of breath, hypoxia, and an ECG consistent with pulmonary embolism and right ventricular strain. She is hypotensive. What is next step? Fibrinolytics.

RISK FACTORS FOR VENOUS THROMBOEMBOLISM (VTE)

- Immobilization.
- Leg fracture or leg surgery.
- Hypercoagulable state (active malignancy, pregnancy, genetic).
- Medications: Oral contraceptives, tamoxifen.

SIGNS AND SYMPTOMS

No sign or symptom is specific for PE.

- Sinus tachycardia (most common rhythm disturbance).
- Dyspnea.
- Cough.
- Tachypnea.
- Pleuritic chest pain.
- Hemoptysis.
- Hypoxia, often in presence of a clear CXR.

DIAGNOSIS

Any of the following three is reasonable:

- **Helical (spiral) CT:** Also called CTPA (CT of pulmonary arteries); to look for embolus in the pulmonary vasculature. Most common. Fast and convenient, fairly sensitive. Downside: IV contrast can damage kidneys.
- **Pulmonary angiogram:** The gold standard for detection of PE. Very sensitive. Downside: Invasive test.

Westermark's sign: Oligemia seen on the CXR distal to the PE. (Rare finding in the times of CT angiograms; however, a favorite topic on rounds with attendings).

- **Ventilation-perfusion scan (V/Q scan):** To look for perfusion defects at site of PE. Does not affect kidneys. Okay for pregnant patients. Downside: long test and not useful in patients with underlying lung disease.
- Other findings:
  - **ECG:** Often normal! Sinus tachycardia is the most common finding. S in lead I, Q and inverted T waves in lead III, when found is characteristic. ECG may show diffuse ST changes and tachycardia (see Figure 2.7-1) (S1Q3T3 is the mnemonic).

Hampton's hump:
Wedge-shaped infiltrate seen on CXR.

  - **CXR:** May show a peripheral infiltrate (Figures 2.7-2 and 2.7-3), representating a pulmonary infarct, or may be normal.
  - **ABGs:** Usually reveal hypoxemia, hypocapnia, and respiratory alkalosis (if big PE).
  - **D-dimer:** Measures products of fibrin degradation (will be elevated).
  - A low D-dimer with low clinical suspicion essentially rules out PE as cause of symptoms.
  - **Leg ultrasonography (venous duplex):** To detect DVT—⊕ will make one more suspicious of PE if symptoms.

Angiography is the gold standard in the diagnosis of:
- Deep venous thrombosis
- Dissecting aortic aneurysm
- Ischemic bowel syndrome
- Pulmonary embolism

TREATMENT

- **Acute:**
  - Anticoagulation with heparin or low-molecular-weight heparin. Usually the only therapy in stable patients.

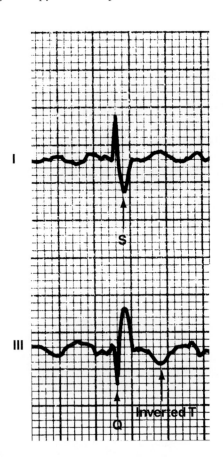

FIGURE 2.7-1. Pulmonary embolism. S_1-Q_3-T_3 pattern.

Pulmonary artery thrombus

wedge-shaped infarct

FIGURE 2.7-2. **Drawing depicting Hampton's hump.**

(Reproduced, with permission, from Schwartz DT. *Emergency Radiology: Case Studies.* New York: McGraw-Hill, 2008: 38.)

FIGURE 2.7-3. **Hampton's hump.**

Note the wedge-shaped infiltrate. Can be mistaken for pneumonia, so a careful history is very important if this finding is seen. (Reproduced, with permission, from Schwartz DT. *Emergency Radiology: Case Studies.* New York: McGraw-Hill, 2008: 38.)

- Thrombolysis **if hemodynamically unstable** or echo shows right ventricular strain (secondary to pumping against a big clotted artery).
- Other options in very specific cases:
  - Interventional pulmonary angiography: Mechanical disintegration or local thrombolysis.
  - Surgery: Embolectomy (if huge clot).
- **Prolonged:**
  - Patients with PEs or deep venous thromboses (DVTs) are orally anticoagulated with warfarin for 6 months.
  - Patients with multiple thromboembolic episodes and patients with an ongoing risk factor may need anticoagulation for indefinite period.

Pneumothorax

Air in the pleural space.

A 20-year-old tall man arrives complaining of sudden onset of severe shortness of breath and pleuritic chest pain. *Think: Primary spontaneous pneumothorax.*

- Spontaneous pneumothorax affects approximately 20,000 persons annually, usually from rupture of a subpleural bleb or pleural necrosis due to lung disease.
- Primary spontaneous pneumothorax occurs in an otherwise healthy person, while secondary spontaneous pneumothorax occurs in patients who have underlying lung disease.

ETIOLOGY

- **Primary spontaneous pneumothorax:**
  - Male smokers
  - Patients tall for weight
- **Secondary spontaneous pneumothorax:**
  - COPD
  - Cystic fibrosis
  - Pneumonia
  - Cancer

SIGNS AND SYMPTOMS

- Chest pain.
- Dyspnea.
- Hyperresonance on affected side.
- ↓ breath sounds on affected side.
- Tracheal deviation *away* from affected side (in tension pneumothorax).

DIAGNOSIS

Upright CXR is ~ 83% sensitive; demonstrates an absence of lung markings where the lung has collapsed.

TREATMENT

- 100% oxygen.
- For pneumothoraces > 20% of lung volume or with hemodynamic compromise, perform tube thoracostomy to remove air.
- Pleurodesis to adhere the visceral and parietal pleura, in cases of recurrent pneumothorax.

Mediastinum

MASSES

- **Anterior (4 Ts):**
  - Thymoma
  - Teratoma
  - Thyroid
  - Terrible lymphoma
- **Middle:**
  - Vascular lesions
  - Lymph nodes
- **Posterior:** Neurogenic tumor

PULMONOLOGY

MEDIASTINITIS

CAUSES

- Esophageal perforation.
- Postmedian sternotomy.
- Inhalation anthrax (hemorrhagic mediastinitis).
- TB, histoplasmosis (chronic).

SYMPTOMS

- Initial symptoms similar to viral syndrome.
- After 1–3 days, fever, and dyspnea develop. Patients die from airway obstruction and hypoxia.

TREATMENT

High-dose penicillin, ciprofloxacin, or doxycycline is recommended.

PNEUMOMEDIASTINUM

CAUSES

- Esophageal rupture is the first possibility to be considered (often associated with left hydropneumothorax).
- **Boerhaave's syndrome:** Ruptured esophagus from violent retching. Associated with very high mortality if not identified and managed surgically.
- Rupture of alveolus, bronchus, or trachea.

TREATMENT

Treat underlying cause.

Physical finding in pneumomediastinum: Hamman's sign: A crunching sound occurring with the heartbeat.

INTERSTITIAL LUNG DISEASE

- A group of diverse disorders involving the parenchyma of the lung that cause alveolitis, interstitial inflammation, and fibrosis or a granulomatous response.
- There are known and idiopathic etiologies (Table 2.7-11).

SYMPTOMS

- Dyspnea (chronic, progressive)
- Exercise intolerance
- Nonproductive cough
- Tachypnea

EXAM FINDINGS

- End-inspiratory crackles
- Clubbing of digits
- Pulmonary hypertension

PULMONOLOGY

TABLE 2.7-11.   Interstitial Lung Disease Causes

KNOWN CAUSES	IDIOPATHIC
Environmental/occupational (dusts, fumes)	Sarcoidosis
Drugs (amiodarone, gold)	Idiopathic pulmonary fibrosis
Radiation	Collagen vascular disease
Infections	Goodpasture's syndrome
Hypersensitivity pneumonitis	Alveolar proteinosis
Pulmonary edema	Amyloidosis
Neoplasms (lymphatic carcinoma, lymphoma)	Bronchiolitis obliterans with organizing pneumonia now known as "Crypotogenic Organizing Pneumonia or COP"
	Neurofibromatosis, tuberous sclerosis
	Lymphangioleiomyomatosis
	Eosinophilic pneumonias
	Lymphocytic interstitial pneumonia

DIAGNOSIS

- Usually requires biopsy.
- High-resolution CT, can be used as diagnostic modality for idiopathic pulmonary fibrosis (IPF).
- CXR (may show diffuse bilateral reticular infiltrates).
- PFTs (mostly demonstrate restrictive abnormalities and reduced gas transfer).

TREATMENT

- Removal/cessation of exposure to known environmental causes. Often, there is no effective treatment.
- Supplemental oxygen as needed.
- Steroids (possibly in combination with cyclophosphamide or azathioprine).
- Lung transplant.

EXAMPLES OF ENVIRONMENTAL LUNG DISEASE

- **Asbestosis:** A diffuse interstitial lung disease caused by dust of mineral silicates. Asbestos exposure is associated with an $\uparrow$ risk of **mesotheliomas** (also lung cancers). Smokers with asbestos exposure are particularly at a high risk for developing lung cancer.
- **Silicosis:** Nodular fibrosis of the lung caused by exposure to silica flour, sand blasting, or the manufacture of abrasive soaps. These patients are at a greater risk of developing pulmonary TB disease.
- **Coal workers' pneumoconiosis:** An occupational hazard of ~ 50% of all coal miners; they develop progressive massive fibrosis, usually involving upper lung fields.
- **Byssinosis (cotton dust exposure):** Patients experience "chest tightness" with an associated $\downarrow$ in FEV_1 with exposure to cotton dust. Clinically behaves like COPD. Treatment is to wear protective equipment and to use bronchodilators.
- **Farmer's lung:** A *hypersensitivity pneumonitis* caused by exposure to spores of thermophilic actinomycetes. Thought to be associated with a suppressor T-cell defect, is IgG mediated. Symptoms include fever, chills, cough, and dyspnea, and episodes occur more frequently during

wet weather. Treat with steroids, and avoid exposure. Long-term complications include pulmonary fibrosis and weight loss.

 A farmer presents with fever, cough, and difficulty breathing after several days of filling his silo with grain. *Think: Hypersensitivity pneumonitis.*

CAUSES OF LUNG FIBROSIS

- *Upper* lung zone fibrosis: Remember the mnemonic **CHARTS**:
  - **C**oal workers' pneumoconiosis
  - **H**istiocytosis, Langerhans' cell; **H**ypersensitivity pneumonitis (chronic)
  - **A**nkylosing spondylitis
  - **R**adiation (usually unilateral, radiation for breast cancer)
  - **T**uberculosis
  - **S**ilicosis, **S**arcoidosis (chronic)
- *Lower* lung zone fibrosis: Remember the mnemonic **I SOAR**:
  - **I**diopathic pulmonary fibrosis (IPF)
  - **S**ystemic sclerosis
  - **O**thers (eg, drug induced)
  - **A**sbestosis
  - **R**heumatoid arthritis

LUNG CANCER

Two types of cancer share a "**s**"entral location:
- **S**mall cell
- **S**quamous cell

TYPES

- **Small cell lung cancer:**
  - Central location.
  - Sensitive to chemotherapy.
  - Surgery is *not* indicated.
  - Poor prognosis with high recurrence after initial response to chemotherapy.
- **Non–small cell lung cancer:**
  - Includes squamous cell, large cell, and adenocarcinoma.
  - Poor response to chemotherapy.
  - Treated with surgery if early stage.
  - Prognosis varies with stage.

 A 61-year-old heavy smoker presents with shoulder pain, ptosis, and anhydrosis. What does he have? Pancoast tumor (metastasis to supraclavicular lymph node in lung cancer).

EPIDEMIOLOGY

- Leading cause of cancer death in both men and women in the United States.
- Cases have been decreasing in men, but increasing in women.
- Smoking is by far the most important causative factor in the development of lung cancer.

ETIOLOGY

- Smoking
- Passive smoke exposure
- Radon gas exposure
- Asbestos
- Arsenic
- Nickel

SIGNS AND SYMPTOMS

- Cough.
- Hemoptysis: Common with central tumors.
- Dyspnea: Results from significant endobronchial obstruction with collapse of distal lung, pleural effusion, lymphangitic spread of tumor within the lung.
- Symptoms from mediastinal involvement either from spread of the tumor or large mediastinal lymphadenopathy:
  - Hoarseness (recurrent laryngeal nerve paralysis).
  - Dysphagia.
  - Superior vena cava syndrome.
  - Associated (paraneoplastic) syndromes (see Table 2.7-12)

Bronchoalveolar cancer, a type of adenocarcinoma, is not linked to smoking and is more common in women.

Chronic cough is the most common symptom of lung cancer.

TABLE 2.7-12. Syndromes Associated with Lung Cancer

Horner's syndrome	Sympathetic nerve paralysis produces enophthalmos, ptosis, miosis, amd ipsilateral anhidrosis.
Pancoast's syndrome	Superior sulcus tumor injuring the eighth cervical nerve and the first and second thoracic nerves and ribs, causing shoulder pain radiating to arm.
Superior vena cava syndrome	Tumor causing obstruction of the superior vena cava and subsequent venous return, producing facial swelling and plethora, cough, headaches, epistaxis, syncope. Symptoms worsened with bending forward and on awakening in the morning.
Syndrome of inappropriate antidiuretic hormone (SIADH)	Ectopic antidiuretic hormone release in the setting of plasma hyposmolarity, producing hyponatremia without edema. Seen in small cell lung cancer.
Eaton-Lambert syndrome	Presynaptic nerve terminals attacked by antibodies, decreasing acetylcholine release. Treated by plasmapheresis and immunosuppression, 40% associated with small cell lung cancer, 20% have other cancer, 40% have no cancer.
Trousseau's syndrome	Venous thrombosis associated with metastatic cancer.
PTH-like hormone	Results in high calcium, low phosphate; seen in squamous cell lung cancer.

PULMONOLOGY

TABLE 2.7-13. **Distinction Between Small and Non–Small Cell Lung Cancer**

CHARACTERISTIC	SMALL CELL LUNG CANCER	NON–SMALL CELL LUNG CANCER
Histology	Small, dark nuclei; scant cytoplasm.	Copious cytoplasm, pleomorphic nuclei.
Ectopic peptide production (causing paraneoplastic syndromes)	▪ ACTH—causes a Cushing syndrome ▪ ADH—causes SIADH (low Na+) ▪ Eaton-Lambert syndrome ▪ Gastrin—can cause stomach ulcer ▪ Calcitonin—can cause low Ca+ ▪ ANF	▪ PTHrP (PTH related peptide). Presents with hypercalcemia. Classically in squamous subtype.
Response to radiotherapy	80–90% will shrink	30–50% will shrink
Response to chemotherapy	Very responsive to chemo	Somewhat responsive to chemo
Surgical resection for	Not indicated	Stages I, II, IIIA
Included subtypes	Small cell only	Adenocarcinoma, sqamous cell, large cell, bronchoalveolar
5-year survival rate all stages	5%	10% in later stages; up to 90% in early stages

ACTH, adrenocorticotropic hormone; ADH, antidiuretic hormone (also known as arginine vasopressin [AVP]); ANF, atrial natriuretic factor; PTH, parathyroid hormone.

TREATMENT

The two main types of lung cancer, small cell and non–small cell cancer, have different responses to radiotherapy, chemotherapy, and surgery (see Table 2.7-13). Generally, small cell—always chemo, never surgery; non–small cell—surgery if cancer is local, chemo only if there is metastatic disease.

HOW TO PRESENT A CHEST RADIOGRAPH (CXR)

- First, confirm that the CXR belongs to your patient.
- If possible, compare to a previous film.
- Then, present in a systematic manner:
  1. *Technique:* Rotation, anteroposterior (AP) or posteroanterior (PA), penetration, inspiratory effort.
  2. *Bony structures:* Look for rib, clavicle, scapula, and sternum fractures.
  3. *Airway:* Look for tracheal deviation, pneumothorax, pneumomediastinum.
  4. *Pleural space:* Look for fluid collections, which can represent hemothorax, chylothorax, pleural effusion.

5. *Lung parenchyma:* Look for infiltrates and consolidations: These can represent pneumonia, pulmonary contusions, hematoma, or aspiration. The location of an infiltrate can provide a clue to the location of a pneumonia:
   - Obscured right (R) costophrenic angle = Right lower lobe.
   - Obscured left (L) costophrenic angle = Left lower lobe.
   - Obscured R heart border = Right middle lobe.
   - Obscured L heart border = Left upper lobe.
6. *Mediastinum:* Look at size of mediastinum—a widened one (> 8 cm) goes with aortic dissection. Look for enlarged cardiac silhouette (more than one-half thoracic width at base of heart), which may represent congestive heart failure (CHF), cardiomyopathy, or pericardial effusion.
7. *Diaphragm:* Look for free air under the right hemidiaphragm (suggests bowel perforation). Look for stomach, bowel, or nasogastric tube (NGT) above diaphragm (suggests diaphragmatic rupture).
8. *Tubes and lines:*
   - Identify all tubes and lines.
   - An endotracheal tube should be 2 cm above the carina. A common mistake is right mainstem bronchus intubation.
   - A chest tube (including the most proximal hole) should be in the pleural space (not in the lung parenchyma).
   - An NGT should be in the stomach and uncoiled.
   - The tip of a central venous catheter (central line) should be in the superior vena cava (not in the right atrium).
   - The tip of a Swan-Ganz catheter should be in the pulmonary artery.
   - The tip of a transvenous pacemaker should be in the right ventricle.

A sample CXR presentation may sound like:

This is the CXR of Mr. Jones. The film is an AP view with good inspiratory effort. There is an isolated fracture of the eighth rib on the right. There is no tracheal deviation or mediastinal shift. There is no pneumo- or hemothorax. The cardiac silhouette appears to be of normal size. The diaphragm and heart borders on both sides are clear; no infiltrates are noted. There is a central venous catheter present, the tip of which is in the superior vena cava.

Rheumatology

Rheumatology is a broad discipline covering diseases of the joints, connective tissue, and certain immunological disorders. Also covered in this chapter are conditions that are not typically classified as rheumatologic, but nonetheless affect the musculoskeletal system. Table 2.8-1 discusses laboratory data commonly used in rheumatology.

LOWER BACK PAIN

Leading causes of back pain: **ACTIONS.**

- Arthritis (rheumatoid, osteoarthritis, ankylosing spondylitis).
- Congenital anomalies (spina bifida, spondolysis [not covered here]).
- Trauma (strains, sprains, fractures, and lumbar disk herniation).
- Infection (abscess).
- Osteoporosis (secondary fracture, compression).
- Neoplasms (primary or metastatic).
- Spinal stenosis.

TABLE 2.8-1. Laboratory Data Commonly Used in Rheumatology

FINDING	SIGNIFICANCE
ESR	Determined by filling a tube with whole blood and measuring the rate of sedimentation of red cells—changes in the rate are seen with ↑ plasma proteins. Certain proteins called *acute-phase reactants* (negatively charged proteins) are produced at an ↑ rate during an inflammatory response. These proteins cause RBCs to adhere to one another like stacks of coins called **rouleaux,** which fall through the plasma faster than free RBCs. This is a very nonspecific test. An ↑ ESR is seen in infections, tissue infarctions, malignancies, collagen vascular diseases, and states of ↑ physiologic stress (pregnancy, extreme exercise).
ANA	Found in many rheumatologic disorders, such as: ■ SLE ■ Rheumatoid arthritis ■ Scleroderma ■ Polymyositis and dermatomyositis
RF	This is an IgM antibody directed against the Fc portion of IgG. Found mainly in rheumatoid arthritis but also in **vasculitides.**
Complement levels	Complement levels drop when there is ↓ production in the liver or ↑ loss—either through the formation of immune complexes or from glomerular disease. Complement levels can be low with: ■ Liver disease (viral hepatitis) ■ SLE nephritis ■ Glomerulonephritis (C3 is the most reduced) ■ Bacterial endocarditis ■ Serum sickness ■ Rheumatoid arthritis with vasculitis

ANA, antinuclear antibody; ESR, erythrocyte sedimentation rate; IgG, immunoglobulin G; IgM, immunoglobulin M; RBC, red blood cell; RF, rheumatoid factor; SLE, systemic lupus erythematosus.

An athlete presents with nonspecific lower back pain of 2 months' duration. On examination he does not have any restriction of movement, no neurological signs, and ⊖ straight leg-raising test. *Think: Acute low back pain.* **Next step:** Education, conservative management.

Lumbar Disk Herniation

■ Disk herniation is a common cause of chronic lower back pain.
■ L4–L5 and L5–S1 are the most common sites affected.
■ Herniation occurs when the nucleus pulposus prolapses through the annulus fibrosis.
■ More common in men and overweight individuals.

The nucleus pulposus is a thick gel. Herniation of the nucleus pulposus is like toothpaste being squeezed out of the tube.

SIGNS AND SYMPTOMS

■ Occurs due to activities that involve sudden movement or heavy lifting.
■ Pain is worse with coughing, sneezing, Valsalva, and spinal flexion.
■ Pain (sciatica) and paresthesia with a dermatomal distribution.
■ Specific signs depend on nerve root involved:

	Sensory Loss/ Pain Distribution	Motor Deficit	Reflex
L4	Anterior thigh	Impaired dorsiflexion and inversion at the ankle (anterior tibialis)	Knee jerk
L5	Lateral calf and first web space	Extends big toe (extensor hallucis longus)	—
S1	Lateral and plantar aspect of foot	Foot plantar flexion and eversion (peroneus longus and brevis)	Ankle jerk

TREATMENT

■ Nonsteroidal anti-inflammatory drugs (NSAIDs) and epidural injection for symptomatic relief.
■ Surgical treatment is indicated only for refractory pain and/or neurological deficits.

Vertebral Compression Fracture

■ The most common manifestation of osteoporosis.
■ Also seen in patients on long-term steroids and in patients with lytic bony metastases.
■ Thoracic spine is the most common site affected (see Figure 2.8-1).

SIGNS AND SYMPTOMS

■ Height loss.
■ Sudden back pain after mild trauma.
■ Local radiation of pain—the extremities are rarely affected (unlike a herniated disk).

FIGURE 2.8-1. **Compression fracture of osteoporosis.**

Note the anterior collapse of the vertebra. (Reproduced, with permission, from Wilson FC, Lin PP. *General Orthopedics*. New York: McGraw-Hill, 1997: 489.)

DIAGNOSIS

- Plain radiographs of the lumbosacrum will not show compression fracture until there is loss of 25–30% bone height.
- Magnetic resonance imaging (MRI) and computed tomography (CT) are more sensitive.

TREATMENT

- Symptomatic relief with NSAIDs.
- Vertebroplasty:
  - Usually reserved for fractures with > 50% loss of bone height.
  - Consists of an orthopedic cement (polymethylmethacrylate) that is injected into the vertebral body.
  - Restores height and relieves pain.
- Prevention of osteoporosis:
  - Weight-bearing exercises.
  - Estrogen replacement therapy.
  - Calcium supplementation to ↑ bone mass.
  - Calcitonin to inhibit bone resorption.
  - Bisphosphonates to inhibit osteoclast activity.

Bisphosphonates such as alendronate (Fosamax) irritate gastric mucosa, so advise patients to eat beforehand and stay upright for 30 minutes after taking it.

Spinal Metastasis and Cauda Equina Syndrome

- Metastatic lesions invade the spinal bone marrow, leading to compression of the spinal cord.
- Typically involves the thoracic spine.
- Cauda equina syndrome occurs when the compression occurs below spinal cord (which typically ends at around L1) at the lumbar and sacral nerve roots.
- The most common primary tumors involved include breast, lung, prostate, kidney, lymphoma, and multiple myeloma.

Spinal cord compression is an emergency. Missed diagnosis can lead to permanent paralysis.

A multiple myeloma patient suddenly becomes incontinent of urine and has leg weakness. **Next step:** MRI and start steroids. Cord compression found: Get emergent neurosurgical and radiation consultation.

A 60-year-old man presents with severe back pain that has point tenderness. He says he has some numbness in his inner legs. **Next step:** Start steroids and send for emergent spine MRI.

Any cancer patient who develops back pain should be investigated for spinal metastases.

SIGNS AND SYMPTOMS

- Back pain that is worse at night.
- **Lower extremity weakness.**
- Hyperreflexia.
- Upward Babinski sign.
- **Urinary incontinence.**
- ↓ rectal sphincter tone.
- Cauda equina syndrome classically has **saddle anesthesia** and bladder/bowel incontinence.

Common causes of spinal cord compression:
- Multiple myeloma
- Lymphoma
- Metastatic lung, prostate, and breast cancer

DIAGNOSIS

MRI is the preferred imaging technique.

Saddle anesthesia: Loss of sensation over the buttocks, perineum, and thighs. Seen with cauda equina syndrome.

TREATMENT

Glucocorticoids are used to reduce inflammation and edema. Radiation therapy should be started as soon as possible. Surgery is indicated only if radiation fails to improve the symptoms or if compression is due to actual bone fragment (radiation will not shrink bone).

Osteoarthritis (OA)

- Degeneration of articular cartilage followed by new and abnormal bone formation; more common in women.
- Involves distal interphalangeal joint (DIP), proximal interphalangeal joint (PIP), thumb base, hip, knee, and spine.

ETIOLOGY

- Primary disease: Idiopathic.
- Secondary disease: Known underlying etiology such as trauma, metabolic (hemachromatosis, Wilson's disease), endocrine (acromegaly), or congenital (congenital hip dislocation).

SIGNS AND SYMPTOMS

- Joint pain worse with use and relieved with rest.
- Morning stiffness that resolves within 20 minutes.
- Painless nodules on the hand (see Figure 2.8-2):
    - **Heberden's nodes** at the DIPs.
    - **Bouchard's nodes** at the PIPs.
- Loss of range of motion (eg, ↓ internal rotation of hip).
- Joint effusions and crepitus.
- Periarticular muscle wasting and weakness from disuse.

FIGURE 2.8-2. Heberden's and Bouchard's nodes of osteoarthritis.

(Reproduced, with permission, from Wilson FC, Lin PP. *General Orthopedics.* New York: McGraw-Hill, 1997: 413.)

DIAGNOSIS

- Lab findings are normal.
- X-ray will show joint space narrowing, osteophyte formation, and subchondral cysts.
- Synovial fluid analysis shows noninflammatory picture (white cell count < 2000).

TREATMENT

- NSAIDs for symptomatic relief.
- Intra-articular injection of lidocaine, Hyaluronan, steroids provides temporary relief.
- Joint replacement as necessary.
- Weight loss.
- Strengthen periarticular muscles.

CONNECTIVE TISSUE DISORDERS

See Table 2.8-2 for synovial fluid characteristics.

Rheumatoid Arthritis (RA)

- A systemic inflammatory disease primarily affecting the synovial membranes.
- Pannus (granulation tissue) develops in the joint spaces and erodes into the articular cartilage and bone.

TABLE 2.8-2. Synovial Fluid Characteristics

	NONINFLAMMATORY (EG, OA)	INFLAMMATORY (EG, RA, SLE, GOUT, PSEUDOGOUT, SARCOIDOSIS)	SEPTIC (EG, BACTERIAL)	HEMORRHAGIC (EG, TRAUMA, TUBERCULOSIS, COAGULOPATHY)
Color	Clear/yellow	Yellow/white	Yellow/white	Red
Clarity	Transparent	Transluscent/opaque	Opaque	Opaque
Viscosity	High	Variable	Low	Variable
WBC	< 2000	2000–100,000	> 100,000	Variable
Differential	< 25% PMN	> 50% PMN	> 95% PMN	NA
Culture	⊖	⊖	⊕	Variable

PMN, polymorphonuclear neutrophil; WBC, white blood cell count.

Common deformities in RA:
- **Ulnar deviation** of the digits.
- **Boutonniere deformity:** Hyperextension of the DIP and flexion of the PIP (Figure 2.8-3A).
- **Swan neck:** Flexion of the DIP and extension of the PIP (Figure 2.8-3B).

Note that in drug-induced SLE there is no kidney or central nervous system involvement.

SIGNS AND SYMPTOMS

- Synovitis is characterized by joint swelling, warmth, erythema, and reduction in both active and passive range of movement.
- Early symptoms are nonspecific: Malaise, anorexia, fatigue, vague musculoskeletal complaints.
- Hypertrophy of synovial tissue.
- **Prolonged morning stiffness; pain worse in morning, too.**
- Joint pain—most common joints affected: PIP, metacarpophalangeal (MCP), wrist, knees, ankles.
- Joint subluxation results from ligament laxity and muscle weakness, causing deformity such as swan neck, Boutonniere, Z shape.
- Subcutaneous painless rheumatic nodules.
- Instability of cervical spine due to bone erosion.
- Extra-articular involvement also occurs. Common manifestations include vasculitis, pleuritis, pulmonary nodules, and secondary amyloidosis.

DIAGNOSIS

At least four out of the following seven criteria must be present to diagnose rheumatoid arthritis; criteria 1 through 4 must have been present for ≥ 6 weeks:

1. Morning stiffness for ≥ 1 hour.
2. Arthritis of three or more joint areas.
3. Arthritis of hand joints (see Figure 2.8-3).
4. Symmetric arthritis.
5. Rheumatoid nodules.
6. ⊕ serum rheumatoid factor (see Table 2.8-3 for common serology of rheumatologic conditions).
7. Radiographic changes.

A B

FIGURE 2.8-3. **Boutonniere (A) and swan neck (B) deformities of rheumatoid arthritis.**

(Reproduced, with permission, from Knoop KJ, Stack LB, Storrow AB, et al. *Atlas of Emergency Medicine*, 3rd ed. New York: McGraw-Hill, 2010: 384-385. Photo contributors: E. Lee Edstrom, MD and Cathleen M. Vossler, MD.)

TABLE 2.8-3. Common Serology of Rheumatologic Conditions

	ANTIBODY	HLA
SLE	Anti-ds (60–70%) (indicates disease activity)	DR2, DR3
	Anti-SM (Smith) (25%)	
	Anticardiolipin	
	Lupus anticoagulant	
DIL	Antihistone (sensitive, use to rule out DIL)	DR3
Sjögren's	Anti-SSA(Ro)	
	Anti-SSB(La)	
Ankylosing spondylitis		B27
Reiter's		B27
MCTD		Anti-U₁ RNP
Poly/dermatomyositis	Anti-Jo (polymyositis)	DR3
	Anti-Mi2 (dermatomyositis)	
	Anti-PM1	
Systemic sclerosis	Anti-topoisomerase-1 (SCL-70)	
	Antinucleolar	
CREST	Anticentromere	
RA	Rheumatoid factor	DR4
		(associated with severe disease)
Behçet's		B5

CREST, calcinosis, Raynaud's phenomenon, esophageal dysmotility, sclerodactyly, and telangiectasia; DIL, drug-induced lupus; MCTD, mixed connective tissue disease; RA, rheumatoid arthritis.

LABORATORY

- Rheumatoid factor (RF) is ⊕ in 80% of patients with RA.
- Anticyclic citrullinated peptide (anti-CCP): Sensitivity 50–75%; specificity 90–95%.
- Anemia of chronic disease.
- Elevated erythrocyte sedimentation rate (ESR).
- X-ray: Soft tissue swelling, juxta-articular osteopenia, subluxation, erosion.

TREATMENT

- Once diagnosis is established, treatment with disease-modifying antirheumatic drugs (DMARDs; Table 2.8-4) should be initiated. DMARDs have been shown to slow or even reverse joint damage. They should be started within 3 months of diagnosis.
- NSAIDs, glucocorticoid injections, and/or low-dose steroids for symptomatic relief.
- Physical therapy to maintain strength and range of motion.

Rheumatoid arthritis: Pain improves with use. **Osteoarthritis:** Pain worsens with use.

OA can cause morning stiffness but is it usually short-lived (in contrast to RA).

311

OA affects the **O**uter joints on the hand—the DIPs. RA affects the inner joints—MCPs and PIPs.

OA is not a systemic inflammatory disease; therefore, lab studies should be normal.

If the WBC count is low in an RA patient, think of **Felty's syndrome:**
- Rheumatoid arthritis
- Splenomegaly
- Leukopenia

TABLE 2.8-4. Disease-Modifying Antirheumatic Drugs (DMARDs)

DRUGS	TOXICITY	MONITORING PARAMETERS
Methotrexate	Stomatitis, pneumonitis, hepatic fibrosis, marrow suppression	Blood counts (CBC), liver function tests
Leflunamide	Gastrointestinal disturbances, alopecia, mouth ulcers	Blood counts, liver function tests
Minocycline	Skin pigmentation (brown-black)	None
Gold	Rash, stomatitis, marrow suppression, proteinuria	CBC, urinalysis
Hydroxychloroquine	Retinal toxicity	Eye exam
Sulfasalazine	Marrow suppression, hepatitis	Blood counts, liver function tests
Cyclosporine	Hypertension, hirsutism, gingival hyperplasia, nephrotoxicity	Blood pressure, renal function
Azathioprine	Marrow suppression, hepatitis	CBC

Systemic Lupus Erytematosus (SLE)

- A chronic inflammatory disease that can affect virtually every organ system, including kidney, skin, joints, lungs, central nervous system (CNS).
- Classified as an autoimmune disorder with elaboration of characteristic autoantibodies.
- Can present with overlapping rheumatologic syndromes (though 90% have skin and joint involvement).
- Associated with HLA-DR2 and -DR3.

EPIDEMIOLOGY

- Female-to-male ratio: 9:1.
- People of African descent > whites.
- More common in African-Americans.

SIGNS AND SYMPTOMS

- Fever, fatigue, weight loss.
- Anemia (often Coombs' ⊕).
- Alopecia.
- Arthralgias (symmetric).
- Photosensitive rash.
- Raynaud's phenomenon.
- Serositis (pleuritic, pericarditis).
- Nephritis/nephrotic syndrome.
- Recurrent abortions (antiphospholipid syndrome).
- Purpura.

DIAGNOSIS

American College of Rheumatology (ACR) criteria: ≥ 4 of the following at any given time (sensitivity and specificity ~ 96%; mnemonic: **MD SOAP BRAIN**):

- **M**alar rash: "Butterfly" distribution; spares nasolabial folds.
- **D**iscoid rash: Raised erythematous patches; scaling; may scar.
- **S**erositis: Pleuritis/pericarditis.
- **O**ral ulcers: Usually painless.
- **A**rthritis, systemic, more than two joints.
- **P**hotosensitivity.
- **B**lood disorder: Any cell line can be affected.
- **R**enal disorder: Multiple types.
- **A**ntinuclear antibody (ANA).
- **I**mmunologic disorder: Autoantibodies, false-⊕ syphilis tests (rapid plasma reagin [RPR], Venereal Disease Research Laboratory [VDRL]).
- **N**eurologic disorder: Seizures, psychosis, "lupus cerebritis."

Ultraviolet light causes flare-ups, so many SLE patients are sensitive to sunlight.

LABS

- Autoantibodies:
  - **ANA**—present in about 95%.
  - **Anti-Smith (Sm)**—specific for SLE.
  - **Anti-dsDNA**—specific; associated with renal disease if high.
  - **Anticardiolipin** and **lupus anticoagulant**—associated with recurrent fetal loss, thrombocytopenia, heart disease; congenital heart block in the fetus. (*Note:* Lupus anticoagulant is a misnomer—it is a pro-thrombotic state, though it paradoxically causes an elevated partial thromboplastin time.)
- Flares can be associated with transaminitis, anemia, elevated ESR, proteinuria, hematuria, and granular casts in urine, Low complement C3, C4.

TREATMENT

- Avoid stress or medical procedure/surgery during flare (exacerbates SLE).
- NSAIDs.
- Antimalarials (chloroquines): Improves skin rash and arthritis.
- Glucocorticoids with severe disease/end-organ damage.
- Steroid-sparing threapy: Cyclophosphamide/azathioprine reserved for severe disease.
- Avoid drugs known to cause SLE-like syndrome.

SLE mean survival rate (from diagnosis):
- 85% at 5 years
- 80% at 10 years
- 75% at 20 years

PROGNOSIS

- **Poorer prognosis:**
  - Hypocomplementemia C3, C4.
  - ⊕ anti-dsDNA.
  - Nephritis/nephrotic syndrome.
  - Hypoalbuminemia.
  - Cr > 1.5.
- **Better prognosis:** ⊕ antiU₁RNP.

An SLE patient has arthritic pain despite being on NSAIDs. **Next step:** Start hydroxychloroquine.

Drug-Induced Lupus (DIL)

An entity distinct from SLE—it is an idiopathic reaction to certain drugs. Distinguished by:

- Complete resolution of disease once offending drug is discontinued.
- Presence of serum antihistone antibodies (very sensitive).
- Lack of renal or CNS involvement.

ETIOLOGY

- Procainamide: Most common offender—used in the treatment of atrial fibrillation in patients with Wolff-Parkinson-White syndrome.
- Hydralazine: Second most common offender—used to treat preeclampsia.
- Isoniazid: Used to treat tuberculosis (TB).
- Quinidine: Used to treat malaria and leg cramps.
- Methyldopa: Old antihypertensive drug, still used in obstetrics.
- Chlorpromazine: Antiemetic also associated with dystonic reactions.
- Penicillamine: Used to treat Wilson's disease.
- Alpha-interferon: Experimental, used to treat multiple sclerosis (MS) and other autoimmune and viral conditions.

TREATMENT

- Discontinue the offending drug.
- Supportive therapy.
- May need steroids for severe cases.

Drugs associated with DIL—

H&P, IQ CAMP

Hydralazine
Procainamide
Isoniazid
Quinidine
Chlorpromazine
Alpha-interferon
Methyldopa
Penicillamine
Take H&P. If you're smart (in the high IQ CAMP), you'll discontinue these drugs in patients with a malar rash.

Scleroderma (Systemic Sclerosis)

An autoimmune disorder characterized by widespread small vessel fibrosis secondary to overproduction of collagen and other extracellular matrix proteins.

SIGNS AND SYMPTOMS

- Raynaud's phenomenon (vasospasm of arteries in hands in response to cold or emotional stress, resulting in discoloration of hands).
- Thickened, tight skin.
- Nailfold capillaries—giant loops formed by abnormal capillaries at nailfold.
- Dysphagia due to esophageal fibrosis especially the lower two-thirds.
- Renal artery fibrosis.
- Pulmonary hypertension and pulmonary fibrosis.
- Telangiectasias.
- Cardiac conduction disease/pericardial effusion.
- In the limited form of scleroderma, symptoms are generally limited to the **CREST syndrome:**
  - Calcinosis (calcium deposition forming nodules)
  - Raynaud's phenomenon
  - Esophageal dysmotility
  - Sclerodactyly (stiffness of skin of fingers)
  - Telangiectasias

LABORATORY

- ANA ⊕ in 95%.
- Anti SCl-70 (topoisomerase antibody).
- Antibody to centromere—specific to CREST variant.

- Antibody to nucleolar Ag.
- Normochromic, normocytic anemia.
- Elevated ESR.
- ↓ vital capacity on pulmonary function tests (restrictive lung disease). May get ↓ DL_{CO} if pulmonary fibrosis.

TREATMENT

- Penicillamine—may inhibit collagen cross-linking.
- Captopril—helps control the renal hypertension.
- Calcium channel blockers—diminish the Raynaud's phenomenon.
- Steroids—rarely effective in altering the disease course.

Sarcoidosis

- A systemic illness with no known cause, primarily affecting the lungs.
- Characterized by noncaseating granulomas.
- More common among blacks and women.

A 40-year-old black woman presents with dyspnea, malaise, visual disturbances, and a rash. Chest x-ray shows bilateral hilar adenopathy. *Think: Sarcoidosis.*

SIGNS AND SYMPTOMS

Almost any part of the body can be affected. Some typical extrapulmonary findings are:

- Skin—erythema nodosum (erythematous nodes on extensor surfaces of lower extremities, also seen in other conditions), lupus pernio on the face.
- Kidney—hypercalciuria (macrophages ↑ metabolism of vitamin D to 1,25-dihydroxyvitamin D).
- Eyes—uveitis (inflammation of uveal tract, iris, ciliary body, choroid).
- Cardiac—conduction defects.
- Nervous—Bell's palsy (self-limited 7th nerve palsy of unknown etiology).
- Lofgren's syndrome—triad of erythema nodosa, arthritis, and bilateral hilar lymphadenopathy (good prognosis).

STAGING

I: Bilateral hilar adenopathy.
II: Hilar adenopathy plus lung parenchymal involvement.
III: Lung parenchymal involvement alone.
IV: Pulmonary fibrosis.

DIAGNOSIS

Requires transbronchial biopsy to prove existence **of noncaseating granulomas,** but not sufficient on its own to make diagnosis; requires clinical, laboratory, and radiographic adjuncts.

In sarcoidosis, remember, when you go from stage II to stage III, you actually lose the hilar adenopathy.

315

LABORATORY

Diagnosis cannot be made or excluded on the basis of laboratory findings alone. Common laboratory findings include:

- Lymphocytosis on bronchoalveolar lavage.
- Eosinophilia.
- False-⊕ RF and ANA.
- Elevated angiotensin-converting enzyme (ACE).
- Skin anergy to common antigens.
- **Kveim test:** Splenic tissue from a patient known to have sarcoidosis is injected intradermally to the patient being tested. The test is ⊕ if the patient develops a granulomatous reaction at the site and biopsy shows noncaseating granulomas.
- Elevated 24-hour urine calcium.
- Chest x-ray shows **bilateral hilar adenopathy** and perihilar calcifications (see Figure 2.8-4).
- Elevated ESR.

TREATMENT

Corticosteroids.

PROGNOSIS

- Most patients have resolution of their disease within 2 years.
- Death from pulmonary failure occurs in a minority of patients.

Sjögren's Syndrome

A lymphocytic infiltrate in salivary and lacrimal glands, causing ↓ secretions from these glands, usually in association with other rheumatological diseases (eg, RA).

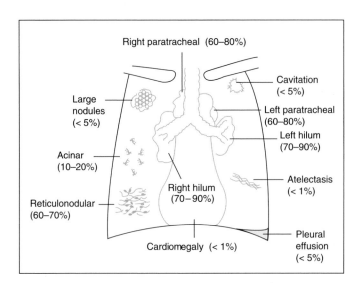

FIGURE 2.8-4.   Abnormal CXR findings in sarcoidosis.

(Reproduced, with permission, from Fauci AS et al. [eds.]. *Harrison's Principles of Internal Medicine*, 14th ed. New York: McGraw-Hill, 1998: 1925.)

ETIOLOGY

- Autoimmune.
- Found in many with coexisting connective tissue diseases (any).

SIGNS AND SYMPTOMS

- Dry mouth, dry eyes (keratoconjuctivitis sicca).
- Can have any symptoms associated with other connective tissue disorders.

LABS

- ⊕ RF in 90%.
- ⊕ ANA in 70%.
- ⊕ La (SS$_B$) and Ro (SS$_A$).
- DR3 association.

DIAGNOSIS

- Biopsy of minor salivary glands would show sialadenitis with lymphocytic infiltration.
- Schirmer's test.
- Typical symptoms.

Both polymyositis and dermatomyositis are more common in women.

TREATMENT

- Treat symptoms with artificial tears, sialogogues (ie, sucking candies that increase saliva production). May use cyclosporine eye drops.
- Corticosteroids.

PROGNOSIS

Risk of lymphoma > 40%.

Polymyositis and Dermatomyositis

- Connective tissue disease causing proximal muscle weakness.
- Associated with HLA-DR3.
- Dermatomyositis has similar manifestations to polymyositis plus skin involvement.

Seronegative arthritis—

PAIR

Psoriatic
Ankylosing spondylitis
Inflammatory bowel disease
Reiter's syndrome

 A 57-year-old woman complains of difficulty getting out of a chair and difficulty combing her hair. *Think: Polymyositis.*

ETIOLOGY

Unknown; many viruses implicated (coxsackie, influenza).

SIGNS AND SYMPTOMS

- Weakness first occurring in legs.
- Difficulty with squatting, kneeling, rising from chair, climbing stairs.
- Dysphagia, dysphonia.

Polymyositis and dermatomyositis can be distinguished from myasthenia gravis by the lack of ocular involvement (ptosis).

- Abnormal ECG (with advanced disease).
- With dermatomyositis: Purple-red papular/scaly photosensitive rash on face, neck ("V sign," "shawl sign"); erythema, scaling on extensor surfaces of joints (Gottron's papules; very specific); periorbital edema, heliotropic rash.

DIAGNOSIS

Four criteria:

1. Muscle weakness.
2. ↑ creatine phosphokinase (CPK)/aldolase.
3. Muscle biopsy showing T-cell infiltrate with myonecrosis.
4. Electromyogram (EMG) shows myopathy: Increased spontaneous activity, with low amplitude, short duration myopathic potentials on voluntary activation.

LABS

- ⊕ ANA.
- Elevated CPK, lactic dehydrogenase (LDH), aspartate transaminase (AST), aldolase.
- ESR is elevated in only ~50% of cases.
- One-third have **myositis-specific antibodies:**
  - **Anti-Jo:** One-third with pure myositis.
  - **Anti-Mi2:** Dermatomyositis specific.
  - **Anti-PM1.**
- CXR may show interstitial pulmonary disease.

TREATMENT

- Glucocorticoids (for polymyositis or dermatomyositis): 80% respond within 6 weeks.
- If poor response to glucocorticoids, high suspicion of malignancy.
- Methotrexate, azathioprine if steroid resistant.

PROGNOSIS

- Approximately 15% have malignancy, especially with dermatomyositis.
- Insidious, progressive disease.

SERONEGATIVE ARTHRITIDES

- Includes ankylosing spondylitis, psoriatic arthritis, ulcerative colitis, and Reiter's syndrome.
- Many (not all) associated with HLA-B27 genotype.
- Unlike SLE, RA, and scleroderma, these have *asymmetric* arthritis and often have spinal involvement (sacroiliitis, spondylitis).

Ankylosing Spondylitis

Chronic systemic inflammatory disorder affecting primarily the axial skeleton, but can affect multiple organs.

The rash of dermatomyositis involves the upper eyelids; the rash of SLE does not.

Ankylosing spondylitis:
- Anterior uveitis
- Apical lung fibrosis
- Aortitis
- Aortic insufficiency
- Atrioventricular conduction defect
- Amyloidosis
- Achilles entesopathy

Both azathioprine and methotrexate suppress the bone marrow. Azathioprine is also hepatotoxic.

SIGNS AND SYMPTOMS

- Peak onset of symptoms between ages 20 and 30.
- Affects men to women 3:1.
- Low back pain with reduced range of motion most common presenting symptom.
- Worse at night, better with exercise/worse with inactivity.
- Spinal ankylosis is a late manifestation of the disease.
- Highly variable disease course (may be self-limiting with spontaneous remission).
- Extra-articular involvement: Uveitis, neurological symptoms, pulmonary, renal, genitourinary (GU) abnormalities, gastrointestinal (GI), cardiac.

 A young man presents with stiffness in the lower back that improves with exercise. *Think: Ankylosing spondylitis.*

DIAGNOSIS

- Pelvic radiograph: Sacroiliitis is the hallmark of ankylosing spondylitis.
- Osteitis and bone erosions at sites of osseous attachment of ligaments and tendons (enthesopathy).
- Spine radiograph: Syndesmophytes—vertical bridging between vertebrae and ossification of spinal ligaments seen in late disease ("bamboo spine"; see Figure 2.8-5).
- Elevated ESR, C-reactive protein (CRP).
- HLA-B27.

TREATMENT

- Exercise/physical therapy.
- Smoking cessation: Ankylosing spondylitis patients may develop costochondritis with restrictive pulmonary problems, worsened by development of chronic obstructive pulmonary disease (COPD).
- Avoid falls (high risk of vertebral fracture and cauda equina syndrome).
- NSAIDs.
- For advanced disease, sulfasalazine, DMARDs, and newer drugs such as anti–tumor necrosis factor therapy are being utilized.

 The brittle spine of ankylosing spondylitis is prone to fracture even with minimal trauma. Patients should be restricted from high-risk activities such as skydiving, bungee jumping, and contact sports.

Reactive Arthritis

An HLA-B27-associated syndrome involving the musculoskeletal, genitourinary, and ocular systems. Occurs in two forms:

1. Sexually transmitted (1–2 weeks after exposure); more common in men.
2. Post-dysentery (most commonly due to *Salmonella*, *Shigella*, *Yersinia*, and *Campylobacter*); more common in women and children.

SIGNS AND SYMPTOMS

- Conjunctivitis.
- Urethritis/cervicitis.
- Arthritis: Asymmetric, lower extremities.
- Oral ulcerations.
- Balanitis.

 Reactive arthritis: "Can't see, can't pee, can't climb a tree."

FIGURE 2.8-5. **Bamboo spine of ankylosing spondylitis.**

Note the bridging syndesmophytes. (Reproduced, with permission, from Wilson FC, Lin PP. *General Orthopedics.* New York: McGraw-Hill, 1997: 454.)

LABORATORY

- Elevated ESR.
- Urethral culture may reveal *Chlamydia trachomatis*.

TREATMENT

- NSAIDs for arthritis.
- Doxycycline for urethritis/cervicitis.

Behçet's Syndrome

Autoimmune disease associated with HLA-B5, characterized by oral and genital ulceration and eye symptoms.

SIGNS AND SYMPTOMS

- Aphthous (oral) ulcers
- Genital ulcers
- Deep vein thrombophlebitis
- Arthritis (nondeforming)
- Uveitis
- Colitis
- Psychiatric disturbances

Behçet's syndrome:
"Though I enjoyed the experience, I was afterward *beset* with oral and genital ulcers."

DIAGNOSIS

Must have recurrent oral ulcers plus two of the following:

- Recurrent genital ulcers.
- Eye lesions.
- Skin lesions.
- $\oplus$ pathergy test: Abnormal inflammatory skin reaction to scratch or intradermal saline injection.

LABORATORY

- Elevated ESR.
- Hypergammaglobulinemia.
- Cryoglobulinemia.
- **Pathergy test:** Inflammatory reaction of skin to any scratches.

TREATMENT

- Colchicine or interferon-α for arthritis.
- Aspirin or antiplatelet agents for thrombophlebitis.
- Steroids for uveitis and CNS manifestations.

Behçet's ulcers pain the male but spare the female (painless in women).

Gonococcal Septic Arthritis

A disseminated gonococcal infection; more common in women than men.

ETIOLOGY

- *Neisseria gonorrhoeae.*
- More likely during pregnancy and menstruation.

SIGNS AND SYMPTOMS

- After 1–4 days of a **migratory polyarthritis,** 60% of patients develop a tenosynovitis and 40% a purulent monarthritis.
- Patients will sometimes have fever but, surprisingly, urethritis is rarely seen.
- Most patients develop a characteristic skin lesion—**small necrotic pustules**—over their extremities, usually the fingers and toes.

DIAGNOSIS

- Synovial fluid shows elevated WBCs.
- Gram stain and blood culture are $\oplus$ in < 50% of cases.
- Joint cultures are usually $\ominus$.

TREATMENT

- Very sensitive to antibiotic therapy (eg, ceftriaxone).
- Surgical drainage is not usually necessary.

Polyarteritis Nodosa (PAN)

Systemic necrotizing vasculitis of small and medium-sized muscular arteries.

 A 50-year-old woman complains of abdominal pain, fever, and joint pains. On lab work she is found to have acute renal failure with RBC casts in the urine. *Think: PAN (multisystem involvement).* **Next step:** Angiography. Biopsy shows characteristic vasculitis.

SIGNS AND SYMPTOMS

- Nonspecific symptoms predominate: Fever, weight loss, malaise.
- Specific symptoms depend on organ involved. Most common ones are:
  - Glomerulonephritis, arthritis, mononeuritis multiplex.
  - Other systems that may be involved are GI, skin, cardiac, GU, and CNS. Note conspicuous absence of pulmonary involvement.

LABORATORY

- Red cell casts in urine.
- One-third of patients have hepatitis B antigenemia.
- Diagnosis is made by tissue biopsy of affected organ.

TREATMENT

- Prednisone.
- Cyclophosphamide.

PAN—spares the lungs. **Churg-Strauss**—lung symptoms predominate.

Churg-Strauss Disease

Medium-vessel arteritis, also known as allergic angiitis and granulomatosis; it is very similar to PAN except that the pulmonary findings predominate.

SIGNS AND SYMPTOMS

- Bronchospasm (asthma).
- Eosinophilia.
- Fever.
- Erythematous maculopapular rashes, palpable purpura, and cutaneous nodules.
- Red casts in urine.

TREATMENT

Steroids; if steroids fail, consider azathioprine and cyclophosphamide.

Wegener's Granulomatosis

Chronically relapsing small-artery vasculitis of upper and lower respiratory tracts and glomerulonephritis.

- Kidney: Glomerulonephritis.
- Lungs: Hemoptysis, pulmonary infiltrates.
- Nasopharynx: Sinusitis, otitis.
- Arthralgias/arthritis.
- Fever.
- Weight loss.

DIAGNOSIS

- Granulomatous vasculitis on lung biopsy.
- $\oplus$ circulating antineutrophil cytoplasmic antibody (c-ANCA) titer.
- Exclusion of Goodpasture's syndrome, tumors, and infectious disease.

TREATMENT

Steroids, cyclophosphamide.

Takayasu's Arteritis

- An arteritis of unknown (possibly autoimmune) etiology that is seen commonly in young people of Asian descent.
- Usually affects medium and large-sized arteries.
- More common in women.

SIGNS AND SYMPTOMS

- Loss of pulses in arms and carotids bilaterally.
- Raynaud's phenomenon.
- Signs of transient brain ischemia such as blindness and hemiplegia.
- Abdominal pain, atypical chest pain.

DIAGNOSIS

- Arteriography shows narrowing of aorta +/– aneurysm.
- Magnetic resonance angiography (MRA) is helpful if arteriography is not available.

TREATMENT

- Steroids
- Methotrexate

Temporal Arteritis (Giant Cell Arteritis)

Inflammation of medium and large-sized arteries, commonly the temporal artery. See the Neurology chapter.

Goodpasture's is the other disease that involves both lungs and kidney. Its triad is:
- Glomerulonephritis
- Pulmonary hemorrhage
- Anti-GBM Ab

Takayasu's is also called *pulseless disease* and *aortic arch syndrome*.

JOINT DISORDERS

Gout

- Inflammation and severe joint pain (arthralgia) secondary to urate crystal deposition.
- Caused by either overproduction or underexcretion of uric acid.

EPIDEMIOLOGY

- Men > women.
- Typical age of onset: 45.
- For serum urate > 9–10 mg/dL, incidence of attack 5%/year.

ETIOLOGY

- ↑ production of uric acid:
  - Idiopathic.
  - Leukemia/tumor lysis syndrome.
  - Hemolytic anemia.
  - Strenuous exercise.
  - Excessive fructose ingestion.
  - Glucose-6-phosphate dehydrogenase (G6PD) deficiency.
  - Lesch-Nyhan syndrome.
  - High-protein diet.
  - Nicotinic acid.
- ↓ excretion:
  - Aspirin
  - Chronic renal disease
  - Lead nephropathy
  - EtOH ingestion
  - DKA
  - Thiazide diuretics

Gout: *Small* joints, ⊖ birefringence, needle-shaped
Pseudogout: *Large* joints (eg, knee), ⊕ birefringence, rhomboid-shaped

SIGNS AND SYMPTOMS

- Rapid onset of extreme joint pain and swelling.
- Fifty percent of first attacks are in the great toe (podagra; see Figure 2.8-6).
- **Tophi:** Aggregates of urate crystals and giant cells, which may cause tissue erosion.

Fifty percent of first gout attacks involve first metatarsophalangeal joint.

DIAGNOSIS

- **Joint aspirate:**
  - Negatively birefringent needle-shaped urate crystals in joint aspirate.
  - Large number of PMNs (5000–7000).
  - ↓ viscosity of joint fluid (low hyaluronate).
- **Labs:**
  - ↑ WBC count, proteinuria, elevated ESR, elevated uric acid, isosthenuria.
  - Twenty-four-hour urinary uric acid level: > 750 mg indicates overproducer.

Aspirin is *contraindicated* in acute gout because it ↓ urate excretion.

TREATMENT

- **Acute attack:**
  - Colchicine: May be poorly tolerated secondary to GI effects, cytopenias.
  - NSAIDs, particularly indomethacin.
  - Steroids can be used if NSAIDS or colchicine are contraindicated.
- **Chronic:**
  - Initiate allopurinol and/or probenecid treatment only after acute attack is resolved; otherwise, may prolong or worsen attack.
  - Allopurinol: Use in overproducers and those with renal insufficiency.
  - Probenecid, sulfinpyrazone, uricosurics: ↑ excretion of uric acid. Do not use in patients with chronic renal insufficiency.

A man comes in with swollen, painful joint. What is the first step? Joint fluid aspiration and analysis.

FIGURE 2.8-6. Podagra.

(Reproduced, with permission, from Fauci AS et al. [eds.]. *Harrison's Principles of Internal Medicine*, 14th ed. New York: McGraw-Hill, 1998: 2162.)

Pseudogout

Deposition of calcium pyrophosphate dihydrate (CPPD) crystals in joint spaces causing chondrocalcinosis.

ETIOLOGY

- Acute inflammatory reaction to the deposition of CPPD in joint spaces.
- Changes related to age that make the synovial fluid environment more hospitable to CPPD growth.
- Associated with hemochromatosis, hypothyroidism, hyperparathyroidism, diabetes mellitus.

SIGNS AND SYMPTOMS/DIAGNOSIS

- Similar to gout: Affected joints are painful and red.
- Unlike gout:
  - Large joints are affected (knees, wrists, shoulder).
  - The crystals are rhomboid (gouty crystals are needle-shaped).
  - Radiographs demonstrate calcification in the articular cartilage.
  - There is ⊕ **birefringence** of crystals.

TREATMENT

- NSAIDs can alleviate symptoms.
- Aspirating synovial fluid shortens the duration of the attacks.
- No therapy is available to remove CPPD crystals.

Nongonococcal Septic Arthritis

- Nongonococcal septic arthritis is seen when there is previous joint damage or bacteremia.
- It is monarticular and affects the large joints (knee, hip, shoulder, and wrist).

ETIOLOGY

- **Young adults:**
  - *Staphylococcus aureus*, beta-hemolytic strep, and gram-⊖ bacilli.
  - Lyme disease must also be considered.
- **Sickle cell anemia patients:** *Salmonella* and *S aureus* (equal).
- **IV drug users and immunocompromised:** Gram-⊖ organisms such as *E coli* and *Pseudomonas aeruginosa*, as well as *S aureus*.

RISK FACTORS

- Rheumatoid arthritis
- Prosthetic joints
- Immunodeficiency
- Age
- IV drug abuse

Nongonococcal septic arthritis: Patients will often describe previous **trauma** to the joint.

SIGNS AND SYMPTOMS

- Pain, swelling, and warmth over the joint.
- Limited range of motion.
- Fever.

DIAGNOSIS

- Blood cultures are ⊕ in 50% of cases.
- ESR and CRP will be elevated.
- Gram stain can pick up 75% of *S aureus* infections.
- **Arthrocentesis** is both diagnostic and therapeutic. Joint fluid will reveal an elevated white count (need > 50,000–100,000 cells/mm³), predominantly polymorphonucleocytes and a low glucose level. The arthrocentesis releases fluid, thereby lowering pressure within the joint capsule and alleviating pain. Arthrocentesis should be avoided if the overlying skin is infected or if there is bacteremia because the procedure introduces a portal of entry for bacteria into the joint.

IV drug abuser with septic joint: Must do echo to rule out endocarditis.

TREATMENT

- Systemic antibiotics.
- Serial arthrocentesis may be necessary if synovial fluid rapidly accumulates.
- Surgical drainage is needed for septic hip and for septic joints that do not improve with intravenous antibiotics within 72 hours.

Avascular Necrosis (AVN) of the Hip

The limited blood supply to the head of the femur makes this site particularly vulnerable to AVN.

ETIOLOGY

Seen with a variety of conditions such as trauma, long-term steroid therapy, excessive radiation, alcoholism, sickle cell disease, and Gaucher's disease.

Arthrocentesis should never be attempted in hemophiliacs until the clotting disorder is corrected with the appropriate blood product.

SIGNS AND SYMPTOMS

Pain, often referred to the **knee,** exacerbated by internal rotation of the hip.

AVN of the hip in children is called Legg-Calvé-Perthes disease.

DIAGNOSIS

MRI or bone scan is needed for early detection of the disease. Plain radiographs will be ⊕ only in the late stage.

TREATMENT

Total hip replacement.

Costochondritis

Painful swelling of the costochondral articulations at the anterior chest wall. Chest pain often confused with pulmonary embolism or myocardial infarction.

ETIOLOGY

Associated with:

- Recent upper respiratory tract infection.
- Trauma.
- Overuse.

SIGNS AND SYMPTOMS

- Typically affects the second through fifth costochondral joints.
- Pain is sharp, worse with deep breathing and movement; may radiate to the shoulders and arms.
- Pain is reproducible with palpation.

DIAGNOSIS

Diagnosis is clinical. Can do a chest x-ray to look for metastatic lesions to the sternal bone marrow, which can produce similar symptoms; however, chest x-ray is usually normal.

TREATMENT

- NSAIDs.
- Avoid overuse of muscles.

In patients with risk factors for MI, be sure to obtain ECG.

Carpal Tunnel Syndrome

- Painful compression of the median nerve as it passes through the carpal tunnel (see Figure 2.8-7).
- More common in women.

ETIOLOGY

- Anything that ↑ pressure within the carpal tunnel can cause it.
- Most common causes are trauma to carpal bones and flexor tenosynovitis.
- Can be secondary to systemic illnesses such as RA, sarcoidosis, acromegaly, hypothyroidism, diabetes.

SIGNS AND SYMPTOMS

- Muscle weakness and atrophy—mostly in the thenar eminence.
- **Phalen's sign:** Presence of paraesthesias along median nerve distribution after holding wrist flexed at 90 degrees for 30 seconds.
- **Tinel's sign:** Pain radiating down the fingers following percussion over the carpal tunnel.

1. Carpal Tunnel   2. Sensory Spread   3. Phalen Test
of Median Nerve

FIGURE 2.8-7.   **Carpal tunnel syndrome.**

1. The flexor retinaculum in the wrist compresses the median nerve to produce hypoesthesia in the radial 3½ digits. 2. Percussion on the radial side of the palmaris longus tendon produces tingling in the 3½ digital region (Tinel's sign). 3. Phalen test. Hyperflexion of the wrist for 60 seconds may produce pain in the median nerve distribution; this is relieved by extension of the wrist. (Reproduced, with permission, from DeGowin DL, Brown DD. *DeGowin's Diagnostic Examination*, 7th ed. New York: McGraw-Hill, 2000: 720.)

TREATMENT

- Rest with wrist splint worn as much as possible and elevation of the hand to reduce inflammation.
- Steroids injected into carpal tunnel are suitable for temporary situations.
- Surgical division of the flexor retinaculum.

Neurology

Abrupt onset of new neurologic deficits (see Table 2.9-1) caused by cerebro-vascular disease, which can be ischemic or hemorrhagic in nature.

TYPES OF STROKE

- **Stroke:** Cerebral vascular event resulting in infarcted cerebral tissue, regardless of the presence or absence of neurologic deficits.
- **Stroke in evolution:** Neurologic deficits continue to fluctuate or ↑ over time.
- **Completed stroke:** Neurologic deficits have remained stable for 24–72 hours.
- **Transient ischemic attack (TIA):** Neurologic deficit resolving completely in 24 hours (usually within 30 minutes) and resulting in no apparent infarcted tissue on magnetic resonance imaging (MRI).
- **Crescendo TIAs:** Two or more TIAs within 24 hours—highly predictive of impending stroke, constitutes a medical emergency.

COMMON STROKE SEQUELAE

- **Anosognosia:** The inability to identify body dysfunction—patients are unaware of their neurological deficits. From the Greek *nosos* (disease), *gnosis* (knowledge).
- **Aphasia:** A defect in comprehension or expression of spoken or written language.
- **Broca's aphasia:** A deficit in speech and written expression. Most typically occurs in Brodman's area 44 or 45—the left frontal region for 90% of the population (think: Broca's area = Broken expression).
- **Wernicke's aphasia:** Patients tend to articulate a fluent nonsense with natural rhythm, and comprehension is impaired. Results from injury to Brodman's area 22—posterior part of the superior temporal gyrus of dominant hemisphere. Patients are aware they are speaking, but they do not know what they are saying (Wernicke's is Wordy, Word salad).
- **Apraxia:** Disturbance in the ability to perform previously mastered motor tasks (ie, forgetting how to ride a bike = apraxia).
- **Dysarthria:** Disturbance in the articulation of speech. Possible injured areas are vast, including the trigeminal nerve motor branch (V), facial nerve (VII), glossopharyngeal nerve (IX), vagus nerve (X), and hypoglossal nerve (XII).
- **Dysphagia:** Difficulty swallowing.

EPIDEMIOLOGY (SOURCES: WORLD HEALTH ORGANIZATION AND AMERICAN STROKE ASSOCIATION)

- **Worldwide:**
  - There were over 20.5 million strokes in 2001; 5.5 million of these were fatal.
  - High blood pressure contributes to over 12.7 million strokes.
- **United States:**
  - Stroke is the third leading cause of death, behind heart disease and cancer. It is the number one cause of long-term disability.
  - Each year, about 700,000 people suffer a stroke. About 500,000 of these are first attacks, and 200,000 are recurrent attacks.
  - At all ages, more women than men have a stroke.
  - African-Americans have a two- to threefold greater risk of ischemic stroke and are more likely to die of stroke.

Top 5 Leading Causes of Death in United States

"CORONers CAN STROKE POLEs ACCIDENTally"

1. **Coron**ary artery disease
2. **Can**cer
3. **CVA (Stroke)**
4. Chronic obstructive **"Pole"** munary disease
5. **Accident**s

TABLE 2.9-1. Neurological Deficits in Stroke

ARTERY OCCLUSION	DEFICIT	OTHER
Middle cerebral	■ Contralateral hemiparesis (face and hand more affected). ■ Contralateral hemisensory deficit. ■ Homonymous hemianopsia (blindness affecting the right or the left half of the visual fields of both eyes) opposite to occluded artery. ■ If dominant MCA affected (left side in 92–94% of people), patient will be aphasic. ■ If nondominant MCA affected, confusion, constructional apraxia, contralateral body neglect.	
Anterior cerebral (see Figure 2.9-1)	■ Contralateral weakness of leg or foot. ■ Broca's aphasia. ■ Incontinence. ■ Abulia (lack of motivation).	
Internal carotid	■ Presentation similar to MCA occlusion.	
Posterior cerebral (see Figure 2.9-2)	■ Homonymous hemianopsia of contralateral visual field (occipital cortex). ■ Other visual field defects including vertical gaze and oculomotor nerve palsy. ■ If dominant hemisphere affected, anomia (difficulty naming objects) or alexia (inability to read) may occur.	Pupillary reflexes spared.
Posterior inferior cerebellar	Clinical: Sudden onset of: ■ Nausea/vomiting. ■ Vertigo. ■ Hoarseness. ■ Ataxia. ■ Ipsilateral palate and tongue weakness. ■ Contralateral disturbance of pain and temperature sensation. ■ Dysphagia, dysarthria, and hiccup. ■ Ipsilateral Horner's syndrome (ptosis, miosis, hemianhidrosis, and apparent enophthalmos).	1. Motor system typically spared. 2. Lateral medullary (Wallenberg's) syndrome. Horner's syndrome: **HORNE** **H**—hemianhidrosis (loss of sweating). **O**—one eye (usually unilateral). **R**—relaxed eyelid (ptosis). **N**—narrow pupil (miosis). **E**—enophthalmos (sunken eyes).
Anterior inferior cerebellar	Definition: Infarction of lateral portion of pons. Clinical: ■ Ipsilateral facial weakness. ■ Gaze palsy. ■ Deafness. ■ Tinnitus.	No Horner's syndrome, dysphagia, or dysarthria.

(continued)

NEUROLOGY

TABLE 2.9-1.   Neurological Deficits in Stroke *(continued)*

ARTERY OCCLUSION	DEFICIT	OTHER
Lacunar	Lenticulostriate branches of the middle cerebral artery (midbrain) become occluded as a result of chronic hypertension. ■ Symptoms may present gradually over several days. ■ CT or MRI may not detect stroke. Presentations: ■ Pure motor hemiparesis: Affecting face, arm, leg without other disturbances. ■ Pure sensory stroke: Hemisensory loss. ■ Ataxic hemiparesis: Pure motor hemiparesis combined with ataxia. ■ Clumsy hand dysarthria: Dysarthria, dysphagia, facial weakness, and weakness/clumsiness of contralateral hand.	

> **Risk Factors for Ischemic Stroke—**
>
> *"Ischemic strokes have only a DASH of tissue perfusion"*
>
> **D**iabetes
> **A**trial fibrillation
> **S**moking
> **H**ypertension/
>   **H**ypercoagulability/
>   **H**yperlipidemia/
>   **H**eart attack (recent)

■ There is a high risk of a stroke within 6 years after a heart attack.
■ Eight percent of ischemic strokes and 38% of hemorrhagic strokes result in death within 30 days.
  ■ **Ischemic penumbra:** The tissue surrounding an infarcted zone that is dysfunctional but not infarcted and that may recover full functionality if the hypoxic state resolves. The volume of the ischemic penumbra is often greater than that of the infarcted core, and thus its salvage can dramatically reduce the degree of permanent deficit.
■ Almost a quarter of people who have an initial stroke die within a year.

FIGURE 2.9-1.   CT of ischemic stroke of the anterior cerebral artery (ACA).

Note that the lesion is hypodense. (Reproduced, with permission, from Johnson MH. CT evaluation of the earliest signs of stroke. *The Radiologist* 1(4): 89–199, 1994.)

FIGURE 2.9-2. Low attenuation area within the cerebellum posteriorly on the right (arrowheads) suggestive of infarct in right PICA distribution.

Risk Factors for Hemorrhagic Stroke—

"Hemorrhagic strokes leave you with a bloody HAT"

Hypertension
AVM/**A**neurysm/
   Anticoagulated
Trauma

RISK FACTORS

- Ischemic:
  - Hypertension (HTN)
  - Smoking
  - Diabetes mellitus (DM)
  - Dyslipidemia
  - Atrial fibrillation
  - Hypercoagulable state
  - Recent myocardial infarction (MI)
- Hemorrhagic:
  - Hypertension
  - Arteriovenous malformation (AVM)
  - Trauma
  - Ruptured aneurysm
  - Bleeding diathesis/anticoagulation

CLASSIFICATION AND ETIOLOGY

- Ischemic stroke:
  - Thrombotic:
    - Large-vessel disease—atherosclerosis usually located at bifurcation of carotid, vertebrobasilar system, or middle cerebral artery. A disease process that starts with a **T** but does not **T**ravel.
    - Small-vessel disease—microatheroma or lipohyalinosis usually due to HTN or DM, causing lacunar infarcts in subcortical tissues.
    - Similar pathophysiology to acute myocardial infarction, where a damaged vessel becomes occluded with thrombus.
  - **Embolic:** Usually of cardiac origin (60%), source often unknown, sometimes carotid (artery-to-artery embolus).
  - **Hypoperfusion:** Shock, etc.; most affect *watershed* areas (most commonly parasagittal strips of cortex).
- Hemorrhagic stroke:
  - **Subarachnoid:** Head trauma most common, aneurysms, AV malformations.

For stroke: The strongest risk factor is **hypertension,** with **smoking** as a close second.

Watershed injury describes ischemic injury to brain tissue located at distal end of cerebrovascular tree, usually due to a low-flow state.

TIAs used to be defined as any stroke whose symptoms resolved completely within 24 hours. With the advent of MRI and the ability to detect "silent" infarctions, the definition has narrowed toward including only those cases with no detectable infarcts.

NEUROLOGY

NEUROLOGY

Risk of stroke after TIA:
- First month: 4–8%
- First year: 12–14%
- At 5 years: 24–29%

The initial CT should be done *without* contrast as fresh blood is radiolucent relative to old blood and normal cerebral tissue. Contrast-enhanced CT or MRI is useful subsequently to reveal regions of infarct.

- **Intracerebral:** Hypertension, amyloid, bleeding disorders, trauma, tumors.
- **Metabolic stroke:**
  - Not necessarily related to vasculature/territories.
  - Usually secondary to cerebral energy failure (hypoglycemia).
  - Often resolves without deficits.
- **Venous stroke:**
  - Usually from thrombosis of cerebral veins/dural sinus.
  - Does not obey territories.
  - Often hemorrhagic.

PATHOPHYSIOLOGY

- **Ischemic stroke:**
  - Occlusion of artery feeding brain causes oxygen depletion and damage to neurons.
  - The ensuing ischemia results in release of inflammatory cytokines, which ↓ flow by increasing viscosity. These cytokines further damage neuronal function.
  - With reperfusion of ischemic area, oxygen free radicals are produced, which also damage neurons.
- **Hemorrhagic stroke** (see Figure 2.9-3): The extravasation of blood into the central nervous system (CNS) resulting from subarachnoid hemorrhage (SAH), HTN, or bleeding into a prior ischemic stroke.

SIGNS AND SYMPTOMS

- Thrombotic strokes often show relatively slow progressive onset, often during sleep.
- Embolic strokes present suddenly, often in discrete steps ("stuttering onset"), most often during waking hours.

FIGURE 2.9-3. **Head CT demonstrating intracerebral hemorrhagic.**

- Hemorrhagic strokes evolve over minutes, invariably during waking hours.
- Twenty percent of stroke patients have a history of at least one TIA.

DIAGNOSIS/WORKUP

- A noncontrast computed tomography (CT) scan is useful for quick diagnosis and localization. It can also be helpful to exclude hemorrhagic strokes. Will pick up ~ 90% of bleeds; the remaining 10% will be picked up with lumbar puncture.
- MRI/magnetic resonance angiography (MRA) for further study and follow-up.
- Carotid ultrasound to screen for carotid stenosis.
- Cardiac echocardiography may be used to screen for embolic source. Transesophageal echo (TEE) is most sensitive. A bubble study may be performed to evaluate for a patent foramen ovale (PFO). According to the American Stroke Association, PFO is present in up to 20% of the population, increasing the risk of cerebrovascular accident (CVA) by 25%. Also need to look for atrial/aortic thrombus or dilated atria.
- Electrocardiogram (ECG) to look for atrial fibrillation.

TIAs preceding thrombotic strokes tend to present with similar symptoms because the transient ischemia is locked to the distribution of the stenotic artery. Conversely, TIAs preceding embolic strokes tend to have more variable presentation.

TREATMENT

- **TIA:**
  - Main "treatment" involves assessment of risk factors, and diagnostic studies to see if there is a correctable cause for brain ischemia (eg, critical carotid stenosis).
  - Beyond that, patients should be started on a daily aspirin or alternative antiplatelet agent.
- **General measures for stroke:**
  - Correct hypoxemia (supplemental oxygen), hypoglycemia (D50), hypotension (IVF), and hyperthermia (acetaminophen).
  - Deep venous thrombosis (DVT) prophylaxis (compression stockings, low-molecular-weight subcutaneous injections).
  - Regular turning of comatose patients to prevent decubitus ulcers.
  - NPO initially, then parenteral feeding for those without intact gag reflex to avoid risk of aspiration. Of note, the gag reflex is absent (at baseline prior to CVA) in up to 25% of the population.
- **Ischemic stroke:**
  - Monitor blood pressure. Do not treat acutely unless other acute conditions such as concurrent MI, aortic dissection, hypertensive encephalopathy, congestive heart failure (CHF), or acute renal failure (ARF) are present.
  - Treat systolic blood pressure (SBP) > 220, diastolic blood pressure (DBP) > 110, or mean arterial pressure (MAP) > 130. Start with labetalol 10 mg IV. Do not ↓ the MAP more than 20%. MAP = (Systolic + 2 x Diastolic)/3.
  - For patients who present **within 3 hours** of symptom onset, IV tissue plasminogen activator (t-PA) is an FDA-approved option, currently considered standard of care. Patients must have a moderate-sized stroke and have no contraindications to thrombolytic therapy.
  - Investigational therapies include intra-arterial t-PA and mechanical clot retrieval via aspiration catheter introduced through the groin.
  - Anticoagulation is not indicated acutely; there is little evidence to support its use in any given case, although you will still see it being used. Often reserved for refractory cases and posterior circulation stroke.

Remember, decreasing the systemic perfusion pressure (BP) causes a corresponding ↓ in cerebral perfusion pressure in ischemic stroke and can be detrimental, as it can extend the area of infarct. Be **very** careful when lowering BP in stroke.

NEUROLOGY

There has been no advantage shown of alternative antiplatelet agents such as clopidogrel or ticlopidine over aspirin. Use of these alternative agents should be reserved for those who have a true allergy to aspirin, or those who have had their stroke while on aspirin.

- Aspirin or other antiplatelet agent both acutely and once daily following hospital discharge.
- **Hemorrhagic stroke:**
  - Elevate head of the bed 30 degrees.
  - Provide a quiet environment, analgesia, and sedation as needed.
  - Treat elevated intracranial pressure with hyperventilation, hyperosmolar agents (mannitol, glycerol), and steroids as needed.
  - Prevent straining (Valsalva) with antitussives and stool softeners as needed.
  - Nimodipine 60 mg for SAH (to reduce vasospasm).
  - BP control (more important in hemorrhagic than ischemic stroke).

BRAIN HERNIATION

- The movement of brain tissue into a space that it does not normally occupy, which can lead to coma and death.
- It is usually caused by a mass/lesion; can be caused by a bleed.

CLASSIFICATION

- **Transtentorial herniation:** The upper thalamic region herniates downward through the tentorium.
  - *Uncal herniation* is a common type of transtentorial herniation in which the gyrus moves through the anterior section of the tentorial opening.
  - The third nerve is often affected by the brain tissue that is displaced.
  - Patients often present with an enlarged pupil on the ipsilateral side of the herniation as well as a contralateral hemiparesis.
  - This is often followed by coma.
- **Subfalcine herniation:** The cingulate gyrus herniates across the midline.
  - Clinically, this may compromise blood flow through the anterior cerebral artery and can present as a headache.
  - Anterior cerebral artery infarction is a complication of this type of herniation.
- **Central herniation:** The entire cerebral hemisphere herniates across the tentorium as a result of ↑ intracranial pressure.
- **Tonsillar herniation:**
  - Result of ↑ pressure in the posterior fossa, causing parts of the cerebellum to herniate through the foramen magnum.
  - This type of herniation results in compression of the lower brain stem, which contains the respiratory center and leads to central respiratory failure.

CNS INFECTIONS

Rabies

A rapidly progressing viral infection affecting the human nervous system; usually from raccoons or bats.

EPIDEMIOLOGY

- Fewer than 10 cases per year in the United States.
- Fifty percent of cases from raccoon bites.
- Other cases transmitted by dogs, skunks, foxes, coyotes, bats, and bobcats.
- Rare cases from tissue transplantation (cornea).
- First unvaccinated patient to survive a human rabies infection: Jeanna Giese in 2004.

A patient with encephalitis, hydrophobia, and aerophobia should have rabies virus workup.

SIGNS AND SYMPTOMS

Two phases:

- *Prodromal phase*: Pain, paresthesias, gastrointestinal (GI)/respiratory symptoms, irritability, apprehension, **hydrophobia** (aversion to swallowing water because of pain), aerophobia (fear of fresh air).
- *Excitation phase*: Hyperventilation, hyperactivity, disorientation, and seizures. Patient becomes increasingly lethargic. Further involvement of cardiac and respiratory nerves leads to death.

RABIES

Respiratory failure
Aerophobia/
   Apprehension/
   Aversion to water
Bad pains
Irritability
Excitation
Seizures

DIAGNOSIS

- Fluorescent antibody staining, polymerase chain reaction (PCR).
- Presence of Negri bodies postmortem in brain tissue.

TREATMENT

- Wash affected area thoroughly with soap and water.
- No antiviral therapy available.
- Supportive treatment:
  - Rabies immunoglobulin (passive immunization).
  - Human diploid cell rabies vaccine (active immunization—because of long incubation period, early injections provide sufficient time for protective immunity).
  - Active and passive immunization are administered in different parts of body so that immunoglobulin (passive) does not neutralize the vaccine (active).
  - Isolation of patient.
  - Preexposure prevention with vaccine should be used for high-risk individuals like zookeepers and veterinarians.

Rabies is universally fatal unless vaccine is given prior to the onset of symptoms. Immunize for:
- Raccoon bites
- Skunk bites
- Bat exposure (bite may be too small to see)
- Fox bites
- Bite from feral dog or cat

Bacterial Meningitis

Acute infection of the subarachnoid space and leptomeninges.

CAUSES (IN DESCENDING ORDER)

- *Streptococcus pneumoniae* (40–60%).
- *Neisseria meningitidis* (young adults).
- *Listeria monocytogenes* (immunocompromised hosts and very young or old). ("*Listeria* affects those with tumbling motility.")
- Gram-⊖ bacilli.
- *Haemophilus influenzae* (unimmunized adults). ("*Hae*, I was going to get vaccinated, but my chance *flu* by.")
- Group B strep (neonates). Penicillin is given to birthing mothers to treat this normal flora in 25% of women.

Kernig's sign: Extending the knee with the thigh at right angles causes pain in back and hamstring.

Brudzinski's sign: Forced neck flexion results in flexion at the knee and hip.

"*Neisseria* sucks down sugar and poops protein"
↓ Glucose   ↑ Protein

Why is glucose low in bacterial meningitis?
Low glucose in CNS is caused mainly by bacterial inhibition of glucose transport into the CSF, less so by bacterial consumption. The value should be compared to a concurrently determined blood glucose level.

When meningitis is suspected on clinical grounds, do not wait for results of lab tests or imaging studies: Treat empirically!

PATHOPHYSIOLOGY

- Bacteria commonly colonize the nasopharynx, which can then enter the bloodstream.
- Via the blood, the bacteria make their way into the cerebrospinal fluid (CSF) through the choroid plexus.
- Most signs and symptoms are secondary to the body's own inflammatory response.
- Bacteremia, sinusitis, otitis, and direct trauma could predispose to meningitis.

SIGNS AND SYMPTOMS

- Triad of headache, stiff neck, and fever (95%).
- Mental changes such as confusion, lethargy, or coma in 80%.
- Seizures occur in 10–30%.
- Nausea, vomiting, and photophobia are common complaints.
- Look for classic maculopapular rash of meningococcemia—occurs on days 1–3 of illness in 30–60% of infected patients; prominent in areas of the skin subjected to pressure.

DIAGNOSIS

- Blood culture is ⊕ in 50–60%.
- Lumbar puncture (LP; see Table 2.9-2):
  - Neutrophil count, protein, and opening pressure ↑.
  - Monocytes may predominate in cases of *Listeria*.
- Glucose ↓.
- Check Gram stain for presence of microorganisms.
- Cerebrospinal fluid (CSF) culture ⊕ in 80%.
- CT before LP to rule out abscess as source of meningeal irritation/ infection and mass effect. These pose risk of herniation during LP.

TREATMENT

- Good empiric coverage includes third-generation cephalosporin and vancomycin.
- Empiric treatment with antibiotics based on age. This is adjusted once the Gram stain or sensitivity results are completed.

TABLE 2.9-2. CSF Findings in Meningitis and Abscess

	WBCs	Diff.	Protein	Glucose	Opening Pressure
Bacterial meningitis	Very high	Polys	High	Low	High
Viral meningitis	High	Lymphs/monos	Norm	Norm	Norm/high
TB/fungal meningitis	High	Lymphs/monos	High	Low	High
Brain abscess	Norm/high	Polys	High	Low	Very high

- *Streptococcus pneumoniae:* Vancomycin + cefotaxime or ceftriaxone.
- *N. meningitidis:* Penicillin G or ceftriaxone.
- If patient is at risk for *Listeria* (old, young, or immunocompromised), you must add ampicillin.
- "Amp up" the coverage for those with tumbling motility.
- Add steroids before antibiotics if *S. pneumoniae* is the cause (↓ neurologic sequelae).

Viral Meningitis

- Also called aseptic meningitis.
- ↑ incidence in summer, early fall.
- Most commonly caused by enterovirus.
- More common than bacterial.
- Course is more benign.
- Signs and symptoms are similar to bacterial, but less pronounced (patient does not appear toxic).
- CSF shows normal to low protein, normal to high glucose, and lymphocytosis. Cultures and PCR can usually identify the cause.
- Treatment is supportive except in cases of varicella or herpes, in which antiviral therapy might be useful.

For CSF findings, remember: Viruses utilize proteins to replicate (low protein), utilize intracellular glucose (normal to high "extracellular" glucose), and are perceived as an immunological threat, (high lymphocyte count).

NEUROLOGY

Botulism

A paralytic disease caused by the toxin of *Clostridium botulinum*, resulting in presynaptic destruction of neuromuscular junction.

Etiology

- Ingestion of improperly prepared home-processed foods, canned foods.
- Wound contamination.

Pathophysiology

- Toxin blocks the release of acetylcholine at the peripheral nerve endings.
- Usual incubation period is 18–36 hours.
- A **descending** paralysis ensues, leading to respiratory failure and death.

Signs and Symptoms

- **Neurologic:** Dry mouth, diplopia, dysphagia, dysarthria, **descending weakness** of the extremities and muscles of ventilation.
- **GI:** Nausea, vomiting, diarrhea, abdominal cramps.
- Patient will generally be afebrile.

Descending weakness: Botulism; tick disease; and Guillain-Barré syndrome, Miller Fischer variant.

Diagnosis

Detection of neurotoxin by serology, only in specialized labs.

Treatment

- **Ingestion:**
  - Antitoxin.
  - Whole bowel irrigation (requires either alert patient or protected airway).
  - Toxic ingestion of substance not adsorbed to charcoal (charcoal has greateast utility only in iron, lead, lithium, and zinc [**Lead LiFe Z**ealously]).

Signs of Botulism—

"5 Ds"

Dry mouth
Diplopia
Dysphagia
Dysarthria
Descending weakness

Botulinum spores in honey can replicate in the gut of a newborn (who does not have normal bacterial flora yet) and cause botulism. (Typically on exam: "Baby ate honey, then became hypotonic . . .")

- **Wound contamination:** Drainage of lesion, antitoxin, and penicillin.
- **For both:**
  - Intubation with ventilatory support.
  - Prevention.
  - The toxin can be inactivated after 10 minutes in boiling water. The spores, however, can withstand boiling temperatures for several hours.

SEIZURE DISORDERS

- **Seizure:** Abnormal and excessive neuronal discharge causing a transient disturbance of cerebral function.
- **Epilepsy:** Two or more unprovoked seizures.
- One percent of population has disease.
- A range of effects can be seen, from the asymptomatic to overt convulsions.

CLASSIFICATION

- **Partial:** Focal, only part of cortex involved.
- **Simple:** No loss of consciousness (LOC), no postictal state.
- **Complex:** Postictal state present, LOC may or may not be present.
- **Generalized:** Always associated with LOC, whole cortex is involved.
- **Absence (petit mal):** Brief episode of nonresponsiveness to external or internal stimuli; motor tone is preserved.
- **Tonic-clonic (grand mal):** Generalized convulsion—brief tonic phase (stiffening) followed by clonic phase (rhythmic jerking).
- **Status epilepticus:** A long continuous seizure lasting 30 minutes or two or more seizures in a row without a lucid interval. *Emergency:* must implement the ABCs (airway, breathing, and circulation) of cardiopulmonary resuscitation (CPR).

Loss of bowel or bladder function and tongue biting are important clues in the diagnosis of a seizure.

ETIOLOGY

- Fever (affects 2–5% of 6- to 60-month-old kids); long-term risk 2.4% (baseline population risk of epilepsy = 1%).
- Idiopathic.
- Head trauma—an isolated seizure following trauma does not imply epilepsy. Risk of sequelae depends on severity of injury/hypoxia.
- Stroke.
- Mass lesions.
- Meningitis/encephalitis (infectious).
- Metabolic: Hypoglycemia, hyponatremia, hyperosmolarity, hypocalcemia, uremia, hepatic encephalopathy, porphyria, drugs, eclampsia, hyperthermia.
- Brain malformation/dysplastic cortex.

3-Hz spike and wave is the pathognomonic EEG pattern of absence seizures.

DIAGNOSIS

- Electroencephalogram (EEG).
- CT or MRI to rule out any lesions.
- Routine blood tests and toxicology screen to rule out metabolic or drug-induced seizures.

TREATMENT

- Address underlying cause if appropriate.
- Anticonvulsant therapy: Check for therapeutic levels in known epileptics.
- Benzodiazepines to break ongoing seizure.
- Phenytoin, carbamazepine, and valproic acid are common preventive medications for seizure.

Isoniazid (INH) causes seizures refractory to anticonvulsant therapy. They are treated with pyridoxine (vitamin B_6).

BRAIN NEOPLASMS

See Table 2.9-3.

TABLE 2.9-3. CNS Tumors

TUMOR	DESCRIPTION
Astrocytoma	■ Most common neuroectodermal tumor (also **most common intracranial tumor** in general). ■ Those occurring in adults are usually high grade—poor prognosis. ■ **Glioblastoma multiforme (GBM)** is an aggressive anaplastic type.
CNS lymphomas	■ Originate from B cells that have entered the CNS. ■ Commonly affects eyes, spinal cord, or leptomeninges. ■ Presents with headache, vision problems, and behavioral/personality changes. ■ Diagnose by identifying malignant lymphocytes. ■ Treatment with chemotherapy, radiation, and steroids.
Oligodendrogliomas	■ Tend to calcify. ■ More benign and better prognosis than astrocytoma. ■ Epileptogenic.
Ependymoma	■ In adults, characteristically found in spinal canal. ■ In children, most common location in fourth ventricle. ■ With excision, 5-year survival rate is 80%.
Meningiomas	■ Most common mesodermal tumor. ■ Usually benign and slow growing, but usually discovered at large size. ■ Clinically, may present as a cranial nerve palsy.
Schwannomas	■ Most common cranial nerve tumor. ■ Vestibular (acoustic) neuromas are eighth cranial nerve tumors. Anyone with unilateral deafness should have this ruled out. ■ Associated with neurofibromatosis type 1 > type 2.
Pituitary tumors	See Endocrinology chapter.
Metastatic tumors to CNS	■ 80,000 per year. ■ More common than primary tumors. ■ Metastases common from lung, breast, and malignant melanoma.

ETIOLOGY

- Exposure to ionizing radiation.
- Hereditary syndromes (ie, neureofibromatosis—six or more café au lait spots; tuberous sclerosis—facial angiofibromas, subungual fibromas, and ash leaf spot).
- HIV (lymphoma is typically of the B-cell subtype).

EPIDEMIOLOGY

- Kills > 13,000 per year.
- Originates from brain, spinal cord, or meninges.
- Most common:
  - Glial origin (50–60%)
  - Meningiomas (25%)
  - Schwannomas (8%)

SIGNS AND SYMPTOMS

In migraines, prolonged headache may be followed several hours later by vomiting. In brain tumors, acute headache is followed immediately by vomiting.

- Headache (40%); usually the result of ↑ intracranial pressure:
  - Present upon awakening and disappears within 1 hour (but can take any form).
  - Can wake patient from sleep.
  - Worse while lying supine.
  - New headache in middle-aged or older person.
  - Change in headache character in person with chronic headaches.
- Nausea or vomiting especially on awakening.
- Irritability, apathy.
- Sometimes vision loss, weakness of extremities.
- Seizures, focal neurologic deficits.
- Lethargy, weight loss more common with metastatic disease (patients are cachetic secondary to the ↑ metabolic demands of the tumor).

DIAGNOSIS/WORKUP

- MRI/CT for detection of mass and preliminary diagnosis.
- Biopsy for histology and definitive diagnosis.
- Positron-emission tomography (PET) scans and EEG occasionally have some diagnostic role.

TREATMENT

- Corticosteroids to ↓ edema and intracranial pressure.
- Surgical resection, if possible.
- Radiation and perhaps chemotherapy for high-grade tumors.

NEUROPATHIES

Forty to fifty percent of patients with ocular myasthenia gravis go on to develop generalized myasthenia gravis.

Myasthenia Gravis

PATHOPHYSIOLOGY

Autoimmune disease in which antibodies against the postsynaptic nicotinic acetylcholine receptor prevent acetylcholine from binding. Therefore, an end-plate potential is ↓ at the neuromuscular junction.

EPIDEMIOLOGY

- Two peaks of incidence:
  - Women ages 20–40.
  - Men older than age 60.
- Twenty percent have thyroid disease.
- Ten percent thymoma, 70% thymic hyperplasia.

SIGNS AND SYMPTOMS

- Muscular weakness and fatigue.
- Ptosis and diplopia (by affecting muscles of eye).
- Proximal muscle weakness.
- Intact reflexes.
- Nasal speech, dysphagia.
- Myasthenic crisis: Severe, life-threatening exacerbation, usually compromising respiratory status, and often requiring ventilatory support.
- Exacerbations in known patients may occur secondary to medication: aminoglycosides, ciprofloxacin, ampicillin, erythromycin, beta blockers, lithium, magnesium, procainamide, verapamil, quinidine, chloroquine, timolol.

DIAGNOSIS

- Myasthenia antibodies on serology.
- **Edrophonium (Tensilon™) test:** Edrophonium, which inhibits acetylcholinesterase, is given to the patient and a set of muscle groups is observed. In order for the test to be ⊕, the patient's muscle strength must improve, which is due to the ↑ availability of acetylcholine at the postsynaptic receptor (typically this test is used in acute setting).
- **Repetitive nerve stimulation** will display a quick reduction in the amplitude of the action potentials in myasthenic patients.
- CT of chest for thymoma/thymic hyperplasia (peak mass of thymus normally is puberty).

LABS AND TESTS

- Antibody presence against acetylcholine receptor (AChR).
- Chest MRI to evaluate any thymus abnormalities.

TREATMENT

- Most patients are able to have normal lives.
- If mild, anticholinesterase drug.
- Thymectomy when indicated (most patients experience long-term improvement; curative for 35%).
- Prednisone as first-line therapy.
- Cyclosporine or azathioprine if prednisone is not effective.
- Plasmapheresis and immunoglobulin therapy can also be useful.
- Patients in crisis should get steroids, pulmonary function tests, ICU admission, but not acetylcholinesterase inhibitors until crisis is under control. (Patients in crisis are unable to clear their secretions, so giving cholinergic agonists may worsen the ability to maintain their airway.)

Guillain-Barré Syndrome

Syndrome of transient immune-mediated **ascending paralysis** usually following a viral upper respiratory tract infection.

Symptoms worsen as day progresses. (This is the opposite of rheumatoid arthritis.)

"E-DRO-PHONE-I-UM" **("ET phone home")** Imagine ET's "tensed" trembling index finger improve as his myasthenia gravis symptom is lessened by edrophonium.

In myasthenia gravis, repetitive muscle use quickly induces fatigue, whereas in Eaton-Lambert syndrome, repetitive muscle use improves muscle strength.

Anterio mediastinum differential (limited and worth knowing)—

The 4 Ts

Thymomas—slow growing, varying sizes

Teratoma—large, round, lobulated

Thyroid, parathyroid—causes tracheal deviation at thoracic outlet

"Terrible" lymphoma—usually causes adjacent pleural effusion

ETIOLOGY

- Most cases are preceded by a respiratory or GI infection.
- *Campylobacter jejuni:* Most frequently associated as molecular mimicry occurs between human gangliosides and *C jejuni* lipo-oligosaccharides (LOSs). First our immune systems fight the bacteria LOSs, then our own gangliosides!
- Other potential causes: Herpes simplex virus, cytomegalovirus, Epstein-Barr virus, and *Mycoplasma*.
- Vaccines have been implicated as a potential cause in the past (ie, influenza, rabies vaccines).

PATHOPHYSIOLOGY

An immune-mediated demyelination of axons/axonopathy can also occur.

SIGNS AND SYMPTOMS

- Initial symptoms include paresthesias in the feet (or arms) and leg weakness, which progresses as an ascending motor paralysis, usually over several days.
- Distal muscle weakness is common soon afterward—may last a few weeks.
- Deep, aching pain in back and legs.
- Areflexia.
- Tachypnea.
- Quadriparesis and respiratory muscle paralysis occur in 30% of patients, and one-third of patients will need mechanical ventilation.
- Respiratory muscle paralysis can be fatal.
- Cranial nerves can be involved.

DIAGNOSIS

- CSF shows ↑ protein, but no WBCs.
- Electromyography (EMG) shows signs of demyelination with marked ↓ in action potential conduction velocities.
- The diagnosis is usually made clinically since CSF and EMG testing are often normal in the early course of this syndrome.

TREATMENT

- Most patients will have to be hospitalized.
- Mechanical ventilation for respiratory muscle paralysis.
- Plasma exchange and IV immunoglobulin in selected patients.
- Reassurance. Most patients make a full recovery, although < 5% of patients die from respiratory failure.
- Most cases resolve spontaneously over the course of several weeks to months.

HEADACHE

TOP 10 CAUSES OF HEADACHE

- Chronic headache syndromes (migraine, cluster, tension headaches).
- SAH.
- Meningitis.
- Hypertension.

- Mass lesion.
- Temporal arteritis.
- Trigeminal neuralgia.
- Brain abscess.
- Pseudotumor cerebri.
- Subdural hematoma.

Migraine Headache

PATHOPHYSIOLOGY

- According to the vasogenic theory, cerebral vasoconstriction is followed by vasodilation.
- It is thought that there are genetic and hormonal components to migraines.

EPIDEMIOLOGY

- Sixty percent have family history.
- Twelve percent in the United States affected.
- Females > males.

SIGNS AND SYMPTOMS

- **Migraine with aura** (classic, rarely seen): Patient suffers from aura approximately 1 hour before onset. The focal neurological dysfunction can include photophobia, sonophobia, nausea, vomiting, vertigo, dysarthria, tinnitus, diploplia, weakness, and ataxia. Patient may also complain of scintillating scotoma (65%) or homonymous hemianopsia.
- **Migraine without aura** (common): Photophobia and sonophobia are again noted, along with anorexia, nausea, vomiting, and general malaise. Specific visual findings are usually not involved.
- Both types have prodromal symptoms (60%) 1–2 days before attack. These include lethargy, food craving, depression, and fluid retention.
- Headache phase of migraine may last several hours. It is characterized by a unilateral, throbbing head pain.
- Paresthesias occur over 10–20 minutes, as opposed to those caused by CVA. A CVA produces paresthesias much more acutely. Never miss a stroke!

TREATMENT

- **Nonpharmacologic:** Avoidance of triggers; stress reduction; dark, quiet environment.
- **Acute treatment:**
  - Nonsteroidal anti-inflammatory drugs (NSAIDs).
  - Ergotamine derivatives.
  - 5-HT receptor agonists (sumatriptan—may cause malignant HTN).
  - Antiemetics (metoclopramide IV—watch for dystonic reaction, which is treated with diphenhydramine).
  - Valproic acid, tricyclics, gabapentin.
- **Prophylaxis:** Calcium channel blockers, beta blockers, tricyclics, and serotonergic drugs.

Triggers of migraines include: red wine, chocolate, monosodium glutamate (MSG), lack of sleep, menses, stress.

5-HT receptor agonists can cause coronary vasospasm.

NEUROLOGY

Tension Headache

SIGNS AND SYMPTOMS

- Muscular contractions causing bandlike pain located in head and neck.
- Neck stiffness.
- Usually bilateral.
- No prodrome.
- Worsens as the day progresses.

TREATMENT

- Aspirin or acetaminophen.
- Narcotics if severe.
- Prophylaxis with tricyclics such as amitriptyline.
- Relaxation.

Cluster Headache

A severe vascular headache that clusters in the same area of the head and time of day, usually lasting for several weeks.

 A 38 year-old-man believes he is having a cluster headache. He presents with drooling and right facial nerve paralysis. On exam, he has vesicular lesions on an erythematous base in the ear canal. *Think: "Ramsay Hunt Syndrome"*, *Herpes Zoster infection of the 7th nerve.*

EPIDEMIOLOGY

- Greater incidence in males than females.
- ↑ incidence after alcohol, nitrates, or stress.

SIGNS AND SYMPTOMS

- Unrelenting unilateral facial pain, which tends to occur in clusters.
- Pain so severe it can lead to suicide.
- Headaches are often seasonal.
- Accompanied by ipsilateral autonomic signs, including conjunctival injection, lacrimation, rhinorrhea, nasal congestion, ptosis, miosis, eyelid edema, and facial sweating.

TREATMENT

- **Acute episodes:**
  - High-flow oxygen.
  - Intranasal lidocaine.
  - Ergotamine, sumatriptan, and antiemetics if the above fail.
- **Prophylaxis:** Verapamil, methysergide, high-dose prednisone followed by rapid taper, lithium, or indomethacin.

Headache of Temporal (Giant Cell) Arteritis

Idiopathic inflammation of medium and large arteries, usually the temporal artery, histologically characterized by giant multinucleated cells.

 A 62-year-old woman presents with headache, pain when she chews, and scalp tenderness. *Think: Temporal arteritis.* **Next step:** Treat with steroids. This can save vision.

ETIOLOGY

Thought to be part of a systemic vasculitis that has gone undetected except for the temporal and ophthalmic artery involvement.

EPIDEMIOLOGY

More common in women and persons older than age 60.

SIGNS AND SYMPTOMS

- Unilateral headache in distribution of temporal artery.
- Thickened, tender temporal arteries.
- Ipsilateral visual loss (ophthalmic artery).
- Claudication of the masseter, temporalis, and tongue muscles.
- Scalp tenderness.
- Pulsating temporal artery, also sometimes nodular.

DIAGNOSIS

- Based on the 1990 American College of Rheumatology criteria for classification of temporal arteritis, at least three of the following five items must be present (sensitivity [$\oplus$ in disease] 93.5%, specificity [absent in healthy] 91.2%):
  1. Age of onset > 50 years.
  2. New-onset headache or localized head pain.
  3. Temporal artery tenderness to palpation or reduced pulsation.
  4. Erythrocyte sedimentation rate (ESR) > 50 mm/h.
  5. Abnormal arterial biopsy (necrotizing vasculitis with granulomatous proliferation and infiltration).
- Definitive diagnosis by temporal artery biopsy.
- Anemia is frequently seen.

TREATMENT

- Corticosteroids as soon as suspected; *can lead to blindness if treatment is delayed.*
- NSAIDs for pain relief.

Causes of painful vision loss:
- Optic neuritis
- Giant cell arteritis
- Acute angle-closure glaucoma

More than 50% of patients with temporal arteritis have polymyalgia rheumatica.

NEUROLOGY

Closed-angle glaucoma can be exacerbated by anything that dilates eyes (ie, sympathomimetics, anticholinergics). Treat with timolol or pilocarpine drops or systemic acetazolamide. Avoid atropine and scopolamine!

NEUROLOGY

See Table 2.9-4 for the differential diagnosis for acute vision loss.

TABLE 2.9-4. Differential Diagnosis for Acute Vision Loss

DIFFERENTIAL DIAGNOSIS	DESCRIPTION	TREATMENT
Central retinal artery occlusion	▪ Typically painless loss of vision. ▪ Causes ischemic stroke of retina. ▪ Cherry red spot on fovea.	Dissolve or dislodge embolus.
Retinal detachment	▪ Symptoms include flashes of light. ▪ Floaters. ▪ Vision loss.	Surgery or laser treatment.
Vitreous hemorrhage	▪ Caused by bleeding into vitreous humor. ▪ Common causes are diabetic retinopathy and retinal tears. ▪ Symptoms initially include floaters, which progress to vision loss.	Photocoagulation or vitrectomy.
Optic neuritis	▪ Painful, unilateral vision loss with partial resolution. ▪ Inflammation of optic nerve or absence of clinical findings. ▪ Caused by demyelination. ▪ Visual acuity at its worst in 1 week. ▪ Other symptoms include headache and eye pain with movement. ▪ Many patients have progression to multiple sclerosis.	Steroids.
Temporal arteritis	▪ See description under Headaches.	

Causes of painless vision loss:
- Central retinal artery occlusion (pallor and cherry red spot)
- Central retinal vein occlusion (thunderstorm)
- Retinal detachment (curtain)

Dementia

Loss of cognitive function with normal sensorium.

ETIOLOGY

- Stroke.
- Infection (particularly syphilis, AIDS, Creutzfeldt-Jakob disease).
- Epilepsy.
- Vitamin deficiency (folate [chemo, alcoholics], B_{12} [alcoholics, elderly] thiamine [Wernicke's], niacin [patients on pyridoxine therapy for tuberculosis]).
- Normal pressure hydrocephalus (NPH).
- Neurodegenerative disorders (Alzheimer's, Parkinson's, Huntington's, amyotrophic lateral sclerosis).
- Trauma.
- Toxins.
- Tumors.

DIAGNOSIS/WORKUP

Dementia workup should include complete blood count (CBC), electrolyte panel, vitamin B_{12}, folate, rapid plasma reagin (RPR), and head CT.

TREATMENT

- Treat underlying disorder.
- Optimize sensory function (vision aids, hearing aids).
- Simplify activities of daily living (simplify floor plans, stairs).
- Ensure physical safety (bedrails, companions).

> **Causes of dementia—**
>
> **VINCENT van Gogh was demented**
>
> **V**itamin deficiency
> **I**nfection
> **N**PH
> **C**VA
> **E**pilepsy
> **N**eurodegeneration
> **T**rauma/**T**umors/**T**oxins

Alzheimer's Disease

Slowly progressive dementia characterized by amyloid plaques and neurofibrillary tangles in the neurons of the cerebral cortex (mostly temporal lobe).

EPIDEMIOLOGY

- Older people.
- Family history (apolipoprotein E genotype).
- Higher incidence in patients with Down syndrome.
- Down's syndrome has ↑ incidence of four "A's": **ALL** (acute lymphocytic leukemia), **ASD** (atrial septal defect), **A**lzheimer's, and **A**tlantoaxial instability.

SIGNS AND SYMPTOMS

- Usually present with subtle onset of memory deficits accompanied by a progressive dementia.
- The earliest signs may include the inability to pay bills, go shopping, or other routine daily activities.
- Later on, patients will display aphasia, apraxia, confusion, and hallucinations.
- Patients may become incontinent and mute and require constant assistance with most tasks.

Alzheimer's is the most common cause of dementia.

DIAGNOSIS

- Diagnosis is mainly clinical; other causes of dementia need to be ruled out.
- Cortical atrophy on CT or MRI (see Figure 2.9-4).
- EEG slowing later in disease.

TREATMENT

- Donepezil, tacrine, and selegiline may slow cognitive decline.
- Memantine, vitamin E, exercise, and mental activity may be protective.
- Behavioral symptoms can be treated with neuroleptics, anxiolytics, and antidepressants.

Parkinson's Disease

Complex progressive disorder involving movement and higher cognitive function.

ETIOLOGY

- Degeneration of neurons in the substantia nigra.
- May be secondary to toxins (manganese, carbon monoxide, designer drugs—"ecstasy") and encephalitis.

EPIDEMIOLOGY

Mean age is 55; more common in men (3:2).

FIGURE 2.9-4. **Alzheimer's disease.**

Note the severe frontal atrophy. (Reproduced, with permission, from Lee SH, Rao K, Zimmerman RA [eds.]. *Cranial MRI and CT.* New York: McGraw-Hill, 1999: 194.)

SIGNS AND SYMPTOMS

Signs and symptoms fluctuate:

Remember: Parkinson's is marked by a resting tremor.

- **Pill-rolling resting tremor** (thumb rubs fingers, most prominent at rest).
- **Cogwheel rigidity** (ranging the extremities is awkward, there are alternating moments of brief fluidity followed by coarse rigidity—actually thought to be a tremor of the entire limb).
- **Bradykinesia:** ↓ amplitude and slowing of movements, manifested as micrographia, hypomimia (mask facies), hypophonia.
- Shuffling gait, festinating gait.
- Depression, hallucinations (occurs in 25% of patients, partially secondary to dopaminergic agonist therapy).
- Impaired autonomic dysfunction (gastroparesis, orthostatic hypotension).
- Postural instability usually occurs 8 years into disease process.
- Cognitive decline is a late feature.

DIAGNOSIS

- Clinical presentation.
- Response to levodopa-carbidopa.

TREATMENT

- Amantadine (antiviral) may improve tremor and bradykinesia in early disease by blocking reuptake of dopamine into presynaptic neurons.
- Levodopa: Converted to dopamine in substantia nigra; co-administer with carbidopa (does not cross blood-brain barrier) to block metabolism of levodopa in peripheral tissues.
- Anticholinergics: Block cholinergic inhibition of dopaminergic neurons in substantia nigra; commonly trihexyphenidyl, benztropine mesylate.
- Selegiline: Selective monoamine oxidase MAO-B inhibitor, blocks central metabolism of dopamine.
- Dopamine receptor agonists such as bromocriptine, pergolide, pramipexole.

Normal Pressure Hydrocephalus (NPH)

A distinct clinical syndrome in the setting of hydrocephalus without ↑ intracranial pressure.

ETIOLOGY

Most patients have no clear cause; however, it can sometimes be seen after a CNS event (SAH, meningitis, trauma, tumor).

SIGNS AND SYMPTOMS

Classic triad ("Wet, Wild, and Wobbly"):

- Urinary incontinence.
- Dementia (most refractory to treatment).
- Gait disorder (most responsive to treatment).

DIAGNOSIS

- Normal pressure on lumbar puncture (LP).
- Enlarged ventricles on CT or MRI.
- Temporal horns are normally slitlike, their dilatation is a sensitive indicator of early of mild hydrocephalus.
- Clinical improvement after LP and removal of a volume of CSF.

TREATMENT

- CSF ventricular shunt.
- Choroid plexectomy in some cases.

NPH is one of the few reversible causes of dementia.

FEATURES OF BRAIN DEATH

- Preserved cardiac function.
- No spontaneous respiratory function.
- No cranial nerve reflexes (especially pupils).
- No posturing (decerebrate [predominant extensors] or decorticate [flexors predominate, with fists clenched over the "core" muscles]).
- No evidence of hypothermia (rectal).
- No known reversibility of state (drugs).

Dermatology

Rashes That Can Be Seen on Palms and Soles—

Mrs. E

Meningococcemia
RMSF
Syphilis
Erythema multiforme

TOP CAUSES OF RASH WITH FEVER

- Rubella.
- Measles.
- Staphylococcal scalded syndrome.
- **Toxic shock syndrome.**
- Scarlet fever.
- **Meningococcemia.**
- **Disseminated gonococcal infection.**
- **Bacterial endocarditis.**
- **Rocky Mountain spotted fever (RMSF).**
- Kawasaki's disease.
- **Erythema nodosum.**
- **Hypersensitivity vasculitis.**

IMPORTANT QUESTIONS TO ASK IN ANY SKIN CONDITION

See Tables 2.10-1 and 2.10-2 for definitions of primary and secondary skin lesions and Table 2.10-3 for diagnostic procedures used in dermatology.

1. When did it start?
2. Where did it start?
3. Does it hurt? Itch? Other symptoms?
4. How has it spread?
5. How has each lesion changed over time?
6. What makes it worse (sun, heat, pregnancy, cold, medications, exposures)?
7. Previous treatments?

TABLE 2.10-1. Definitions of Primary Skin Lesions

Macule	A flat, nonpalpable area of skin discoloration (vitiligo, café au lait spot).
Papule	An elevated, palpable solid area of skin < 0.5 cm diameter (acne, lichen planus).
Plaque	An elevated area of skin > 2 cm diameter that has a larger surface area compared to its elevation above the skin (psoriasis, seborrheic keratosis).
Wheal	An elevated, rounded or flat-topped area of dermal edema that disappears within hours (urticaria).
Vesicle	A circumscribed, elevated, fluid-containing lesion of < 0.5 cm diameter (varicella-zoster).
Bullae	A circumscribed, elevated, fluid-containing lesion of > 0.5 cm diameter (pemphigus vulgaris).
Pustule	A circumscribed, elevated, pus-containing lesion (acne, disseminated gonococcal infection).
Nodule	An elevated, palpable solid lesion > 0.5 cm diameter (nodulocystic acne, erythema nodosum).
Petechiae	A red-purple nonblanching macule < 0.5 cm diameter, usually pinpoint in size (meningococcemia).
Purpura	A red-purple nonblanching macule > 0.5 cm diameter (Henoch-Schönlein purpura).
Telangiectasia	A blanchable dilated blood vessel (rosacea, cirrhosis, Osler-Weber-Rendu).

TABLE 2.10-2. Definitions of Secondary Skin Lesions

Scale	An accumulation of dead, exfoliating epidermal cells.
Crust	Dried serum, blood, or purulent exudate that accumulates on the skin surface (scab).
Erosion	A superficial loss of epidermis, leaving a denuded, moist surface; heals without scarring because doesn't penetrate through dermal-epidermal junction.
Excoriation	A linear erosion produced by scratching.
Ulcer	A loss of epidermis extending into dermis; heals with scarring because it penetrates into dermis.
Scar	Replacement of normal skin with fibrous tissue as a result of healing.
Atrophy	Thinning of skin.
Lichenification	Thickening of epidermis with accentuation of normal skin markings.

TABLE 2.10-3. Diagnostic Procedures Used in Dermatology

Diascopy	Pressing of a glass slide firmly against a red lesion will determine if it is due to capillary dilatation (blanchable) or to extravasation of blood (nonblanchable).
KOH preparation	Used to identify fungus and yeast. Scrape scales from skin, hair, or nails and treat with a 10% KOH solution to dissolve tissue material. Septated hyphae are revealed in fungal infections, and pseudohyphae and budding spores are revealed in yeast infections.
Tzanck preparation	Used to identify vesicular viral eruptions. Scrape the base of a vesicle and smear cells on a glass slide. Multinucleated giant cells will be identified in herpes simplex, herpes zoster, and varicella infections.
Scabies preparation	Scrape skin of a burrow between fingers, side of hands, axilla, or groin. Mites, eggs, or feces will be identified in scabies infection.
Use of Wood's lamp	Certain conditions will fluoresce when examined under a long-wave ultraviolet light ("black" lamp). Tinea capitis will fluoresce green or yellow on hair shaft.
Patch testing	Detects type IV delayed hypersensitivity reactions (allergic contact dermatitis). Nonirritating concentrations of suspected allergen are applied under occlusion to the back. Development of erythema, edema, and vesicles at site of contact 48 hours later indicates an allergy to offending agent.
Biopsy	Type of biopsy performed depends on the site of lesion, the type of tissue removed, and the desired cosmetic result. Shave biopsy is used for superficial lesions. Punch biopsy (3–5 mm diameter) can remove all or part of a lesion and provides tissue sample for pathology. Elliptical excisions provide more tissue than a punch biopsy and are used for deeper lesions or when the entire lesion needs to be sent to pathology.
Therapeutic modalities	Cryosurgery, curettage and electrodesiccation, phototherapy.

DERMATOLOGY

Urticaria, angioedema, anaphylaxis, and atopic dermatitis are examples of type I hypersensitivity reactions occurring in the skin.

Immediate Type I Hypersensitivity Reactions (IgE Mediated)

- Immunologic reaction mediated by immunoglobulin E (IgE) and mast cells, characterized by vasodilation and transudation of fluid.
- As the antigen binds to IgE on the mast cell surface, the mast cell degranulates and releases histamine and prostaglandin, causing vasodilation, ↑ capillary permeability, and smooth muscle contraction.
- **Urticaria** (hives/wheals): Leakage of plasma into the dermis causes a swelling after exposure to allergen. Wheals usually last < 24 hours and may recur on future exposure to the antigen.
- **Angioedema:** A deeper involvement of subcutaneous tissues with less demarcated swelling, usually characterized by swelling of the eyelids, lips, and tongue (see Figure 2.10-1). A deficiency of C1 esterase can cause hereditary angioedema.
- **Anaphylaxis** is the most severe systemic form of type I hypersensitivity reaction, characterized by bronchoconstriction and hypotension.

TREATMENT

- Antihistamines (H_1 and H_2 blockers).
- Corticosteroids.
- Airway protection (if needed).
- Epinephrine (for anaphylaxis).

Hypersensitivity (Leukocytoclastic) Vasculitis

- A group of vasculitides in which immune complexes lodge in small blood vessels, resulting in inflammation; fibrinoid necrosis; and painful, palpable purpura.
- Can be caused by drugs, infectious agents, or other sources.
- Gastrointestinal (GI) tract, kidney, and joints affected.

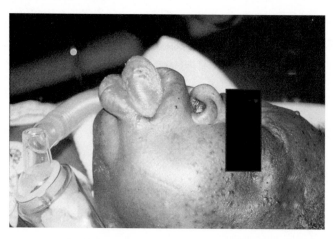

FIGURE 2.10-1.   Angioedema.

Also see Color Insert. Note severe tongue, lip, and peri-orbital swelling. In addition, patient has a tracheostomy to maintain the airway. (Reproduced, with permission, from Knoop KJ, Stack LB, Storrow AB, et al. *Atlas of Emergency Medicine*, 3rd ed. New York: McGraw-Hill, 2010: 112. Photo contributor: W. Brian Gibler, MD.)

DERMATOLOGY

- Henoch-Schönlein is a classic example (associated with strep infection + penicillin; small-vessel vasculitis with purpura of lower extremities/buttocks; IgA deposits in glomeruli).
- Common causes: Idiopathic, infection, sulfonamides and penicillin, neoplasms, connective tissue disorders (systemic lupus erythematosus [SLE], Sjögren's, rheumatoid arthritis, Wegener's granulomatosis).

SIGNS AND SYMPTOMS

- Pruritus and pain, associated with fever and malaise.
- **"Palpable purpura"** —multiple, scattered, nonblanchable red papules distributed over lower extremities, arms, and buttocks (see Figure 2.10-2).
- May be crusted due to necrosis of tissue overlying the blood vessel.

DIAGNOSIS

Biopsy.

TREATMENT

- Eliminate and/or treat causative agent.
- Systemic corticosteroids/immunosuppressive agents.

FIGURE 2.10-2. **Henoch-Schönlein purpura.**

Also see Color Insert. (Reproduced, with permission, from Knoop KJ, Stack LB, Storrow AB, et al. *Atlas of Emergency Medicine,* 3rd ed. New York: McGraw-Hill, 2010: 361. Photo contributor: Kevin J. Knoop, MD, MS.)

An acute or chronic relapsing pruritic type I (IgE) immediate hypersensitivity inflammatory reaction where scratching and rubbing → further lichenification of skin (often described as the "itch that rashes").

RISK FACTORS

- Family history
- Lots of allergies
- Asthma
- ↑ IgE
- **Exacerbating factors:**
  - Scratching, **stress,** infection, wool, skin dehydration, pregnancy, menstruation, and foods (milk, eggs); symptoms are usually worse in winter.
  - Usually improves with age.

SIGNS AND SYMPTOMS

- Pruritus.
- **Infantile eczema:** Red, exudative, crusty, and oozy lesions primarily affecting the face (cheeks) and extensor surfaces; spares diaper area; may clear by 2 years of age.
- **Juvenile and adult eczema:** Dry, lichenified pruritic plaques distributed over flexural areas (antecubital, popliteal, neck).

COMPLICATIONS

Secondary bacterial and viral infections with *Staphylococcus*, herpes simplex virus, and molluscum contagiosum.

TREATMENT

- Topical corticosteroids (mainstay of therapy).
- Avoid scratching (will provoke the rash).
- Lubricate dry skin.

Allergic triad:
- **Atopic dermatitis**
- **Allergic rhinitis**
- **Asthma**

Atopic dermatitis: Affected areas—**FACE**
Flexor surfaces get **A**dults. **C**hildren get **E**xtensor surfaces.

Dermatitis resulting from skin contact with a substance causing a delayed (type IV) hypersensitivity immune response.

TRIGGERS

- Poison ivy, oak, sumac.
- Nickel (jewelry).
- Formaldehyde.
- Rubber.
- Chemicals in shoes.

SIGNS AND SYMPTOMS

Intensely pruritic rash with linear, papular, erythematous lesions with **indistinct margins in the distribution of the exposure** (if allergic to watch band, there is a bandlike rash in the same spot around wrist).

DERMATOLOGY

DIAGNOSIS

History and physical usually enough; can biopsy.

TREATMENT

- Avoid exposure.
- If severe, use topical or systemic steroids/antihistamines.

IRRITANT CONTACT DERMATITIS

Dermatitis resulting from exposure to substances that cause physical, mechanical, or chemical irritation to the skin.

TRIGGERS

Common exposures after daily repetitive use of soapy water, cleansers, rubbing alcohol.

SIGNS AND SYMPTOMS

- Erythematous pruritic chapped skin, dryness, fissuring.
- Most commonly affects hands.

DIAGNOSIS

History and physical, but patch testing may be necessary to differentiate from allergic contact dermatitis.

TREATMENT

Goal is to restore normal epithelial barrier and then protect.

- ↓ exposure to soap and water.
- Emollients.
- Severe cases: Topical corticosteroids.

MISCELLANEOUS INFLAMMATORY CONDITIONS

Pityriasis Rosea

- A common self-limiting eruption of a single **herald patch** (see Figure 2.10-3) followed by a generalized secondary eruption within 2 weeks.
- The rash lasts around 2–6 weeks.

 A young person presents with a pruritic, spotted rash on the trunk that began as one solitary larger patch. *Think: Pityriasis rosea.*

ETIOLOGY

Herpes simplex virus type 7 is suspected.

DERMATOLOGY

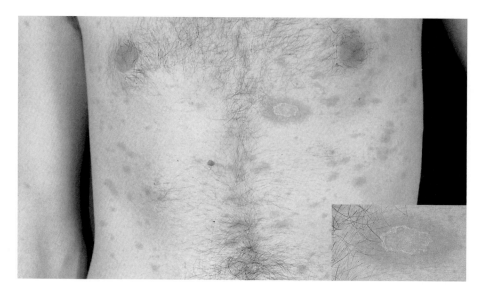

FIGURE 2.10-3. Pityriasis rosea.

Also see Color Insert. Papules and small erythematous plaques; note herald patch, an erythematous plaque with scale in central portion of lesion and collarette on border. (Reproduced, with permission, from Wolff K, Johnson RA, Suurmond D. *Fitzpatrick's Color Atlas & Synopsis of Clinical Dermatology*, 5th ed. New York: McGraw-Hill, 2005: 119.)

EPIDEMIOLOGY

- Affects children and young adults, primarily ages 10–40.
- Clusters of cases in spring and fall.

SIGNS AND SYMPTOMS

- Mild pruritus (present in 75% of cases).
- A 2- to 10-cm solitary, oval erythematous **herald patch** with a collarette of scale precedes the generalized eruption in 80% of patients.
- Within days, multiple smaller pink oval scaly patches appear over trunk and upper extremities.
- Secondary eruption occurs in a **Christmas tree** distribution, oriented parallel to the ribs.

TREATMENT

- Symptomatic.
- No treatment shortens disease course.
- Can use topical steroids, antihistamines if needed.
- Ultraviolet B (UVB) phototherapy or sunlight can help.

Psoriasis

- Chronic, noninfectious hyperproliferative inflammatory disorder characterized by thick adherent scales.
- Often presents with multiple exacerbations and remissions.

 A 35-year-old man presents with salmon-colored papules covered with silvery white scale on his scalp, elbows, and knees. *Think: Psoriasis.*

↑ epidermal cell proliferation, forming thick adherent scales.

RISK FACTORS

- Trauma.
- Infection.
- Emotional stress.
- Drugs (lithium, beta blockers, iodine, and antimalarials).

SIGNS AND SYMPTOMS

- Mild pruritus.
- Well-demarcated, thick, **"salmon-pink" plaques** with an adherent silver-white scale.
- Distributed bilaterally over **extensor surface** of extremities, often on elbows and knees, and trunk and scalp.
- Nails are commonly involved: Pitting of nails, oil spots (yellow-brown spots under nail plate), onycholysis (separation of distal nail plate from nail bed), subungual hyperkeratosis (thickening of epidermis under nail plate).
- Can occur at site of injury (**Koebner phenomenon**).
- Pinpoint capillary bleeding occurs if scale is removed (**Auspitz sign**).

COMPLICATIONS

Psoriatic arthritis, a destructive arthritis of the distal interphalangeal joints of hands and feet (**rheumatoid factor** ⊖).

TREATMENT

- **Mild psoriasis:** Topical meds (tar, anthralin, steroids, calcipotriene).
- **Severe:** Systemic therapy—usually phototherapy or immunosuppressants (UVB phototherapy, PUVA [psoralin + UVA], retinoids, methotrexate, cyclosporine, infliximab).

Erythema Nodosum

An inflammatory disorder of subcutaneous fat (panniculitis) characterized by painful erythematous nodules on lower legs; likely immune reaction.

 A 23-year-old woman presents with a cough, and a chest x-ray shows mediastinal lymphadenopathy. She has painful skin nodules on the skin of the tibia. *Think: Erythema nodosum* as a manifestation of sarcoidosis.

ETIOLOGY

- Idiopathic.
- Drugs (sulfonamides, oral contraceptives).
- Infection (strep, tuberculosis, histoplasmosis, coccidiomycosis).
- Autoimmune (sarcoid, inflammatory bowel disease).

SIGNS AND SYMPTOMS

- Nodules scattered over lower legs, bilaterally but not symmetrically (see Figure 2.10-4).
- Can be associated with fever, malaise, arthralgias.

TREATMENT

Removal/treatment of cause; steroids if necessary.

Erythema Multiforme

A general name used to describe an immune complex–mediated hypersensitivity reaction to different causative agents.

Note: Erythema multiforme, Stevens-Johnson syndrome, and toxic epidermal necrolysis are considered by many to be part of the same spectrum of disease.

CAUSES

- **Drugs** (penicillins, sulfonamides, barbiturates, nonsteroidal anti-inflammatory drugs [NSAIDs], thiazides, phenytoin).
- **Viruses** (usually herpes simplex virus, but also hepatitis A and B).
- **Bacteria** (*Streptococcus*, *Mycoplasma*)
- **Fungi**.
- Malignancy, radiotherapy, pregnancy.

FIGURE 2.10-4. Erythema nodosum.

Also see Color Insert. (Reproduced, with permission, from Wolff K, Johnson RA, Suurmond D. *Fitzpatrick's Color Atlas & Synopsis of Clinical Dermatology*, 5th ed. New York: McGraw-Hill, 2005: 149.)

DERMATOLOGY

Although characterized by **target lesions,** multiforme refers to the wide variety of lesions that may be present, including papules, vesicles, and bullae (see Figure 2.10-5). Affected sites include dorsa of hands, palms and soles, penis (50%), feet, and face.

TREATMENT

Discontinue offending agent and treat any underlying infections (eg, oral acyclovir to prevent herpes outbreak).

Stevens-Johnson Syndrome

- Erythema multiforme with systemic illness (fever, malaise) and multiple mucous membrane involvement (oral, vaginal, conjunctival) (see Figure 2.10-6).
- Extensive target-like lesions and mucosal erosion covering < 10% body surface area.
- Ocular involvement may result in scarring, corneal ulcers, or uveitis; 5% mortality.
- May evolve to toxic epidermal necrolysis.

Stevens-Johnson syndrome and toxic epidermal necrolysis are severe variants of erythema multiforme that are potentially life threatening.

Toxic Epidermal Necrolysis

Widespread full-thickness necrosis of skin covering > 30% body surface area.

FIGURE 2.10-5. Erythema multiforme.

Also see Color Insert. (Reproduced, with permission, from Wolff K, Johnson RA, Suurmond D. *Fitzpatrick's Color Atlas & Synopsis of Clinical Dermatology,* 5th ed. New York: McGraw-Hill, 2005: 141.)

DERMATOLOGY

FIGURE 2.10-6. Stevens-Johnson syndrome.

Also see Color Insert. (Reproduced, with permission, from Knoop KJ, Stack LB, Storrow AB, et al. *Atlas of Emergency Medicine*. 3rd ed. New York: McGraw-Hill, 2010: 344. Photo contributor: Alan B. Storrow, MD.)

SIGNS AND SYMPTOMS

- Prodrome of fever and influenza-like symptoms.
- Pruritus, pain, tenderness, and burning.
- Classic target-like lesions symmetrically distributed on dorsum of hand, palms, soles, face, and knees. Many cases have mucosal lesions—painful erythematous erosions on lips, buccal mucosa, conjunctiva, and anogenital region.
- Initial **target lesions** can become confluent, erythematous, and tender, with bullous formation and subsequent loss of epidermis.
- Epidermal sloughing may be generalized, resembling a second-degree burn, and is more pronounced over pressure points.
- ⊕ **Nikolsky's sign** (sloughing of skin with gentle pressure).

DIAGNOSIS

Biopsy.

COMPLICATIONS

- Secondary skin infections.
- Fluid and electrolyte abnormalities.
- Dehydration.
- Death (30% mortality).

DERMATOLOGY

- Removal and/or treatment of causative agent (suppressive therapy with acyclovir to prevent recurrences of herpes simplex virus).
- Hospitalization for severe disease, fluids (like burn victims) and steroids.

Decubitus Ulcers

Any pressure-induced ulcer that occurs secondary to external compression of the skin, resulting in ischemic tissue necrosis; may extend to underlying subcutaneous tissue, muscle, joints, or bones. Many patients who develop these are in the hospital.

RISK FACTORS

Immobility, malnutrition, elderly, diabetes, ↓ level of consciousness.

STAGES

- **I**—nonblanching erythema of intact skin.
- **II**—partial-thickness skin loss involving epidermis and/or dermis (superficial ulcer).
- **III**—full-thickness skin loss involving epidermis and dermis (deep, crateriform ulcer). May involve damage to subcutaneous tissue, extending down to but not through fascia.
- **IV**—full-thickness skin loss with extensive damage to muscle, bone, or other supporting structures.

COMPLICATIONS

Osteomyelitis, bacteremia, sepsis.

TREATMENT

- **Prophylaxis:**
  - Mobilizing patients as soon as possible.
  - Repositioning patients every 2 hours.
  - Pressure-reducing devices (foam, air, or liquid mattresses).
  - Correction of nutritional status.
- **Local wound care:**
  - Proper cleansing with mild agents.
  - Moisturizing to maintain hydration and promote healing.
  - Polyurethane, hydrocolloid, or absorptive dressings, and topical antibiotics for wound.
  - Necrotic tissue may require surgical debridement, flaps, and skin grafts.
  - Antibiotics if infection.

> Decubitus ulcers develop over bony prominences: sacrum, ischial tuberosities, iliac crests, greater trochanters, heels, elbows, knees, occiput. Can develop at any site that can be compressed against a hard surface.

DERMATOLOGY

See Table 2.10-4 for commonly tested infectious causes of fever and rash.

TABLE 2.10-4. **Fever and Rash—Commonly Tested Infectious Causes**

DISEASE	ETIOLOGY	SKIN FINDING(S)	RASH CHARACTERISTICS	OTHER CLINICAL FINDINGS
Measles	Paramyxovirus	Blanching erythematous maculopapular rash that becomes confluent.	Rash starts at hairline and behind ears → centrifugally to face → neck/trunk, extremities.	Koplik's spots, fever, cough, coryza, conjunctivitis.
Rubella	Rubella virus	Similar to measles but patient doesn't look as "sick."	By second day, facial exanthem fades.	Prominent postauricular, posterior cervical lymph nodes.
Varicella (chickenpox)	Varicella-zoster virus	Pruritic vesicular lesions in successive crops; vesicles evolve to pustules and crust over time.	First lesions begin on face/scalp → trunk/back.	Herpes zoster (shingles): Painful vesicular lesions; does **not** cross midline.
Erythema infectiosum (fifth disease)	Parvovirus B19	Erythematous macules and papules giving lacy "reticulated" appearance.	"Slapped cheek" in children.	
Roseola infantum ("exanthem subitum")	HHV-6, HHV-7	Multiple blanchable macules and papules trunk → extremities (after high fever prodrome).	Rash spares face.	Primarily in infants. High fever 3–4 days prior to appearance of rash.
Infectious mononucleosis	Epstein–Barr virus	Generalized maculopapular rash in 100% of patients with administration of ampicillin/amoxicillin.		Splenomegaly.
Scarlet fever	Group A *Streptococcus*	Coarse, erythematous, blanching rash; circumoral pallor; strawberry tongue; linear petechiae in skin folds (Pastia's lines).	Rash fades in several days → desquamation of skin.	Rash appears 1–3 days after strep pharyngitis.
Acute rheumatic fever	Group A *Streptococcus*	Erythema marginatum (transient macular rash with central clearing found on proximal extremities).	Subcutaneous nodules on bony prominences.	

DERMATOLOGY

Erysipelas

- Erysipelas, erysipeloid, and necrotizing fasciitis are variants of cellulitis.
- An acute onset of superficial spreading cellulitis, arising in inconspicuous breaks in skin (see Figure 2.10-7).

ETIOLOGY

Group A beta-hemolytic *Streptococcus pyogenes*.

SIGNS AND SYMPTOMS

- Pain.
- An **erythematous, shiny area** of warm and tender skin with a well demarcated and indurated advancing border.
- **Face is most commonly involved,** but can affect any area, especially sites of chronic edema.

DIAGNOSIS

Gram stain reveals gram-⊕ cocci in chains.

TREATMENT

Penicillin: If allergic, use vancomycin or macrolide.

Cellulitis

An acute deep infection of dermis and subcutaneous tissue characterized by erythema, tenderness, and warmth of involved area.

ETIOLOGY

- *Staphylococcus aureus.*
- Group A beta-hemolytic *Streptococcus pyogenes.*
- *Haemophilus influenzae.*

RISK FACTORS

Abrasion, burn, surgery, bites, neuropathy, immunocompromise.

FIGURE 2.10-7. Erysipelas.

Also see Color Insert. (Reproduced, with permission, from Fauci AS et al [eds]. *Harrison's Principles of Internal Medicine*, 17th ed. New York: McGraw-Hill, 2008: 885.)

A 54-year-old man with insulin-dependent diabetes presents with a warm, erythematous, slightly tender rash with poorly demarcated borders that began on his calf yesterday and has now spread up his leg. *Think: Cellulitis.*

A detailed history is particularly important to reveal the portal of entry in cellulitis.

SIGNS AND SYMPTOMS

- Warmth and tenderness of infected site.
- Erythematous, edematous, **shiny area of warm and tender skin** with poorly demarcated, **nonelevated** border.

TREATMENT

- Penicillin: If penicillin allergic or methicillin-resistant *S aureus* (MRSA), use vancomycin.
- For *H influenzae*, use third-generation cephalosporin.

Toxic Shock Syndrome (TSS)

A toxin-mediated disease characterized by acute onset of fever, hypotension, diarrhea, and generalized skin and mucous erythema, followed by failure of multiple organ systems.

EPIDEMIOLOGY

- Ages 20–30.
- ↑ incidence in women using high-absorbency tampons and in patients with burns, ulcers, surgical wounds, and nasal packs.

ETIOLOGY

S aureus producing TSS toxin-1 (TSST-1) or group A beta-hemolytic streptococci (rare).

SIGNS AND SYMPTOMS

- Acute onset of fever, hypotension, tingling sensation in hands and feet, myalgia, headache, confusion, disorientation, and diarrhea.
- A generalized erythematous macular eruption occurs most intensely at affected site followed by desquamation of palms and soles 1–2 weeks after onset of illness with edema of face, hands, and feet.
- Erythema of oral mucosa, bulbar conjunctiva, vagina, and tympanic membrane.

TREATMENT

- Admission to intensive care unit.
- Removal of potential foreign bodies.
- Antibiotics (anti-staph) and supportive care.

Meningococcemia (*Neisseria* Meningitis)

A potentially fatal disease resulting from meningococcal bacteremia, usually affecting children 6 months to 1 year old, asplenic, or compliment-deficient patients.

SIGNS AND SYMPTOMS

- Acutely ill patient often with discrete **pink macules, papules,** and **petechiae,** which can be distributed over trunk, extremities, and palate (see Figure 2.10-8) (see Table 2.10-1 for definitions of primary skin lesions).
- With fulminant disease, patients have **purpura,** ecchymosis, and confluent area of gray-black necrosis.
- Signs of meningeal irritation (eg, nuchal rigidity).

DIAGNOSIS

- Blood cultures reveal meningococci.
- Cerebrospinal fluid (CSF) culture is usually ⊕.

COMPLICATIONS

- Meningitis (50–90%).
- **Waterhouse-Friderichsen syndrome** (fulminant meningococcemia with adrenal hemorrhage).

TREATMENT

- Admission to intensive care unit.
- Vancomycin and ceftriaxone IV at first clinical suspicion of meningococcemia.

Meningococcemia is fatal if untreated. Treat empirically prior to completion of tests if suspected on clinical grounds.

Rocky Mountain Spotted Fever (RMSF)

A potentially life-threatening disease due to *Rickettsia rickettsii,* transmitted via female *Dermacentor* tick (American dog tick in the eastern United States or the Rocky Mountain wood tick in the western United States).

EPIDEMIOLOGY

Mostly in children, southeastern states.

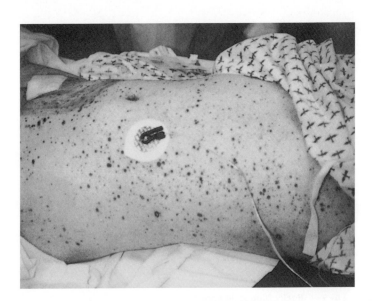

FIGURE 2.10-8. Meningococcemia.

Also see Color Insert. (Reproduced, with permission, from Knoop KJ, Stack LB, Storrow AB, et al. *Atlas of Emergency Medicine,* 3rd ed. New York: McGraw-Hill, 2010: 423. Photo contributor: Kevin J. Knoop, MD, MS.)

DERMATOLOGY

- Sudden onset of high **fever (> 102°F)**, myalgia, severe headache, rigors, nausea, and photophobia within first 2 days of tick bite.
- Rash within a few days, consisting of small, pink **blanchable macules** that **first appear peripherally** on wrists, forearms, ankles, **palms,** and **soles** (see Figure 2.10-9) and then **spread centrally to trunk,** proximal extremities, and face. Finally evolve to deep red papules.

DIAGNOSIS

Indirect fluorescent antibody (IFA) assay.

COMPLICATIONS

Some patients develop long-term sequelae lasting > 1 year, including paraparesis; hearing loss; peripheral neuropathy; bladder/bowel incontinence; and cerebellar, vestibular, and motor dysfunction.

TREATMENT

- **Doxycycline** is considered the drug of choice.
- **Chloramphenicol** for pregnant patients, children younger than 8 years (due to concern of staining the teeth), and severe disease.

Herpes Zoster

- An acute dermatomal viral infection caused by reactivation of latent varicella-zoster virus that has remained dormant in a sensory root ganglion.
- The virus travels down the sensory nerve, resulting initially in dermatomal pain, followed by skin lesions.
- Usually occurs in people > 50 or immunocompromised.
- Skin lesions are vesicles unilaterally along dermatome that ultimately crust over.

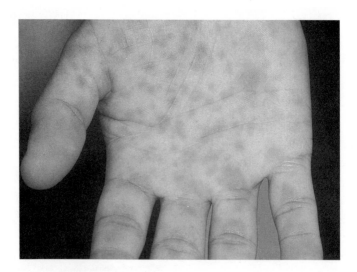

FIGURE 2.10-9. **Rocky Mountain spotted fever.**

Also see Color Insert. (Reproduced, with permission, from Knoop KJ, Stack LB, Storrow AB, et al. *Atlas of Emergency Medicine.* 3rd ed. New York: McGraw-Hill, 2010: 372. Photo contributor: Daniel Noltkamper, MD.)

DERMATOLOGY

SIGNS AND SYMPTOMS

See Figure 2.10-10.

DIAGNOSIS

Confirmed by **Tzanck preparation** revealing multinucleated giant cells, and culture of lesions.

COMPLICATIONS

- **Postherpetic neuralgia** (more common in the elderly and may persist for weeks to years after infection).
- **Herpes zoster ophthalmicus:** Lesions on nasal tip or eye indicate zoster involvement of nasociliary branch of ophthalmic nerve, resulting in uveitis, conjunctivitis, retinitis, optic neuritis, or glaucoma. An ophthalmic consult is necessary.
- **Ramsay Hunt syndrome:** Lesions on external surface of ear or auditory canal indicate zoster involvement of facial and auditory nerve, resulting in facial paralysis, hearing loss, changes in taste perception, ear pain, and vertigo.
- **Herpetic whitlow is HSV of fingers** (see Figure 2.10-11). Occurs in medical personnel exposed to patient's secretions (even without clinical herpes; virus may be shed in saliva). Treat with wet-to-dry dressing. Do not open vesicles or infection will spread.

TREATMENT

Antivirals (valacyclovir, famcyclovir); analgesia.

Patients with zoster can infect nonimmune contacts with chickenpox. Exposed nonimmune contacts should be treated with varicella-zoster immune globulin (VZIG).

FIGURE 2.10-10. Varicella-zoster virus infection: herpes zoster in T8–T10 dermatome.

Note typical dermatomal distribution of rash. **Also see Color Insert.** (Reproduced, with permission, from Wolff K, Johnson RA, Suurmond D. *Fitzpatrick's Color Atlas & Synopsis of Clinical Dermatology*, 5th ed. New York: McGraw-Hill, 2005: 823.)

FIGURE 2.10-11.   **Herpes simplex virus infection: herpetic whitlow.**

Also see Color Insert. (Reproduced, with permission, from Wolff K, Johnson RA, Suurmond D. *Fitzpatrick's Color Atlas & Synopsis of Clinical Dermatology,* 5th ed. New York: McGraw-Hill, 2005: 805.)

> A 24-year-old medical student working in the ICU held a patient's endotracheal tube with his ungloved hand to keep it from falling out. Two weeks later he has a vesicular lesion on an erythematous base that is extremely painful. *Think: Herpetic whitlow.*

CUTANEOUS FUNGAL INFECTIONS

See Table 2.10-5.

Lyme Borreliosis (Lyme Disease)

- A multisystem disease transmitted by the bite of an *Ixodes* genus deer tick infected with a spirochete *Borrelia burgdorferi.*
- Characterized by three stages of disease: localized, disseminated, and chronic.
- Occurs more in summer, northeastern United States.

SIGNS AND SYMPTOMS

- Acute onset of fever, chills, myalgia, weakness, headache, and photophobia.
- **Erythema chronicum migrans** (ECM) develops at site of tick bite in most patients within 1 month (an expanding erythematous annular plaque with a central clearing) (see Figure 2.10-12).

FIGURE 2.10-1. **Angioedema.**

(Reproduced, with permission, from Knoop KJ, Stack LB, Storrow AB, et al. *Atlas of Emergency Medicine*, 3rd ed. New York: McGraw-Hill, 2010: 112. Photo contributor: W. Brian Gibler, MD.)

FIGURE 2.10-2. **Henoch-Schönlein purpura.**

(Reproduced, with permission, from Knoop KJ, Stack LB, Storrow AB, et al. *Atlas of Emergency Medicine*, 3rd ed. New York: McGraw-Hill, 2010: 361. Photo contributor: Kevin J. Knoop, MD, MS.)

FIGURE 2.10-3.   Pityriasis rosea.

Papules and small erythematous plaques; note herald patch, an erythematous plaque with scale in central portion of lesion and collarette on border. (Reproduced, with permission, from Wolff K, Johnson RA, Suurmond D. *Fitzpatrick's Color Atlas & Synopsis of Clinical Dermatology*, 5th ed. New York: McGraw-Hill, 2005: 119.)

FIGURE 2.10-4.   Erythema nodosum.

(Reproduced, with permission, from Wolff K, Johnson RA, Suurmond D. *Fitzpatrick's Color Atlas & Synopsis of Clinical Dermatology*, 5th ed. New York: McGraw-Hill, 2005: 149.)

FIGURE 2.10-5.   Erythema multiforme.

(Reproduced, with permission, from Wolff K, Johnson RA, Suurmond D. *Fitzpatrick's Color Atlas & Synopsis of Clinical Dermatology*, 5th ed. New York: McGraw-Hill, 2005: 141.)

FIGURE 2.10-6. Stevens-Johnson syndrome.

(Reproduced, with permission, from Knoop KJ, Stack LB, Storrow AB, et al. *Atlas of Emergency Medicine.* 3rd ed. New York: McGraw-Hill, 2010: 344. Photo contributor: Alan B. Storrow, MD.)

FIGURE 2.10-7. Erysipelas.

(Reproduced, with permission, from Fauci AS et al [eds]. *Harrison's Principles of Internal Medicine,* 17th ed. New York: McGraw-Hill, 2008: 885.)

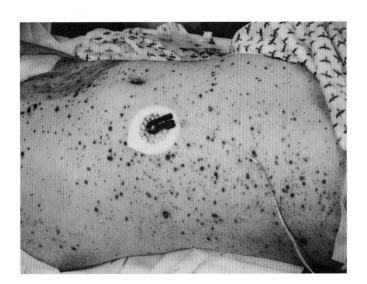

FIGURE 2.10-8. Meningococcemia.

(Reproduced, with permission, from Knoop KJ, Stack LB, Storrow AB, et al. *Atlas of Emergency Medicine,* 3rd ed. New York: McGraw-Hill, 2010: 423. Photo contributor: Kevin J. Knoop, MD, MS.)

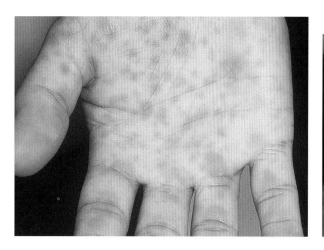

FIGURE 2.10-9. **Rocky Mountain spotted fever.**

(Reproduced, with permission, from Knoop KJ, Stack LB, Storrow AB, et al. *Atlas of Emergency Medicine.* 3rd ed. New York: McGraw-Hill, 2010: 372. Photo contributor: Daniel Noltkamper, MD.)

FIGURE 2.10-10. **Varicella-zoster virus infection: herpes zoster in T8–T10 dermatome.**

Note typical dermatomal distribution of rash. (Reproduced, with permission, from Wolff K, Johnson RA, Suurmond D. *Fitzpatrick's Color Atlas & Synopsis of Clinical Dermatology,* 5th ed. New York: McGraw-Hill, 2005: 823.)

FIGURE 2.10-11. **Herpes simplex virus infection: herpetic whitlow.**

(Reproduced, with permission, from Wolff K, Johnson RA, Suurmond D. *Fitzpatrick's Color Atlas & Synopsis of Clinical Dermatology,* 5th ed. New York: McGraw-Hill, 2005: 805.)

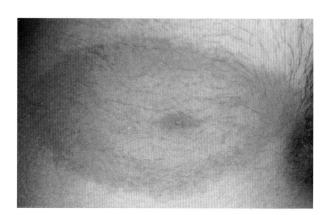

FIGURE 2.10-12. **Erythema chronicum migrans rash of Lyme disease.**

(Reproduced, with permission, from Fauci AS et al. [eds.]. *Harrison's Principles of Internal Medicine,* 17th ed. New York: McGraw-Hill, 2008: 1056.)

TABLE 2.10-5. Cutaneous Fungal Infections

	DERMATOPHYTES	CANDIDIASIS	PITYRIASIS (TINEA) VERSICOLOR
Definition	Group of noninvasive fungi that infect keratinized tissue of epidermis, nails, and hair resulting in tinea infection.	Superficial yeast infection found on mucosal surfaces typically in moist occluded areas.	Chronic asymptomatic scaling condition characterized by well-demarcated patches with variable pigmentation usually on the trunk.
Etiology	*Trichophyton, Microsporum,* and *Epidermophyton.*	*Candida albicans* (most often). **Predisposing factors:** Diabetes, obesity, heat, maceration, steroid use (systemic and topical); invasive disseminated candidiasis in immunocompromised hosts.	*Plasmodium ovale* (aka *Malassezia furfur*).
Types	■ Tinea pedis (athlete's foot). ■ Tinea cruris (jock itch). ■ Tinea corporis (ringworm). ■ Onychomycosis (nail infection).	■ Genital (balanitis, vulvovaginitis). ■ Diaper dermatitis. ■ Oropharynx (thrush). ■ Nail (chronic paronychia). ■ Intertrigo.	
Diagnosis	■ **KOH → multiple septated hyphae.** ■ **Wood's lamp** → bright green fluorescence in hair shaft (tinea capitis).	**KOH → pseudohyphae** (elongated yeast without true septations).	KOH → round yeast and elongated pseudohyphae (**"spaghetti and meatballs"**).
Treatment	■ Prevention (well-ventilated, cotton clothing). ■ Topical antifungals (not for hair or nails). ■ Systemic antifungals (if no response to topicals).	■ Keep areas dry. ■ Topical antifungals (nystatin, azole, imidazole creams), oral antifungals for recurrent infections.	Topical agents (selenium sulfide shampoo, azole creams).

DERMATOLOGY

DIAGNOSIS

- Serology: IgM titers are elevated in acute disease and peak 3–6 weeks after exposure.
- IgG levels peak when arthritis develops.
- May have false-⊖ results in first 4 weeks and false-⊕ results with other spirochetal infection and in patients with some autoimmune disorders (systemic lupus erythematosus, rheumatoid arthritis).

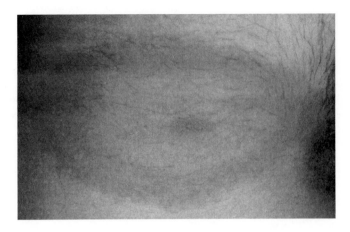

FIGURE 2.10-12. Erythema chronicum migrans rash of Lyme disease.

Also see Color Insert. (Reproduced, with permission, from Fauci AS et al. [eds.]. *Harrison's Principles of Internal Medicine,* 17th ed. New York: McGraw-Hill, 2008: 1056.)

COMPLICATIONS

- Sixty percent of untreated cases with disseminated infection develop arthritis (mediated by immune complex formation) 4–6 weeks following tick bite.
- May also develop **neurologic** (meningitis, encephalitis, or Bell's palsy) and cardiac involvement (carditis, atrioventricular block).

TREATMENT

Amoxicillin or doxycycline.

Acne Vulgaris

- Inflammation of pilosebaceous units of certain areas of the body including face, trunk, upper arms, and upper back caused by *Propionibacterium acnes* within the follicle.
- Typically seen in adolescents and up to 25 years.
- **Comedones** are the result—open (blackheads) and closed (whiteheads).
- Nodules or cysts are seen in more severe cases.

TREATMENT

- Goal is to remove plugging and treat infection (combination treatment is best).
- **Mild:** Topical antibiotics (clindamycin, erythromycin), benzoyl peroxide, topical retinoids.
- **Moderate:** Consider adding oral antibiotic (eg, minocycline) or oral contraceptives in females.
- **Severe:** Isotretinoin (Accutane).

Seborrheic Keratosis

- The most common benign tumor of the elderly.
- Develop from proliferating epidermal cells.
- Appear as waxy, stuck-on, tan-brown, verrucous lesions.

- **Sign of Leser-Trelat** is the association of multiple seborrheic keratoses with internal malignancy, usually adenocarcinoma of the gastrointestinal tract. No treatment is necessary.

Basal Cell Carcinoma

- The **most common** type of skin cancer due to a malignancy of the epidermal basal cells.
- Basal cells invade locally but almost never metastasize.
- Usually affect ages > 40 years.
- Whites generally affected.
- Risks are fair skin with chronic sun exposure, or radiation therapy.
- Diagnosed with biopsy and treated with excision.

 A 47-year-old white man presents with pearly, painless, ulcerated nodules with **overlying telangiectasias**. *Think: Basal cell carcinoma.*

FINDINGS

- **Nodular type:** A single translucent, **"pearly,"** waxy nodule or papule with **telangiectasias** and a **rolled border,** distributed on face and neck.
- **Superficial spreading type:** Multiple erythematous scaly plaques with a well-defined border distributed primarily on trunk; no relation to sun exposure.
- **Sclerosing type:** Yellowish white sclerotic waxy plaques with poorly defined borders, resembling scar tissue or morphea.
- **Pigmented type:** May have any of the above characteristics with pigmentation and is easily confused with malignant melanoma.

Squamous Cell Carcinoma

- A tumor of malignant keratinocytes accounting for the second most frequent type of skin cancer.
- Growth may be an **actinic keratosis** or de novo.
- Related to sun exposure, radiation exposure, immunosuppression, human papillomavirus, and xeroderma pigmentosum.

FINDINGS

- An erythematous scaling plaque that may be eroded or ulcerated with crust.
- Usually on sun exposed area of lips, cheeks, ears, scalp.
- **Biopsy:** Reveals malignant keratinocytes invading the dermis with keratin pearls.

TREATMENT

Excision or radiation if surgery can't be done.

Dysplastic nevus is a premalignant precursor to malignant melanoma.

DERMATOLOGY

Malignant Melanoma

- Melanoma is the malignant proliferation of melanocytes (pigment cells).
- It is the deadliest skin cancer.
- It may arise from normal-appearing skin (70%) or from a preexisting melanocytic nevi (mole) (30%).
- **Prognosis is based on the thickness of the primary tumor,** measured histologically according to the depth of invasion from the surface to the deepest part of the tumor (Breslow's classification) or according to the depth of penetration in relation to the different layers of the dermis (Clark's classification).
- Risks are sun exposure, fair skin and family history.

Melanomas can be brown, black, white, or blue.

CLINICAL VARIANTS

- **Superficial spreading melanoma:** Accounts for 70% of melanomas; characterized by horizontal growth. May develop as a new mole or as a change in a preexisting mole. It appears as an elevated plaque with irregular borders and variegated colors, but evolves into a nodule with bleeding and ulceration.
- **Nodular melanoma:** Characterized only by a vertical growth. Develops as a blue, gray, or black papule or nodule that may ulcerate or bleed. Associated with a poor prognosis because it metastasizes early.
- **Lentigo maligna melanoma:** Accounts for 10% of melanomas and occurs on sun-exposed areas of the skin in elderly patients. A slow-growing macule that gradually forms irregular borders, indistinct edges, or variable shades of color. May be present for years as a macule (lentigo maligna) before development of melanoma.
- **Acral lentiginous melanoma:** Accounts for < 5% of melanomas, and is common in black and Asian people. Develops as a flat, variably pigmented macule on the palms, soles, and nail beds that enlarges peripherally during its and then becomes nodular.

Suspicious features of malignant melanoma include the
ABCDEE's:
Asymmetry
Border (irregular)
Color (variegated and mottled)
Diameter (> 0.6 cm)
Elevation
Enlargement

TREATMENT

- Surgical excision with margins of at least 1 cm, depending on depth of lesion for local disease.
- Interferon may be added in high risk as adjuvant therapy.

PROGNOSIS

Deep tumors and node involvement are high risk.

On exam, a patient is found to have an asymmetrical, variegated 7-mm lesion with an irregular border. *Think: Malignant melanoma.*
Next step: Biopsy. **Treatment:** Resection.

Health Maintenance and Evidence-Based Medicine

Leading Causes of Death in the United States

1. Heart disease (26.6%).
2. Cancer (22.8%).
3. Stroke (5.9%).
4. Chronic obstructive pulmonary disease (COPD; 5.3%).
5. Unintentional injury (4.8%).
6. Diabetes mellitus (3.1%).

Note: Death rates for 2005. *National Vital Statistics Reports* 56(10): 2008.

Annual Exams

HISTORY AND COUNSELING

- **Health maintenance:**
  - Nutrition.
  - Exercise (recommend 30 minutes of aerobic exercise 3×/wk).
  - Weight gain/loss.
- **Accident prevention:**
  - Safety belt/helmet use.
  - Smoke detectors.
  - Firearm safety.
- **Toxic habits:**
  - Alcohol consumption (CAGE criteria; see Alcohol section).
  - Tobacco use.
  - Illicit drug use.
- **Sexuality:**
  - Contraception.
  - Sexually transmitted disease (STD) prevention.
- **Domestic violence:**
  - Elder abuse.
  - Spousal abuse.

The only cancer screenings that are effective:
- Breast cancer (mammogram).
- Cervical cancer (Pap smear).
- Colon cancer (sigmoidoscopy/ colonoscopy).
- Prostate cancer (prostate-specific antigen [PSA]— controversial).

TESTS AND EXAMS

- **Breast cancer screening protocol:**
  1. Ages 20–39 years:
     - Monthly breast self-exam (BSE).
     - Clinical breast examination (CBE) every 1–3 years.
  2. Ages 40–49 years:
     - Monthly BSE.
     - CBE every year.
     - Mammogram every 1–2 years.
  3. Ages 50–64 years:
     - Monthly BSE.
     - CBE every year.
     - Mammogram annually.
  4. Age 65 years and over:
     - Monthly BSE.
     - CBE every year.
     - Mammogram every 2 years.

- **Cervical cancer screening protocol:**
  - Perform Pap smear beginning within 3 years of first sexual activity or 18 years of age until the age of 65.
  - Perform every 2–3 years if three consecutive ⊖ Pap smears.
- **Colon cancer screening:**
  - Rectal exam yearly after age 50 years.
  - Occult blood in stool yearly after age 50 years.
  - Flexible sigmoidoscopy every 5 years after age 50 years, or colonoscopy every 8–10 years.
- **Prostate screening (controversial!):**
  - PSA and digital rectal exam yearly starting at age 50.
  - No screening after age 75.
- **Cardiovascular:**
  - Lipid profile starting at 25 years, every 5 years.
  - Blood pressure every 2 years.

CLASSIFICATION OF HYPERTENSION IN ADULTS

- Normal: < 120/80 mmHg.
- Prehypertension: 120–139/80–89 mmHg.
- Stage 1 hypertension: 140–159/90–99 mmHg.
- Stage 2 hypertension: > 160/100 mmHg.

AGE-RELATED CHANGES

- Height: ↓ as bone mass is lost with age.
- Vision and auditory screening at 65 years and older.

Adult Vaccinations

- **Tetanus:**
  - *Who:* Everyone.
  - *When:* Diphtheria, tetanus, and acellular pertussis (DTaP) series in childhood, booster every 10 years (or if > 5 years with a dirty wound).
- **Hepatitis A:**
  - *Who:* Travelers to countries with high /intermediate endemicity, men who have sex with men, illicit drug users, chronic liver disease, occupational risk, food handlers, clotting disorders.
  - *When:* Two doses 6–12 months apart, first dose takes 4 weeks to work effectively (any age).
- **Hepatitis B:**
  - *Who:* Everyone.
  - *When:* One series of three injections (time 0, 1 month, and 6 months) (any age).
- **Influenza:**
  - *Who:* Health care workers, age > 65, the chronically ill, and household contacts of these people.
  - *When:* Annually, autumn (new vaccine each year based on prediction of prevalent strains).
- **Pneumococcal (streptococcal) pneumonia:**
  - *Who:* Age > 65 or chronically ill.
  - *When:* Once every 5 years up to two doses.

Vaccinations for AIDS patients:
- Influenza
- Hepatitis B
- *Haemophilus influenzae*
- Childhood vaccines, if missed

HEALTH MAINTENANCE

- **Measles, mumps, rubella (MMR):**
    - *Who:* All persons born after 1956 who lack evidence of immunity to measles.
    - *When:* First one at age 12–15 months, second one between 4 and 6 years, then a booster during adulthood if not previously received or not immune.
- **Varicella:**
    - *Who:* Healthy adults with no history of varicella infection or previous vaccination.
    - *When:* Two doses of varicella vaccine delivered 4–8 weeks apart are recommended.
- **Human papillomavirus:**
    - *Who:* Females 49 years and younger.
    - *When:* 0, 2, and 6 months.

Raloxifene mimics estrogenic effects on osteoclasts but has no effect on breast, endometrium, or lipid profile. Useful for prevention of osteoporosis in women at high risk for breast cancer. Other benefits are lost.

HEALTH PROMOTION IN WOMEN

Hormone Replacement Therapy (HRT)

- Indicated in women with moderate to severe postmenpausal symptoms including vasomotor and urogenital symptoms.
- **Benefits:** ↓ risk of:
    - Osteoporosis.
    - Senile dementia.
    - Urinary incontinence, urinary tract infections (UTIs), and vaginal atrophy (local estrogen also effective).
    - Reduces hot flashes.
- ↑ **risks:**
    - Coronary artery disease and stroke: Recent trials (Heart and Estrogen/Progestin Replacement Study [HERS and HERS II]) show ↑ risk.
    - Endometrial cancer: Associated with unopposed estrogen use. Can be prevented by using estrogen-progestin combination.
    - Breast cancer: Women with estrogen receptor–⊕ breast cancer worsen with HRT. Increases risk as well.
    - Venous thromboembolism.

Estrogen:
- Inhibits osteoclast bone resorption.
- Elevates high-density lipoprotein (HDL), lowers low-density lipoprotein (LDL), but raises triglycerides.

Domestic Violence

EPIDEMIOLOGY

- Lifetime prevalence 20% for women.
- In the United States, ~ 2000 women die each year as a direct result of injuries.

SIGNS AND SYMPTOMS

- Frequent or unexplained injuries.
- Depression.
- Suicide attempts.
- Anxiety.
- Chronic pain.
- Substance abuse.
- Headaches.

How to ask about domestic violence:
- "Have you ever been hit, hurt, or threatened by your partner?"
- "Have you ever been a victim of domestic violence?"
- "Many of my patients with your symptoms have experienced physical violence. Has this happened to you?"

SCREENING

- Women should be routinely asked about domestic violence due to its high prevalence.
- Routine screening of women by physicians is thought to yield ⊕ results in about half of all cases.

TREATMENT

- Treat medical conditions.
- Assess safety of patient's current situation.
- Provide information (shelters, social agencies).
- Reassure patient that no one deserves to be abused.

Depression

EPIDEMIOLOGY

- Debilitating mood disorder that has a lifetime prevalence of about 15%.
- Incidence higher in women.
- Mean age is 40 years.

RISK FACTORS

- Family history of depression, suicide, substance abuse.
- Presence of chronic disease.
- Personal history of substance abuse.
- Lack of support system.

SIGNS AND SYMPTOMS

- Depressed mood with sadness.
- Weight loss.
- Guilt.
- Fatigue.
- Insomnia or hypersomnia.
- Anhedonia.
- Psychomotor agitation or retardation.
- Difficulty concentrating or suicidal ideation, for at least 2 consecutive weeks.

TREATMENT

- All patients should be asked specifically about suicidal intent.
- Patients who are actively suicidal require inpatient evaluation by a psychiatrist.
- Evaluate for antidepressant medication.

Differential diagnosis of depression:
- Bereavement
- Substance abuse
- Hypothyroidism
- Medication side effect
- Organic brain disease

How to ask about depression:
- "Have you been feeling overwhelmingly sad lately?"
- "Have you lost pleasure in the things you used to enjoy?"

How to ask about suicidal intent:
- "Have you ever thought that life was not worth living?"
- "Have you ever thought about killing yourself?"
- "Have you ever made a plan to kill yourself?"

SUBSTANCE ABUSE

Alcohol Abuse

- Associated with failure to fulfill work or social obligations, physical danger because of alcohol use, or recurrent legal problems due to alcohol use.

Cancers due to alcohol use:
- **Head and neck cancers**
- **Esophageal and gastric cancers**
- **Pancreatic cancer**
- **Liver cancer**
- **Breast cancer**

What order do you want to give a chronic alcoholic vitamin replacement therapy to prevent neurologic deterioration? Thiamine, then glucose and folate.

Alcohol and benzodiazepine withdrawal are **life threatening.** Opioid and cocaine withdrawal are not.

■ Alcohol dependence is at least three of the following: tolerance, withdrawal, taking more than intended, desire to cut down, time spent obtaining alcohol, aspects of life sacrificed.

SCREENING

CAGE questions:

1. Have you ever tried to **C**ut down your drinking?
2. Have you ever been **A**ngry/**A**nnoyed when people ask about your drinking?
3. Have you ever felt **G**uilty about your drinking?
4. Have you ever had an **E**ye-opener (drink on waking up in the morning)?

SYSTEMIC EFFECTS

See Table 2.11-1.

WITHDRAWAL SYNDROME

- Can range from mild anxiety and tremor to alcohol withdrawal seizures and delirium tremens.
- **Alcohol withdrawal is life threatening.**
- Treat with benzodiazepine taper.
- Usual onset is 12–48 hours after last drink.

DELIRIUM TREMENS

- Tachycardia, fever, hallucinations.
- Five to thirty percent mortality if untreated.
- Treatment: Sedation with benzodiazepines and intensive care.

TABLE 2.11-1. **Systemic Effects of Alcohol Abuse**

	ACUTE	CHRONIC
Central nervous system (CNS)	CNS depression, amnesia, fragmented sleep.	Peripheral neuropathy, Wernicke's and Korsakoff's syndromes (thiamine deficiency), cerebellar degeneration, alcoholic dementia.
Cardiovascular system	Decreased myocardial contractility, peripheral vasodilation.	Hypertension, cardiomyopathy, ↑ HDL cholesterol.
Gastrointestinal system	Esophageal and gastric inflammation, acute pancreatitis.	Mallory-Weiss tear, esophageal varices, portal hypertension, chronic pancreatitis.
Liver	Impaired gluconeogenesis.	Alcohol-induced hepatitis, cirrhosis.
Hematopoietic system	Macrocytosis.	Thrombocytopenia, hypersplenism, ↓ platelet aggregation.
Genitourinary system	Erectile dysfunction.	Testicular atrophy, amenorrhea, ovarian atrophy, ↑ risk of spontaneous abortion, fetal alcohol syndrome.

HEALTH MAINTENANCE

Tobacco Use

- Single largest cause of preventable death in the United States.
- About 450,000 people in the United States die each year from tobacco-related disease:
    - 40% cardiovascular
    - 35% due to cancer
    - 20% respiratory
    - 5% cerebrovascular

TOBACCO-RELATED DISEASE

Smoking:

- Promotes atherosclerosis, thrombosis, arrhythmias.
- Reduces oxygen-carrying capacity of the blood.
- Reduces elasticity in the lungs and causes COPD and emphysema.
- During pregnancy associated with increased risk of spontaneous abortion, fetal death, and sudden infant death syndrome.
- Smokeless tobacco products cause oral and head and neck cancers.

 A 50-year-old man complains of pain in legs with walking. Straight leg raising test indicates claudication. **Next step:** Smoking cessation counseling.

SMOKING CESSATION

Counseling should be a primary focus of all physician encounters with smokers:

- Identify all smokers and tobacco users by routine questioning during history.
- Instruct all tobacco users to stop, giving personalized advice and support (eg, " If you stop smoking, your cough will improve").
- Evaluate each patient for readiness and motivation. If the patient is not motivated, reinforce that support for smoking cessation will be available when the patient is ready.
- Formulate a plan with the patient, including a quit date, nicotine replacement or other pharmacologic therapy, and follow-up appointment for support.
- **Pharmacotherapy:**
    - Nicotine patches are associated with a 40% quit rate.
    - Bupropion is associated with a 55% quit rate.
    - Chantix (varenicline): Oral preparation works by partially activating the nicotine receptors in the brain. Typically given for 12 days.
    - Combination is associated with a 66% quit rate.
    - Ongoing counseling may improve abstinence.

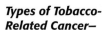

Types of Tobacco-Related Cancer—

CANCER PLUS

Colon
A
Neck
Cervix
Esophagus
Renal
Pancreas
Lung
Urogenital (bladder)
Stomach

The most effective way to extend life expectancy in a healthy patient is smoking cessation.

Opioid Use

SIGNS AND SYMPTOMS OF USE AND OVERDOSE

- Depressed mental status.
- Respiratory depression.
- Pupillary constriction (or dilation with profound respiratory depression).
- Overdose can cause death.

A patient on opioids for true pain control has little risk of developing opiate dependence.

TREATMENT OF OVERDOSE

- Naloxone is an opioid antagonist that rapidly reverses toxicity, but is short acting (< 30 min).
- Use is both diagnostic and therapeutic.
- Respiratory support if respiration is depressed.

OPIATE WITHDRAWAL SYNDROME

- Not life threatening, except in very young and very old, but may → relapse, using street drugs, and exposure to needle sharing with its attendant risks such as acquisition of HIV and hepatitis C.
- **Signs and symptoms:** Nausea, vomiting, diarrhea, mydriasis, piloerection, muscle pain.
- **Treatment of withdrawal and addiction:**
  - Symptomatic relief for withdrawal.
  - Long-acting opioid (eg, methadone) for treatment of addiction.

A significant percentage of patients presenting with cocaine chest pain will have biochemical evidence for a myocardial infarction.

Sympathomimetics (Cocaine and Speed)

SIGNS AND SYMPTOMS

Syndrome of catecholamine excess: Agitation, tachycardia, hypertension, hyperthermia, psychosis, seizures, chest pain.

TREATMENT

- Benzodiazepines to control excess sympathetic discharge and anxiety.
- Cooling measures to control hyperthermia.
- Nitroglycerin and heparin to control chest pain.

Beta blockers are relatively contraindicated in patients with cocaine use due to the risk of unopposed alpha-adrenergic tone, which may worsen vasoconstriction.

INJURY PREVENTION

Motor Vehicle Injuries

- **Statistics:**
  - Cause 30% of all deaths between ages 15 and 25.
  - Disproportionately affect the young, so responsible for more years of life lost than any other single cause.
  - Alcohol is implicated in 44% of all traffic fatalities.
  - Seatbelt use is associated with an 89% reduction in mortality, and concurrent airbag use further reduces mortality.
  - Motorcycle use is associated with a fatality rate 20 times greater than that of passenger cars.
  - Helmet use reduces motorcycle fatalities by 37% and reduces the incidence of head injury by 67%.

- **Screening:**
  - Ask all patients about seatbelt use, airbag availability, helmet use, child safety seat use, and alcohol use.
  - Intervene when patients show behaviors that put others in danger (eg, adult does not provide toddler with a child safety seat).

Falls

Most common cause of injuries.

RISK FACTORS

- Elderly
- Disabled
- Alcohol

PREVENTION

- Assess gait of each patient.
- Assess vision of each patient.
- Provide corrective devices or referral for identified impairment.
- Counsel alcohol cessation.

NUTRITIONAL DISORDERS

Malnutrition

- Marasmus: Starvation.
- Kwashiorkor: Protein deficiency.
- Essential fatty acids: Linoleic and linolenic acids.

RISK FACTORS

- Low socioeconomic class.
- Nursing home and hospitalized patients.

COMPLICATIONS

- Anemia.
- Anasarca.
- Poor wound healing.
- Decubitus ulcer.
- Infection.
- Death.

Obesity

Body mass index (BMI) > 30 kg/m^2.

COMPLICATIONS

- Atherosclerosis.
- Metabolic syndrome.
- Type 2 diabetes.
- Sleep apnea.
- Osteoarthritis.
- Gout.

- Venous stasis.
- Biliary disease.
- Endometrial cancer.
- Postmenopausal breast cancer.

TREATMENT

- Behavior modification, exercise.
- Low-calorie diet with < 25% of calories from fat.
- Goal: 10% weight loss over 6 months.
- If the above fail, consider:
    - Pharmacologic therapy.
    - Bariatric surgery (for BMI > 40 m² or > 35 m² with comorbid disease).

Vitaminoses

See Table 2.11-2.

TABLE 2.11-2. Syndromes of Vitamin Deficiency and Excess

VITAMIN	DEFICIENCY	EXCESS
Vitamin A	**Early:** Night blindness. **Late:** Keratomalacia, blindness.	**Acute:** Gastrointestinal symptoms, headache, papilledema. **Chronic:** Joint pain, hair loss, fissured lips, anorexia, weight loss, hepatomegaly.
Vitamin C	**Scurvy:** Petechial hemorrhage, ecchymoses, gum bleeding, poor wound healing, anemia.	Uricosuria, kidney stones.
Vitamin E	Areflexia, decreased proprioception, gait abnormality.	Potentiates oral anticoagulants.
Vitamin K	Prolonged bleeding time.	Attenuates oral anticoagulants.
Niacin	**Pellagra:** Chronic wasting, dermatitis, dementia, diarrhea.	Gastrointestinal symptoms, flushing, pruritus, hepatotoxicity.
Thiamine (vitamin B₁)	- Beriberi (dry). - Peripheral neuropathy. - Wernicke's encephalopathy (horizontal nystagmus followed by lateral rectus palsy, fever, ataxia, encephalopathy, death). - Korsakoff's syndrome (retrograde amnesia, confabulation).	
Pyridoxine (vitamin B₆)	- Seizures. - Glossitis, cheilosis. - Gastrointestinal symptoms. - Weakness. - Peripheral neuropathy.	

Heat Exhaustion

- Normal core temperature, symptoms due to dehydration and salt loss.
- Characterized by headache, nausea and vomiting, weakness, irritability, and cramps.
- Treat with oral or IV hydration with salt-containing fluids, and patient should rest in a cool environment.

Heatstroke

- Failure of thermoregulation.
- Associated with elevated core temperature and central nervous system (CNS) dysfunction such as altered mental status, focal deficits, hemiplegia, and posturing.
- Exertional heatstroke is a result of exercise or physical labor in a high-heat-index environment.
- Classic or nonexertional heatstroke is usually seen in elderly or nonacclimated patients during summer heat waves.
- **Treatment:** Rapid cooling by cooling blanket, evaporation, ice packs to axilla and groin, or gastric or peritoneal lavage is critical to prevent rhabdomyolysis, multiorgan failure, and death.

Cold-Related Illness

Risk factors: Overwhelming cold exposure, extremes of age, intoxication, homeless, chronic illness, iatrogenic.

FROSTBITE

- Caused by exposure of the skin to freezing temperatures; usually seen on the extremities, nose, and ears.
- As the body reduces cutaneous blood flow in freezing temperatures to maintain the core body temperature, capillary blood becomes more viscous, and ice crystals form in the extracellular space. This causes direct tissue injury and osmotic pressures that cause intracellular dehydration.

TREATMENT

- Rapid rewarming with clean water at 40–42°C.
- Tetanus prophylaxis.
- Debridement of tissues and prophylactic antibiotics remains controversial.

HYPOTHERMIA

Core (rectal) temperature:

- Mild: 32–35°C.
- Moderate: 28–32°C.
- Severe: < 28°C.

SIGNS AND SYMPTOMS

- Shivering.
- Poor judgment.
- Paradoxical undressing.

What would a hypothermic patient show on electrocardiogram? Osborn wave

- Cardiac dysrhythmias.
- Osborne wave: A convex, upward deflection of the J point on electrocardiogram.

TREATMENT

- **Rewarming** by:
  - Warming blanket.
  - Warm packs to groin and axillae.
  - Infusion of **warmed IV fluid.**
- For severely hypothermic or pulseless patients: Warm-fluid lavage of bladder, stomach, peritoneum, and pleural space.

MEDICAL ETHICS

See Table 2.11-3.

TABLE 2.11-3. Principles of Medical Ethics

PRINCIPLE	DEFINITION
Autonomy	- Ability to function independently and to make decisions about one's care free from the undue influence or bias of others. - All patients are considered autonomous if they have the ability to understand the situation as evaluated with competency examination by psychiatrist (capacity) and are not a danger to self or others (suicidal, homicidal, demented, delirious).
Nonmalfeasance	- The principle of *primum non nocere,* or first, do no harm.
Beneficence	- The principle of doing good. - The practice of doing whatever is best for the patient without the consideration of the patient's wishes is called *paternalism.*
Distributive justice	- The principle of equal and fair allocation of benefit. Patients of different race, gender, and disability should be treated differently only on the basis of medical need and projected benefit.
Advance directives	- Oral or written instructions from a patient to family members and health care professionals about health care decisions. - May include living wills, designation of a health care proxy, specific instructions about which therapies to accept or decline including intubation, surgery or medical treatments, and Do Not Resuscitate (DNR) orders. A DNR order applies only to advanced cardiac life support (ACLS) resuscitation, and does not include intubation and ventilation unless specifically addressed.

HEALTH MAINTENANCE

- Practice of incorporating the best available evidence from the medical literature for a diagnostic test or treatment into daily patient care.
- Best evidence obtained from randomized clinical trials.

STEPS

1. Identify a clinical problem.
2. Formulate a question.
3. Search for the best evidence.
4. Appraise the evidence.
5. Apply the information to the clinical problem.

SOURCES OF MEDICAL EVIDENCE

- **Randomized controlled clinical trial:** *This is the strongest type of evidence.* The selected population is randomized to receive either the treatment in question or a placebo (or the current standard of care), and the outcome is measured. The ideal randomized controlled trial is triple-blinded, meaning that the treating physician, the patient, and the investigators do not know which treatment has been given until the analysis is complete. These studies can establish cause and effect.
- **Cohort study:** The selected population is identified as being exposed or not exposed, and is monitored for subsequent effects. These studies are used when the exposure cannot be assigned for logistical or ethical reasons.
- **Case control study:** Populations with and without a given outcome are selected, and historical (retrospective) data is collected on exposure to a given agent or treatment.
- **Meta-analysis:** Evaluates the data of many trials that address the same question, and attempts to combine the information. These studies are best used when the clinical problem is infrequent and large randomized trials cannot be done.

If a disease has a high incidence with a low prevalence, it is a disease that causes rapid fatality. If a disease has a high prevalence with a low incidence, it is a chronic disease with a low fatality.

Statistical Concepts

See Table 2.11-4 for statistical concepts and Table 2.11-5 for sensitivity and specificity vs. positive and negative predictive value.

Types of Prevention

- **Primordial:** Deals with underlying conditions → exposure to causative factors.
- **Primary:** Deals with limiting the incidence of disease by controlling causes and risk factors.
- **Secondary:** The detection and amelioration of disease in a preclinical and presymptomatic stage.
- **Tertiary:** Prevention of future negative effects of the existing disease.

By screening a population, the death rate of a cancer dropped from 1% to 0.4%. How many people are needed to screen to save one life? NNT = $1 / (\text{control rate} - \text{experimental rate})$; $1 / (0.01 - 0.004) = 167$

TABLE 2.11-4. **Statistical Concepts**

CONCEPT	DEFINITION
Sensitivity	▪ Measures the ability of a test to accurately detect true-positive results: TP / (TP + FN) (true positive test results/all patients with the disease). ▪ The more sensitive a test, the less likely the test is to fail to detect a positive result. This is sometimes called a true-positive rate (TPR).
Specificity	▪ Measures the ability of a test to accurately detect true-negative results: TN / (FP + TN) (true negative test result/all patients without the disease). ▪ The more specific a test, the less likely the test is to fail to detect a negative result. This is sometimes called a true-negative rate (TNR).
Positive predictive value	▪ Measures the chance that a patient with a positive test result in truth has the disease: TP / (TP + FP) (true positives/test positives). **Depends on disease prevalence.**
Negative predictive value	▪ Measures the chance that a patient with a negative test result in truth does not have the disease: TN / (TN + FN) (true negatives/test negatives). **Depends on disease prevalence.**
Likelihood ratio	▪ Measures the fixed relationship between the chance of given test result in a patient with the disorder and the chance of the same test result in a patient without the disorder. ▪ Likelihood ratio for a positive test result is expressed as: sensitivity/(1-specificity) or true-positive rate (TPR)/false-positive rate (FPR). ▪ Likelihood ratio for a negative test result is expressed as: (1-sensitivity)/specificity or false-negative rate (FNR)/true-negative rate (TNR). ▪ A test with known likelihood ratios can help a clinician with decision making; the pretest likelihood that a patient has a disease can be either improved with a high positive likelihood ratio (< 2) or reduced with a low negative likelihood ratio (> 0.5).
Confidence interval	▪ Range around a sample mean that contains the true population mean to any desired degree of probability (frequently 95%).
Number needed to treat	▪ Measures the number of patients with a given disease that a clinician would need to treat with the tested therapy in order to see one beneficial event or prevent one adverse event. **Calculating numbers needed to treat NNT:** Number needed to treat = 1 / (control group rate – experimental group rate)
Prevalence	▪ Number of individuals with a given disease in a population at one point in time (number with disease/number in population).
Incidence	▪ Number of new events (new cases of disease) over a specific period of time (number of new events/number in population).

HEALTH MAINTENANCE

	DISEASE PRESENT	**DISEASE ABSENT**	
Test Positive	True Positive (TP)	False Positive (FP)	Positive predictive value = TP / (TP + FP)
Test Negative	False Negative (FN) Sensitivity = TP / (TP/FN)	True Negative (TN) Specificity = FP / (FP + TN)	Negative predictive value = FN / (FN + TN)

Awards and Opportunities for Students Interested in Medicine

- General Awards
- Research Awards
- Summer Externships
- Year-Long Fellowships
- For Minority Students
- Ethnic
- For Women
- Awards and Links to Medical Subspecialty Societies
- Evidence-Based Medicine Links

The Columbia University College of Physicians and Surgeons web site has an excellent web site with a list of resources for medical students, which is a great place to start your search for opportunities: *www.cumc.columbia.edu/dept/ps/affairs/subject1.html.*

The Paul & Daisy Soros Fellowships for New Americans

The fellowships are grants for $20,000 for up to 2 years of graduate study in the United States. The recipients are chosen on a national competitive basis. Thirty fellowships will be awarded each year.

A New American is an individual who (1) is a resident alien (i.e., holds a green card) or (2) has been naturalized as a U.S. citizen or (3) is the child of two parents who are both naturalized citizens.

The purpose of The Paul & Daisy Soros Fellowships for New Americans is to provide opportunities for continuing generations of able and accomplished New Americans to achieve leadership in their chosen fields. The program is established in recognition of the contributions New Americans have made to American life and in gratitude for the opportunities the United States has afforded the donors and their family. *Contact:* 400 West 59th Street, New York, NY 10019. Phone: 212-547-6926; fax: 212-548-4623; *www.soros.org/initiatives/map.*

AMERICAN ASSOCIATION FOR THE HISTORY OF MEDICINE OSLER MEDAL

The medal is awarded for the best unpublished essay on a medico-historical subject written by a student in a school of medicine or of osteopathy in the United States or Canada. Essays appropriate for consideration by the committee may pertain either to the historical development of a contemporary medical problem or to a topic within the health sciences of a discrete past period. The essay should demonstrate either original research or an unusual appreciation and understanding of the problem or situation discussed. Winner will receive $500 in travel money to deliver paper at the American Association for the History of Medicine.

Coe Memorial Scholarship

For medical students who are from the Auburn, New York, area. *Contact:* Norstar Trust Company, Coe Memorial Scholarship Fund, 120 Genesee St., Auburn, NY 13021.

Country Doctor Scholarship Program

$10,000 annually, $40,000 aggregate

Georgia residents qualify for funding to obtain primary care medical degrees such as internal medicine, general surgery, OB/GYN, pediatrics, and family practice. In return, the student must practice in a Georgia board-approved town of 15,000 or less population. *Contact:* Joe B. Lawley, PhD, State Medical Education Board, 270 Washington St. SW, 7th Floor, Room 7093, Atlanta, GA 30334.

ILLINOIS HOSPITAL ASSOCIATION SCHOLARSHIP

$500 award for students who are Illinois residents with demonstrated financial need and academic acheievement. *Contact:* Scholarship, The Illinois Hospital Association, Center for Health Affairs, 1151 East Warrenville Rd., P.O. Box 3015, Naperville, IL 60566.

New York Academy of Medicine: David E. Rogers Fellowship Program

The David E. Rogers Fellowship Program is national fellowship for medical students in support of a project initiated during the summer between the first and second years of medical school. Ten fellowships of $2,500 will be awarded. The fellowship is meant to enrich the educational experiences of medical students through projects that couple medicine with the needs of underserved or disadvantaged patients or populations. For more information, contact the Rogers Fellowship at *rogers@nyam.org* or the New York Academy of Medicine. Contact your school's financial aid office for more info.

DoctorsCare Internationale Foundation Scholarships

DoctorsCare is an independent nonprofit organization created to promote scientific research, education, and medical health programs that contribute toward improving the health of mankind. The foundation has funds for annual grants for needy men and women in the field of medicine. Applications may be obtained by sending a self-addressed, stamped envelope to: Grants Department, Doctors Care Internationale Foundation, P.O. Box 1111, Houston, TX 77251-1111.

WILDERNESS SOCIETY CHARLES S. HOUSTON AWARD

Award for a project proposal that is likely to result in a substantive contribution to the field of wilderness or environmental medicine. The applicant will conduct his project during the calendar year and present results at the Annual Meeting of the Society. Award: $1,500; www.ddcf.org/page.asp?page Id=12.

U.S. Department of Health and Human Services Innovations in Health Award

An annual competition for innovative proposals for health promotion and disease prevention. The proposal must be concerned with disease prevention or health promotion. It could describe a community risk-reduction effort; a project for a whole community or a special population group, such as the aged or children; a health promotion program at the worksite; or a preventive approach for community education, such as primary and secondary school programs. Awards range from $250 to $3,000; www.medicalreservecorps.gov/HomePage.

Life and Health Insurance Medical Research Fund Medical Scientist Scholarship

A 5-year scholarship program for an MD/PhD student who will have completed 2 years of medical school before July and is usually not already funded. $16,000 per year; http://mstp.uci.edu/currentstudents/fellowships.php.

AMERICAN ACADEMY OF MEDICAL ETHICS WILLIAM LILEY ESSAY CONTEST

An essay contest for medical students and residents on a topic designated by the Academy. $250–$2,000 prizes; http://ps.cpmc.columbia.edu/affairs/awards/awrd0087.html.

Paul W. Mayer Scholarship in Medicine and Biology

Sponsored by the Alliance for Engineering, this is a scholarship to encourage student excellence in the field of biomedical engineering. Grant is $200. Contact your school's financial aid office for more info.

Jerry L. Memorial Pettis Scholarship

Sponsored by the American Medical Association Education and Research Foundation, this scholarship will be awarded to a junior or senior medical student with a demonstrated interest in the communication of science. Financial need of nominees will not be a consideration. *Contact:* American Medical Association Education and Research Foundation, 515 North State Street, Chicago, IL 60610. Phone: 312-464-5357; fax: 312-464-5973; *www.ama-assn.org/medsci/erf/toc.htm.*

STUDENT PAPER COMPETITION IN MEDICAL INFORMATICS

Students are invited to submit papers expressing original ideas in the broad areas of medical informatics and computer applications in medical care for the SCAMC (Symposium on Computer Applications in Medical Care). Awards consist of the Martin N. Epstein Award of $1,000 and two cash prizes of $600 and $400 for second and third place. Contact your school's financial aid office for more info.

American College of Legal Medicine Schwartz Award

Each year the ACLM presents the Schwartz Award for the outstanding paper on legal medicine. The award provides a $1,000 honorarium, transportation, accommodations, and meals at the ACLM annual meeting. Contact your school's financial aid office for more info.

Medical History Society of New Jersey Stephen Wickes Prize in the History of Medicine

Any currently enrolled undergraduate, graduate, or professional student is eligible to submit

CLASSIFIED

an original essay on a historical subject in the medical or allied fields. The topic may be historical aspects of a current problem, or it may deal with a specific subject in a defined period of the past. Prize: $100. Contact your school's financial aid office for more info.

NORTHEASTERN OHIO UNIVERSITY COLLEGE OF MEDICINE WILLIAM CARLOS POETRY COMPETITION

The Human Values in Medicine at Northeastern Ohio Universities College of Medicine is sponsoring this annual poetry-writing competition for students attending schools of medicine or osteopathy in the United States. Prize: $100–$300. Contact your school's financial aid office for more info.

New York Academy of Medicine: The Paul Klemperer Fellowship in the History of Medicine and the Audrey and William H. Helfand Fellowship in the Medical Humanities

Each year the New York Academy of Medicine offers the Paul Klemperer Fellowship and the Audrey and William H. Helfand Fellowship to support work in history and the humanities as they relate to health, medicine, and the biomedical sciences. The Klemperer Fellowship supports research using the Academy Library as a historical resource. It is intended specifically for a scholar in residence in the collections of the Academy Library.

The Helfand Fellowship more broadly supports work in the humanities, including both creative projects dealing with health and the medical enterprise, and scholarly research in a humanistic discipline — other than history of medicine — as applied to medicine and health. Although residence is not obligatory, preference in the selection process will be given applicants whose projects require use of the resources of the Academy Library and who plan to spend time at the Academy. The Helfand Fellowship and the Klemperer Fellowship each provide stipends of up to $5,000 to support travel, lodging, and incidental expenses for a flexible period between June 1, 2001, and May 31, 2002. Besides completing research or a creative project, each Fellow will be expected to make a presentation at the Academy and submit a final report on the project. Applications are accepted from anyone — regardless of citizenship, academic discipline, or academic status — who wishes to use the Academy's collections for historical research or for a scholarly or creative project in the medical humanities. *Contact*: Fellowship Program Coordinator, New York Academy of Medicine, 1216 Fifth Avenue, Room 612, New York, NY 10029. Phone: 212-822-7204; fax: 212-996-7826.

Agency for International Development Internship

Sponsoring Agency: A.I.D.

Two-week educational program (over Christmas holiday) for graduate students from the Caribbean and South and Central America, which may lead to summer placement in transnational corporations over summer. Program focuses on U.S. foreign policy and Latin American indebtedness. Travel costs to seminar in Baton Rouge paid.

ALPHA OMEGA ALPHA ESSAY AWARD

The purpose of these $500–$750 awards is to stimulate medical students to address general topics in medicine and to enable the society to recognize in a tangible way excellent and thoughtful presentations. The topic of the essay may be any nontechnical aspect of medicine, including medical education, medical ethics, philosophy as related to medicine, reflections on illness, science, and the culture and history of medicine.

American Bureau for Medical Advancement in China

Open to fourth-year students. Several university teaching hospitals in Taiwan offer clinical clerkships to qualifying students. Electives of 2 months are optimal, although shorter ones will be considered. It is expected that students will be able to provide for their own transportation and room and board, but Warner-Lambert has provided a grant to accommodate several partial scholarships.

American College of Nutrition

Award based on original scientific work in Clinical Nutrition. Award: $500 plus transportation to meeting.

AMERICAN COLLEGE OF PREVENTIVE MEDICINE

$1,000 award for the best paper on preventive medicine–oriented topics; papers concerned with women's health issues encouraged.

National Council on Aging— Geriatric Fellowship

Sponsored by Travelers Insurance Aging, Inc., this program is designed to increase students' technical knowledge of geriatrics and to help sensitize them to social and personal problems facing older people. A fellowship of $3,000 will be provided.

Joseph and Rose Kennedy Institute of Ethics National Humanities in Medicine Seminar

This seminar was established to achieve three purposes: to provide selected medical students with an intensive experience in research and writing in the history of medicine, or philosophy of medicine, or literature and medicine; to encourage these students to develop programs of research and writing in a discipline of the humanities, which they will carry out during subsequent years of professional education and training and during careers as clinicians and humanists; and to link these students with other humanists in medicine across generational and disciplinary boundaries. Each student will receive a stipend of $1,200 to cover room and board. Students will be reimbursed for round-trip airfares to and from their school or home.

ACP-ASIM MEDICAL STUDENT ABSTRACT COMPETITION

Wanted: Students involved in research projects through their medical schools or community service programs they want to share with others, or who have come across as interesting case during an internal medicine rotation or through an internal medicine preceptorship program. If you are a medical student member of the ACP-ASIM, you are invited to submit an abstract to the annual Medical Student Abstract Competition. Ten winners will be awarded an expense-paid trip to the annual session. Abstracts may be submitted electronically using our online form at *www.acp.org*.

Medical Student Membership in the American College of Physicians–American Society of Internal Medicine

ACP-ASIM membership entitles you to special discounts on various college products, free attendance at ACP-ASIM annual session (the annual scientific meeting) and local chapter meetings, and a subscription to IMpact, the medical student newsletter.

AMA Political Action Committee (AMPAC)

AMPAC is a bipartisan group that serves to advance the interest of medicine within Congress, specifically by supporting candidates for office that are friendly to medicine. They also provide numerous programs to educate physicians, medical students, and their families on political activism. The board directs the programs and activities of this extremely important political action committee. Adding medical students to the leadership of this group will provide for better medical student representation within the group, as well as greater student involvement in this important process. Terms are for 2 years. Contact the American Medical Association for more information.

AMA FOUNDATION LEADERSHIP AWARD PROGRAM

This award is an exciting opportunity to advance your leadership skills within organized medicine. Medical students who have demonstrated strong non-clinical leadership skills in medicine or community affairs and have an interest in further developing these skills within organized medicine are eligible. The objective of the award program is to encourage involvement in organized medicine and continue leadership development among the country's brightest and most energetic medical students and residents. Twenty-five medical students will be selected. Travel expenses for award winners, including airfare and 3 nights' lodging, will be paid for directly by the AMA Foundation to attend the 2001 AMA National Leadership Development Conference. For applications, call 1-800-AMA-3211, ext. 4751 or 4746.

American Medical Student Association (AMSA)

International Health Opportunities; *www.amsa.org/global/ih/ihopps.cfm.*

AMA-MSS Councils

The medical student section of the AMA (AMA-MSS) has several councils for which it seeks medical students. Application involves a current curriculum vitae, an essay on why you want to be a member of an AMA Council, which council(s) you prefer, what you consider to be your major strengths and qualifications for the position, and what benefits you feel are likely to result from your participation.

- Council on Constitution and Bylaws
- Council on Ethical and Judicial Affairs
- Council on Legislation
- Council on Long-Range Planning and Development
- Council on Medical Education
- Council on Medical Service
- Council on Scientific Affairs

EDITORIAL POSITIONS WITH MEDICAL STUDENT JAMA

MS/JAMA is the 7- to 8-page medical student section of the *Journal of the American Medical Association* (JAMA) that appears in the first JAMA of every month, September through May, and is also produced each month on the MS/JAMA web site. As a regular section of a major medical journal, produced by and for medical students, MS/JAMA represents a unique opportunity to train to become journal editors, writers, and contributors. The MS/JAMA web site is located at *www.ama-assn.org/msjama.*

AMA-MSS Committee Application

Medical students are sought to serve on the following AMA-MSS committees:

- Committee on Computers and Technology (formerly Computer Projects Committee)
- Committee on Long-Range Planning
- Legislative Affairs Committee
- Minority Issues Committee
- Ad Hoc Committee on Community Service and Advocacy
- Ad Hoc Committee on Membership Recruitment and Retention
- Ad Hoc Committee on MSS Programs and Activities
- Ad Hoc Committee on Scientific Issues Committee (CSI)
- Ad Hoc Committee on International Health and Policy

All applications must be completed and submitted with a CV to: American Medical Association, Department of Medical Student Services, 515 North State Street, Chicago, IL 60610. Fax: 312-464-5845.

National Tay-Sachs & Allied Disease Foundation

The primary objective of these awards is to stimulate interest in the field of lysosomal storage diseases. The research may be basic, applied, or clinical and should be performed under the direction of an investigator experienced in the field. Stipend: $1,500.

NEW YORK ACADEMY OF MEDICINE: THE GLORNEY-RAISBECK MEDICAL STUDENT GRANTS IN CARDIOVASCULAR RESEARCH PROGRAM

Three grants of $3,000 will be provided to support projects in either clinical or basic research initiated during the summer. Competition is open to MD candidates in a metropolitan area medical school in New York City, Long Island, Westchester County, or New Jersey. The award will be paid directly to the sponsoring medical school for distribution to the recipient. The deadline for submission of applications is March. *Contact:* Fellowship Program Coordinator, New York

Academy of Medicine, 1216 Fifth Avenue, Room 612, New York, NY 10029. Phone: 212-822-7204; fax: 212-996-7826.

New York Academy of Medicine: The Louis L. Seaman Medical Student Research Grants in Microbiology

Four grants of $2,500 will be provided to support summer research projects in the field of microbiology. Competition is open to MD students in a metropolitan area medical school in New York City, Long Island, Westchester County, or New Jersey. The award will be paid directly to the student, but is contingent on the submission of a written report on the project. *Contact:* Fellowship Program Coordinator, New York Academy of Medicine, 1216 Fifth Avenue, Room 612, New York, NY 10029. Phone: 212-822-7204; fax: 212-996-7826.

American Medical Association Education and Research Foundation Seed Research Grants

Up to $2,500 support for medical students for small research projects or, in some instances, to provide interim funding prior to large grant approvals from other sources. Grants will be awarded in two cycles during the school year: (1) September through November and (2) January through March. *Contact:* American Medical Association Education and Research Foundation, 515 North State Street,

Chicago, IL 60610. Phone: 312-464-5357; fax: 312-464-5973; *www.ama-assn.org/medsci/erf/toc.htm.*

WEIS CENTER FOR RESEARCH GEISINGER CLINIC

Three-month program designed to expose medical students to career opportunities in research. Primary emphasis is at the cellular/molecular level of cardiovascular function. Stipend: $800/month.

John A. Hartford/AFAR Medical Student Geriatric Scholars Program

To encourage medical students, particularly budding researchers, to consider geriatrics as a career, the Medical Student Geriatric Scholars Program awards short-term scholarships through a national competition. The program provides an opportunity for these students to train at an acclaimed center of excellence in geriatrics. Each scholar receives a $3,000 stipend. Students in the New York metropolitan area can apply for funding through the Farr Fox and Leslie R. Samuels Foundation/ AFAR Medical Student Geriatric Scholars Program. Contact American Federation for Aging Research (AFAR), 1414 Avenue of the Americas, 18th Floor, New York, NY 10019. Phone: 212-752-2327; fax: 212-832-2298; e-mail: *amfedaging@aol.com.*

Glenn Foundation/AFAR Scholarships for Research in the Biology of Aging

Inaugurated in 1994, this scholarship program was designed to attract potential scientists and clinicians to aging research. Provides PhD and MD students the opportunity to conduct a 3-month research project. Students will work in an area of biomedical research in aging under the auspices of a mentor. Each scholarship carries an award of $5,000. *Contact:* American Federation for Aging Research (AFAR), 1414 Avenue of the Americas, 18th Floor, New York, NY 10019. Phone: 212-752-2327; fax: 212-832-2298; e-mail: *amfedaging@aol.com.*

MERCK/AFAR RESEARCH SCHOLARSHIPS IN GERIATRIC PHARMACOLOGY FOR MEDICAL STUDENTS

To develop a corps of physicians with an understanding of medication use in the elderly, the Merck Company Foundation and AFAR created the Merck/ AFAR Research Scholarships in Geriatric Pharmacology. Medical students will have the opportunity to undertake a 2- to 3-month full-time research project in geriatric pharmacology. Up to nine $4,000 scholarships will be awarded in 2001. *Contact:* American Federation for Aging Research (AFAR), 1414 Avenue of the Americas, 18th Floor, New York, NY 10019. Phone: 212-752-2327; fax: 212-832-2298; e-mail: *amfedaging@aol.com.*

American Oil Chemists' Society

Graduate students in any area of science dealing with fats and lipids who are doing research toward an advanced degree, and who are interested in the area of science and technology fostered by this Society, are eligible. Must be a graduate student who has not yet received his or her degree or begun employment prior to the AOCS meeting he/she is to attend. The award will provide funds equal to travel costs, hotel accommodations, and stipend to permit attendance at the national meeting of the AOCS held in the spring.

Biomedical Synergistics Institute—Ninth International Conference

Award for those individuals in training who submit the best original paper dealing with the Institute enhancement of human functioning. Papers published previously are not eligible for awards. Four student award categories with each receiving a prize of $250. The All Functioning Categories winner will receive a $1,000 prize.

AAA PRESLEY–CARL ZEISS YOUNG INVESTIGATOR AWARD

Recognizes excellence in research using light and/or electron microscopy. Must be a graduate student, medical student, postdoc (within 5 years of receiving PhD), or medical resident. $500 prize and certificate. Contact the Advisory Commit-

tee of Young Anatomists (ACYA) at 301-571-8314 or *exec@anatomy.org.*

AAA Zeiss Student Research Award

Recognizes excellence in research using state-of-the-art imaging methods, such as confocal and/or electron microscopy. Must be a graduate student or medical student. $500 prize and certificate. Contact the Advisory Committee of Young Anatomists (ACYA) at 301-571-8314 or *exec@anatomy.org.*

AAA/Genentech Student Research Award

Recognizes excellence in research using molecular biological techniques in the study of morphological changes at the cellular and/or whole animal level. Must be a graduate student, medical student, postdoc (within 5 years of receiving PhD), or medical resident. $500 prize and certificate. Contact the Advisory Committee of Young Anatomists (ACYA) at 301-571-8314 or *exec@anatomy.org.*

ALPHA OMEGA ALPHA RESEARCH FELLOWSHIPS

The purpose of the fellowships is to stimulate interest in research among medical students. Areas of research may include clinical investigation, basic research, epidemiology, and the social sciences, as related to medicine. The program is de-

signed to stimulate students who have not had prior research experience. Fellowship is for $2,000.

American Medical Association Education and Research Foundation

Open to third- and fourth-year medical students who have completed the required clerkships in medicine, surgery, and pediatrics. The program consists of 4- to 6-week clerkships in general, pediatric, and surgical nutrition. Scholarships are only for students who do not have clinical nutrition clerkships available at their own schools. Students accepted into the program will receive a $700 award to defray living and traveling costs.

American College of Sports Medicine National Student Research Award

The National Student Research Award recognizes the most outstanding research project of the year at the graduate/professional student level. An important consideration for the award is the extent of the student's participation in the project. Each applicant must be enrolled in a graduate or professional program in the areas of clinical or basic exercise science or sports medicine at an accredited university, be principal author of a submitted and accepted abstract for presentation at the ACSM annual meeting, and be a member of ACSM or one of its regional chapters at the time of application and at the time the award is presented. The New Investigator and National Student Research awards provide support for the recipients to attend the annual meeting and present their research. Registration fees, travel expenses, lodging, banquet tickets, and framed certificates (presented at the annual awards banquet) are awarded to the recipients. *Contact:* American College of Sports Medicine, Graduate Scholarships for Minorities and Women, 401 W. Michigan St., Indianapolis, IN 46202-3233. Phone: 317-637-9200; fax: 317-634-7817; *www. acsm.org/.*

AMERICAN ACADEMY OF ALLERGY ASTHMA AND IMMUNOLOGY SUMMER FELLOWSHIP GRANT

Summer fellowship grants of $2,000 will be awarded to outstanding medical students who wish to pursue research in the following areas: physiology of allergic diseases, pharmacology of allergy and inflammation, basic cellular and molecular immunology, AIDS, and other topics pertinent to the understanding of allergic and immune mechanisms of disease. Eligibility: Full-time medical students residing in the United States or Canada who have successfully completed at least 8 months of medical school by the time the fellowship starts. Past Summer Fellowship Grant recipients are not eligible. *Contact:* American Academy of Allergy Asthma and Immunology, 611 East Wells Street, Milwaukee, WI 53202-3889. Phone: 414-272-6071; fax: 414-272-6070; *www.aaaai.org/.*

SUMMER EXTERNSHIPS

National Institute of Health Summer Research Award

www.training.nih.gov/.

Africa with Crossroads

Sponsoring agency: Operation Crossroads Africa

For senior medical school students who would like to work on a 5- to 7-week project in Africa that might focus on one of the following themes: (1) the community health approach, (2) diagnosis and treatment of tropical diseases, (3) preventive approaches to tropical diseases, and (4) the use of paramedics. Each project will also involve some labor. No stipend. The sponsoring agency will assist students in finding funds for transportation.

AMERICAN LIVER FOUNDATION STUDENT RESEARCH FELLOWSHIPS

To gain exposure in the research laboratory and possibly consider liver research a career option. Award is $2,500 per month for 3 months. *Contact:* American Liver Foundation, 1425 Pompton Avenue, Cedar Grove, NJ 07009. Phone: 201-857-2626; *www.liverfoundation.org/.*

Mucopolysaccharidosis Society Summer Fellowship

Eight-week summer fellowship for study of mucopolysaccharide diseases. Stipend: $1,500.

Utica College of Syracuse Summer Clerkships

Both of the following programs offer students clinical experience augment their classroom university instruction, reinforce clinical skills, and create interest in their future choice of both medical specialty and geographic area of practice: The summer clerkships (2–8 weeks) are designed for students who have completed either 1 or 2 years of training. Preference is given to second-year students. Stipend is $250/2 weeks. The clinical electives are credit courses offered on a year-round basis in 22 specialties for third- and fourth-year medical students.

MEMORIAL SLOAN-KETTERING CANCER CENTER SUMMER FELLOWSHIP

Sponsored by National Cancer Institute and Eugene W. Kettering Education Fund.

Eight-week summer fellowship offered to medical students in

401

their first 2 years. Objective of program is the educational enrichment of medical students by offering experience in research and clinical oncology and enhancement of their knowledge of cancer and promotion of future interest in the field. *Contact:* Chuck Ferrero, Box 187, Memorial Sloan-Kettering Cancer Center, 1275 York Ave., NY 10012 (212) 639-8457; *www. mskcc.org/mskcc/html/2637.cfm.*

Simon Kramer Externship in Radiation Oncology

Sponsored by the Thomas Jefferson Hospital, Philadelphia, this fellowship provides a unique opportunity for the medical student to obtain a 6-week experience in the Department of Radiation Therapy and Nuclear Medicine at Jefferson. Flexible beginning date; stipend of $1,200.

New York State Legislative Fellow

Fellows work as regular legislative staff members of the offices to which they are assigned. The work is full time, demanding, and is intended to use and develop the expertise of Fellows while offering an exclusive view of legislative procedures.

EDUCATION AND RESEARCH FOUNDATION OF THE SOCIETY OF NUCLEAR MEDICINE AWARDS

The purpose of the Student Fellowship Program is to provide financial support for students wishing to spend time in clinical or basic research activities in a nuclear medicine division for a 3-month period with a stipend of $3,000.

Student Fellowship Award Foundation of the Society of Nuclear Medicine

This fellowship provides financial support for students to spend elective quarters and/or summers in departments of nuclear medicine assisting in clinical and basic research activities.

Roswell Park Memorial Research Institute (Buffalo, NY) Summer Oncology Program

Provides direct support for students in the health professions engaged in research during the summer. Fellowships are awarded for an 8-week period. Research is restricted to topics in oncology. Participation in this program is limited to students completing their first or second year of study.

RUTGERS UNIVERSITY SUMMER SCHOLARSHIPS

Ten scholarships are available for this year's Summer School of Alcohol Studies to medical students. Award covers university fees, tuition, room, and meals ($975); weekend meals and travel are not included. However, a $200 stipend for related expenses will also be given to each scholarship recipient.

New York Academy of Medicine HIV Professional Development Project

Two-month internship in HIV-focused health care and social service settings. 35 hours/week, $10/hr.

Case Western Reserve University—Pathology

For those who have completed their sophomore year in medical school. This is a 12-month fellowship with a $12,000 stipend. The time will be divided between diagnostic pathology on the autopsy service and research related to the immunological and biochemical characterization of human cancer.

CLENDENING, LOGAN TRAVELING FELLOWSHIP

Sponsoring agency: University of Kansas Medical Center

This fellowship is open to registered medical students of any recognized medical school in the United States or Canada. The fellowship is of the value of $1,500. Applicants may elect to travel anywhere in the world for the purpose of studying any aspect of medical history of interest to them.

Costep of the U.S. Public Health Service

U.S. Public Health Service offers opportunities in Indian Health Services, Health Resources, and Services Administration, NIH, Food and Drug

Administration, CDC, Alcohol, Drug Abuse and Mental Health Administration, etc. U.S. citizenship and at least one year of medical school required. Positions are available all year round. $2,000/month plus travel costs. Information is available in Student Affairs; for application, call 1-800-279-1605 or 301-594-2633.

Cystic Fibrosis Foundation Student Traineeships

The Cystic Fibrosis Foundation announces student traineeships which are offered to introduce students to research related to CF. Applicants must be students in or about to enter a doctoral program (MD, PhD, or MD/PhD). Each applicant must work with a faculty sponsor on a research project related to CF. The award is $1,500, of which $1,200 is designated as a stipend for the trainee, and the remaining $300 may be used for laboratory expenses. For an application, write to: Office of Grants Management, Cystic Fibrosis Foundation, 6931 Arlington Road, Bethesda, MD 20814, or call 1-800-FLIGHT CF.

AMA-MSS GOVERNMENT RELATIONS INTERSHIP PROGRAM APPLICATION

The Department of Medical Student Services, in conjunction with the Washington office of the American Medical Association, is pleased to offer assistance to students seeking to increase their involvement and education in national health policy and in the national legislative activities of organized medicine.

Through the Government Relations Internship Program, stipends of $2,500 are available to assist selected students who are completing health policy internships in the Washington, DC, area. To be eligible for the program, students must be AMA members who have secured a policy internship in the Washington, DC, area. Through the program, students may also apply for an internship at the AMA's Washington office (two positions available), or at the Health Care Financing Administration in Baltimore, Maryland (one position available). Students participating in the program generally arrange their internships with congressional offices, specialty societies, or federal agencies in the DC area. A list of possible internship contacts is available.

The Betty Ford Center Summer Institute for Medical Students

Provides experiential education in chemical dependency and its treatment, primarily by student participation in the patient and family rehabilitation process. Five groups of 12 students will participate in the 5-day summer school program. Each session four Family Program participants follow the weekly schedule of family members, and eight students selected for the Inpatient Program are assigned to one of four inpatient treatment units. Program activities include lectures, meals, group therapy sessions, peer groups, exercise sessions, meditation, medallion ceremonies, and Alcoholics and Narcotics Anonymous meetings. Students are asked to maintain a focused journal. A basic set of books and a reference manual is provided to each student. Scholarships to this very special program include the cost of all materials, lodging, and meals. A travel stipend is also included. A total of 60 scholarships will be awarded. Students may apply to attend one of four summer sessions. For application information, write: Betty Ford Center Training Department, 39000 Bob Hope Drive, Rancho Mirage, CA 92270. Phone: 619-773-4108; toll free: 1-800-854-9211, ext. 4108; fax: 619-773-1697.

The Albert Schweitzer Fellowship

Provides complete funding for medical students who will work in Lambaréné, Gabon, as junior physicians, supervised by Schweitzer Hospital medical staff. Prior completion of clerkships in medicine, pediatrics, and surgery are required; some background or coursework in tropical medicine or parasitology is important but not a prerequisite. Because all patient encounters occur in French, a working knowledge of that language is absolutely essential. For more information, contact: The Albert Schweitzer Foundation, 330 Brookline Avenue, Boston, MA 02215.

HOWARD HUGHES MEDICAL INSTITUTE RESEARCH SCHOLARS TRAINING

Students in good standing in a medical school in the United States who have completed the second year but have not yet received the MD are eligible. The program is for at least 9 months and usually 1 year at NIH. Salary program $16,800, and other benefits are included. *Contact:* 1-800-424-9924.

American Diabetes Association, Inc. Medical Scholars Program Awards

The goal of the program is to produce new leaders in diabetes research by supplying physicians-in-training the opportunity to contribute to the process of discovery in basic or clinical research laboratories. Award is $30,000 for 1 year. Eligibility: Students must have completed at least 2 years of medical school. *Contact:* American Diabetes Association, Inc. Research Department, 1701 North Beauregard Street, Alexandria, VA 22311. Phone: 703-549-1500, ext. 2376; fax: 703-549-1715; *www.diabetes.org/research/.*

Pew Charitable Trust/ Rockefeller University Fellowships in Human Nutrition

One-year program designed to give hands-on laboratory experience and mastering of new methods in biomedical science for application to problems in human nutrition. Students should have completed their third year by July 1. Stipend: $14,700. Pierce, Chester Research Symposium.

UNIVERSITY OF PITTSBURGH PATHOLOGY FELLOWSHIP

One-year fellowship for medical students who have completed their second year and wish to spend an additional year of in-depth study of pathology in research (pathology, molecular biology, genetics, etc.) and practice before going on to the third year. The stipend is $11,000, and a scholarship for the next year of medical school (up to the state tuition rate at Pittsburgh) will be provided.

Association of Pathology Chairman Student Fellowship

Year-long full-time fellowship in participating schools for students after the second year of medical school. Intended to give students an in-depth research and/or clinical experience in pathology between the basic science and clinical years. Support varies by school, as do openings for students not from that school.

New York City Health Research Training Program

This is a practicum in public health research. The student participates in a project under the direct supervision of a preceptor. The projects are submitted by preceptors from within the Health Department or from outside agencies such as hospitals, medical schools, or other health-related institutions. A seminar series is part of the program. Work-study students are preferred. However, some alternative support is available for those not eligible for work-study. Full time in summer, part time during school year.

NEW YORK CITY URBAN FELLOWS PROGRAM

Year-long program offering the opportunity and challenge of an intensive field experience in urban government. Fellows work closely with city officials on long- and short-term projects and attend weekly seminars to gain an academic perspective on the workings and problems of local government. $17,000 stipend and insurance.

National Institutes of Health Summer Research Fellowship

With the guidance of a preceptor from one of the Institutes, students conduct research in a selected area of laboratory investigation. Program offers practical experience in research procedures and lectures and seminars designed to enhance education and investigative skills. Program runs a minimum of 8 weeks.

National Institutes of Health Clinical Electives Program

Medical students are invited to apply for clinical electives of 8 weeks with opportunities research and clinical experience with physician-scientists in Bethesda.

OSLER LIBRARY FELLOWSHIP PROGRAM

A fellowship program for historians, physicians, and students conducting research in the history of medicine. Intended to serve those who need to establish temporary residence in order to undertake research in the Osler Library.

Henry Luce Foundation Scholars Program

This program provides an intensive year-long experience in Asia designed to broaden the scholar's professional perspectives and to sharpen their perceptions of Asia, America, and themselves. The support consists of airfare, stipend, medical insurance, etc.

Echoing Green Foundation Fellowship

One-year fellowship providing entrepreneurial people with the opportunity to develop and implement an innovative public service project (health, environment, youth service, international development, etc.). Students must develop a proposal. Stipend is $25,000 per year.

HEALTH RESEARCH GROUP MEDICAL STUDENT FELLOWSHIP

One-year fellowship in Washington researching and monitoring federal health agencies, congressional lobbying, publication of consumer-oriented educational manuals, etc.

Rosalie B. Hite Cancer Center Research Fellowship

Sponsoring agency: University of Texas System

Fellowship open to graduate students or research workers in the area of cancer research. Selection of Fellows is on the basis of academic excellence of the candidate and applicability of the proposed program to the problems of cancer research. Graduate work is to be under the supervision of a faculty member of a component of the University of Texas at Houston, affiliated with the Graduate School of Biomedical Sciences Sciences degree-granting program.

Charles A. Dana Foundation Clinical Research Training Program

Sponsoring agency: University of Pennsylvania School of Medicine

Opportunity for medical students to participate in a year-long in-depth clinical research training experience under the guidance of selected faculty who are accomplished investigators in the fields of epidemiology, clinical research methodology, and the delivery of health care services. Training will be provided in clinical research methods, clinical epidemiology, biostatistics, and scientific communication. Stipend of $11,000 plus expenses.

CHARLES A. AND ANNE MORROW LINDBERGH FOUNDATION

A foundation dedicated to furthering Charles and Anne Morrow Lindbergh's shared vision of a balance between technological advancement and environmental preservation. Lindbergh grants are made in the following categories: agriculture; aviation/aerospace; conservation of natural resources—including animals, plants, water, and general conservation (land, air, energy, etc.); education—including humanities/education, the arts, and intercultural communication; exploration; health—including biomedical research, health and population sciences, and adaptive technology; and waste minimization and management. A Jonathan Lindbergh Brown Grant may be given to a project to support adaptive technology or biomedical research that seeks to redress imbalance between an individual and his or her human environment. Grants are made to individuals as well as educational and publication programs. *Contact: www.lindbergh-foundation.org.*

National Medical Fellowship—Commonwealth Fund

This program is designed to encourage academically gifted minority medical students to pursue careers in academic medicine and biomedical research. Open to those students who have completed their junior year. Duration is 8–12 weeks. Students have the option to participate in the summer or during the academic year. Fellowship award is for $5,000, with $2,000 earmarked for mentor to offset expenses during the research period.

National Institute of Arthritis and Musculoskeletal and Skin Diseases (NIAMS)

The Minority Travel Award Program provides travel funds for minority students and faculty members from minority institutions for attendance at national scientific meetings. *Contact: www.nih.gov/niams.*

NIH PREDOCTORAL FELLOWSHIP AWARDS FOR MINORITY STUDENTS

The National Research Service Award Predoctoral Fellowship for Minority Students will provide up to 5 years of support for research training leading to the PhD or equivalent research degree; the combined MD/PhD degree; or other combined professional degree and research doctoral degree in biomedical, behavioral sciences, or health

services research. These fellowships are designed to enhance the racial and ethnic diversity of the biomedical, behavioral, and health services research labor force in the United States. Accordingly, academic institutions are encouraged to identify and recruit students from underrepresented racial and ethnic groups who can apply for this fellowship. Support is *not* available for individuals enrolled in medical or other professional schools *unless* they are also enrolled in a combined professional doctorate/PhD degree program in biomedical, behavioral, or health services research. *Contact: www.nih.gov.*

National Medical Fellowships, Inc.

NMF offers awards and fellowships to American Blacks, mainland Puerto Ricans, Mexican-Americans, and American Indians who are U.S. citizens enrolled in accredited schools of allopathic or osteopathic medicine in the United States. Funding is variable, yearly, and renewable. *Contact:* National Medical Fellowships, Inc., 254 West 31st Street, 7th Floor, New York, NY 10001. Phone: 212-714-1007.

Metropolitan Life Award Program for Academic Excellence in Medicine

This program recognizes and rewards third-year minority medical students for outstanding academic achievement and demonstrated leadership. $2,500 need-based

awards to underrepresented minorities. Nominated by dean's office.

AMERICAN COLLEGE OF SPORTS MEDICINE MINORITY SCHOLARSHIP

The American College of Sports Medicine annually awards graduate scholarships for minorities and females of up to $1,500 each to be used to cover college or university tuition and/or fees. The purpose of these scholarships is to provide partial support toward the education of graduate and/or medical students with outstanding promise and a strong interest in research and scholarly activities as they pursue a career in sports medicine or exercise science. Scholarships are renewable for up to 4 years based on their research and professional activities and satisfactory academic progress in full-time study toward a graduate degree. Students who are not currently ACSM members are eligible to apply. Free student membership in the American College of Sports Medicine is also provided each year of an awardee's graduate scholarship. *Contact:* American College of Sports Medicine, Graduate Scholarships for Minorities and Women, 401 W. Michigan St., Indianapolis, IN 46202-3233. Phone: 317-637-9200; fax: 317-634-7817; *www.acsm.org/.*

Congressional Black Caucus Foundation, Inc. Scholarships

Offers grant money for doctoral study to minority students. *Con-*

tact: Congressional Black Caucus Foundation, Inc., 1004 Pennsylvania Avenue SE, Washington, DC 20003. Phone: 1-800-784-2577 or 202-675-6730; fax: 202-547-3806.

American Indian Graduate Center Grants

Grants of $250–$10,000 are available for American Indian students who are members of a federally recognized American Indian tribe or Alaska Native group, or possess one-fourth degree federally recognized Indian blood with financial need after exhausting available aid at their school financial aid office. *Contact*: American Indian Graduate Center, 4520 Montgomery Blvd. NE, Suite 1-B, Albuquerque, New Mexico 87109. Phone: 505-881-4584.

ETHNIC

DR. ANTHONY BAGATELOS MEMORIAL SCHOLARSHIP

Grant money available for Greek descent/Greek Orthodox faith with intentions to practice medicine within the nine-county area surrounding San Francisco Bay. Applications may be obtained by contacting: Annunciation Greek Orthodox Cathedral, 245 Valencia St., San Francisco CA 94103.

Chinese American Physicians Society (CAPS)

CAPS is offering 8 to 10 scholarships of $1,000–$2,000 each annually to two categories of medical students. The first is the Dr. Lester Chen Memorial Scholarships to students of Asian descent from the San Francisco Bay area. The other is the CAPS Scholarships to all medical students in need of financial aid regardless of their hometown, sex, race, or color. The applicants are judged according to their academic achievements, financial needs, community service records, and essays. Special credit is also given to those who are willing to serve the Chinese communities after their graduation. The deadline for submitting the completed application is usually the first Friday in October. Due to the huge number of requests for applications and our shortage of manpower, we can no longer send out the application by mail unless a self-addressed stamped envelope is enclosed with the request. Please obtain the applications from the student financial aid office of your medical school starting from April 1 each year. You can also print a copy of the published scholarship application from our web site. If you need more information about the scholarship program, please contact Chinese American Physicians Society, Lawrence M. Ng, MD, Executive Director, 345 Ninth Street, Suite 204, Oakland, CA 94607-4206. Phone: 510-895-5539 (voice and fax); e-mail: *scholarship@caps-ca.org*.

JAPANESE MEDICAL SOCIETY SCHOLARSHIP AWARD

$1,500–$5,000 grants to students of Japanese ancestry who are enrolled or accepted in a U.S. medical school. Applications may be obtained by contacting: Japanese Medical Society of America, Inc. Scholarship Committee, One Henry Street, Englewood Cliffs, NJ 07632.

JEWISH VOCATIONAL SERVICE ACADEMIC SCHOLARSHIP

For Jewish medical students living in Chicago. Applications are accepted December 1 through March 1. *Contact*: Jewish Vocational Service, One South Franklin Street, Chicago, Illinois 60606. Phone: 312-346-6700, ext. 2214.

Hellenic Medical Society Scholarship

Awards for medical students of Hellenic heritage from New York, New Jersey, Pennsylvania, Connecticut; must be a second-year student enrolled at an accredited U.S. school. *Contact*: Hellenic Medical Society of New York, 401 East 34th Street, New York NY 10016.

AAUW Educational Foundation International Fellowship

This is a grant for foreign students to pursue graduate studies in the United States. *Contact:* American Association of University Women, 1111 Sixteenth St. NW, Washington, DC 20036. Phone: 1-800-326-AAUW; fax: 202-872-1425; e-mail: *info@aauw.org.*

AMWA CARROLL L. BIRCH AWARD

Sponsored by the Chicago Branch of the American Medical Women's Association, the award is presented for the best original research paper written by a Student Life Member of AMWA. Women must be enrolled in an accredited U.S. medical or osteopathic medical school to apply. The recipient of the award receives a cash prize of $500 and a plaque presented at AMWA's annual meeting. An article noting the award winner will appear in one of the Association's publications, and an abstract may be published in AMWA's journal. Contact your school's financial aid office for more info.

AMWA Bed and Breakfast Program

The program assists students who are traveling for a residency or job interview or physician members attending an out-of-town conference. Our members contact the national office with details of the trip. The national office responds by sending the traveler a listing of volunteers in the destination area. There is an administrative fee of $10 for students and $15 for physicians.

BPW Career Advancement Scholarship for Women

Grants of $500–$1,000 for women over 25 in their third or fourth year of studies with critical need for assistance. *Contact:* Scholarships/Loans Business and Professional Women's Foundation, 2012 Mass Ave. NW, Washington, DC 20036. Phone: 202-293-1200, ext. 169.

AWARDS AND LINKS TO MEDICAL SUBSPECIALTY SOCIETIES

American Society of Clinical Oncology Medical Student Rotation: *www.ascocancerfoundation.org/TACF/Awards/Award+Opportunities*

American College of Rheumatology Research and Education Foundation/Abbott Medical Student Clinical Preceptorship: *www.rheumatology.org/ref/awards/summerclinical.asp*

ACR Research and Education Foundation: *www.rheumatology.org/ref/awards/index.asp*

Agency for Healthcare Research and Quality: *www.ahrq.gov/fund/funding.htm*

Alliance for Lupus Research: *www.lupusresearch.org/grants_03.html*

American Autoimmune Related Diseases Association: *www.aarda.org/programs.html*

American Diabetes Association: *www.diabetes.org/main/professional/research/research.jsp*

Arthritis Foundation: *www.arthritis.org/research/default.asp*

Arthritis National Research Foundation: *www.curearthritis.org*

Crohn's and Colitis Foundation: *www.ccfa.org/science/research/*

Johnson & Johnson/Society for the Arts in Healthcare: *www.thesah.org*

Juvenile Diabetes Research Foundation: *www.jdrf.org/index.cfm?fuseaction=home.viewPage&page_id=8AC28525-1BC5-4E79-9A9079E0DE3C5739*

Lupus Research Institute: *www.lupusresearchinstitute.org/research_grants.jsp*

National Multiple Sclerosis Society: *www.nationalmssociety.org/research.asp*

National Psoriasis Foundation: *www.psoriasis.org/research/*

Robert Wood Johnson Foundation: *http://rwjfpfsp.stanford.edu/*

SLE Foundation, Inc.: *www.lupusny.org*

Scleroderma Foundation: *www.scleroderma.org/research/researchhome.htm*

Sjogren's Syndrome Foundation: *www.sjogrens.com/research/*

www.acponline.org/journals/ ebm/ebmmenu.htm: Reviews the evidence for current medical practice.

www.ebem.org: Evidence-based emergency medicine home page.

cebm.jr2.ox.ac.uk: NHS Research and Development Centre of Evidence Based Medicine.

www.update-software.com/co-chrane.htm: Web site for the Cochrane Library, the most well-known site for critically appraised topics or evidence-based reviews.

www.ebando.com: Bandolier: online publication on evidence-based health care.

www.shef.ac.uk/~scharr/ir/net-ting.html: Netting the evidence: A ScHARR introduction to evidence-based practice on the Internet.

www.ti.ubc.ca/pages/letter.html: Therapeutics Letter: Evidence-based review of pharmaceutical products.

www.ncbi.nlm.nih.gov/PubMed: Pub Med, a MEDLINE search engine through the National Library of Medicine.

igm.nlm.nih.gov: Grateful Med, a MEDLINE search engine through the National Library of Medicine.

www.cdc.gov: The Centers for Disease Control and Prevention: Contains full text issues of *Morbidity and Mortality Weekly Report.*

www.nejm.org: New England Journal of Medicine.

www.jwatch.org: Journal Watch.

www.bmj.com/index.shtml: British Medical Journal.

jama.ama-assm.org: Journal of the American Medical Association.

CLASSIFIED

Preface

The *Lab Manual for Health Assessment in Nursing*, 5th edition, can be used as a laboratory manual and study guide for the fifth edition of *Health Assessment in Nursing*. Each chapter corresponds to a chapter in the textbook, and contains a **chapter pretest**, **interactive learner activities**, a **nursing interview guide**, a **physical assessment guide**, and a **chapter posttest** with **multiple choice questions**, **critical thinking activities**, and a **case study**.

The Lab Manual can assist you with comprehending theoretical content, applying this content to acquiring history and physical assessment skills, and preparing for tests.

How to Use This Lab Manual

Before beginning study in each textbook chapter, take the **Chapter Pretest**. This test is designed to assess the information you may already know from a prior course. It tests basic information related to the content framework or the anatomy and physiology basic to each chapter. (Answers are located at the back of the book.) If you answer most of the questions correctly, proceed to the next section. Otherwise, review the basic framework content or anatomy and physiology found at the very beginning of the appropriate chapter.

Next, read the chapter and then participate in the **Learner Activities**. These activities are designed to assist you with learning the assessment skills covered in each chapter and will increase your understanding and retention of chapter content. These activities actively involve you as a learner and also offer you opportunities to work with lab partners or peers in your class.

Then you can interview your lab partner, peer, or family member using the **Nursing Interview Guide** and record your subjective findings. After practicing the physical examination on your lab partner, peer, or client, you can document your findings on the **Physical Assessment Guide**. Both of these tools serve as a guide to remind you of the steps involved in performing a thorough nursing history and physical examination. The completed guides can also be handed in to your nursing instructor to be evaluated for accuracy and completeness of client data. The Nursing Interview Guide and Physical Assessment Guide for each chapter are also available on thePoint website for those who prefer to do these electronically.

To test your comprehension of the content provided, take the **Chapter Posttest**. Again, the test answers are provided at the back of the lab manual for self-checking.

You can test your critical thinking abilities by answering the questions in the **Critical Thinking Activity**.

Test your analysis abilities by using the **Case Study** activity. For this activity, you are given an opportunity to work through the steps of analyzing the data, identifying abnormal data and strengths, assembling cue clusters, drawing inferences, making possible nursing diagnoses, identifying defining characteristics, confirming or ruling out diagnoses, and documenting conclusions. Blank **diagnostic analysis charts** will guide your thinking and are provided at the end of this book as well as on thePoint website for *Health Assessment in Nursing*, for those who prefer an electronic format.

Finally, use the **Self-Reflection Activity** that is available on thePoint website to identify the degree to which you have met each of the **Chapter Learning Objectives**. This self-evaluation will help you identify those parts of the chapter you need to review to fully comprehend it.

We believe this lab manual will assist you to actively learn the content and skills needed to effectively perform a Client Nursing History and Physical Examination.

Best wishes and happy learning!

Janet R. Weber
Jane H. Kelley
Ann D. Sprengel

Contents

369 0240640

KU-627-880

Lab Manual for

Health Assessment in Nursing

FIFTH EDITION

Alistair Mackenzie Library
Wishaw General Hospital
50 Netherton Street
Wishaw
ML2 0DP

JANET R. WEBER, RN, EdD
Professor
Director RN-BSN Program
Department of Nursing
Southeast Missouri State University
Cape Girardeau, Missouri

JANE H. KELLEY, RN, PhD
Adjunct Professor
School of Nursing
Indiana Wesleyan University
Louisville, Kentucky

ANN D. SPRENGEL, RN, EdD
Professor
Director of Undergraduate Studies
Department of Nursing
Southeast Missouri State University
Cape Girardeau, Missouri

*Special acknowledgment to Wesley L. Weber for the original book cover graphic design
that clearly illustrates the complex, evolving nature of assessment.*

Wolters Kluwer | Lippincott Williams & Wilkins
Health
Philadelphia · Baltimore · New York · London
Buenos Aires · Hong Kong · Sydney · Tokyo

ALISTAIR MACKENZIE LIBRARY
Barcode: 3690240640
Class no: WY 100 WEB

Acquisitions Editor: Chris Richardson
Product Manager: Helen Kogut
Editorial Assistant: Zachary Shapiro
Production Project Manager: Cynthia Rudy
Design Coordinator: Holly McLaughlin
Illustration Coordinator: Doug Smock
Manufacturing Coordinator: Karin Duffield
Prepress Vendor: Aptara, Inc.

5th edition

Copyright © 2014 Wolters Kluwer Health | Lippincott Williams & Wilkins.

Copyright © 2010 Wolters Kluwer Health | Lippincott Williams & Wilkins. Copyright © 2007, 2003 by Lippincott Williams & Wilkins. All rights reserved. This book is protected by copyright. No part of this book may be reproduced or transmitted in any form or by any means, including as photocopies or scanned-in or other electronic copies, or utilized by any information storage and retrieval system without written permission from the copyright owner, except for brief quotations embodied in critical articles and reviews. Materials appearing in this book prepared by individuals as part of their official duties as U.S. government employees are not covered by the above-mentioned copyright. To request permission, please contact Lippincott Williams & Wilkins at Two Commerce Square, 2001 Market Street, Philadelphia, PA 19103, via email at permissions@lww.com, or via our website at lww.com (products and services).

9 8 7 6 5 4 3 2 1

Printed in the United States

ISBN: 978-1-4511-4281-5

Care has been taken to confirm the accuracy of the information presented and to describe generally accepted practices. However, the author(s), editors, and publisher are not responsible for errors or omissions or for any consequences from application of the information in this book and make no warranty, expressed or implied, with respect to the currency, completeness, or accuracy of the contents of the publication. Application of this information in a particular situation remains the professional responsibility of the practitioner; the clinical treatments described and recommended may not be considered absolute and universal recommendations.

The author(s), editors, and publisher have exerted every effort to ensure that drug selection and dosage set forth in this text are in accordance with the current recommendations and practice at the time of publication. However, in view of on-going research, changes in government regulations, and the constant flow of information relating to drug therapy and drug reactions, the reader is urged to check the package insert for each drug for any change in indications and dosage and for added warnings and precautions. This is particularly important when the recommended agent is a new or infrequently employed drug.

Some drugs and medical devices presented in this publication have Food and Drug Administration (FDA) clearance for limited use in restricted research settings. It is the responsibility of the health care provider to ascertain the FDA status of each drug or device planned for use in his or her clinical practice.

LWW.com

DRC0913

Preface

The *Lab Manual for Health Assessment in Nursing*, 5th edition, can be used as a laboratory manual and study guide for the fifth edition of *Health Assessment in Nursing*. Each chapter corresponds to a chapter in the textbook, and contains a **chapter pretest, interactive learner activities**, a **nursing interview guide**, a **physical assessment guide**, and a **chapter posttest** with **multiple choice questions, critical thinking activities**, and a **case study**.

The Lab Manual can assist you with comprehending theoretical content, applying this content to acquiring history and physical assessment skills, and preparing for tests.

How to Use This Lab Manual

Before beginning study in each textbook chapter, take the **Chapter Pretest**. This test is designed to assess the information you may already know from a prior course. It tests basic information related to the content framework or the anatomy and physiology basic to each chapter. (Answers are located at the back of the book.) If you answer most of the questions correctly, proceed to the next section. Otherwise, review the basic framework content or anatomy and physiology found at the very beginning of the appropriate chapter.

Next, read the chapter and then participate in the **Learner Activities**. These activities are designed to assist you with learning the assessment skills covered in each chapter and will increase your understanding and retention of chapter content. These activities actively involve you as a learner and also offer you opportunities to work with lab partners or peers in your class.

Then you can interview your lab partner, peer, or family member using the **Nursing Interview Guide** and record your subjective findings. After practicing the physical examination on your lab partner, peer, or client, you can document your findings on the **Physical Assessment Guide**. Both of these tools serve as a guide to remind you of the steps involved in performing a thorough nursing history and physical examination. The completed guides can also be handed in to your nursing instructor to be evaluated for accuracy and completeness of client data. The Nursing Interview Guide and Physical Assessment Guide for each chapter are also available on thePoint website for those who prefer to do these electronically.

To test your comprehension of the content provided, take the **Chapter Posttest**. Again, the test answers are provided at the back of the lab manual for self-checking.

You can test your critical thinking abilities by answering the questions in the **Critical Thinking Activity**.

Test your analysis abilities by using the **Case Study** activity. For this activity, you are given an opportunity to work through the steps of analyzing the data, identifying abnormal data and strengths, assembling cue clusters, drawing inferences, making possible nursing diagnoses, identifying defining characteristics, confirming or ruling out diagnoses, and documenting conclusions. Blank **diagnostic analysis charts** will guide your thinking and are provided at the end of this book as well as on thePoint website for *Health Assessment in Nursing*, for those who prefer an electronic format.

Finally, use the **Self-Reflection Activity** that is available on thePoint website to identify the degree to which you have met each of the **Chapter Learning Objectives**. This self-evaluation will help you identify those parts of the chapter you need to review to fully comprehend it.

We believe this lab manual will assist you to actively learn the content and skills needed to effectively perform a Client Nursing History and Physical Examination.

Best wishes and happy learning!

Janet R. Weber
Jane H. Kelley
Ann D. Sprengel

Contents

Alistair Mackenzie Library
Wishaw General Hospital
50 Netherton Street
Wishaw
ML2 0DP

Copyright © 2014. Wolters Kluwer Health | Lippincott Williams & Wilkins. Lab Manual for Health Assessment in Nursing, 5e.

Nurse's Role in Health Assessment: Collecting and Analyzing Data

Chapter Overview

The role of the nurse in assessment and diagnosis is more prevalent today than ever before in the history of nursing. Assessment is the first and most critical phase of the nursing process. If data collection is inadequate or inaccurate, incorrect nursing judgments may be made that adversely affect the remaining phases of the process: diagnosis, planning, implementation, and evaluation. The data collected is analyzed and synthesized to identify nursing diagnoses, collaborative problems, make referrals, make judgments about the effectiveness of nursing interventions, and evaluate client care outcomes. The nursing process should be thought of as circular, not linear.

Activities and quizzes follow to enhance your learning about the initial step of the nursing process.

Chapter Learning Objectives

1. Explain how assessment skills are needed for every situation the nurse encounters.
2. Differentiate between a holistic nursing assessment and a physical medical assessment.
3. Describe how assessment fits into the total nursing process.
4. List and describe the steps of the nursing process: subjective data collection; objective data collection; validation of data, documentation of data, and analysis of data.
5. Describe the steps of the analysis phase of the nursing process.
6. Compare and contrast the four basic types of nursing assessment: (a) initial comprehensive, (b) ongoing or partial, (c) focused/problem-oriented, and (d) emergency.
7. Explain how the nurse's role in assessment has changed over the past century. Discuss what the nurse's role might be 25 years from now.

CHAPTER PRETEST

Activity A MATCHING

Match the terms in the left column with the correct descriptions in the right column.

Term

_____ **1.** Nursing assessment

_____ **2.** Nursing diagnoses

_____ **3.** Planning

_____ **4.** Implementation

_____ **5.** Evaluation

_____ **6.** Nursing diagnosis

_____ **7.** Subjective data

_____ **8.** Objective data

_____ **9.** Collaborative problem

_____ **10.** Referral problem

Description

a. Developing a plan of nursing care and outcome criteria

b. Carrying out the plan of care

c. Sensations or symptoms that can be verified only by the client (e.g., pain)

d. Problem that requires the attention or assistance of other health care professionals

e. Assessing whether outcome criteria have been met and revising the plan of care if necessary

f. Collection of subjective and objective data

g. Clinical judgment about individual, family, or community responses to actual or potential health problems and life processes

h. Physiologic complications that nurses monitor to detect their onset or changes in status

i. Analysis of subjective and objective data to make a professional nursing judgment

j. Findings directly observed or indirectly observed through measurements (e.g., body temperature)

Activity B LEARNER ACTIVITIES

After reading Chapter 1 in the textbook, participate in the following learning activities.

1. Assess your lab partner's dietary intake for yesterday and his or her satisfaction with the intake.

2. Share with your lab partner the last time you went to a physician. Describe your reason for seeing the physician. What examinations did the physician perform? What conclusions were made? Discuss how the focus of a nursing assessment would differ from the physician's assessment. Discuss how the conclusions would differ.

3. Write down everything you can observe about your lab partner without asking them any questions. Now make a judgment based on that observation, and validate the observation with your partner by asking them questions. For example, "You look tired today. Do you feel tired? Describe to me your patterns of sleeping and resting."

4. Role-play how Florence Nightingale would have performed a nursing assessment in her era. Then role-play how a nurse today would approach that assessment from a different perspective (e.g., type of equipment used, type of questions asked). Next, brainstorm with your lab partner how a nursing assessment might change in the future—20 years from now.

CHAPTER POSTTEST

Activity C MULTIPLE CHOICE QUESTIONS

Choose the one best answer for each of the following multiple choice questions.

_____ **1.** A medical examination differs from a comprehensive nursing examination in that the medical examination focuses primarily on the client's

    a. physiologic status.

    b. holistic wellness status.

    c. developmental history.

    d. level of functioning.

Copyright © 2014. Wolters Kluwer Health | Lippincott Williams & Wilkins. Lab Manual for Health Assessment in Nursing, 5e.

_____ **2.** The result of a nursing assessment is the

   a. prescription of treatment.

   b. documentation of the need for a referral.

   c. client's physiologic status.

   d. formulation of nursing diagnoses.

_____ **3.** Although the assessment phase of the nursing process precedes the other phases, the assessment phase is

   a. continuous.

   b. completed on admission.

   c. linear.

   d. performed only by nurses.

_____ **4.** When a client first enters the hospital for an elective surgical procedure, the nurse should perform an assessment termed

   a. entry.

   b. exploratory.

   c. focused.

   d. comprehensive.

_____ **5.** An assessment of a client who already has a complete recorded database in the system and returns to the health care agency with a specific health concern is referred to as a(n)

   a. ongoing or partial assessment.

   b. focused or problem-oriented assessment.

   c. emergency assessment.

   d. initial comprehensive assessment.

_____ **6.** To prepare for the assessment of a client visiting a neighborhood health care clinic, the nurse should first

   a. discuss the client's symptoms with other team members.

   b. plan for potential laboratory procedures.

   c. review the client's health care record.

   d. determine potential health care resources.

_____ **7.** The nurse is preparing to meet a client in the clinic for the first time. After reviewing the client's record, the nurse should

   a. analyze data that have already been collected.

   b. review any past collaborative problems.

   c. avoid premature judgments about the client.

   d. consult with the client's family members.

_____ **8.** Before beginning a comprehensive health assessment of an adult client, the nurse should explain to the client that the purpose of the assessment is to

   a. arrive at conclusions about the client's health.

   b. document any physical symptoms the client may have.

   c. contribute to the medical diagnosis.

   d. validate the data collected.

_____ **9.** To arrive at a nursing diagnosis or a collaborative problem, the nurse goes through the steps of analysis of data. After proposing possible nursing diagnoses, the nurse should next

   a. cluster the data collected.

   b. draw inferences and identify problems.

   c. document conclusions.

   d. check for the presence of defining characteristics.

Copyright © 2014. Wolters Kluwer Health | Lippincott Williams & Wilkins. Lab Manual for Health Assessment in Nursing, 5e.

____ **10.** The depth and scope of nursing assessment has expanded significantly over the past several decades primarily because of

    a. the growing elderly population with chronic illness.

    b. rapid advances in biomedical knowledge and technology.

    c. an increase in the number of baccalaureate programs in nursing.

    d. an increase in the number of nurse practitioners.

Activity D **CRITICAL THINKING ACTIVITIES**

1. Discuss ways in which expanding technology will change the future role of the nurse in health assessment.

2. Compare and contrast a nursing assessment with a medical assessment.

Activity E **CASE STUDY**

Read the following case study. What would you like to know about this client that you do not know from reading the case study? Write down all the questions you think you may want to ask this client to collect this additional data. Next write down all the observations you would want to make to gather additional data. Compare your answers with two to three students in your class. What did you learn from the other students?

Mrs. GM, a 35-year-old Caucasian, comes into the emergency room with nausea and vomiting. She is pale and is holding her abdomen. Her boyfriend accompanies her and says she has been unable to eat for 2 days. Her vital signs are temperature 98.6°F, pulse 98/minute, BP 130/80 mm Hg, respirations 20 breathes/minute.

How Well Did You Do?

After you have read the chapter and completed the exercises in this chapter, visit thePoint to access the Self-Reflection Activity. This activity will help you identify to what degree you have met each of the chapter objectives. You can then review the chapter for objectives you have met partially or not at all.

Other tools to help you, like the Diagnostic Reasoning Guides, Nursing Interview Guides, Physical Assessment Guides, and NCLEX-Style Chapter Review Questions, are also available on thePoint.

Copyright © 2014. Wolters Kluwer Health | Lippincott Williams & Wilkins. Lab Manual for Health Assessment in Nursing, 5e.

CHAPTER 2

Collecting Subjective Data: The Interview and Health History

Chapter Overview

Let the pages of this chapter help you review information about the health history interview techniques related to obtaining subjective data during the nursing assessment. Subjective data may be sensed or reported by the client or significant other people, such as family or friends or health care personnel. Subjective data often are not observable or measurable.

Chapter Learning Objectives

For Interviewing:
1. Describe the three phases of an interview.
2. Describe the use of nonverbal communication during an interview.
3. Describe the use of effective verbal communication during a client interview.
4. Describe the types of verbal communication that should be avoided in client interviews.
5. Describe how communication should be varied to communicate with elderly clients.
6. Describe how ethnicity can affect communication.
7. Describe appropriate ways to modify communication with clients who have emotional conditions.

For Taking the Health History:
8. Identify the major categories of a complete health history.
9. Describe the key sources of biographic data.
10. Describe the types of biographic data to be collected.
11. Obtain an accurate nursing history of a client, omitting (at this time) the review of body systems.
12. Use the COLDSPA format to collect information about a health concern.
13. Construct a genogram to identify patterns within family history.
14. Identify the information to be obtained in a review of body systems.
15. Describe the relationship of the lifestyle and health practices profile with health status.
16. Analyze data from the subjective data collected in the client interview to formulate valid nursing diagnoses, collaborative problems, and/or referrals.

CHAPTER PRETEST

Activity A **MULTIPLE CHOICE QUESTIONS**

Choose the one best answer for each of the following multiple choice questions.

_____ **1.** During an interview, the nurse collects both subjective and objective data from an adult client. Subjective data would include the client's
  a. perception of pain.
  b. height.
  c. weight.
  d. temperature.

_____ **2.** During an interview with an adult client, the nurse can keep the interview from going off course by
  a. using open-ended questions.
  b. rephrasing the client's statements.
  c. inferring information.
  d. using closed-ended questions.

_____ **3.** The nurse has interviewed a Hispanic client with limited English skills for the first time. The nurse observes that the client is reluctant to reveal personal information and believes in a hot–cold syndrome of disease causation. The nurse should
  a. indicate acceptance of the client's cultural differences.
  b. request a family member to interpret for the client.
  c. use slang terms to identify certain body parts.
  d. remain in a standing position during the interview.

_____ **4.** For a nurse to be therapeutic with clients when dealing with sensitive issues such as terminal illness or sexuality, the nurse should have
  a. advanced preparation in this area.
  b. experience in dealing with these types of clients.
  c. knowledge of his or her own thoughts and feelings about these issues.
  d. personal experiences with death, dying, and sexuality.

_____ **5.** The nurse is interviewing a client in the clinic for the first time. The client appears to have a very limited vocabulary. The nurse should plan to
  a. use very basic lay terminology.
  b. have a family member present during the interview.
  c. use standard medical terminology.
  d. show the client pictures of different symptoms, such as the "faces pain chart."

_____ **6.** The nurse is interviewing a client in the clinic for the first time. When the client tells the nurse that he smokes "about two packs of cigarettes a day," the nurse should
  a. look at the client with a frown.
  b. tell the client that he is spending a lot of money foolishly.
  c. provide the client with a list of dangers associated with smoking.
  d. encourage the client to quit smoking.

_____ **7.** During a client interview, the nurse uses nonverbal expressions appropriately when the nurse
  a. avoids excessive eye contact with the client.
  b. remains expressionless throughout the interview.
  c. uses touch in a friendly manner to establish rapport.
  d. displays mental distancing during the interview.

____ **8.** During the interview of an adult client, the nurse should
  a. use leading questions for valid responses.
  b. provide the client with information as questions arise.
  c. read each question carefully from the history form.
  d. complete the interview as quickly as possible.

____ **9.** While interviewing a client for the first time, the nurse is using a standardized nursing history form. The nurse should
  a. maintain eye contact while asking the questions from the form.
  b. read the questions verbatim from the form.
  c. ask the client to complete the form.
  d. ask leading questions throughout the interview.

____ **10.** The nurse is interviewing a 78-year-old client for the first time. The nurse should first
  a. assess the client's hearing acuity.
  b. establish rapport with the client.
  c. obtain biographic data.
  d. use medical terminology appropriately.

Activity B LEARNER ACTIVITIES

After reading Chapter 2 in the textbook, participate in the following learning activities.

1. Obtain permission to observe client interviews in a clinic. Observe the clients' nonverbal communications. Notice the different nonverbal responses of clients. Notice differences between male and female, elderly and young, and ethnically different clients.

2. Use the COLDSPA mnemonic with peers or friends who are experiencing pain or other symptoms.

3. Review Box 2-1: COMMUNICATION TO AVOID, p. 15 in the textbook. Experiment using these poor techniques to interview your lab partner. What is the outcome when you use each technique that is to be avoided?

4. Practice with a peer or lab partner collecting information from a selected portion of the health history. First, use the structural form and questions for the section. Next, repeat data collection for the section, but this time do not use any structured questions. Use only broad open-ended questions, such as "Tell me about what you have been doing when you experience the symptom" and "Can you think of anything else?"

Activity C INTERVIEWING AND RECORDING ASSESSMENT FINDINGS

After reading Chapter 2 in the textbook, use the following Nursing Interview Guide to interview and record your subjective findings for a health history of a lab partner, peer, or client. Your instructor may ask you to turn this in to be evaluated. Forms are also available on thePoint *website.*

Nursing Interview Guide to Collect Subjective Data From the Client	
Questions	**Findings**
Biographical Data	
Name	
Gender	
Address, phone number	
Date and place of birth	
Nationality or ethnicity	
Marital status	
Religious or spiritual practices	
Primary and secondary languages spoken, written, and read; birth language	

Copyright © 2014. Wolters Kluwer Health | Lippincott Williams & Wilkins. Lab Manual for Health Assessment in Nursing, 5e.

Nursing Interview Guide to Collect Subjective Data From the Client (continued)

Questions	Findings
Educational level	
Occupation and working status	
Who lives with the client? Identify significant others	
Caregivers and support people for the client	
Reason for Seeking Health Care	
1. What is your major health care or concern?	
2. Are you comfortable with seeking care from this organization? Past experiences good or not?	
History of Present Health Concern (use COLDSPA when appropriate)	
1. Character of symptom or condition	
2. Onset (when did it begin; better? worse? same?)	
3. Location (where and does it radiate?)	
4. Severity (on scale of 1–10?)	
5. Pattern (what makes it better? worse?)	
6. Associated factors (other associated symptoms? Effect on leisure or exercise?)	
Past Health History	
Problems at birth?	
Childhood illnesses?	
Immunizations to date?	
Acute or chronic adult illnesses (physical, emotional, mental)?	
Surgeries?	
Pregnancies? Births? Miscarriages? Abortions?	
Accidents? Injuries?	
Prolonged pain or pain patterns?	
Medications	
Allergies?	
Family Health History	
Recall as many genetic relatives as possible (parents, grandparents, siblings) with age, longevity, chronic illnesses (i.e., heart disease, stroke, diabetes, cancer, arthritis, Alzheimer's).	
Review of Systems	
Skin, hair, and nails: Skin color, temperature, condition, excessive sweating, rashes, lesions, balding, dandruff, condition of nails	
Head and neck: Headache, swelling, stiffness of neck, difficulty swallowing, sore throat, enlarged lymph nodes	

Copyright © 2014. Wolters Kluwer Health | Lippincott Williams & Wilkins. Lab Manual for Health Assessment in Nursing, 5e.

Nursing Interview Guide to Collect Subjective Data From the Client (continued)

Questions	Findings
Eyes: Vision, eye infections, redness, excessive tearing, halos around lights, blurring, loss of side vision, moving black spots/specks in visual fields, flashing lights, double vision, and eye pain	
Ears: Hearing, ringing or buzzing, earaches, drainage from ears, dizziness, exposure to loud noises	
Mouth, throat, nose, and sinuses: Condition of teeth and gums; sore throats; mouth lesions; hoarseness; rhinorrhea; nasal obstruction; frequent colds; sneezing or itching of eyes, ears, nose, or throat; nose bleeds; snoring	
Thorax and lungs: Difficulty breathing, wheezing, pain, shortness of breath during routine activity, orthopnea, cough or sputum, hemoptysis, respiratory infections	
Breasts and regional lymphatics: Lumps or discharge from nipples, dimpling or changes in breast size, swollen or tender lymph nodes in axilla	
Heart and neck vessels: Last blood pressure, ECG tracing or findings, chest pain or pressure, palpitations, edema	
Peripheral vascular: Swelling, or edema, of legs and feet; pain; cramping; sores on legs; color or texture changes on the legs or feet	
Abdomen: Indigestion, difficulty swallowing, nausea, vomiting, abdominal pain, gas, jaundice, hernias	
Male genitalia: Excessive or painful urination, frequency or difficulty starting and maintaining urinary stream, leaking of urine, blood noted in urine, sexual problems, perineal lesions, penile drainage, pain or swelling in scrotum, difficulty achieving an erection and/or difficulty ejaculating, exposure to sexually transmitted infections	
Female genitalia: Sexual problems; sexually transmitted diseases; voiding problems (e.g., dribbling, incontinence); reproductive data such as age at menarche, menstruation (length and regularity of cycle), pregnancies, and type of or problems with delivery, abortions, pelvic pain, birth control, menopause (date or year of last menstrual period), and use of hormone replacement therapy	
Anus, rectum, and prostate: Bowel habits, pain with defecation, hemorrhoids, blood in stool, constipation, diarrhea	
Musculoskeletal: Swelling, redness, pain, stiffness of joints, ability to perform activities of daily living, muscle strength	
Neurologic: General mood, behavior, depression, anger, concussions, headaches, loss of strength or sensation, coordination, difficulty speaking, memory problems, strange thoughts and/or actions, difficulty learning	

Copyright © 2014. Wolters Kluwer Health | Lippincott Williams & Wilkins. Lab Manual for Health Assessment in Nursing, 5e.

Nursing Interview Guide to Collect Subjective Data From the Client (continued)	
Questions	**Findings**
Lifestyle and Health Practices Profile	
Description of Typical Day "Please tell me what an average or typical day is for you. Start with awakening in the morning and continue until bedtime."	
Nutrition and Weight Management • "What do you usually eat during a typical day? Please tell me the kinds of foods you prefer, how often you eat throughout the day, and how much you eat." • "Do you eat out at restaurants frequently?" • "Do you eat only when hungry? Do you eat because of boredom, habit, anxiety, depression?" • "Who buys and prepares the food you eat?" • "Where do you eat your meals?" • "How much and what types of fluids do you drink?"	
Activity Level and Exercise • "What is your daily pattern of activity?" • "Do you follow a regular exercise plan? What types of exercise do you do?" • "Are there any reasons why you cannot follow a moderately strenuous exercise program?" • "What do you do for leisure and recreation?" • "Do your leisure and recreational activities include exercise?"	
Sleep and Rest • "Tell me about your sleeping patterns." • "Do you have trouble falling asleep or staying asleep?" • "How much sleep do you get each night?" • "Do you feel rested when you awaken?" • "Do you nap during the day? How often and for how long?" • "What do you do to help you fall asleep?"	
Substance Use • "How much beer, wine, or other alcohol do you drink on the average?" • "Do you drink coffee or other beverages containing caffeine (e.g., cola)? If so, how much and how often?" • "Do you now or have you ever smoked cigarettes or used any other form of nicotine? How long have you been smoking/did you smoke? How many packs per week? Tell me about any efforts to quit." • "Have you ever taken any medication *not prescribed* by your health care provider? If so, when, what type, how much, and why?" • "Have you ever used, or do you now use, recreational drugs? Describe any usage." • "Do you take vitamins or herbal supplements? If so, what?"	

Copyright © 2014. Wolters Kluwer Health | Lippincott Williams & Wilkins. Lab Manual for Health Assessment in Nursing, 5e.

Nursing Interview Guide to Collect Subjective Data From the Client (continued)	
Questions	**Findings**
Self-Concept and Self-Care Responsibilities • "What do you see as your talents or special abilities?" • "How do you feel about yourself? About your appearance?" • "Can you tell me what activities you do to keep yourself safe, healthy, or to prevent disease?" • "Do you practice safe sex?" • "How do you keep your home safe?" • "Do you drive safely?" • "How often do you have medical checkups or screenings?" • "How often do you see the dentist or have your eyes (vision) examined?"	
Social Activities "What do you do for fun and relaxation?" • "With whom do you socialize most frequently?" • "Are you involved in any community activities?" • "How do you feel about your community?" • "Do you think that you have enough time to socialize?" • "What do you see as your contribution to society?"	
Relationships "Who is (are) the most important person(s) in your life? Describe your relationship with that person." • "What was it like growing up in your family?" • "What is your relationship like with your spouse?" • "What is your relationship like with your children?" • "Describe any relationships you have with significant others." • "Do you get along with your in-laws?" • "Are you close to your extended family?" • "Do you have any pets?" • "What is your role in your family? Is it an important role?" • "Are you satisfied with your current sexual relationships? Have there been any recent changes?"	
Values and Belief System "What is most important to you in life?" • "What do you hope to accomplish in your life?" • "Do you have a religious affiliation? Is this important to you?" • "Is a relationship with God (or another higher power) an important part of your life?" • "What gives you strength and hope?"	

Nursing Interview Guide to Collect Subjective Data From the Client (continued)	
Questions	**Findings**
Education and Work • "Tell me about your experiences in school or about your education." • "Are you satisfied with the level of education you have? Do you have future educational plans?" • "What can you tell me about your work? What are your responsibilities at work?" • "Do you enjoy your work?" • "How do you feel about your coworkers?" • "What kind of stress do you have that is work related? Any major problems?" • "Who is the main provider of financial support in your family?" • "Does your current income meet your needs?"	
Stress Levels and Coping Styles • "What types of things make you angry?" • "How would you describe your stress level?" • "How do you manage anger or stress?" • "What do you see as the greatest stressors in your life?" • "Where do you usually turn for help in a time of crisis?"	
Environment • "What risks are you aware of in your environment such as in your home, neighborhood, on the job, or any other activities in which you participate?" • "What types of precautions do you take, if any, when playing contact sports, using harsh chemicals or paint, or operating machinery?" • "Do you believe you are ever in danger of becoming a victim of violence? Explain."	

CHAPTER POSTTEST

Activity D MULTIPLE CHOICE QUESTIONS

Choose the one best answer for each of the following multiple choice questions.

_____ 1. During an interview with an adult client for the first time, the nurse can clarify the client's statements by
   a. offering a "laundry list" of descriptors.
   b. rephrasing the client's statements.
   c. repeating verbatim what the client has said.
   d. inferring what the client's statements mean.

_____ 2. During an interview between a nurse and a client, the nurse and the client collaborate to identify problems and goals. This occurs during the phase of the interview termed
   a. introductory.
   b. ongoing.
   c. working.
   d. closure.

Copyright © 2014. Wolters Kluwer Health | Lippincott Williams & Wilkins. Lab Manual for Health Assessment in Nursing, 5e.

_____ 3. The nurse is preparing to interview an adult client for the first time. The nurse observes that the client appears very anxious. The nurse should
  a. allow the client time to calm down.
  b. avoid discussing sensitive issues.
  c. set time limits with the client.
  d. explain the role and purpose of the nurse.

_____ 4. The nurse is beginning a health history interview with an adult client who expresses anger at the nurse. The best approach for dealing with an angry client is for the nurse to
  a. allow the client to ventilate his or her feelings.
  b. offer reasons why the client should not feel angry.
  c. provide structure during the interview.
  d. refer the client to a different health care provider.

_____ 5. The nurse is planning to interview a client who is being treated for depression. When the nurse enters the examination room, the client is sitting on the table with shoulders slumped. The nurse should plan to approach this client by
  a. providing the client with simple explanations.
  b. offering to hold the client's hand.
  c. using a highly structured interview process.
  d. expressing interest in a neutral manner.

_____ 6. The nurse is planning to interview a client who has demonstrated manipulative behaviors during past clinic visits. During the interview process, the nurse should plan to
  a. give the client rules with which he must agree to comply.
  b. provide structure and set limits with the client.
  c. tell the client that the nurse is aware of his past behaviors.
  d. approach the client in an authoritative manner.

_____ 7. During a client interview, the nurse asks questions about the client's past health history. The primary purpose of asking about past health problems is to
  a. determine whether genetic conditions are present.
  b. summarize the family's health problems.
  c. evaluate how the client's current symptoms affect his or her lifestyle.
  d. identify risk factors to the client and his or her significant others.

_____ 8. While interviewing an adult client about her nutrition habits, the nurse should
  a. ask the client for a 3-day recall of food intake.
  b. review the ChooseMyPlate information with the client.
  c. ask the client about limitations to activity.
  d. encourage the client to drink three to four glasses of water daily.

_____ 9. While interviewing an adult client about the client's stress levels and coping responses, an appropriate question by the nurse is
  a. "Do you feel stress at work?"
  b. "How often do you feel stressed?"
  c. "Is stress a problem in your life?"
  d. "How do you manage your stress?"

Copyright © 2014. Wolters Kluwer Health | Lippincott Williams & Wilkins. Lab Manual for Health Assessment in Nursing, 5e.

Activity E CASE STUDY

Read the following case study. Then, work through the steps of analyzing the case study data. First identify abnormal data and strengths in **subjective and objective findings**, assemble **cue clusters**, draw **inferences**, make possible **nursing diagnoses**, identify **defining characteristics**, **confirm or rule out** the diagnoses, and **document** your conclusions. Use the blank diagnostic analysis charts provided at the end of this book (also available on the Point website) to guide your thinking. Propose nursing diagnoses that are specific to the client in the case study. Identify collaborative problems, if any, for this client. Finally, identify data, if any, that point toward a medical problem requiring a referral.

Stacey Kline is a 29-year-old graphic artist. She is single and lives in a one-bedroom apartment in the city. She has an extensive social network in the city and goes out to clubs and bars until at least midnight about four nights a week. Her work is very fulfilling for her, and she rates her stress level as moderate. She eats two meals a day (usually out), drinks "a lot" of coffee, smokes a pack of "light" cigarettes a day, and drinks whenever she goes out with friends. Stacey does not have a serious boyfriend at present, but she is taking birth control pills "to prevent a disaster with some guy I don't care about." She has a good supportive relationship with her family, who live 15 minutes away. She visits them at least twice a week. She is a Roman Catholic and tries to go to Mass every other week. She says her faith is important to her but it does not rule her life.

How Well Did You Do?

After you have read the chapter and completed the exercises in this chapter, visit thePoint to access the Self-Reflection Activity. This activity will help you identify to what degree you have met each of the chapter objectives. You can then review the chapter for objectives you have met partially or not at all.

Other tools to help you, like the Diagnostic Reasoning Guides, Nursing Interview Guides, Physical Assessment Guides, and NCLEX-Style Chapter Review Questions, are also available on thePoint.

Copyright © 2014. Wolters Kluwer Health | Lippincott Williams & Wilkins. Lab Manual for Health Assessment in Nursing, 5e.

CHAPTER 3

Collecting Objective Data: The Physical Examination

Chapter Overview

Nursing assessment includes both the collection of subjective data (discussed in Chapter 2) and the collection of objective data (discussed in this chapter). Objective data include information about the client that the nurse directly observes during interaction with the client and information elicited through physical assessment (examination) techniques. This chapter can help you review the reasons and techniques to obtain objective assessment data (data that are observable and/or measurable) on clients.

Chapter Learning Objectives

1. Describe the ways to prepare the physical environment and make it conducive to a physical examination.
2. Explain the ways to prepare a client for a physical examination.
3. Describe the various positions used to perform a physical examination.
4. Demonstrate the correct method used for inspection during a physical examination.
5. Explain the purpose and differences between light, deep, and bimanual palpation.
6. Demonstrate the correct direct, indirect, and blunt percussion techniques used during a physical examination.
7. Explain the correct use of a stethoscope and the purpose of the bell and the diaphragm.
8. Survey the various pieces of equipment used to perform a physical examination.

CHAPTER PRETEST

Activity A **MATCHING**

Match the terms in the left column with the correct description in the right column.

Term

_____ **1.** Sims' position

_____ **2.** Sitting position

_____ **3.** Supine position

_____ **4.** Standing position

_____ **5.** Prone position

_____ **6.** Lithotomy position

_____ **7.** Fingerpads

_____ **8.** Ulnar surface or palm of hand

_____ **9.** Dorsal surface of hand

_____ **10.** Bell of stethoscope

_____ **11.** Diaphragm of stethoscope

Description

a. Part of examiner's hand used to feel for temperature

b. Side-lying position used during the rectal examination

c. Position used during much of the physical examination including examination of the head, neck, lungs, chest, back, breast, axilla, heart, vital signs, and upper extremities

d. Back-lying position used for examination of the abdomen (with one small pillow under the head and another under knees); this position also allows easy access for palpation of peripheral pulses

e. Larger end of stethoscope used to detect breath sounds, normal heart sounds, and bowel sounds

f. Position used to examine male genitalia and to assess gait, posture, and balance

g. Part of examiner's hand used to feel for fine discriminations: pulses, texture, size, consistency, shape, and crepitus

h. Client lies on abdomen with head turned to side; may be used to assess back and mobility of hip joint

i. Part of examiner's hand used to feel for vibration, thrills, or fremitus

j. Smaller end of stethoscope used to detect low-pitched sounds (abnormal heart sounds and bruits)

k. Back-lying position with hips at edge of examining table and feet supported in stirrups; used for examination of female genitalia, reproductive tract, and rectum

Activity B **LEARNER ACTIVITIES**

After reading Chapter 3 in the textbook, participate in the following learning activities.

1. Recall a time when you were about to have a physical examination. Remember the anxieties and concerns you were feeling. What were your greatest fears? Share these feelings with your lab partner.

2. Now practice verbally preparing your lab partner for a physical examination. Explain the privacy, confidentiality, time, positioning, and purpose of the examination.

3. Inspect the forearm of your lab partner. Do you have sufficient lighting? Explain. Now use Table 3-2, p. 46 in the textbook to use various parts of your hand to palpate pulses, texture, shape, and temperature of the forearm.

4. Practice indirect percussion (see Fig. 3-6, textbook p. 49) on your lab partner to determine the various percussion tones listed in Table 3-3, p. 48 in the textbook. Use studs in walls to percuss flat and dull tones. Fill a milk carton partway with water and percuss it. Now percuss an empty milk carton and notice the difference. Blow or puff out your cheeks and palpate percuss over one of them. What different types of percussion notes are you hearing?

5. Use Table 3-1, pp. 33–40 in the textbook, EQUIPMENT NEEDED FOR PHYSICAL EXAMINATIONS, to identify the equipment pieces needed. Find each of these pieces of equipment in your learning lab and discuss its purpose and how to use it with your lab partner. (The use of some of the equipment will be discussed in the forthcoming chapters [i.e., ophthalmoscope in eye chapter, otoscope in ear chapter]). Do not attempt to use the equipment until you have seen a demonstration and understand the basic safety principles for using the equipment.

Copyright © 2014. Wolters Kluwer Health | Lippincott Williams & Wilkins. Lab Manual for Health Assessment in Nursing, 5e.

CHAPTER POSTTEST

Activity C MULTIPLE CHOICE QUESTIONS

Choose the one best answer for each of the following multiple choice questions.

____ 1. Before beginning a physical assessment of a client, the nurse should first
   a. wash both hands with soap and water.
   b. determine whether the client is anxious.
   c. ask the client to remove all clothing.
   d. request a family member to be present.

____ 2. To alleviate a client's anxiety during a comprehensive assessment, the nurse should
   a. begin with intrusive procedures first to get them completed quickly.
   b. explain each procedure being performed and the reason for the procedure.
   c. remain in the examination room while the client changes into a gown.
   d. ask the client to sign a consent for the physical examination.

____ 3. While performing a physical examination on an older adult, the nurse should plan to
   a. complete the examination as quickly as possible.
   b. ask the client to change positions frequently.
   c. provide only minimal teaching related to health care.
   d. use minimal position changes.

____ 4. During a comprehensive assessment, the primary technique used by the nurse throughout the examination is
   a. palpation.
   b. percussion.
   c. auscultation.
   d. inspection.

____ 5. While examining a client, the nurse plans to palpate temperature of the skin by using the
   a. fingertips of the hand.
   b. ulnar surface of the hand.
   c. dorsal surface of the hand.
   d. palmar surface of the hand.

____ 6. During palpation of a client's organs, the nurse palpates the spleen by applying pressure between 2.5 and 5 cm. The nurse is performing
   a. light palpation.
   b. moderate palpation.
   c. deep palpation.
   d. very deep palpation.

____ 7. While performing a physical examination on an adult client, the nurse can detect the density of an underlying structure by using
   a. inspection.
   b. palpation.
   c. Doppler magnification.
   d. percussion.

____ **8.** When the nurse places one hand flat on the body surface and uses the fist of the other hand to strike the back of the hand flat on the body surface, the nurse is using

   a. firm percussion.
   b. direct percussion.
   c. indirect percussion.
   d. blunt percussion.

____ **9.** An adult client visits a clinic and tells the nurse that she suspects she has urinary tract infection. To detect tenderness over the client's kidneys, the nurse should instruct the client that he or she will be performing

   a. moderate palpation.
   b. deep palpation.
   c. indirect percussion.
   d. blunt percussion.

____ **10.** The most commonly used method of percussion is

   a. direct percussion.
   b. mild percussion.
   c. indirect percussion.
   d. blunt percussion.

____ **11.** During a comprehensive assessment of the lungs of an adult client with a diagnosis of emphysema, the nurse anticipates that during percussion the client will exhibit

   a. hyperresonance.
   b. tympany.
   c. dullness.
   d. flatness.

____ **12.** While percussing an adult client during a physical examination, the nurse can expect to hear flatness over the client's

   a. lungs.
   b. bone.
   c. liver.
   d. abdomen.

____ **13.** During a comprehensive assessment of an adult client, the nurse can best hear high-pitched sounds by using a stethoscope with a

   a. 1-inch bell.
   b. 1½-inch diaphragm.
   c. 15-inch flexible tubing.
   d. 1-inch diaphragm.

Activity D **CRITICAL THINKING ACTIVITIES**

1. When might you use deep palpation during a physical examination? Bimanual palpation? Direct percussion? Indirect percussion?

2. Explain how the universal precautions (see Box 3-1, pp. 41–43 in textbook) and infection control guidelines would apply to the physical examination techniques of inspection, percussion, palpation, and auscultation.

3. Describe how you would prepare yourself to perform a total physical examination of a client of the opposite sex. Describe how you would prepare the client both emotionally and physically.

4. Mr. SM, a 60-year-old Hispanic man, comes to the ER in a wheelchair being pushed by his son. He states "I just fell off a step ladder in my garage and cannot walk."

How would you use the following physical assessment techniques to gather more data on Mr. SM's legs and feet?

- Inspection
- Percussion
- Palpation
- Auscultation

Compare your answers with a lab partner.

How Well Did You Do?

After you have read the chapter and completed the exercises in this chapter, visit thePoint to access the Self-Reflection Activity. This activity will help you identify to what degree you have met each of the chapter objectives. You can then review the chapter for objectives you have met partially or not at all.

Other tools to help you, like the Diagnostic Reasoning Guides, Nursing Interview Guides, Physical Assessment Guides, and NCLEX-Style Chapter Review Questions, are also available on thePoint.

Copyright © 2014. Wolters Kluwer Health | Lippincott Williams & Wilkins. Lab Manual for Health Assessment in Nursing, 5e.

CHAPTER 4

Validating and Documenting Data

Chapter Overview

After you collect assessment data, what do you do with them? How do you know that they are reliable information? Validation of data is the process of confirming or verifying that the subjective and objective data you have collected is reliable and accurate. How does this data become part of the client's record? Health care agencies have individual policies and procedures for documentation of client data. Electronic Health Records (EHRs) may be used by a variety of health care providers to focus on the total health (emotional, physical, social, spiritual) of the client to share data with other health care providers (i.e., dieticians, physical therapists, laboratories) to promote collaboration of all those *involved in the client's care*. The primary reason for documentation of assessment data is to promote effective communication among multidisciplinary health team members to facilitate safe and efficient client care. Use the following activities to review and enhance the validation and documentation process.

Chapter Learning Objectives

1. Define validation of data.
2. Describe the steps of the validation process.
3. Describe conditions or situations that require data to be rechecked and validated.
4. Discuss several ways to validate data.
5. Describe the purposes of documenting assessment data.
6. Describe the general guidelines and rules for documenting data.
7. Describe various types of standardized assessment forms used for documenting data.
8. Document assessment findings, using a variety of assessment forms (e.g., narrative progress notes, flow sheets).
9. Discuss the significance of documentation as specified by your state nurse practice act and TJC standards.

CHAPTER PRETEST

Activity A MULTIPLE CHOICE QUESTIONS

Choose the one best answer for each of the following multiple choice questions.

_____ 1. If the nurse makes an error while documenting findings on a client's record, the nurse should
   a. erase the error and make the correction.
   b. obliterate the error and make the correction.
   c. draw a line through the error and have it witnessed.
   d. draw a line through the error, writing "error" and initialing.

_____ 2. The nurse is preparing to document assessment findings in a client's record. The nurse should
   a. write in complete sentences with few abbreviations.
   b. avoid slang terms or labels unless they are direct quotes.
   c. record how the data were collected.
   d. use the term "normal" to describe nonpathologic findings.

_____ 3. The nurse has assessed the breath sounds of an adult client. The best way for the nurse to document these findings on a client is to write
   a. "bilateral lung sounds clear."
   b. "the client's lung sounds were clear on both sides."
   c. "client's lung sounds were auscultated with stethoscope and were clear on both sides."
   d. "after listening to client's lung sounds, both lungs appeared clear."

_____ 4. An example of an objective finding in an adult client is
   a. a client's symptom of pain.
   b. family history data.
   c. genetic disorders.
   d. vital signs.

_____ 5. While recording the subjective data of an adult client who complains of pain in his lower back, the nurse should include the location of the pain and the
   a. cause of the pain.
   b. client's caregiver.
   c. client's occupation.
   d. pain relief measures.

_____ 6. One disadvantage of the open-ended assessment form is that it
   a. does not allow for individualization.
   b. asks standardized questions.
   c. requires a lot of time to complete.
   d. does not provide a total picture of the client.

_____ 7. The nurse is recording admission data for an adult client using a cued or checklist type of assessment form. This type of assessment form
   a. prevents missed questions during data collection.
   b. covers all the data that a client may provide.
   c. clusters the assessment data with nursing diagnoses.
   d. establishes comparability of data across populations.

Copyright © 2014. Wolters Kluwer Health | Lippincott Williams & Wilkins. Lab Manual for Health Assessment in Nursing, 5e.

____ **8.** One advantage for an institution to use an integrated cued/checklist type of assessment data form is that it

    a. allows a comprehensive and thorough picture of the client's symptoms.

    b. may be easily used by different levels of caregivers, which enhances communication.

    c. provides for easy and rapid documentation across clinical settings and populations.

    d. includes the 11 health care patterns in an easily readable format.

____ **9.** An assessment form commonly used in long-term care facilities is the nursing minimum data set. One primary advantage to this type of assessment form is that it

    a. establishes comparability of nursing data across clinical populations.

    b. clusters all the nursing and medical diagnoses in one place.

    c. allows for individualization for each client in the health care setting.

    d. uses a flowchart format for easy documentation of objective data.

____ **10.** In some health care settings, the institution uses an assessment form that assesses only one part of a client. These types of forms are termed

    a. progressive.

    b. specific.

    c. checklist.

    d. focused.

____ **11.** The nurse is planning to assess a newly admitted adult client. While gathering data from the client, the nurse should

    a. validate all data before documentation of the data.

    b. document the data after the entire examination process.

    c. record the nurse's understanding of the client's problem.

    d. use medical terms that are commonly used in health care settings.

Activity B LEARNER ACTIVITIES

After reading Chapter 4 in the textbook, participate in the following learning activities.

1. Observe your lab partner for 1 to 2 minutes. Then document your observations in objective terms (i.e., height, weight, age, gender, hair and skin color, mood, attitude, well-being status). Next validate your observations with your lab partner. Did you learn anything new about them?

2. Interview your lab partner to determine how his or her physical and mental health has been during the past month. Do this beginning with five basic questions:

    a. How have you felt during the past month?

    b. Have you had any major illnesses during this time?

    c. Have you had any minor illnesses during this time?

    d. Rate your current health on a scale of 1 to 10 (with 1 being poor and 10 being great).

    e. How would you like your health to improve?

Document your subjective data findings.

Copyright © 2014. Wolters Kluwer Health | Lippincott Williams & Wilkins. Lab Manual for Health Assessment in Nursing, 5e.

CHAPTER POSTTEST

Activity C MATCHING

Identify the following items as either subjective (S) or objective (O) data by writing "S" or "O" on each line.

_____ **1.** Describes severe right-sided headache

_____ **2.** Reddened, raised, indurated area on deltoid area of left arm

_____ **3.** Cannot eat seeds or uncooked grains without abdominal discomfort

_____ **4.** Passing flatus

_____ **5.** Bowel sounds present in all four quadrants

_____ **6.** Complains of lower back pain on movement

_____ **7.** Pattern of request for pain medication every 2 hours

_____ **8.** Pale, clammy, and diaphoretic

_____ **9.** Feels nauseated and dizzy

_____ **10.** Emesis of 200 mL light beige thin liquid

Activity D CRITICAL THINKING ACTIVITIES

1. Discuss the possible results of failing to document data. How could this affect the client? The nurse?

2. Discuss a variety of ways to validate client data obtained during a nursing history interview.

3. The entry below was made on a client admitted to a medical unit. The entry leaves a lot of unanswered questions for the nurse. Correct this entry by adding hypothetical details as needed to present a complete and accurate entry that precisely describes the client's current condition.

Mrs. Jones arrives in room 2344. Headache; flushed, cool skin; pale; nausea and vomiting; temperature normal; blood pressure 136/85 mm Hg; pulse rapid; respirations rapid. Swollen extremity. Requesting pain medication.

How Well Did You Do?

After you have read the chapter and completed the exercises in this chapter, visit thePoint to access the Self-Reflection Activity. This activity will help you identify to what degree you have met each of the chapter objectives. You can then review the chapter for objectives you have met partially or not at all.

Other tools to help you, like the Diagnostic Reasoning Guides, Nursing Interview Guides, Physical Assessment Guides, and NCLEX-Style Chapter Review Questions, are also available on thePoint.

Copyright © 2014. Wolters Kluwer Health | Lippincott Williams & Wilkins. Lab Manual for Health Assessment in Nursing, 5e.

Thinking Critically to Analyze Data and Make Informed Nursing Judgments

Chapter Overview

Initially, sorting through subjective and objective assessment data may seem to be an overwhelming task. This analysis of data (diagnostic phase) is the second step of the nursing process. This phase requires the nurse to use critical thinking skills to differentiate normal findings from abnormal findings, to draw inferences, to make nursing diagnoses, and to confirm or rule out conclusions. The end result of this phase is the identification of a nursing diagnosis (health promotion, actual, or risk), collaborative problem, or the need for referral to another health care professional.

Chapter Learning Objectives

1. Describe how critical thinking relates to diagnostic reasoning.
2. Determine your own ability to think critically.
3. Describe seven essential critical thinking characteristics.
4. List the six essential components of the diagnostic phase of the nursing process.
5. List the seven distinct steps used in this textbook to perform data analysis.
6. Define and give examples of wellness, risk, and actual nursing diagnoses.
7. Define and give examples of collaborative problems.
8. Explain why experienced expert nurses have an advantage over novice nurses in making accurate diagnoses.
9. Discuss the common "pitfalls" of diagnostic reasoning.
10. Explain the ways to increase the accuracy of your diagnostic reasoning skills.

CHAPTER PRETEST

Activity A MATCHING

Match the terms in the left column with the correct description in the right column.

Term

____ **1.** Critical thinking

____ **2.** Intuition

____ **3.** Health promotion nursing diagnosis

____ **4.** Collaborative problem

____ **5.** Risk nursing diagnosis

____ **6.** Actual nursing diagnosis

____ **7.** Syndrome nursing diagnosis

____ **8.** Knowledge

____ **9.** Cognitive abilities

____ **10.** Analysis of data

____ **11.** Diagnostic phase

Description

a. A nursing diagnosis that indicates the client has an opportunity to enhance a health status

b. Certain physiologic complications that nurses monitor to detect their onset or change in status

c. Aptitude involving the act or process of knowing, including both awareness and judgment

d. The fact or condition of knowing something with familiarity gained through experience or association

e. Quick and ready insight

f. The way in which one processes information using knowledge, past experience, intuition, and cognitive abilities to formulate conclusions or diagnoses

g. Diagnostic phase of the nursing process

h. A nursing diagnosis that indicates the client does not currently have a problem but is at high risk for developing it

i. A nursing diagnosis that indicates the client is currently experiencing the stated problem or has a dysfunctional pattern

j. Analysis of data

k. Clinical judgments that describe a specific cluster of nursing diagnoses that occur together and have similar nursing interventions to resolve the situation

Activity B LEARNER ACTIVITIES

After reading Chapter 5 in the textbook, participate in the following learning activities.

1. Review Box 5-1, "ESSENTIAL ELEMENTS OF CRITICAL THINKING," p. 66 in the textbook. Rate yourself on a scale of 1 to 5 for each element (5 being that you possess a high degree of that element) to determine your level of critical thinking. Discuss with your peers ways to improve your critical thinking based on these critical thinking elements.

2. Interview your lab partners to assess their current level of well-being for the day. Use the seven steps described in the textbook to analyze the data you collect to draw conclusions. Can you identify any nursing diagnoses or collaborative problems? Do they need to be encouraged to see a health care provider?

3. Review the diagnostic reasoning pitfalls in Chapter 5. Discuss with your lab partner which pitfall(s) you made while attempting to diagnose your lab partner. What will you do in the future to avoid this pitfall when diagnosing your clients?

CHAPTER POSTTEST

Activity C MULTIPLE CHOICE QUESTIONS

Choose the one best answer for each of the following multiple choice questions.

____ **1.** One characteristic of a nurse who is a critical thinker is the ability to

    a. form an opinion quickly.

    b. offer advice to clients.

    c. be right most of the time.

    d. validate information and judgments.

Copyright © 2014. Wolters Kluwer Health | Lippincott Williams & Wilkins. Lab Manual for Health Assessment in Nursing, 5e.

_____ **2.** Before the nurse analyzes the data collected, the nurse should

    a. determine collaborative problems with the health care team.

    b. group the data into clusters or groups of problems.

    c. generate possible hypotheses for the client's problems.

    d. perform the steps of the assessment process accurately.

_____ **3.** The nurse is caring for an adult client who tells the nurse "For weeks now, I've been so tired. I just can't get to sleep at night because of all the noise in my neighborhood." An actual nursing diagnosis for this client is

    a. fatigue related to excessive noise levels as manifested by the client's statements of chronic fatigue.

    b. sleep deprivation related to noisy neighborhood and inability to sleep.

    c. chronic fatigue syndrome related to excessive levels of noise in neighborhood.

    d. readiness for enhanced sleep related to control of noise level in the home.

_____ **4.** A common error for beginning nurses who are formulating nursing diagnoses during data analysis is to

    a. formulate too many nursing diagnoses for the client and family.

    b. include too much data about the client in the history.

    c. obtain an insufficient number of cues and cluster patterns.

    d. quickly make a diagnosis without hypothesizing several diagnoses.

_____ **5.** When formulating a nursing diagnosis, the format that is most useful to clearly document the client's problem is

    a. NANDA label (for problem) + related to + etiology + AMB (as manifested by) + defining characteristics.

    b. NANDA label + defining characteristics + AMB (as manifested by) the etiology.

    c. NANDA label + definition + defining characteristics + AMB (as manifested by) etiology.

    d. NANDA label + definition + etiology + AMB (as manifested by) + defining characteristics.

_____ **6.** Select the following nursing diagnosis that is correctly stated.

    a. Risk for Impaired Skin Integrity related to immobility, bedrest, pain in legs, and the client states "I will not go to Physical therapy."

    b. Risk for Impaired Skin Integrity related to immobility as manifested by constant bedrest and the inability to ambulate the client twice a day.

    c. Risk for Impaired Skin Integrity related to immobility secondary to right-sided paralysis, dehydration, and reluctance to participate in physical therapy as manifested by reddened coccyx and very dry skin.

    d. Risk for Impaired Skin Integrity related to bedrest, lack of time to ambulate client, right-sided paralysis, and reluctance to participate in physical therapy as manifested by reddened coccyx and very dry skin.

_____ **7.** Which of the following sequences describes the correct order of steps for analyzing data?

    a. Identify abnormal data and strengths, cluster data, draw inferences, propose possible nursing diagnoses, check for the presence of defining characteristics, confirm or rule out nursing diagnoses, document conclusions.

    b. Identify abnormal data and strengths, cluster data, draw inferences, check for the presence of defining characteristics, propose possible nursing diagnoses, confirm or rule out nursing diagnoses, document conclusions.

    c. Identify abnormal data and strengths, draw inferences, cluster data, check for the presence of defining characteristics, propose possible nursing diagnoses, confirm or rule out nursing diagnoses, document conclusions.

    d. Identify abnormal data and strengths, draw inferences, cluster data, check for the presence of defining characteristics, confirm or rule out nursing diagnoses, propose possible nursing diagnoses, document conclusions.

____ **8.** Which of the following is a collaborative problem?

    a. Risk for skin breakdown

    b. Risk for osteoporosis

    c. Risk for stress

    d. Risk for rape trauma syndrome

Activity D CRITICAL THINKING ACTIVITY

Mrs. Phillips, age 65, has smoked three packs of cigarettes a day for 40 years. She complains of difficulty fixing her own meals, bathing and dressing herself, and an inability to climb a short flight of stairs due to shortness of breath. She lives in a second floor apartment building that does not have an elevator. Her constant cough is congested-sounding, respiratory rate of 26 beats/minute, a shallow breathing pattern, an oral temperature of 37.7°C (99.8°F), blood pressure of 140/92 mm Hg, height 160 cm (5 ft 3 in), weight 57 kg (127 lb).

From the case study above, identify a cue cluster and possible diagnostic conclusion(s) (health promotion [wellness], risk, or actual nursing diagnosis). Describe your critical thinking process. Identify the collaborative problems for which the client is at risk.

How Well Did You Do?

After you have read the chapter and completed the exercises in this chapter, visit thePoint to access the Self-Reflection Activity. This activity will help you identify to what degree you have met each of the chapter objectives. You can then review the chapter for objectives you have met partially or not at all.

Other tools to help you, like the Diagnostic Reasoning Guides, Nursing Interview Guides, Physical Assessment Guides, and NCLEX-Style Chapter Review Questions, are also available on thePoint.

Copyright © 2014. Wolters Kluwer Health | Lippincott Williams & Wilkins. Lab Manual for Health Assessment in Nursing, 5e.

Assessing Mental Status and Substance Abuse

Chapter Overview

Your evaluation of the client's mental status and psychosocial developmental level will provide you with information regarding the client's level of cognitive functioning and emotional stability. These data will be useful to you to determine the reliability of the client's responses throughout the rest of the examination. That is why it is important to begin your examination with an assessment of the client's mental status and developmental level.

Chapter Learning Objectives

1. Discuss the concepts of mental health, mental disorders, and factors that affect both.
2. Discuss the risk factors for mental health disorders and substance abuse across cultures and ways to reduce one's risks.
3. Prepare and interview a client for an accurate history of their mental status and risk for substance abuse.
4. Perform an accurate mental health and risk for substance abuse assessment.
5. Correctly use the SLUMS (St. Louis University Mental Status) Examination tool to assess the client's mental status.
6. Correctly use the Glasgow Coma Scale (GCS) for clients who are at high risk for rapid deterioration.
7. Explain when and how to use the CAGE Self-Assessment Tool to assess alcohol dependence.
8. Correctly use the Alcohol Use Disorders Identification Test (AUDIT): Interview Version to interview a client for risk of alcohol abuse.
9. Correctly use the Confusion Assessment Method (CAM) to assess for confusion.
10. Correctly use the Depression Questionnaire to assess for depression.
11. Describe the seven warning signs to assess for Alzheimer disease.
12. Correctly use the modified SAD Persons Suicide Risk tool to assess for suicide risk.
13. Differentiate between normal and abnormal findings of a mental health status and substance abuse assessment.
14. Analyze data from the interview and physical assessment of mental status and substance abuse risk to formulate valid nursing diagnoses, collaborative problems, and/or referrals.

CHAPTER PRETEST

Activity A MATCHING

Match the terms in the left column with the correct description in the right column. Some descriptions may be used more than once.

Term

____ **1.** Mental health

____ **2.** Alert

____ **3.** Lethargy

____ **4.** Obtunded

____ **5.** Stupor

____ **6.** Coma

____ **7.** Mental disorder

____ **8.** Sedentary lifestyle, substance abuse, exposure to violence

____ **9.** WHO definition of health

____ **10.** Personality and spirituality

Description

a. Slow response, mumbles and incoherent, opens eyes to loud voice

b. Awakens to painful stimuli and then goes back to sleep; has motor response of withdrawal, groans or mumbles

c. Unresponsive to all stimuli

d. Awake and oriented

e. Necessary for total health

f. Opens eyes and answers questions but falls back asleep

g. State of complete physical, mental, and social well-being and not merely the absence of disease or infirmity

h. Underlying psychobiologic dysfunction

i. Factors affecting mental health

Activity B LEARNER ACTIVITIES

After reading Chapter 6 in the textbook, participate in the following learning activities.

1. Go to a community shopping mall during a busy time of the day. Sit and observe those who pass by, noting their hygiene, behaviors, facial expressions, mannerisms, and speech. Document a variety of hygiene observations, facial expressions, mannerisms, and speech.

2. Pair up with a peer and take turns role-playing the various levels of consciousness (LOC): lethargy, obtunded, stupor, and coma. While one person portrays these various levels as the client, use the Glasgow Coma Scale to assess and record the client's LOC.

Activity C INTERVIEWING AND RECORDING ASSESSMENT FINDINGS

After reading Chapter 6, use the following Nursing Interview Guide to interview and record your subjective findings for an assessment of mental status and risk for substance abuse. Your instructor may ask you to turn this in to be evaluated. Forms are also available on thePoint website.

Nursing Interview Guide to Collect Subjective Data From the Client	
Questions	**Findings**
Biographic Data	
1. Name, address, phone numbers.	
2. Age stated by client.	
3. Marital status.	
4. Place of employment.	
5. Educational level.	
Present History	
1. Most current health concern at this time.	
2. Reason for seeking health care?	

Copyright © 2014. Wolters Kluwer Health | Lippincott Williams & Wilkins. Lab Manual for Health Assessment in Nursing, 5e.

Nursing Interview Guide to Collect Subjective Data From the Client (continued)	
Questions	**Findings**
(Apply COLDSPA here as appropriate)	
Past Health History	
1. Head injuries, meningitis, encephalitis, stroke? Effects on health?	
2. Past medical diagnoses, surgeries.	
3. Past counseling services received? Results?	
4. Headaches? Describe.	
5. Served in active duty in armed forces?	
6. Breathing difficulties?	
7. Heart palpitations?	
8. Exposure to environmental toxins?	
Family History	
1. Family history of mental health problems?	
2. Family history of psychiatric disorders, dementia, brain tumors?	
Lifestyle and Health Practices	
1. Describe typical activities in a day.	
2. Energy level with ADLs?	
3. Typical eating habits?	
4. Alcohol consumption? Type? Amount? Frequency?	
5. Use the CAGE self-assessment tool (see Box 6-1, p. 79 in the textbook) to detect at risk clients.	
6. Use the AUDIT Questionnaire (see Assessment Tool 6-1, pp. 93–94 in the textbook) to assess alcohol-related disorders. Calculate score.	
7. Any use of recreational drugs (i.e., marijuana, tranquilizers, barbiturates, cocaine, methamphetamines)?	
8. Sleep patterns.	
9. Typical bowel elimination patterns.	
10. Exercise patterns.	
11. Use of prescribed or OTC drugs.	
12. Religious practices and activities?	
13. Role in family and community?	
14. Relationships with others (family members, coworkers, neighbors)?	
15. Perception of self and relationship with others?	
16. View of one's future? Life goals?	

Copyright © 2014. Wolters Kluwer Health | Lippincott Williams & Wilkins. Lab Manual for Health Assessment in Nursing, 5e.

Activity D **PERFORMING PHYSICAL ASSESSMENT**

Use the following Physical Assessment Guide to assess a peer, friend, or family member for mental health status and risk for substance abuse. Column 1 may be used to guide your examination. Column 2 may be used by your instructor to provide you feedback regarding ways to enhance your skills. Forms are also available on thePoint *website.*

Physical Assessment Guide to Collect Objective Client Data

Questions	Findings
When time is limited, use the Saint Louis University Mental Status (SLUMS) examination (Assessment Tool 6-3, p. 95 in the textbook). Report client's SLUMS score and client's level of education. Otherwise, complete observations 1–10 below.	
1. Observe level of consciousness. Ask for name, address, and phone number as appropriate. If no response: • Call name louder. • Next shake gently. • If still no response, apply painful stimulus. Use the Glasgow Coma Scale (GCS) (see Assessment Tool 6-2, p. 93 in the textbook) for clients who are at high risk for rapid deterioration of consciousness.	
2. Note posture, gait, and body movements.	
3. Observe behavior and the client's affect.	
4. Note dress, grooming, and hygiene.	
5. Observe facial expression.	
6. Observe speech.	
7. Note mood, feelings, and expressions. Use Depression Questionnaire (Box 6-2, p. 81 in the textbook) if depression is suspected. Use the Geriatric Depression scale (Box 32-3, p. 797 in the textbook) for older adults.	
8. Note thought processes and perceptions.	
9. Observe for any destructive or suicidal tendencies.	
10. Observe the following cognitive abilities: • Orientation to person, time, and place • Concentration and attentiveness • Recent memory • Remote memory • Memory to learn new information • Abstract reasoning • Judgment • Visual and constructional ability	
11. Use the Alcohol Use Disorders Identification Test (AUDIT): Interview Version to interview a client for risk of alcohol abuse (see Assessment Tool 6-1, p. 93 in the textbook).	
12. Use the Confusion Assessment Method (CAM) to assess for confusion (see Assessment Tool 6-4, p. 96 in the textbook).	
13. Use the modified SAD Persons Suicide Risk tool to assess for suicide risk (see Assessment Guide 6-1, p. 83 in the textbook).	
Analysis of Date	
1. Formulate nursing diagnoses.	
2. Formulate collaborative problems.	
3. Make necessary referrals.	

Copyright © 2014. Wolters Kluwer Health | Lippincott Williams & Wilkins. Lab Manual for Health Assessment in Nursing, 5e.

CHAPTER POSTTEST

Activity E MULTIPLE CHOICE QUESTIONS

Choose the one best answer for each of the following multiple choice questions.

_____ 1. The nurse assesses a client using the Glasgow Coma Scale. Which of the following indicators will be used to determine the score?

   a. Eye opening, and appropriateness of verbal and motor responses.

   b. Ability to recall recent and remote memories, and to use abstract reasoning.

   c. Assessment of the 12 cranial nerves.

   d. Naming of objects, recall of three words, and ability to redraw a design.

_____ 2. The client's daughter asks the nurse why the nurse is asking her mother depression-related questions. The nurse explains that even though the client has symptoms of dementia, the Geriatric Depression Scale is being used because

   a. depression and dementia are one in the same disorder.

   b. finding out why she is depressed will help determine the cause of her dementia.

   c. depression often mimics signs and symptoms of dementia.

   d. it is the most accurate tool to determine the stage of dementia.

_____ 3. The nurse documents findings from the client's Mini-Mental State Examination. The following information will be documented as a result of this test.

   a. Mood, feelings, expressions, and perceptions.

   b. Orientation, memory, and cognitive function.

   c. Energy level, satisfaction, and social participation.

   d. Appropriateness of dress, grooming, and eye contact.

_____ 4. As part of assessing the client's level of consciousness, the nurse asks questions related to person, place, and time. Which of these statements is true?

   a. Orientation to person is usually lost first and orientation to time is usually lost last.

   b. Orientation to time is usually lost first and orientation to person is usually lost last.

   c. Orientation to person is usually lost first and orientation to place is usually lost last.

   d. Orientation to time is usually lost first and orientation to place is usually lost last.

_____ 5. When the nurse asks the client to explain similarities and differences between objects, what cognitive ability is being tested?

   a. Judgment.

   b. Concentration.

   c. Memory to learn new information.

   d. Abstract reasoning.

_____ 6. After using the SLUMS tool to test a client's mental status, the nurse calculates a score of 12. The nurse should make

   a. the nursing diagnosis: Disturbed thought processes related to substance abuse.

   b. the nursing diagnosis: Ineffective decision making related to loss of memory.

   c. a referral to the primary health care provided for further evaluation.

   d. a referral for the family and client to seek mental health counseling.

_____ 7. The CAGE assessment is used by the nurse to determine if further assessment is needed. The nurse may assess that it is highly likely the client has a problem and would seek additional assessments if the client

   a. answered "yes" to one of the four CAGE questions.

   b. answered "yes" to three of the four CAGE questions.

   c. answered "no" to all of the four CAGE questions.

   d. answered "no" to three of the four CAGE questions.

Copyright © 2014. Wolters Kluwer Health | Lippincott Williams & Wilkins. Lab Manual for Health Assessment in Nursing, 5e.

____ **8.** A female client is assessed to have a score of 6 points on the AUDIT. This would alert the nurse that this client

    a. has a hazardous alcohol consumption.

    b. is a heavy drinker.

    c. is an at risk drinker.

    d. is not at any risk for alcohol harm.

Activity F **CRITICAL THINKING ACTIVITY**

Explain some "normal variations" that may be observed in the mental status exam of different clients from various cultures.

Activity G **CASE STUDY**

Read the following case study. Then, work through the steps of analyzing the case study data. First identify abnormal data and strengths in **subjective and objective findings**, assemble **cue clusters**, draw **inferences**, make possible **nursing diagnoses**, identify **defining characteristics**, **confirm or rule out** the diagnoses, and **document** your conclusions. Use the blank diagnostic analysis charts provided at the end of this book (also available on thePoint website) to guide your thinking. Propose nursing diagnoses that are specific to the client in the case study. Identify collaborative problems, if any, for this client. Finally, identify data, if any, that point toward a medical problem requiring a referral.

Mrs. Carroll, a 54-year-old, sixth grade mathematics teacher, comes to a wellness screening and expresses concern that she has had difficulty recalling her students' names over the past semester. She also misplaces objects more frequently than in the past. Both her memory and misplacing things are getting worse. She has no history of stroke, meningitis, or head injury and no family history of Alzheimer's. Her brother had bipolar disorder. She is able to perform activities of daily living but it is getting more difficult to grade math papers at night. She tires more easily than in the past. She awakens two times a night but is able to return to sleep within 30 minutes. She reports having a good appetite and a daily well-formed bowel movement. She is active in her church community and walks 3 miles, four times a week. She enjoys quilting. Mrs. Carroll has positive relationships with her husband and two daughters.

    Mental status: Alert and oriented to person, place, day, and time. Clean and neat appearance. Has direct eye contact with pleasant cooperative disposition. Speech clear with moderate tone. Somewhat anxious over forgetting names and location of objects. Looking forward to retirement in 8 years. Able to name familiar objects in room. Expressed clear, realistic and logical thought processes about the past and future. Recalls breakfast and past dates of family member's birthdays. Repeated four unrelated words after 5 minutes, one word after 10 minutes, unable to repeat any words after 12 minutes. Explained the meaning of common proverbs, explained what she would do in an emergency situation in her classroom. Correctly drew the face of a clock. Scored 28 on the Saint Louis University Mental Status (SLUMS) Examination.

How Well Did You Do?

After you have read the chapter and completed the exercises in this chapter, visit thePoint to access the Self-Reflection Activity. This activity will help you identify to what degree you have met each of the chapter objectives. You can then review the chapter for objectives you have met partially or not at all.

    Other tools to help you, like the Diagnostic Reasoning Guides, Nursing Interview Guides, Physical Assessment Guides, and NCLEX-Style Chapter Review Questions, are also available on thePoint.

Copyright © 2014. Wolters Kluwer Health | Lippincott Williams & Wilkins. Lab Manual for Health Assessment in Nursing, 5e.

CHAPTER 7

Assessing Psychosocial, Cognitive, and Moral Development

Chapter Overview

This chapter will help you become more familiar with the developmental theories presented in Chapter 7 of the textbook which focuses on the *growth* (addition of new skills or components) and *development* (refinement, expansion or improvement of existing skills or components) of an individual throughout the lifespan. You will expand your knowledge about the developmental concepts of Sigmund Freud (1856–1939), Erik Erikson (1902–1994), Jean Piaget (1896–1980), and Lawrence Kohlberg (1927–1987). Having a basic understanding of the significant contributions made by these theorists of the psychosexual, psychosocial, cognitive, and moral development of humans is fundamental to performing a holistic nursing assessment.

Chapter Learning Objectives

1. Describe major theories of development: Freud (psychosexual), Erikson (psychosocial), Piaget (cognitive), and Kohlberg (moral).
2. Interview a client for an accurate nursing history of psychosocial, cognitive, and moral development.
3. Assess a client's psychosocial, cognitive, and moral development using both subjective and objective data collection.
4. Differentiate between normal and abnormal findings of psychosocial, cognitive, and moral development.
5. Describe findings frequently seen when assessing the older client's psychosocial, cognitive, and moral development.
6. Analyze data from the interview and objective assessment of psychosocial, cognitive, and moral development to formulate valid nursing diagnoses, collaborative problems, and/or referrals.

CHAPTER PRETEST

Activity A   MATCHING

Match the terms in the left column with the correct description in the right column.

Term

_____ **1.** Freud's theory

_____ **2.** Erikson's theory

_____ **3.** Piaget's theory

_____ **4.** Kohlberg's theory

_____ **5.** Middle adult

_____ **6.** Assimilation

_____ **7.** Concrete operational

_____ **8.** Accommodation

_____ **9.** Preoperational

_____ **10.** Sensorimotor

Description

a. Growth and development of intellectual structures

b. Generativity versus stagnation

c. Adaptive process whereby information is incorporated into an already existing *schema*

d. Ability to make a mental representation for something not present using language

e. Id, ego, and superego

f. Creation of a new *schema* or the modification of an old one

g. Thoughts are demonstrated by physical manipulation of objects/stimuli

h. Developmental tasks correspond to biophysical maturity and societal expectations

i. Begins to think and reason logically about objects in the environment

j. Viewed *justice* (or fairness) as the goal of moral judgment

Activity B   LEARNER ACTIVITIES

After reading Chapter 7 in the textbook, participate in the following learning activities.

1. Study Table 7-4: LAWRENCE KOHLBERG'S STAGES OF MORAL DEVELOPMENT on page 105 in your textbook. Within what stage do you think the majority of people you know fall? Why? Discuss with your lab partner to see if the results are similar.

2. Study Table 7-3: JEAN PIAGET'S STAGES OF COGNITIVE DEVELOPMENT on pages 103–104 in your textbook. Think of a child you know who is in each stage of cognitive development within this model. Give examples of the child's behavior that provides rationale for your selection.

Activity C   INTERVIEWING AND RECORDING ASSESSMENT FINDINGS

After reading Chapter 7 in the textbook, use the following Nursing Interview Guide to interview and record your subjective findings for an assessment of psychosocial, cognitive, and moral development of a lab partner, peer, or client. Your instructor may ask you to turn this in to be evaluated. Forms are also available on thePoint *website.*

Nursing Interview Guide to Collect Subjective Data From the Client	
Questions	**Findings**
How old are you?	
Where were you born? How long have you been in this country?	
Where is your place of birth? Tell me about the places where you have lived. When?	
With what cultural group(s) do you most identify? What is your primary language? When do you speak it? Are you fluent in other languages?	
What is your highest level of formal education?	
Discuss your history of employment. If a person states that he is retired, inquire from what occupation(s). How do you presently make a living and maintain your everyday needs?	

Copyright © 2014. Wolters Kluwer Health | Lippincott Williams & Wilkins. Lab Manual for Health Assessment in Nursing, 5e.

Nursing Interview Guide to Collect Subjective Data From the Client (continued)

Questions	Findings
History of Present Health Concerns	
Describe how you are feeling right now. What concerns do you have about your health? Describe any changes you have recently experienced in your health.	
Discuss any concerns you have about your body weight.	
What major stressors are you currently experiencing? How do you cope with stress? When you are having a problem, how do you usually handle them? Does this work? To whom do you turn when you are having a conflict/crisis?	
Do you have any troublemaking decisions? Please give me some examples of recent decisions you have had to make.	
Tell me about life changes you have had to make. Need to make? How will you make these changes?	
Personal Health History	
How would you describe yourself to others? What are your strengths? Weaknesses?	
What is the best method of learning for you?	
Have you ever been treated (or currently being treated) for a psychological or psychiatric problem? If so, please explain if this treatment helped you deal with (or is currently helping you deal with) problems?	
Please tell me about any prescribed medications, herbs, or supplements you are currently taking. Please tell me about any over-the-counter medication/herbs you are currently taking. Please tell me about any current medical treatment or therapy you are undergoing.	
Describe any changes you have recently experienced concerning your weight? Eating? Elimination needs? Sleep? Please tell me about any allergies or sensitivities you have.	
Describe any chronic illnesses with which you have been diagnosed. How has your life changed since you were diagnosed?	
Family History	
Whom do you consider to be your family?	
Describe your life growing up as a child.	
Do you have brothers? Sisters? Tell me about them and the relationships you have with them.	
Discuss any significant genetic predisposition or characteristic trait or disorder that you believe you have inherited.	
Lifestyle and Health Practices	
Due to the unique assessment topic of this chapter, questions related to the client's lifestyle and health practices are addressed in the Assessing Developmental Level: Psychosocial Status section below.	

Copyright © 2014. Wolters Kluwer Health | Lippincott Williams & Wilkins. Lab Manual for Health Assessment in Nursing, 5e.

Activity D PERFORMING PHYSICAL ASSESSMENT OF PSYCHOSOCIAL, COGNITIVE, AND MORAL DEVELOPMENT

Use the following Physical Assessment Guide to assess the psychosocial, cognitive, and moral development of a lab partner, peer, or client. Column 1 will serve as a reminder as to what part of the exam you will do next. Column 2 will be used to record your findings. Your instructor may ask you to turn this in to be evaluated. Forms are also available on thePoint *website.*

Physical Assessment Guide to Collect Objective Client Data

Questions	Findings
Assessment of Freud's stages of psychosexual development	
Determine the client's psychosocial level by asking the following suggested questions. Does the **young adult**: • Still live with parent(s) at home? • Accept roles and responsibilities at place of residence? • Have experience of growing up in a single parent home? • Have unresolved issues with parent(s)? • Have a satisfying sexual relationship with a significant other? • Have gainful employment?	
Does the **middle-aged adult**: • Demonstrate nervous mannerisms? • Frequently derive pleasure from selected activities? • Cope effectively with stress? • Have a satisfying sexual relationship? • Believe physical changes of aging have affected any relationships?	
Does the **older adult**: • Engage in sexual activity? • Positively cope with loss? • Believe any changes in cognition have occurred? • Believe any significant changes have occurred in interests/relationships?	
Assessment of Erikson's Psychosocial Development	
Does the **young adult**: • Accept self—physically, cognitively, and emotionally? • Have independence from the parental home? • Express love responsibly, emotionally, and sexually? • Have close or intimate relationships with a partner? • Have a social group of friends? • Have a philosophy of living and life? • Have a profession or a life's work that provides a means of contribution? • Solve problems of life that accompany independence from the parental home?	

Copyright © 2014. Wolters Kluwer Health | Lippincott Williams & Wilkins. Lab Manual for Health Assessment in Nursing, 5e.

Physical Assessment Guide to Collect Objective Client Data (continued)

Questions	Findings
Does the **middle-aged adult**: • Have healthy life patterns? • Derive satisfaction from contributing to growth and development of others? • Have an abiding intimacy and long-term relationship with a partner? • Maintain a stable home? • Find pleasure in an established work or profession? • Take pride in self and family accomplishments and contributions? • Contribute to the community to support its growth and development?	
Does the **older adult**: • Adjust to the changing physical self? • Recognize changes present as a result of aging, in relationships and activities? • Maintain relationships with children, grandchildren, and other relatives? • Continue interests outside of self and home? • Complete transition from retirement at work to satisfying alternative activities? • Establish relationships with others who are his or her own age? • Adjust to deaths of relatives, spouse, and friends? • Maintain a maximum level of physical functioning through diet, exercise, and personal care? • Find meaning in past life and face inevitable mortality of self and significant others? • Integrate philosophical or religious values into self-understanding to promote comfort? • Review accomplishments and recognize meaningful contributions he or she has made to community and relatives?	
Assessment of Piaget's Cognitive Development	
Determine the clients cognitive level by asking the following questions: Does the **young adult**: • Assume responsibility for independent decision making? • Realistically self-evaluate strengths and weaknesses? • Identify and explore multiple options and potential outcomes? • Seek assistance as necessary? • Place decisions into long-range context? • Make realistic plans for the future? • Seek career mentors?	
Does the **middle-aged adult**: • Differentiate discrepancies among goals, wishes, and realities? • Identify factors that give life meaning and continuity? • Effectively share knowledge and experience with others? • Separate emotional (affective) issues from the cognitive domain for decision making? • Seek new ways to improve/add to knowledge? • Adapt quickly to change and new knowledge?	

Copyright © 2014. Wolters Kluwer Health | Lippincott Williams & Wilkins. Lab Manual for Health Assessment in Nursing, 5e.

Physical Assessment Guide to Collect Objective Client Data (continued)	
Questions	Findings
Does the **older adult**: • Maintain maximal independence with activities of daily living? • Problem-solve ways to find satisfaction with life? • Determine realistic plans for future, including own mortality?	
Assessment of Kohlberg's Moral Development	
Determine the client's moral level by asking the following suggested questions. Does the **young adult**: • State priorities to be considered when making a moral decision? • Perceive being approved by family? • Perceive being approved by peers? • Perceive being approved by supervisor/teachers/authority figures? • Perceive being approved by significant other? • Consider self to be a "good person"? Why or why not? • Able to judge the intentions of others?	
Does the **middle-aged adult**: • State priorities to be considered when making a moral decision? • Focus more on law and order or individual rights when making a decision? • Express willingness to stop unhealthy behavior and change lifestyle patterns to foster a higher level of wellness?	
Does the **older adult**: • State priorities to be considered when making a moral decision? • View rules and laws as changeable using legal means? • Make decisions consistently on internalized rules and in terms of conscience? • Believe in equality for every person?	

CHAPTER POSTTEST

Activity E MULTIPLE CHOICE QUESTIONS

Choose the one best answer(s) for each of the following multiple choice questions.

____   1. The nurse completes her interview of a 39-year-old female client who seems happily married with four healthy children who are doing very well in school and who works part time as a college professor. The nurse would be able to conclude that this client is in which of the following psychosocial developmental stages?

   a. Intimacy.

   b. Isolation.

   c. Generativity.

   d. Stagnation.

Copyright © 2014. Wolters Kluwer Health | Lippincott Williams & Wilkins. Lab Manual for Health Assessment in Nursing, 5e.

_____ **2.** Which of the following statements is true regarding developmental theories?

a. All developmental theories encompass all aspects of human development.

b. Developmental theory often reflects the culture/life experiences of the theorist.

c. Theories can explain all human developmental behaviors.

d. Developmental theories explain exact expected behaviors of human beings.

e. Theories provide developmental facts applicable to all cultures.

_____ **3.** Which of the following statements best describes Sigmund Freud's view of human behavior?

a. The individual person is constantly evolving throughout his lifespan.

b. A person is generally not aware of the underlying reasons for his behavior.

c. A person's conscious level is the largest and most influential level of awareness.

d. The ego serves as the moral component of an individual's personality.

_____ **4.** Sigmund Freud postulated that

a. homosexuality developed only during the _anal_ stage.

b. homosexuality developed from a female's successfully completing the _Electra_ complex.

c. puberty allows sexual impulses to reappear.

d. the _id_ controls the adolescent years.

_____ **5.** The client frequently chews his nails to the point that his fingers are bleeding. When questioned about this, he has attacked people who question him about his nail biting and bit them. Freud would interpret this as which of the following?

a. The patient needs to be fed before any questioning takes place.

b. The patient needs to be assessed for being current with all immunizations.

c. The _id_ is controlling this patient's behavior.

d. The patient has latent sexual phallic impulses.

_____ **6.** Each of Erik Erikson's central developmental tasks is composed of opposing viewpoints. Erikson thus theorized that

a. the accomplishment of each developmental task must be completed by a defined biologic age.

b. positive resolution of a developmental task in one stage is not always necessary for positive resolution of a developmental task in a subsequent stage.

c. the person must accomplish a healthy balance between these opposing viewpoints in order to progress to the next psychosocial stage.

d. if a task is only partially resolved, then the person can still successfully accomplish subsequent stages.

_____ **7.** A 50-year-old patient tells the nurse that she enjoys babysitting her grandchildren while their parents are attending night classes at the local college. She also shares that on many days she volunteers at a neighborhood food bank. Erikson would most likely place this patient as

a. feeling ashamed that she never helped her children complete school.

b. feeling lonely and isolated from family and the community.

c. negatively resolving poor relationships with her uneducated children.

d. positively resolving a sense of generativity versus stagnation.

_____ **8.** A 90-year-old patient is crying and states to the nurse, "I've had such a wasted life." The most appropriate response from the nurse will be

a. "I'm sure you have not had a wasted life."

b. "According to Erikson, you are experiencing despair."

c. "You need to focus on something happy right now."

d. "You are feeling like you have had a wasted life...?"

____ **9.** Which of the following statements correctly discuss Jean Piaget's theory of cognitive development? Select all that apply.
   a. Cognitive development occurs as the result of the person's organization and adaptation to the perceived environment.
   b. Wisdom is an adaptive process whereby information is incorporated into an already existing *schema*.
   c. Equilibration occurs when assimilation equals accommodation.
   d. The quality of the person's learning ceases when he attains formal operational thought.
   e. Piaget did not believe absolute ages should be ascribed to each of his stages of cognitive development.

____ **10.** The person who is able to correctly calculate algebraic equations has most likely attained which Piagetian stage of cognitive development?
   a. Invention of new means through mental combinations.
   b. Concrete operational.
   c. Formal operational.
   d. Coordination of tertiary circular reactions.

____ **11.** Which of the following statements is true regarding Piaget's concept of transductive thinking?
   a. This type of thinking is only characteristic of 3 year olds.
   b. This type of thinking is only used by preschoolers.
   c. Transductive thinking can be used by formal operational thinkers.
   d. Transductive thinking is not used by adults.

____ **12.** Lawrence Kohlberg based his theory of moral development on the premise that
   a. moral development is parallel to cognitive development.
   b. moral development is innate; thus, an infant comes into the world with a conscience.
   c. moral development is determined, in part, by decisions that challenge the person.
   d. moral development does not extend beyond adolescence.

____ **13.** The person who has attained Kohlberg's *Conventional* level of moral development is best described as)
   a. making decisions and behaving based on internalized rules and one's own conscience.
   b. desiring to avoid disapproval from others and be considered a respectful, helpful person.
   c. regarding rules and laws as changeable if the correct lines of communication are followed.
   d. slowly becoming aware that people can have different opinions in a moral dilemma.

Activity F CRITICAL THINKING ACTIVITY

Review Table 7-2: ERIK ERIKSON'S STAGES OF PSYCHOSOCIAL DEVELOPMENT on page 101 in your textbook. At which stage of development do you feel you fit into at this current time? Explain your answer.

Activity G   CASE STUDY

Read the following case study. Then, work through the steps of analyzing the case study data. First identify abnormal data and strengths in **subjective and objective findings**, assemble **cue clusters**, draw **inferences**, make possible **nursing diagnoses**, identify **defining characteristics**, **confirm or rule out** the diagnoses, and **document** your conclusions. Use the blank diagnostic analysis charts provided at the end of this book (also available on thePoint website) to guide your thinking. Propose nursing diagnoses that are specific to the client in the case study. Identify collaborative problems, if any, for this client. Finally, identify data, if any, which point toward a medical problem requiring a referral.

D.S. is a 24-year-old female, who presented to Community College Health Services at 11:45 AM on 4/19/13. She is a nursing student in her second year of study in the associate degree program. She states "I keep getting more and more migraine headaches. They occur soon after I arrive for weekly clinical practicum at the hospital and continue for the next 2 days. I have one 12 hour clinical a week on Thursdays." She said she tries to get at least 5 hours of sleep a night, but often gets closer to 3 hours the night before going to the hospital for her learning experience. She described the pain as a "tight band" around the top of her head above her eyebrows and rates the pain as 9/10. "When I take one 400 mg ibuprofen tablet....that might bring it down to about 6/10 the rest of the time that it persists." She states that she continues to one ibuprofen tablet "almost every 4 hours around the clock until it finally goes away." She added, "Now I'm starting to get the same headache just before an exam and you know we have a test every Monday....So far, I've been able to maintain a 'B' in this pediatric nursing class. I'm so bummed...I'm used to getting 'A's." D.S. is a single mother who has never married. She has a 3-year-old daughter who attends a day-long preschool program. D.S. states that she has been living with her mother since the birth of her daughter. "Mom and I haven't always got along and still don't agree on many things...especially about how to discipline my daughter. That's another story! But I understand. I made many errors in judgment throughout my earlier years. I hung out with the wrong crowd. I used [methamphetamine]. Then I decided to turn my life around. It wasn't easy. I went through rehab. I went back and finished high school...Started making new friends. Then I became pregnant....I have had no contact with the father of my daughter since I told him that I was going to have a baby...it's best this way." D.S. adds, "I do my best to take my daughter over the weekends to the park, zoo, parades, and anything else I can afford." D.S. says that her mother works full-time as a bank teller and helps to take care of her granddaughter. D.S. receives financial assistance from a nursing scholarship for single parents.

How Well Did You Do?

After you have read the chapter and completed the exercises in this chapter, visit thePoint to access the Self-Reflection Activity. This activity will help you identify to what degree you have met each of the chapter objectives. You can then review the chapter for objectives you have met partially or not at all.

Other tools to help you, like the Diagnostic Reasoning Guides, Nursing Interview Guides, Physical Assessment Guides, and NCLEX-Style Chapter Review Questions, are also available on thePoint.

Copyright © 2014. Wolters Kluwer Health | Lippincott Williams & Wilkins. Lab Manual for Health Assessment in Nursing, 5e.

CHAPTER 8

Assessing General Status and Vital Signs

Chapter Overview

From the moment you meet the client you develop a general impression of the client's whole being. You will perform a general survey by assessing the client's overall physical development and body build, gender and sexual development, apparent age, skin condition and color, dress and hygiene, posture and gait, level of consciousness, behaviors, body movements, affect, facial expressions, speech, and vital signs.

Chapter Learning Objectives

1. Prepare the client for a survey of general health status.
2. Interview a client for an accurate general survey of their health status.
3. Perform an accurate general survey.
4. Assess accurate vital sign measurements.
5. Assess for the presence of pain as a "fifth vital sign."
6. Describe the findings frequently seen when assessing the older client's general status and vital signs.
7. Differentiate between normal and abnormal general survey and vital sign findings.
8. Analyze data from the interview and a client's general survey and vital signs to formulate valid nursing diagnoses, collaborative problems, and/or referrals.

CHAPTER PRETEST

Activity A   MULTIPLE CHOICE QUESTIONS

Choose the one best answer for each of the following multiple choice questions.

____ 1. A client has an oral temperature of 37.2 °C (99 °F). The nurse interviews the client. Which of the following pieces of interview data could be an influence on this high body temperature?

   a. The client has just run 4.82 km (3 miles) outside before coming to the interview.

   b. The client drinks eight glasses of water a day.

   c. The client has a history of hypothyroidism.

   d. The client reports having a toe infection treated with antibiotics 3 months ago.

____ **2.** An approximate reading of core body temperature can be taken at various anatomic sites. Which of the following would not be a correct place to take a core body temperature?

    a. Under the tongue.

    b. Forehead and temporal artery.

    c. Opening of ear.

    d. Rectum.

    e. Groin.

____ **3.** When assessing a client's pulse, the nurse should be alert to which of the following characteristics?

    a. Rate, rhythm, amplitude and contour, and elasticity.

    b. Rate rhythm, temperature, rigidity, color, and elasticity.

    c. Tenderness, moistness, contour, elasticity, pressure.

    d. Pain, temperature, amplitude and contour, and elasticity.

____ **4.** A client's blood pressure is affected by

    a. cardiac intake, elasticity of the arteries, blood flow, blood cells, and blood thickness.

    b. cardiac intake, elasticity of the veins, blood flow, blood cells, and blood thickness.

    c. cardiac output, distensibility of the veins, blood volume, blood velocity and viscosity.

    d. cardiac output, distensibility of the arteries, blood volume, blood velocity and viscosity.

____ **5.** Osteoporotic thinning and collapse of the vertebrae secondary to bone loss in an elderly client may result in

    a. lordosis

    b. scoliosis

    c. skeletaldosis

    d. kyphosis

Activity B MATCHING

Match the terms in the left column with the correct description in the right column.

Term

____ **1.** 35.5 °C to 37.7 °C (96 °F to 99.9 °F)

____ **2.** 60 to 100 beats/minute

____ **3.** 12 to 20 breaths/minute

____ **4.** Highest pressure exerted on artery walls

____ **5.** Lowest pressure exerted on artery walls

____ **6.** Pain

____ **7.** Skin color, hygiene, posture, gait, physical build, and development

____ **8.** Difference between systolic and diastolic pressure

____ **9.** Less than 120 mm Hg

____ **10.** Less than 80 mm Hg

____ **11.** Normally about 0.8 °C (1.4 °F) higher than the normal oral temperature

____ **12.** More accurate than oral temperature

____ **13.** 5 degrees C (1 degree F) lower than the Oral temperature

Description

a. Normal diastolic blood pressure range

b. Diastolic blood pressure

c. Normal oral temperature

d. Normal systolic blood pressure range

e. Normal respiratory rate

f. Normal pulse

g. Systolic blood pressure

h. Pulse pressure

i. Overall impression

j. Fifth vital sign

k. Tympanic temperature

l. Axillary temperature

m. Temporal artery temperature

Activity C LEARNER ACTIVITIES

After reading Chapter 8 in the textbook, participate in the following learning activities.

1. Go to a public place, such as a store or a shopping mall, find a place to sit and observe those who are passing by. Look for general survey characteristics including physical and sexual development, skin color, dress, hygiene, posture, gait, body build, comfort level, behavior, facial expression, and speech. Record your findings. Compare these findings to the normal and abnormal findings columns in your textbook.

2. Practice taking vital signs on peers, friends, and family members. Try to find a variety of people: obese, thin, elderly, or young. Practice recording your findings on flowcharts.

3. Using COLDSPA to document the most severe pain you have ever experienced. Then, assess your lab partner for his or her worst experience with pain and document his or her experience using COLDSPA. (More in-depth information on pain assessment is provided in Chapter 9.)

Activity D INTERVIEWING AND RECORDING ASSESSMENT FINDINGS

After reading Chapter 8, use the following Nursing Interview Guide to interview and record your subjective findings for a General Survey or overall impression of a lab partner, peer, or client. Your instructor may ask you to turn this in to be evaluated. Forms are also available on thePoint *website.*

Nursing Interview Guide to Collect Subjective Data From the Client	
Questions	**Findings**
Present History	
1. Height?	
2. Weight?	
3. Fever?	
4. Pain? (COLDSPA)	
5. Allergies?	
6. Present health concerns?	
Past History	
1. Weight gains or losses?	
2. Previous high fevers, cause, and treatment?	
3. History of abnormal pulse?	
4. History of abnormal respiratory rate or character?	
5. Usual blood pressure, who checked it last, and when?	
6. History of pain and treatment?	
Family History	
1. Hypertension?	
2. Metabolic/growth problems?	
Lifestyle and Health Practices	
1. Religious affiliation?	

Activity E **PERFORMING A GENERAL SURVEY AND VITAL SIGN ASSESSMENT**

*Use the following Physical Assessment Guide to perform a General Survey and Vital Sign Assessment of a lab partner, peer, or client. Column 1 will serve as a reminder as to what part of the exam you will do next. Column 2 will be used to record your findings. Your instructor may ask you to turn this in to be evaluated. Forms are also available on the*Point *website.*

Physical Assessment Guide to Collect Objective Client Data	
Questions	**Findings**
Overall Impression of the Client	
1. Observe physical development (appears to be chronologic age) and sexual development (appropriate for gender and age).	
2. Observe skin (generalized color, color variation, and condition).	
3. Observe dress (occasion and weather appropriate).	
4. Observe hygiene (cleanliness, odor, grooming).	
5. Observe posture (erect and comfortable) and gait (rhythmic and coordinated).	
6. Observe body build (muscle mass and fat distribution).	
7. Observe consciousness level (alertness, orientation, appropriateness).	
8. Observe comfort level.	
9. Observe behavior (body movements, affect, cooperativeness, purposefulness, and appropriateness).	
10. Observe facial expression (culture-appropriate eye contact and facial expression).	
11. Observe speech (pattern and style).	
Vital Signs	
1. Gather equipment (thermometer, sphygmomanometer, stethoscope, and watch).	
2. Measure temperature (oral, axillary, rectal, tympanic).	
3. Measure radial pulse (rate, rhythm, amplitude and contour, and elasticity).	
4. Monitor respirations (rate, rhythm, and depth).	
5. Measure blood pressure.	
Analysis of Data	
1. Formulate nursing diagnoses (wellness, risk, actual).	
2. Formulate collaborative problems.	
3. Make necessary referrals.	

Copyright © 2014. Wolters Kluwer Health | Lippincott Williams & Wilkins. Lab Manual for Health Assessment in Nursing, 5e.

CHAPTER POSTTEST

Activity F MULTIPLE CHOICE QUESTIONS

Choose the one best answer for each of the following multiple choice questions.

_____ 1. The nurse is assessing an elderly postsurgical client in the home. To begin the physical examination, the nurse should first assess the client's

    a. height and weight.

    b. ability to swallow.

    c. vital signs.

    d. gait.

_____ 2. While caring for an 80-year-old client in his home, the nurse determines that the client's oral temperature is 35.8 °C (96.5 °F). The nurse determines that the client is most likely exhibiting

    a. normal changes that occur with the aging process.

    b. hypothermia that occurs before an infectious process.

    c. a metabolic disorder resulting in circulatory changes.

    d. an immune disorder resulting in low platelet count.

_____ 3. The nurse is preparing to assess the respirations of an alert adult client. The nurse should

    a. explain to the client that he or she will be counting the client's respirations.

    b. observe for equal bilateral chest expansion of 2.54 to 5.08 cm (1 to 2 in).

    c. count for 15 seconds and multiply the number by 4 to obtain the rate.

    d. ask the client to lie in a supine position, which makes counting the respirations easier.

_____ 4. While assessing an older adult client's respirations, the nurse can anticipate that the respiratory pattern may exhibit a

    a. shorter inspiratory phase.

    b. longer inspiratory phase.

    c. shorter expiratory phase.

    d. longer expiratory phase.

_____ 5. The nurse is caring for a client who is having nothing by mouth (NPO) on the first postoperative day. The client's blood pressure was 120/80 mm Hg approximately 4 hours ago, but it is now 140/88 mm Hg. The nurse should ask the client which of the following questions?

    a. "Are you taking any medications for hypertension?"

    b. "Do you have enough blankets to stay warm?"

    c. "Are you having pain from your surgery?"

    d. "What is your typical blood pressure reading?"

_____ 6. A normal pulse pressure range for an adult client is typically

    a. 20 to 40 mm Hg.

    b. 30 to 50 mm Hg.

    c. 40 to 60 mm Hg.

    d. 60 to 80 mm Hg.

_____ 7. The nurse is preparing to assess an adult client in the clinic. The nurse observes that the client is wearing lightweight clothing that is worn and soiled, although the temperature is below freezing outside. The nurse anticipates that the client may be

    a. abusing drugs.

    b. a victim of abuse.

    c. lacking adequate finances.

    d. anxious.

____ **8.** An elderly client is seen by the nurse in the neighborhood clinic. The nurse observes that the client is dressed in several layers of clothing, although the temperature is warm outside. The nurse suspects that the client's cold intolerance is a result of

    a. decreased body metabolism.

    b. neurologic deficits.

    c. recent surgery.

    d. pancreatic disease.

____ **9.** The nurse assesses the client's vital signs as follows: respirations 20 breaths/minute, tympanic temperature 100.9°F, pulse 88 beats/minute, and blood pressure 104/64 mm Hg. The nurse should

    a. record the vital signs.

    b. instruct the patient to drink more fluids.

    c. refer the client to a primary care provider.

    d. administer Tylenol.

____ **10.** The nurse notes which of the following vital sign findings as an abnormal finding in an 88-year-old client?

    a. 55 mm Hg pulse pressure.

    b. Respiratory rate of 22 breaths/minute.

    c. Oral temperature of 37.7 °C (100 °F).

    d. Blood pressure of 140/90 mm Hg.

Activity G CASE STUDY

Read the following case study. Then, work through the steps of analyzing the case study data. First identify abnormal data and strengths in **subjective and objective findings**, assemble **cue clusters**, draw **inferences**, make possible **nursing diagnoses**, identify **defining characteristics, confirm or rule out** the diagnoses, and **document** your conclusions. Use the blank diagnostic analysis charts provided at the end of this book (also available on thePoint website) to guide your thinking. Propose nursing diagnoses that are specific to the client in the case study. Identify collaborative problems, if any, for this client. Finally, identify data, if any, which point toward a medical problem requiring a referral.

Steve Marin is a 36-year-old white man, who comes to the employee health center for advice. He says he has been under a lot of stress lately. He believes he is drinking too much coffee (12 cups daily) and smoking more than usual (2 packs daily). He is neatly and appropriately dressed in a business suit. His posture is erect, and his gait is smooth. His hands are trembling. He has excess subcutaneous fat, distributed primarily around the waist. Mr. Marin appears tired, anxious, and hurried. He is cooperative, maintains good eye contact, and answers questions quickly. His speech is clear but fast paced.

Vital Signs
Oral temperature: 37.04 °C (98.68 °F)
Radial pulse: 92 beats/minute, strong but irregular
Respirations: 23 breaths/minute, shallow, and somewhat labored
Blood pressure: sitting, right arm 180/112 mm Hg, left arm 172/108 mm Hg; standing, 155/100 mm Hg (standing BP taken in either arm due to similarity of sitting BPs). Denies any pain or discomfort.

How Well Did You Do?

After you have read the chapter and completed the exercises in this chapter, visit thePoint to access the Self-Reflection Activity. This activity will help you identify to what degree you have met each of the chapter objectives. You can then review the chapter for objectives you have met partially or not at all.

    Other tools to help you, like the Diagnostic Reasoning Guides, Nursing Interview Guides, Physical Assessment Guides, and NCLEX-Style Chapter Review Questions, are also available on thePoint.

Copyright © 2014. Wolters Kluwer Health | Lippincott Williams & Wilkins. Lab Manual for Health Assessment in Nursing, 5e.

CHAPTER 9

Assessing Pain: The 5th Vital Sign

Chapter Overview

Pain is the fifth vital sign. It is a subjective phenomenon, and the main assessment tool is the client's reporting and describing the pain itself and how the client experiences the pain. The exact words used to describe the experience of pain are used to help in the diagnosis and management of the pain.

Chapter Learning Objectives

1. Identify pain as the fifth vital sign.
2. Explain the pathophysiology of pain.
3. Classify pain into acute and chronic pain.
4. Name the different physiologic responses to pain.
5. Interview a client experiencing pain, collecting subjective and objective data.
6. Perform a physical assessment on a client who is experiencing pain.
7. Analyze data from the client interview and physical assessment of a client experiencing pain to formulate valid nursing diagnoses, collaborative problems, and/or referrals.

CHAPTER PRETEST

Activity A MULTIPLE CHOICE QUESTIONS

Choose the one best answer for each of the following multiple choice questions.

_____ 1. When assessing the client for pain, the nurse should
   a. doubt the client when he or she describes the pain.
   b. assess for underlying causes of pain, then believe the client.
   c. believe the client when he or she claims to be in pain.
   d. assess for the presence of physiologic indicators (such as diaphoresis, tachycardia, etc.), then believe the client.

_____ **2.** Acute pain can be differentiated from chronic pain because

    a. acute pain always scores more on the visual analog scale than chronic pain.

    b. acute pain is associated with a recent onset of illness or injury with a duration of less than 6 months, whereas chronic pain persists longer than 6 months.

    c. acute pain is not treated and left to subside on its own, whereas chronic pain is referred for treatment.

    d. acute pain occurs only in persons aged less than 45 years, whereas chronic pain occurs in persons aged 46 or above.

_____ **3.** One of the body's normal physiologic responses to pain is

    a. hypotension.

    b. pulse rate below 50 beats/minute.

    c. diaphoresis.

    d. hypoglycemia.

_____ **4.** After assessing a client in pain, the nurse

    a. documents the exact description given by the client.

    b. chooses from the list of pain descriptors what best reflects the client's description.

    c. asks the family to describe how they view the client's pain.

    d. documents how he or she best sees the client's pain.

Activity B LABELING ACTIVITIES

Label the areas indicated on the diagram for referred pain. Insert the names of organs which may refer pain to the indicated area.

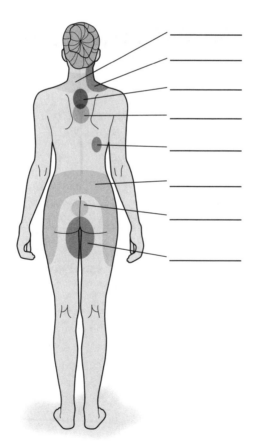

Activity C **LEARNER ACTIVITIES**

After reading Chapter 9 in the textbook, participate in the following learning activities.

1. Clients who describe pain as their main problem are seen on an inpatient or an outpatient basis. Choose a client being seen inpatient who describes pain as his or her main problem. Conduct an interview (collecting subjective and objective data) followed by a focused physical assessment. Document your findings.

2. If possible, also choose a client in an outpatient situation who is experiencing pain and who is referred to a pain clinic for pain management or follow-up. Conduct an interview (collecting subjective and objective data) and a focused physical assessment, and then record your findings. Then discuss the differences you encountered between interviewing an inpatient and an outpatient client.

3. Recall a pain experience you had in the past or are currently experiencing. Have your lab partner be the nurse to assess your current or past pain. Repeat this exercise with you being the nurse and your lab partner being the client.

Activity D **INTERVIEWING AND RECORDING ASSESSMENT FINDINGS**

After reading Chapter 9, use the following Nursing Interview Guide to interview and record your subjective findings for an assessment of pain of a lab partner, peer, or client. Your instructor may ask you to turn this in to be evaluated. Forms are also available on thePoint *website.*

Interview Guide to Collect Subjective Data From the Client	
Questions	**Findings**
Current Symptoms	
1. Are you experiencing pain now or have you had pain in the past 24 hours?	
2. Where is the pain located?	
3. Does it radiate or spread?	
4. Are there any other concurrent symptoms accompanying the pain?	
5. When did the pain start?	
6. What were you doing when the pain first started?	
7. Is the pain continuous or intermittent?	
8. (*Ask for intermittent pain.*) How often do the episodes occur and how long do they last?	
9. Describe in your own words the quality of pain.	
10. What factors relieve your pain?	
11. What factors increase your pain?	
12. Are you on any therapy to manage your pain?	
Past History	
1. Have you had any previous experience with pain?	
Family History	
1. Does anyone in your family experience pain?	
2. How does pain affect your family?	

Copyright © 2014. Wolters Kluwer Health | Lippincott Williams & Wilkins. Lab Manual for Health Assessment in Nursing, 5e.

Interview Guide to Collect Subjective Data From the Client (continued)

Questions	Findings
Lifestyles and Health Practices	
1. What are your concerns about pain?	

2. What are your concerns about the pain's effect on
 	
   a. general activity?
 	
   b. mood/emotions?
 	
   c. concentration?
 	
   d. physical ability?
 	
   e. work?
 	
   f. relations with other people?
 	
   g. sleep?
 	
   h. appetite?
 	
   i. enjoyment of life?	

Activity E PERFORMING PHYSICAL ASSESSMENT OF PAIN

Use the following Physical Assessment Guide to perform a pain assessment on a lab partner, peer, or client. Column 1 will serve as a reminder as to what part of the exam you will do next. Column 2 will be used to record your findings. Your instructor may ask you to turn this in to be evaluated. Forms are also available on thePoint *website.*

Physical Assessment Guide to Collect Objective Client Data

Questions	Findings
General Observations	
1. Observe posture.	
2. Observe facial expression.	
3. Inspect joints and muscles.	
4. Observe skin for scars, lesions, rashes, changes, or discoloration.	
Vital Signs	
1. Measure heart rate.	
2. Measure respiratory rate.	
3. Measure blood pressure.	
Using the client's description of pain and your findings above, continue the assessment. Refer to the physical assessment chapter appropriate for the affected body area.	

Copyright © 2014. Wolters Kluwer Health | Lippincott Williams & Wilkins. Lab Manual for Health Assessment in Nursing, 5e.

CHAPTER POSTTEST

Activity F MULTIPLE CHOICE QUESTIONS

Choose the one best answer for each of the following multiple choice questions.

____ **1.** Which of the following cultural expressions of pain would be likely to be found in a person of Hispanic culture?

    a. Pain is honorable and should be endured.

    b. Pain is part of the preparation for the next life in the cycle of reincarnation.

    c. Pain must be endured to perform gender role duties, but response to it is very expressive.

    d. Pain may be caused by past transgressions and helps to atone and achieve higher spirituality.

____ **2.** Beliefs of health care providers can serve as barriers to an accurate assessment of a client's pain. Which of the following beliefs will **not** be likely to impair the assessment of pain?

    a. Old people have more pain which is to be expected.

    b. Infants can feel pain and may respond with crying or agitation.

    c. A sleeping person feels no pain.

    d. Persons asking for pain medication but who are showing no other evidence of pain are just addicted to the medication.

____ **3.** A popular pain assessment scale for children is:

    a. Visual Analog Scale.

    b. Descriptive Pain Intensity Scale.

    c. FLACC Pain Assessment Scale.

    d. Memorial Pain Assessment Card.

____ **4.** The U.S. government has created guidelines for health care providers caring for clients in pain. Which of the following reflect these guidelines?

    a. Joint Commission Standards for Pain Management.

    b. National Institutes of Health Standards for Pain Treatment.

    c. American Cancer Society Guidelines for Pain Management.

    d. American Pain Society Guidelines for Pain Management.

____ **5.** Pain that is felt in a part of the body that has been removed is called:

    a. Phantom pain.

    b. Referred pain.

    c. Neuropathic pain.

    d. Radiating pain.

____ **6.** Which of the dimensions of pain listed is being assessed by the question "How does the pain treatment you are getting affect your overall mood?"

    a. Physical.

    b. Behavioral.

    c. Cognitive.

    d. Affective.

Copyright © 2014. Wolters Kluwer Health | Lippincott Williams & Wilkins. Lab Manual for Health Assessment in Nursing, 5e.

Activity G CRITICAL THINKING ACTIVITY

A 65-year-old man arrives for a routine yearly health assessment. He describes episodes of "indigestion" that make him "feel really sick and nauseated." He says these episodes started about 2 weeks ago but he doesn't believe they are serious and he just takes an antacid, getting a little relief.

Describe what areas you will focus on for the subjective data collection and what physical assessment you would do for this description of pain. Are there any risk factors you would assess for different possible medical conditions that may cause "indigestion"?

Activity H CASE STUDY

Read the following case study. Then work through the steps of analyzing the case study data. First, identify the abnormal data and strengths in **subjective and objective findings**, assemble **cue clusters**, draw **inferences**, make possible **nursing diagnoses**, identify **defining characteristics**, **confirm or rule out** the diagnoses, and **document** your conclusions. Use the blank diagnostic analysis charts provided at the end of this book (also available on thePoint website) to guide your thinking. Propose nursing diagnoses that are specific to the client in the case study. Identify collaborative problems, if any, for this client. Finally, identify data, if any, that point toward a medical problem requiring a referral.

F.S. is a 38-year-old architect. He is still single and is enjoying his bachelor life. He is a nonsmoker but drinks alcohol—"occasionally two to three drinks." Later he says he has drunk this amount almost daily for the past 10 years. Since his appendectomy around 13 years ago, he has not had any medical examination. "The past few months have been stressful at work and my eating habits have been irregular. Sometimes I have occasional nausea and vomiting." This has advanced from being a mild epigastric upset to constant midepigastric pain radiating to the back. This pain at first was relieved by pain medications, but "now it is not relieved by anything, although I realized that sitting forward helps me to relax a little bit while waiting in the doctor's clinic for my turn." The clinic desk clerk described that Mr. F.S. entered the doctor's clinic walking bent forward with his hands holding his epigastric area. During the examination, he reported severe pain (9/10) with abdominal guarding and with purplish discoloration of the periumbilical area. His respirations were shallow with a rate of 26 beats/minute. Heart rate was 110 beats/minute with a BP 120/80 mm Hg. (He was diagnosed with acute pancreatitis.)

How Well Did You Do?

After you have read the chapter and completed the exercises in this chapter, visit thePoint to access the Self-Reflection Activity. This activity will help you identify to what degree you have met each of the chapter objectives. You can then review the chapter for objectives you have met partially or not at all.

Other tools to help you, like the Diagnostic Reasoning Guides, Nursing Interview Guides, Physical Assessment Guides, and NCLEX-Style Chapter Review Questions, are also available on thePoint.

Copyright © 2014. Wolters Kluwer Health | Lippincott Williams & Wilkins. Lab Manual for Health Assessment in Nursing, 5e.

10

Assessing for Violence

Chapter Overview

Family violence is widespread. It affects families from all socioeconomic groups and ethnicities. Violence may occur across the life span and includes physical abuse, psychological abuse, economic abuse, and/or sexual abuse. Chapter 10 in the textbook and this lab manual chapter help to determine the nature of violence and how to assess victims of violence.

Chapter Learning Objectives

1. Describe how to prepare a physically and emotionally safe environment for a client who has experienced domestic violence.
2. Correctly use domestic violence screening tools provided in the textbook to identify victims of violence across the life span.
3. Describe how to teach clients at risk for violence and how to develop a safety plan.
4. Discuss the significance of accurate and objective documentation of physical findings in clients who have experienced abuse.
5. Accurately document abusive physical findings using injury maps.
6. Analyze data from the client interview and physical assessment of a client at risk for violence and of a client suspected to have suffered abuse to formulate valid nursing diagnoses, collaborative problems, and/or referrals.

CHAPTER PRETEST

Activity A MULTIPLE CHOICE QUESTIONS

Choose the one best answer for each of the following multiple choice questions.

_____ 1. When interviewing a pediatric client and attempting to determine the presence of abuse, the nurse should

   a. confine the interview to yes/no questions to keep the interview simple.

   b. remain calm and accepting in response to any information the client discloses.

   c. ask leading questions to convince the child to offer information.

   d. offer a reward to the child for answering difficult questions.

____ **2.** The nurse is interviewing Mr. Jenkins and, due particularly to his nervous affect and his reaction when his son is mentioned, suspects potential elder abuse. In assessing Mr. Jenkins, the nurse should
  a. focus exclusively on the physical examination, as elder abuse is primarily physical in nature.
  b. make sure that the assessment includes questions to ensure that Mr. Jenkins has access to food and needed medication.
  c. ask to speak to Mr. Jenkins' son directly, to ask him candidly about the potential abuse.
  d. keep in mind that elder abuse is usually reported, indicating that Mr. Jenkins is not likely a victim.

____ **3.** Which of the following is a stage in Walker's cycle of violence?
  a. Reporting the problem.
  b. Hiding the abuse.
  c. Period of reconciliation.
  d. Ending the relationship.

____ **4.** Which of the following is true about violence against women?
  a. Verbal attacks by a husband are not considered violence against a wife.
  b. Wife abuse is an accepted behavior in some societies.
  c. Between married couples, there is no behavior that meets the criteria for rape.
  d. Violence against women is a recent development in the United States.

____ **5.** Johnny is a 5-year-old boy who comes to the clinic for his scheduled injections. Which physical indications would lead you to suspect child abuse?
  a. Bruising on the upper portion of his buttocks.
  b. Regular pattern of circular, coin-sized reddened areas on his back.
  c. Irregular pattern of small, circular reddened areas with healing blisters on various parts of his body.
  d. Crying when he sees the needle for the injection.

____ **6.** Elder abuse can include
  a. nursing home admission.
  b. economic exploitation.
  c. using an elder day-care sitter.
  d. uncontested divorce.

Activity B LEARNER ACTIVITIES

After reading Chapter 10 in the textbook, participate in the following learning activity.

Self-Assessment for Violence: Consider that, statistically, one out of every six persons in your classroom may be a victim of violence. This is a very sensitive topic for anyone to address. Frequently, individuals, including health care professionals, may not recognize that they are victims of abuse. Yet it is essential that health care professionals be aware of their own past experience with violence in order to effectively assess the presence of violence in their clients. Use the screening tool provided in Assessment Tool 10-1 on p. 167 in your textbook to assess for the presence of violence in your own life. If you find that you are a victim of violence, you will want to share this with your nursing instructor or another health care professional.

Copyright © 2014. Wolters Kluwer Health | Lippincott Williams & Wilkins. Lab Manual for Health Assessment in Nursing, 5e.

Activity C INTERVIEWING AND RECORDING ASSESSMENT FINDINGS

After reviewing Chapter 10, use the following guide to interview and record your subjective findings for an assessment of family violence. Refer to Assessment Tool 10-1 in your textbook if any client response is "yes."

Nursing Interview Guide to Collect Subjective Data From the Client	
Questions	**Findings**
Intimate Partner Abuse Screening for Women	
1. Physically hurt by anyone in the past year? By whom?	
2. Fears of others at home or elsewhere? Be sure to acknowledge abuse if present, be supportive, and help the client develop a safety plan.	
Elder Abuse Screening for Geriatric Clients	
1. Activities in a typical day?	
2. Hurt by anyone in the past? Threats from anyone in the past?	
3. Afraid of anyone at home?	
4. Client ever made to do anything he or she did not want to do?	
5. Ever touched without permission?	
6. Belongings taken without permission?	
7. Made to sign papers without understanding them?	
8. Often alone?	
9. Has help ever been refused when needed?	
10. Has anyone ever refused to give or let the client take medications as needed?	
Child Abuse Screening for Children and Adolescents	
Determine developmental level by asking the following:	
1. What is your name? Please spell it.	
2. When is your birthday?	
3. How many eyes do you have? Using the child's or adolescent's answers, formulate developmentally appropriate questions to determine if the child or adolescent was ever abused physically, emotionally, or sexually.	

Copyright © 2014. Wolters Kluwer Health | Lippincott Williams & Wilkins. Lab Manual for Health Assessment in Nursing, 5e.

Activity D **PERFORMING PHYSICAL ASSESSMENT FOR FAMILY VIOLENCE**

Use the following guide to perform an assessment for family violence. Column 1 will serve as a reminder as to what part of the exam you will do next. Column 2 will be used to record your findings. Your instructor may ask you to turn this in to be evaluated. Forms are also available on thePoint *website.*

Assessment Guide to Collect Objective Client Data

Questions	Findings
1. General survey.	
2. Assess mental status.	
3. Evaluate vital signs.	
4. Inspect skin.	
5. Inspect head and neck.	
6. Inspect eyes.	
7. Assess ears.	
8. Assess abdomen.	
9. Assess genitalia and rectal area.	
10. Assess musculoskeletal system.	
11. Assess neurologic system.	

CHAPTER POSTTEST

Activity E **MULTIPLE CHOICE QUESTIONS**

Choose the one best answer for each of the following multiple choice questions.

_____ 1. Before beginning a client interview to assess for the presence of violence, necessary preparations include all except which of the following?

   a. Assure confidentiality of all information revealed.

   b. Choose an environment where the conversation will not be overheard by others.

   c. Discuss legal mandatory reporting requirements.

   d. Provide an appropriate interpreter if the client does not speak English.

_____ 2. A Hispanic mother brings her 2-year-old child to the clinic for a well-child checkup and age-appropriate vaccinations. Which of the following observations indicate potential abuse at home?

   a. Bruising across the lower back and upper buttocks bilaterally.

   b. Symmetrical nickel-sized circular bruising across upper back.

   c. Hand or finger-patterned bruising around upper arm and leg.

   d. Scraped and bruised knee.

_____ 3. Which of the following is **not** a true statement about intimate partner violence?

   a. One in every three women worldwide is a victim of intimate partner violence at some point in her life.

   b. Intimate partner violence is based on the abuser's need to maintain power and control over the victim.

   c. The annual cost in the United States for intimate partner violence exceeds $4 billion for medical and health services, and over $1 billion for lost productivity.

   d. Intimate partner violence is caused by the "victim" refusing her husband's desire for sex.

Copyright © 2014. Wolters Kluwer Health | Lippincott Williams & Wilkins. Lab Manual for Health Assessment in Nursing, 5e.

_____ **4.** Which of the following is true of psychological abuse?

   a. Psychological abuse is easy to define and diagnose.

   b. An abuser may use psychological behaviors such as belittling, exploiting, denigrating, or remaining emotionally unresponsive.

   c. The majority of children experiencing psychological abuse do not use effective coping mechanisms.

   d. Psychological abuse of children does not affect long-term development.

_____ **5.** Which of the following is suggested for family abuse screening?

   a. Universal screening for family and intimate partner violence is recommended.

   b. If there are no obvious signs of abuse, there is no need to screen clients.

   c. Only childbearing-aged and pregnant women should be routinely screened for sexual abuse.

   d. Assess for physical abuse only at the beginning of a couple's new relationship.

Activity F CRITICAL THINKING ACTIVITIES

1. Describe various interview techniques you might attempt to use when you highly suspect that your client is a victim of abuse but he or she is not willing to disclose this information to you.

2. Explain differences in screening for violence in adults, children, and the elderly.

3. Mrs. Smith is a 33-year-old white woman you see in the emergency department with the presenting history of "fell on sidewalk and injured her arm." X-rays revealed a spiral fracture that was inconsistent with her history of falling. Her 10-year-old son who accompanied her has a visible rope burn on his neck. When you question him about your observation, he states, "I hurt my neck when I was playing." When asked if she and her son are alone, she tells you that her husband is waiting in the car. When you ask Mrs. Smith for more details about how these injuries occurred, she begins to cry and says, "There is nothing I can do about this."

With your lab partner, create a safety plan (see Assessment Tool 10-2 on p. 171 in textbook) for Mrs. Smith and her child.

Activity G CASE STUDY

Read the following case study. Then, work through the steps of analyzing the case study data. First, identify abnormal data and strengths in **subjective and objective findings**, assemble **cue clusters**, draw **inferences**, make possible **nursing diagnoses**, identify **defining characteristics**, **confirm or rule out** the diagnoses, and **document** your conclusions. Use the blank diagnostic analysis charts provided at the end of this book (also available on thePoint website) to guide your thinking. Propose nursing diagnoses that are specific to the client in the case study. Identify collaborative problems, if any, for this client. Finally, identify data, if any, that point toward a medical problem requiring a referral.

Tommy Johnson is an 18-month-old boy. His mother brings him to the doctor because he is "being difficult" and refuses to be toilet trained. Mrs. Johnson states, "He is deliberately not going when I put him on the toilet and then soiling his diapers. He is doing it just to be a pest." She tells you that Tommy also refuses to eat and will not drink anything but fruit punch and lemonade from his bottle. While she is explaining this, Tommy just stares at the wall. When asked about their daily activities, she says that he wakes at about 7:00 AM, but usually cries himself back to sleep. When she gets him out of bed, she gives him a bottle and sets him in front of the TV, while she does other things around the house. She tries to feed him lunch but he usually eats very little. The rest of the afternoon is spent napping or watching TV.

   Mrs. Johnson tells you that she did not expect having a child would be this hard. Mr. Johnson no longer lives with his wife and child. He is behind in his child support payments, and Mrs. Johnson tells you that she is struggling to pay the bills.

   You examine Tommy and find that he is frail and thin-looking. It is chilly outside and he is wearing only a thin tee shirt and diaper. Tommy's hair is matted and uncombed. He is in the second percentile for both height and weight. He has multiple bruises on his arms, back, and legs. The bruises are in various stages of healing. Tommy is not meeting the developmental milestones for his age. He also does not interact with you at all while you are examining him.

Copyright © 2014. Wolters Kluwer Health | Lippincott Williams & Wilkins. Lab Manual for Health Assessment in Nursing, 5e.

How Well Did You Do?

After you have read the chapter and completed the exercises in this chapter, visit thePoint to access the Self-Reflection Activity. This activity will help you identify to what degree you have met each of the chapter objectives. You can then review the chapter for objectives you have met partially or not at all.

Other tools to help you, like the Diagnostic Reasoning Guides, Nursing Interview Guides, Physical Assessment Guides, and NCLEX-Style Chapter Review Questions, are also available on thePoint.

Copyright © 2014. Wolters Kluwer Health | Lippincott Williams & Wilkins. Lab Manual for Health Assessment in Nursing, 5e.

11

Assessing Culture

Chapter Overview

The population of the United States has changed a great deal since World War II. The number of immigrants and the number of the countries from which they have come have increased dramatically. The predominant cultures that make up the US population are whites of European descent comprising many varied cultures; African Americans; and Hispanics, from various Latin American countries. However, the Asian American population is rapidly increasing, and there is a substantial group of Native Americans of different tribal affiliations. It is not unusual for both clients and caregivers to be from different cultural groups. Because cultural beliefs and behaviors affect health and health behaviors, it is essential that nurses understand how to interact with people from many different cultures.

Chapter Learning Objectives

1. Explain how culture, genetics, and environment interact to affect health status.
2. Define culture and describe its basic characteristics.
3. Discuss the role of cultural competence of the caregiver in nursing assessment.
4. Describe how the assessment interview needs to be modified to consider cultural variations.
5. Recognize culture-based syndromes and the cultural groups most likely to accept them as diseases.
6. Recognize your own tendency to stereotype.
7. Recognize your own level of ethnocentrism.
8. Recognize your own level of cultural competence.
9. Describe the parts of a cultural assessment.
10. Complete a cultural health assessment on a person of a different culture.
11. Analyze data from the client interview and physical assessment of cultural effects on illness to formulate valid nursing diagnoses, collaborative problems, and/or referrals.

CHAPTER PRETEST

Activity A MATCHING

Match the terms in the left column with the correct descriptions in the right column.

Term

_____ **1.** Culture

_____ **2.** Ethnocentrism

_____ **3.** Ethnicity

_____ **4.** Race

_____ **5.** Minority

Description

a. A socially constructed concept that has meaning for a larger group

b. A shared set of values, beliefs, and learned pattern of behavior

c. The belief that one's beliefs, values, and sanctioned behaviors are superior to others

d. A group with less power or prestige within a society

e. Exists when a socially, politically, or culturally constructed group holds a common set of characteristics not shared by others

Activity B   MULTIPLE CHOICE QUESTIONS

Choose the one best answer for each of the following multiple choice questions.

_____ **1.** Stereotyping is defined as

   a. the belief that one's cultural values are superior to all others.

   b. a worldview that each of us forms values and beliefs based on our own culture.

   c. a culture-bound syndrome found in many cultural groups.

   d. expecting all members of a cultural group to hold the same beliefs and behave in the same way.

_____ **2.** Suzie is a 16-year-old daughter in the Hanes family. She is the youngest of five children. She has had a series of illnesses and does not seem to be regaining her strength. She likes school but is falling behind a bit. Her mother is very attentive to her needs but does not seem overly concerned with the continuing pattern of illness. Which of the following is most likely a Hanes family belief?

   a. Fathers are not involved with their children.

   b. Education is highly valued for sons and daughters.

   c. The family values taking sick roles and caregiver roles.

   d. Self-care is highly valued in the Hanes family.

_____ **3.** Which of the following statements is true about biologic variation?

   a. Both genetics and environment produce biologic variation.

   b. Cultural practices produce biologic variation.

   c. Race is based on physical variations.

   d. Drug metabolism differences are not culture based.

_____ **4.** A culture-bound syndrome seen in the African American community is

   a. empacho.

   b. falling out.

   c. susto.

   d. sickle cell disease.

_____ **5.** Skin color is

   a. darker in persons with tightly curled hair.

   b. a genetic variation associated with distance from the equator.

   c. a valid predictor of intelligence.

   d. a valid characteristic that differentiates racial groups.

Activity C   CHOOSING

Select "Do" or "Don't" by checking the appropriate column for each behavior.

Do	Don't	
		a. Be aware that some nonverbal communication may be insulting to some cultural groups (e.g., direct eye contact).
		b. Assume that a person who looks and behaves much as you do has no cultural differences.
		c. Assume that a negative or hostile communication from a client is directed at you personally as an insult.
		d. Seek feedback and constructive criticism on the transcultural interactions you have with clients.
		e. Recognize and value differences.
		f. Recognize there is variation within all cultural and ethnic groups, often more variation within than between groups.
		g. Seek many opportunities to interact with persons of different cultures, even if it makes you uncomfortable at first.

Copyright © 2014. Wolters Kluwer Health | Lippincott Williams & Wilkins. Lab Manual for Health Assessment in Nursing, 5e.

Activity D LEARNER ACTIVITIES

After reading Chapter 11 in the textbook, participate in the following learning activities.

1. Discuss the purpose and benefits of a cultural assessment. When would you perform the assessment? Explain.

2. Describe the elements of cultural competence. Evaluate yourself and the level of cultural competence you have now. Compare with your lab partner. Working together, make a plan to increase your cultural competence.

3. With your lab partner, make a list of ways in which culture can affect health.

4. Get together with a small group of friends or lab partners to compare beliefs and behaviors related to health and illness. Make a list to see whether there is variation within the groups. Ask each group member the following.

    a. What do you do to stay healthy?

    b. What do you do to feel better when you have a cold?

    c. When do you seek help from a health care professional?

    d. What home remedies do you use? Vitamins/minerals? Herbs? Yoga? Tai chi? Special foods or diets? Alternative or complementary therapies? What home remedies do your family members use?

    e. Do you like to be left alone or have many visitors when you are ill?

    f. What do you believe causes illness?

5. Discuss how family beliefs, habits, roles, and interactions could affect your (or another family member's) health status.

6. Define "culture-bound syndromes." Which clients might experience them?

7. Discuss with your lab partner the aspects of interviewing that have to be considered when assessing a client from a culture different from your own. Choose three of the ways cultural difference can affect interviews. Have each lab partner play a role as a client from a culture that affects the interview (e.g., silence) and role-play the interview. Choose different interview elements and change nurse–client roles for role-play.

8. In a clinical setting with clients from various cultures, observe a nursing assessment of a client from a culture different from your own. What variations in communication do you notice (of nurse or client)? What assessment areas would you wish to modify? Explain your answer. What areas of assessment would you like to add? Explain.

Activity E INTERVIEWING AND RECORDING ASSESSMENT FINDINGS

After reading Chapter 11, use the following Nursing Interview Guide to interview and record your subjective findings for a cultural assessment of a lab partner, peer, or client. Your instructor may ask you to turn this in to be evaluated. Forms are also available on thePoint *website.*

Nursing Interview Guide to Collect Subjective Data From the Client	
Questions	**Findings**
Current Symptoms (Ask Client)	
1. What has brought you to the clinic today?	
2. What do you believe has caused this illness?	
3. What have you done to treat it? Are there family remedies that you usually use for this illness? Have they worked for other family members or for you in the past?	
4. What do you believe that health care providers can do that will help you? (If appropriate, use COLDSPA for symptom analysis)	
5. Are you taking any medications? Do you have allergies or reactions to any medications or foods?	

Copyright © 2014. Wolters Kluwer Health | Lippincott Williams & Wilkins. Lab Manual for Health Assessment in Nursing, 5e.

Nursing Interview Guide to Collect Subjective Data From the Client (continued)

Questions	Findings
Affect and Behaviors (Observe)	
1. Does affect correspond to verbal expressions?	
2. Does pattern of eye contact correspond to the client's culture or to the majority culture?	
3. Does the client divulge information readily or with reluctance?	
4. Does the client seem to accept you (gender, age) as a caregiver?	
5. Does space appear to be an issue with the client?	
6. Are there any other communication patterns that seem to be relevant to this interview?	
Past History (Ask Client)	
1. What has been your experience with health care professionals in the past?	
2. Have you used community caregivers?	
3. Have you had any illnesses like this one before?	
4. Do you have or have you experienced any other illnesses in the past?	
5. What types of illnesses have gotten you to go to a doctor or nurse in the past?	
Family History	
1. How many family members live in the community? In the household?	
2. Are the family members healthy? Have illnesses? Able to provide support to you?	
Lifestyle and Health Practices	
1. Do you believe that exercise is important to health? How much exercise do you get each day? Week?	
2. Do you smoke? Drink alcohol? If yes, how much or how often?	
3. Do you participate in religious practices? Do your beliefs and practices provide strength and comfort? Are they essential to your well-being?	
4. Do you have beliefs that would conflict with treatments or procedures?	
5. What type of diet do you eat? Is it restricted in any way by religious or cultural beliefs? Are there foods that you believe help to make you healthy? Ill?	

(Refer to the textbook for each physiologic system and its potential biomedical variations as you assess the physiologic systems.)

Copyright © 2014. Wolters Kluwer Health | Lippincott Williams & Wilkins. Lab Manual for Health Assessment in Nursing, 5e.

CHAPTER POSTTEST

Activity F **MULTIPLE CHOICE QUESTIONS**

Choose the one best answer for each of the following multiple choice questions.

____ **1.** The nurse and a Hispanic client are developing a transcultural nursing care plan related to hypertension. The nurse will include in the plan
   a. educational materials given to all clients with hypertension.
   b. nutritional information specifically for a Hispanic client.
   c. contact number for the cardiac rehabilitation program at the medical center.
   d. referral to a cardiac specialist.

____ **2.** Risk factors for mental disorders
   a. may be specific to an ethnic group.
   b. are the same for all ethnic groups.
   c. do not affect treatment plans.
   d. are the same as risks for brain injury.

____ **3.** The most effective way for a nurse to learn about an ethnic group within the community in which he/she practices is
   a. study transcultural nursing texts and articles about the group.
   b. interview the traditional healers within the group.
   c. do a community survey of the areas where the ethnic group lives.
   d. spend time with a variety of individuals of that ethnic group.

____ **4.** A client of Chinese origin enters your office to be seen. You can assume
   a. the client will avoid direct eye contact because this conveys respect.
   b. the client will expect a larger interpersonal distance than you are used to.
   c. the client does not speak English.
   d. the client may be well acculturated to your dominant culture, so don't assume.

____ **5.** Which of the following statements is true of cultural groups and magicoreligious beliefs in their health belief systems?
   a. Western majority culture does not have magicoreligious beliefs.
   b. Hispanic culture has religious beliefs but not magicoreligious beliefs.
   c. Afro American culture has magic beliefs but not religious beliefs.
   d. No culture is without an element of magicoreligious beliefs.

____ **6.** Sickle cell disease and other hemoglobinopathies such as thalassemia are often found in persons originating from which geographical regions?
   a. South America.
   b. South Africa.
   c. Mediterranean.
   d. Australia.

____ **7.** Which of the following statement is true of sickle cell disease and other hemoglobinopathies?
   a. Are associated with adapting to high malaria environments.
   b. Are found only in persons of black African origin.
   c. Are associated with Ashkenazi Jewish genes.
   d. Are associated with the Far East.

Copyright © 2014. Wolters Kluwer Health | Lippincott Williams & Wilkins. Lab Manual for Health Assessment in Nursing, 5e.

____ **8.** Which of the following statements is true?

    a. Second generation US citizens from Mexico usually eat a diet primarily based on beans and tortillas.

    b. There is no need to adjust diets according to religious rituals for Italians.

    c. Fasting for Lent or Ramadan is not acceptable for health reasons.

    d. Pork and wine are forbidden in many ethnic groups for religious reasons.

How Well Did You Do?

After you have read the chapter and completed the exercises in this chapter, visit the Point to access the Self-Reflection Activity. This activity will help you identify to what degree you have met each of the chapter objectives. You can then review the chapter for objectives you have met partially or not at all.

    Other tools to help you, like the Diagnostic Reasoning Guides, Nursing Interview Guides, Physical Assessment Guides, and NCLEX-Style Chapter Review Questions, are also available on the Point.

Copyright © 2014. Wolters Kluwer Health | Lippincott Williams & Wilkins. Lab Manual for Health Assessment in Nursing, 5e.

CHAPTER 12

Assessing Spirituality and Religious Practices

Chapter Overview

A large number of Americans profess a belief in God, pray on a regular basis, and frequently use spiritual resources during times of high stress, but how clients use and view spirituality and religion varies immensely. It is important to consider spirituality within the context of client care, but in whatever form spirituality is incorporated into an assessment, the nurse must remain respectful and open. The following activities and questions are provided as a review and to stimulate thoughts regarding spiritual assessment of a client.

Chapter Learning Objectives

1. Describe the difference between spirituality and religion.
2. Explain how understanding spirituality can assist the nurse in identifying the client's coping responses and support systems.
3. Explain how spiritual beliefs can influence one's decision-making relative to health care.
4. Discuss why it is important that nurses be aware of their own spiritual beliefs and biases as they relate to health care.
5. Analyze data from the client interview and physical assessment of the client's spiritual status to formulate valid nursing diagnoses, collaborative problems, and/or referrals.

CHAPTER PRETEST

Activity A   MULTIPLE CHOICE QUESTIONS

Choose the one best answer for each of the following multiple choice questions.

_____ **1.** Shared practices and rituals used to express one's faith can be called
   a. religion.
   b. spirituality.
   c. denomination.
   d. philosophy.

_____ **2.** The path one pursues in the search for life's meaning and purpose.
   a. Religion.
   b. Spirituality.
   c. Denomination.
   d. Philosophy.

____   **3.** While providing spiritual care to clients, nurses must avoid
   a. assessing spiritual needs of clients.
   b. praying with clients as requested.
   c. attempting to convert clients to your own beliefs.
   d. helping clients determine spiritual aspects of responses to illness.

____   **4.** Illness can be affected by which of the following spiritual beliefs?
   a. Beliefs about cause of illness.
   b. Beliefs about meaning of suffering.
   c. Beliefs about dietary practices.
   d. All of the above.

Activity B   LEARNER ACTIVITIES

After reading Chapter 12 in the textbook, participate in the following learning activities.

1. Discuss the purpose and benefits of a spiritual assessment. When would you perform this assessment? Explain.

2. On your own, complete and score yourself on the following assessment tools found in the textbook.
   a. TAKING A SPIRITUAL HISTORY (Assessment Tool 12-1, p. 203).
   b. SELF ASSESSMENT: DAILY SPIRITUAL EXPERIENCES SCALE (Box 12-2, p. 203).
   c. SELF ASSESSMENT: BRIEF RELIGIOUS COPING QUESTIONNAIRE (RCOPE) (Box 12-3, p. 204).

3. With your lab partner, discuss your findings from activity no. 2. Did the tools accurately reflect your beliefs? Why or why not? Which tool did you find most useful in obtaining spiritual information? Were there questions you had difficulty answering? If yes, explain. Were there questions that made you uncomfortable? If yes, explain. Explain how you could make these questions more comfortable for your client.

4. Think about interacting with clients of each of the major world religions, using information from your own experiences and from the textbook Table 12-1: MAJOR WORLD RELIGIONS AND COMMON HEALTH BELIEFS, pp. 201–202. Consider appropriate interview questions based on your knowledge of each of these faiths.

Activity C   INTERVIEWING AND RECORDING ASSESSMENT FINDINGS

After reading Chapter 12, use the following Nursing Interview Guide to interview and record your subjective findings for a spiritual assessment of a lab partner, peer, or client. Your instructor may ask you to turn this in to be evaluated. Forms are also available on thePoint *website.*

Nursing Interview Guide to Collect Subjective Data From the Client	
Questions	**Findings**
Current Symptoms	
1. Affect corresponding to attitude?	
2. Culturally appropriate eye contact when describing spiritual beliefs?	
3. Expresses sense of hope for future and comfort from beliefs?	
4. Ease with which client divulges information?	
5. Perceived stress level?	
6. Presence of spiritual conflicts/struggles?	
7. Display of religious articles?	
8. Desire to participate in usual religious practices?	

Copyright © 2014. Wolters Kluwer Health | Lippincott Williams & Wilkins. Lab Manual for Health Assessment in Nursing, 5e.

Nursing Interview Guide to Collect Subjective Data From the Client (continued)	
Questions	**Findings**
Current Status	
1. What do you believe has caused your illness? Do you believe there is a spiritual cause for the illness?	
2. Would you like to be visited by your own religious figure (pastor, priest, etc.) or someone from pastoral care?	
3. Are there any religious practices that you would like to continue while in the hospital? (e.g., dietary restrictions? Daily prayer rituals?)	
4. Do your spiritual beliefs give you a sense of hope and comfort?	
5. Are you aware of any spiritual conflicts at present?	
Past History	
1. Has your religion helped you cope in the past?	
2. Does your religion encourage you to practice health promotion activities?	
Family History	
1. Do you have strong social and spiritual support systems?	
2. What religion does your family follow? Do all members of your immediate family follow the same religion?	
Lifestyle and Health Practices	
1. How often do you attend religious service/activities?	
2. Do you have a strong connection with one or more religious groups?	
3. Do you see any differences between your beliefs and current health care treatments?	
4. Are you motivated to participate in health promotion activities?	
Analysis of Data	
1. Formulate nursing diagnoses (health promotion, risk, and actual).	
2. Formulate collaborative problems.	
3. Make necessary referrals.	

Copyright © 2014. Wolters Kluwer Health | Lippincott Williams & Wilkins. Lab Manual for Health Assessment in Nursing, 5e.

CHAPTER POSTTEST

Activity D **MULTIPLE CHOICE QUESTIONS**

Choose the one best answer for each of the following multiple choice questions.

_____ 1. During a thorough spiritual assessment, the nurse understands that the questions asked are designed to
   a. encourage the client to explore other religions.
   b. cause the client to question long-held beliefs.
   c. determine if the client and nurse have similar beliefs.
   d. reveal beliefs that might affect client care.

_____ 2. Loss of connection with one's spiritual support most often leads to
   a. a new-found sense of liberation.
   b. spiritual distress.
   c. improved sense of health and well-being.
   d. increased adherence to religious practices.

_____ 3. Knowledge of the client's beliefs in the cause of illness can be useful to the nurse in order to
   a. encourage new beliefs.
   b. dispel religious teachings if they conflict with the nurse's belief system.
   c. promote harmony between health and spirituality.
   d. raise doubt and point out flaws in one's faith.

_____ 4. Because the nurse realizes that spirituality varies, information gained will assist the nurse in
   a. individualizing interventions to meet specific needs.
   b. diagnosing the client with spiritual distress.
   c. teaching strict adherence to rituals and practices to improve outcomes.
   d. providing an overview of widely held beliefs from the major religions.

_____ 5. To give spiritual care to a client, it is not necessary for the nurse to
   a. recognize that depression may result from unmet religious group expectations.
   b. share the same religious beliefs as the client to provide effective spiritual care.
   c. be aware of personal religious beliefs and biases in order to provide effective spiritual care.
   d. prepare to help clients seek a source of strength and hope from their own (clients') religion and spiritual beliefs.

Activity E **CRITICAL THINKING ACTIVITIES**

1. Describe expected assessment findings of a client in spiritual distress.

2. Select a spiritual assessment tool from the textbook (Assessment Tool 12-1, p. 203, Box 12-2, p. 203, or Box 12-3, p. 204) and discuss the benefits/constraints of using this tool to obtain a useful spiritual assessment. How would you use this tool to perform a spiritual assessment?

Copyright © 2014. Wolters Kluwer Health | Lippincott Williams & Wilkins. Lab Manual for Health Assessment in Nursing, 5e.

Activity F CASE STUDY

Read the following case study. Then, work through the steps of analyzing the case study data. First, identify the abnormal data and strengths in **subjective and objective findings**, assemble **cue clusters**, draw **inferences**, make possible **nursing diagnoses**, identify **defining characteristics**, **confirm or rule out** the diagnoses, and **document** your conclusions. Use the blank diagnostic analysis charts provided at the end of this book (also available on thePoint website) to guide your thinking. Propose nursing diagnoses that are specific to the client in the case study. Identify collaborative problems, if any, for this client. Finally, identify data, if any, that point toward a medical problem requiring a referral.

Rhonda Logan is a 51-year-old divorced woman, with no children. She teaches in a parochial elementary school, attends church regularly, and is the primary caregiver for an aging father in ill health. Rhonda is seeking health care related to difficulty going to sleep and staying asleep. She also reports frequent headaches, lack of appetite and motivation, and difficulty concentrating.

When interviewed, Rhonda relates that she initiated the divorce 6 months ago, ending a 25-year marriage from an alcoholic, verbally abusive husband. She states that she feels guilty over her decision to divorce because of her religious beliefs. Rhonda states she cannot understand how a loving God would have placed her in such a loveless relationship. She indicates that if she had tried harder to involve Mr. Logan in marriage counseling, perhaps things would have turned out differently. She further reflects that if she had been able to have children or had devoted less time to her father, her ex-husband would not have drunk so much.

During the interview with the nurse, Rhonda revealed that she fears that she may lose her job because of the Church's view on divorce. She states that her students are the only thing that keeps her "sane." Rhonda perceives less support from her colleagues during and after the divorce. She states that she is disappointed in their lack of Christian support during these "dark times." She states that she believes their behavior is hypocritical because she is hurting and most of the faculty is not acting in a caring way. Though she attends church regularly, she reveals that she is "going through the motions" but is feeling less and less connected to her congregation. The analogy that she shared was of an empty eggshell, void on the inside, fragile on the outside, yet looking whole and strong to onlookers. The nurse noted varied changes in her mood, vacillating among anxiety, anger, preoccupation, sadness, and crying.

How Well Did You Do?

After you have read the chapter and completed the exercises in this chapter, visit thePoint to access the Self-Reflection Activity. This activity will help you identify to what degree you have met each of the chapter objectives. You can then review the chapter for objectives you have met partially or not at all.

Other tools to help you, like the Diagnostic Reasoning Guides, Nursing Interview Guides, Physical Assessment Guides, and NCLEX-Style Chapter Review Questions, are also available on thePoint.

Copyright © 2014. Wolters Kluwer Health | Lippincott Williams & Wilkins. Lab Manual for Health Assessment in Nursing, 5e.

Assessing Nutritional Status

Chapter Overview

Nutritional assessment helps the nurse to identify risk factors for obesity and to promote health. The following activities and questions are provided as a review and, also, to stimulate your thoughts regarding nutritional assessment of the client.

Chapter Learning Objectives

1. Discuss the various factors contributing to healthy nutrition, malnutrition, and overnutrition.
2. Interview a client for an accurate nutritional and hydration history.
3. Correctly identify clients across cultures who are at risk for nutritional and hydration excesses or deficits across the lifespan.
4. Assess a client's overall appearance including body build, muscle mass, and fat distribution.
5. Gather the equipment necessary to perform anthropometric measurements.
6. Accurately measure height, weight, waist circumference, mid-arm circumference, triceps skinfold thickness, and mid-arm muscle circumference.
7. Calculate a client's BMI.
8. Describe the findings frequently seen when assessing the nutritional status of older clients.
9. Discuss physical assessment findings that may indicate changes in hydration status.
10. Describe cultural variations seen in nutritional assessment.
11. Analyze the data from the nutritional interview and physical assessment to formulate valid nursing diagnoses, collaborative problems, and/or referrals.

CHAPTER PRETEST

Activity A MATCHING

Match the terms in the left column with the correct description in the right column.

Term

_____ **1.** Body mass index (BMI)

_____ **2.** Visceral fat

_____ **3.** Triceps skinfold

_____ **4.** Mid-arm circumference

_____ **5.** Cachexia

Description

a. Used to evaluate subcutaneous fat stores

b. Used to assess skeletal muscle mass

c. Malnutrition sometimes seen in clients with cancer

d. Excess fat within the abdominal cavity

e. Estimate total body fat

Activity B **LEARNER ACTIVITIES**

After reading Chapter 13 in the textbook, participate in the following learning activities.

1. Interview your lab partner for a nutritional history. Discuss your overall findings with your lab partner. Discuss why each question gives greater insight into the client's nutritional status.

2. Use the SPEEDY CHECKLIST FOR NUTRITIONAL HEALTH (Assessment Tool 13-3, p. 220 in the textbook) to calculate your lab partner's score as well as your own score to determine if there is nutritional risk. Compare and then discuss your findings. Take turns teaching each other about how to reduce risk factors to enhance one's health.

3. Practice taking anthropometric measurements on peers, friends, and family members. Assess a variety of people: obese, thin, elderly, young. Using textbook Tables 13-3 through 13-8, locate your findings on the standardized tables (below, average, or above national standards).

Activity C **INTERVIEWING AND RECORDING ASSESSMENT FINDINGS**

After reading Chapter 13, use the following Nursing Interview Guide to interview and record your subjective findings for an assessment of the nutritional status of a lab partner, peer, or client. Your instructor may ask you to turn this in to be evaluated. Forms are also available on thePoint *website.*

Nursing Interview Guide to Collect Subjective Data From the Client

Questions	Findings
Current Symptoms	
1. Appetite changes?	
2. Weight changes in last 6 months?	
3. Problems with indigestion, heartburn, bloating, gas?	
4. Constipation or diarrhea?	
5. Dental problems?	
Past History	
1. Food allergies?	
2. Conditions/diseases affecting intake or absorption?	
3. Frequency of dieting?	
Family History	
1. Chronic diseases?	
2. Weight issues?	
Lifestyle and Health Practices	
1. Average daily food and beverage intake?	
2. Type of beverages consumed?	
3. Dine alone or with others?	
4. Number of meals and snacks per day?	
5. Food preferences?	
6. Frequency of eating out?	
7. Long work hours?	
8. Sufficient income for food?	

Copyright © 2014. Wolters Kluwer Health | Lippincott Williams & Wilkins. Lab Manual for Health Assessment in Nursing, 5e.

Activity D PERFORMING PHYSICAL ASSESSMENT

Use the following Physical Assessment Guide for the nutritional status assessment of a lab partner, peer, or client. Column 1 will serve as a reminder as to what part of the exam you will do next. Column 2 will be used to record your findings. Your instructor may ask you to turn this in to be evaluated. Forms are also available on thePoint *website.*

Physical Assessment Guide to Collect Objective Client Data	
Questions	Findings
Current Symptoms	
1. Gather equipment (balance beam scale with height attachment, metric measuring tape, marking pencil, and skinfold calipers).	
2. Measure height.	
3. Measure weight (1 kg = 2.205 lb).	
4. Determine BODY MASS INDEX (BMI = weight in kilograms/height in meters squared or use the NIH website: http//nhlbisupport.com/bmi/bmicalc.htm). Compare results to BMI in Table 13-3, on page 218 in the textbook.	
5. Measure waist circumference and compare findings to Table 13-5 on page 230 in the textbook.	
6. Measure MID-ARM CIRCUMFERENCE (MAC) and compare findings to Table 13-6 on page 231 in the textbook.	
7. Measure TRICEPS SKINFOLD THICKNESS (TSF) and compare to Table 13-7 on page 232 in the textbook.	
8. Calculate MID-ARM MUSCLE CIRCUMFERENCE (MAMC), MAMC (cm) = MAC (cm) − (0.314 × TSF). Refer to Table 13-8 on page 233 in the textbook for interpretation.	
Analysis of Data	
1. Formulate nursing diagnoses (wellness, risk, actual).	
2. Formulate collaborative problems.	
3. Make necessary referrals.	

CHAPTER POSTTEST

Activity E MULTIPLE CHOICE QUESTIONS

Choose the one best answer for each of the following multiple choice questions.

_____ 1. The nurse is caring for an adult female client whose BMI is 38.7. The nurse should instruct the client that she is at greater risk for

    a. heart attack.

    b. osteoporosis.

    c. rheumatoid arthritis.

    d. stomach cancer.

_____ 2. Waist circumference guidelines may not be accurate for adult clients who are shorter than 152.4 cm (5 ft) in height. This restriction is also a concern for which other anthropometric measurement?

    a. Ideal weight.

    b. Mid-arm circumference.

    c. Body mass index (BMI).

    d. Triceps skinfold measurements.

_____ 3. Based only on anthropometric measurements, which set of clients listed below are at the greatest risk for diabetes and cardiovascular disease?

    a. Clients with a BMI of 23.

    b. Females with 88.9 cm (35 in) or greater waist circumference.

    c. Males with 88.9 cm (35 in) or greater waist circumference.

    d. Clients with a BMI of 20.

_____ 4. What is the most common measurement used to determine abdominal visceral fat?

    a. Waist circumference.

    b. Body mass index.

    c. Subcutaneous fat determination.

    d. Triceps skinfold thickness.

_____ 5. Because BMI is calculated using only height and weight, the nurse knows that inaccurate findings would most likely occur in a client

    a. with diabetes.

    b. who is 182.8 cm (6 ft) tall.

    c. with osteoarthritis.

    d. who is a bodybuilder.

_____ 6. The nurse documents that a 45-year-old male is 177.8 cm (5 ft 10 in) tall and weighs 97.5 kg (215 lb). He tells the nurse that he "has a good appetite, but doesn't get much exercise because of his busy work schedule." An appropriate NANDA nursing diagnosis for this client is

    a. normal body nutrition related to healthy eating patterns and good appetite.

    b. altered nutrition, more than body requirements related to intake greater than calories expended.

    c. risk for altered nutrition, more than body requirements related to lack of routine exercise.

    d. obesity related to lack of exercise.

_____ 7. The nurse is preparing to measure the triceps skinfold of an adult client. The nurse should

    a. ask the client to assume a sitting position.

    b. measure the triceps skinfold in the dominant arm.

    c. repeat the procedure three times and average the measurements.

    d. pull the skin toward the muscle mass of the arm.

_____ 8. Of the following measurements, which one helps to determine if a client is underweight, normal weight, or obese?

    a. Mid-arm circumference.

    b. Triceps skinfold.

    c. Body mass index.

    d. Waist–hip ratio.

_____ 9. When would a nurse obtain a mid-arm circumference measurement?

    a. To confirm an abnormal albumin level.

    b. To provide percentage of body fat and muscle tissue.

    c. To screen for nutritional excess or deficits.

    d. To assist in determining body mass index.

Copyright © 2014. Wolters Kluwer Health | Lippincott Williams & Wilkins. Lab Manual for Health Assessment in Nursing, 5e.

____ **10.** To quickly identify a client who may be at risk for nutritional problems, the nurse can use which of the following assessments?

    a. Laboratory blood work.

    b. A comprehensive nutritional assessment.

    c. A physical examination.

    d. A nutritional screening tool.

Activity F   CRITICAL THINKING ACTIVITIES

1. Discuss why determining the presence and extent of abdominal visceral fat is significant during an assessment.

2. Describe the procedure you would use to determine the client's body composition.

3. Discuss the expected changes in height and weight associated with the aging process. How does this affect the BMI accuracy? Why?

4. Explain how an obese client may be undernourished in spite of ample weight and intake. What nursing diagnosis might you make?

Activity G   CASE STUDY

Read the following case study. Then, work through the steps of analyzing the case study data. First identify abnormal data and strengths in **subjective and objective findings**, assemble **cue clusters**, draw **inferences**, make possible **nursing diagnoses**, identify **defining characteristics, confirm or rule out** the diagnoses, and **document** your conclusions. Use the blank diagnostic analysis charts provided at the end of this book (also available on thePoint website) to guide your thinking. Propose nursing diagnoses that are specific to the client in the case study. Identify collaborative problems, if any, for this client. Finally, identify data, if any, which point toward a medical problem requiring a referral.

Gina R. is a 43-year-old married woman, who has been newly diagnosed with diabetes mellitus. She is 157.48 cm (5 ft 2 in) tall, weighs 107.04 kg (236 lb), and has elevated blood glucose levels, cholesterol, and triglyceride levels. Gina has a college education and two teenage children, one of whom is away at college. Her husband is on permanent disability resulting from alcohol-induced cirrhosis. Gina works with an enrichment program for parents of preschoolers. Because she works in a rural area, she spends a large amount of time driving between client home visits.

When interviewed, Gina states that 3 years ago she was diagnosed with a brain tumor but was successfully treated with surgery, radiation, and chemotherapy. She remains on a maintenance dose of prednisone, which she reports stimulates her appetite and has caused her to develop diabetes. Gina takes metformin (Glucophage) to reduce her blood sugar. She correctly states that this medication can also suppress appetite and promote weight loss. When questioned about snacks, she reports that she ate half a box of cookies last evening, but clarified this by stating that they were low-fat cookies.

Further interviewing revealed that Gina knows she must lose weight but states it is difficult because she spends much of her day traveling, has little, if any, time to exercise, and works long hours, so she and her husband eat out frequently. She denies smoking or drinking. Gina reports few social contacts due to her husband's illness. She appears very devoted to her children and her client families that she serves. During the interview, she further states that food was her only pleasure and now that too has been taken away due to dietary restrictions. Though often smiling during the interview, Gina shares that life would have been simpler if her husband had died last summer when he was so critically ill.

How Well Did You Do?

After you have read the chapter and completed the exercises in this chapter, visit thePoint to access the Self-Reflection Activity. This activity will help you identify to what degree you have met each of the chapter objectives. You can then review the chapter for objectives you have met partially or not at all.

Other tools to help you, like the Diagnostic Reasoning Guides, Nursing Interview Guides, Physical Assessment Guides, and NCLEX-Style Chapter Review Questions, are also available on thePoint.

Copyright © 2014. Wolters Kluwer Health | Lippincott Williams & Wilkins. Lab Manual for Health Assessment in Nursing, 5e.

CHAPTER 14

Assessing Skin, Hair, and Nails

Chapter Overview

In any kind of physical assessment, the client's skin, hair, and nails are among the most easily observed characteristics that provide clues to the client's general health condition. Diseases and disorders of the skin, hair, and nails may be local or caused by an underlying systemic condition. Remember that skin assessment may be a sensitive topic for some clients as it is highly visible, often influencing one's body image and self-concept. The following questions and exercises are presented to help you review your observation and other assessment skills. You will also be helped, both in your studies and in your practice, by following the directions for performing a skin self-assessment (see Box 14-1, p. 247 in the textbook) and completing the exercises found in this chapter.

Chapter Learning Objectives

1. Describe the structures and functions of the skin, nails, and hair.
2. Discuss the risk factors for skin cancer and METHICILLIN-RESISTANT *STAPHYLOCOCCUS AUREUS* across cultures and ways to reduce one's risks.
3. Interview a client for an accurate nursing history of the skin, nails, and hair.
4. Perform a physical assessment of the skin, nails, and hair using the correct techniques.
5. Teach a client how to perform a self-assessment of the skin, hair, and nails.
6. Differentiate between normal and abnormal findings of the skin, hair, and nails.
7. Describe the findings frequently seen when assessing the older client's skin, hair, and nails.
8. Analyze data from the interview and physical assessment of the skin, hair, and nails to formulate valid nursing diagnoses, collaborative problems, and/or referrals.

CHAPTER PRETEST

Activity A MULTIPLE CHOICE QUESTIONS

Choose the one best answer for each of the following multiple choice questions.

_____ 1. Connecting the skin to underlying structures is/are the

    a. papillae.

    b. sebaceous glands.

    c. dermis layer.

    d. subcutaneous tissue.

_____ 2. The skin plays a vital role in temperature maintenance, fluid and electrolyte balance, and synthesis of vitamin
   a. A.
   b. B$_{12}$.
   c. C.
   d. D.

_____ 3. The only layer of the skin that undergoes cell division is the
   a. innermost layer of the epidermis.
   b. outermost layer of the epidermis.
   c. innermost layer of the dermis.
   d. outermost layer of the dermis.

_____ 4. A client's skin color depends on melanin and carotene contained in the skin, and the
   a. client's genetic background.
   b. volume of blood circulating in the dermis.
   c. number of lymph vessels near the dermis.
   d. vascularity of the apocrine glands.

_____ 5. Hair follicles, sebaceous glands, and sweat glands originate from the
   a. epidermis.
   b. eccrine glands.
   c. keratinized tissue.
   d. dermis.

_____ 6. The apocrine glands are dormant until puberty and are concentrated in the axillae, the perineum, and the
   a. areola of the breast.
   b. entire skin surface.
   c. soles of the feet.
   d. adipose tissue.

_____ 7. Short, pale, and fine hair that is present over much of the body is termed
   a. vellus.
   b. dermal.
   c. lanugo.
   d. terminal.

_____ 8. A primary function of hair in the nose and eyelashes is to serve as a
   a. response to cold.
   b. filter for dust.
   c. pigment producer.
   d. response to fright.

_____ 9. The nails, located on the distal phalanges of the fingers and toes, are composed of
   a. ectodermal cells.
   b. endodermal cells.
   c. keratinized epidermal cells.
   d. stratum cells.

_____ 10. Squamous cell carcinoma is associated with
   a. overall amount of sun exposure.
   b. intermittent exposure to ultraviolet rays.
   c. precursor lesions.
   d. an increase in the rates of melanoma.

Copyright © 2014. Wolters Kluwer Health | Lippincott Williams & Wilkins. Lab Manual for Health Assessment in Nursing, 5e.

Activity B LABELING ACTIVITIES

Label the following skin structures. Match your answer with Figure 14-1 in the textbook on page 240.

A

B

Label the following nail structures. Match your answer with Figure 14-2 in the textbook on page 241.

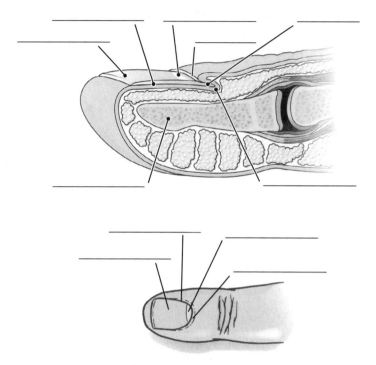

Activity C LEARNER ACTIVITIES

After reading Chapter 14 in the textbook, participate in the following learning activities.

1. Review the information in Evidence-Based Health Promotion and Disease Prevention 14-2: Skin Cancer in the textbook on page 246. Then, determine your own risk for skin cancer. Next, identify and discuss the ethnic groups that are at highest risk for skin cancer.

2. Practice recording the descriptions of various common skin lesions on your own arms and legs (freckles, warts, moles, and sores) by examining the color, size, configuration, and shape of any lesion you find. (Refer to Table 14-1, p. 258; Figures 14-1 to 14-6, pp. 240, 241, 249–251 and Abnormal Findings 14-1 to 14-6, pp. 263–269 in your textbook.) Record your findings and compare to the normal and abnormal findings in your textbook. Share any suspicious findings with your instructor or primary health care provider.

3. Use BOX 14-1, SELF-ASSESSMENT: HOW TO EXAMINE YOUR OWN SKIN, on page 247 in your textbook to examine your own skin. Record your findings and compare to the normal and abnormal findings in your textbook. Share any suspicious findings with your instructor or primary health care provider.

4. Find an 80-year or older elderly client, friend, or relative who will let you examine his or her skin, hair, and nails. Record your findings. Find a young client, friend, or relative who will let you examine his or her skin, hair, and nails. Record your findings and compare the elderly person's findings with those of the younger person's findings. Use your textbook to differentiate between normal and abnormal findings. Refer the clients as necessary.

Activity D INTERVIEWING AND RECORDING ASSESSMENT FINDINGS

After reading Chapter 14, use the following Nursing Interview Guide to interview and record your subjective findings for an assessment of the skin, hair, and nails of a lab partner, peer, or client. Your instructor may ask you to turn this in to be evaluated. Forms are also available on thePoint *website.*

Nursing Interview Guide to Collect Subjective Data From the Client

Questions	Findings
Current Symptoms	
1. Skin problems (rashes, lesions, dryness, oiliness, drainage, bruising, swelling, pigmentation)	
2. Changes in lesion appearance	
3. Feeling changes (pain, pressure, itch, tingling)	
4. Hair loss or changes	
5. Nail changes	
6. Body odor problems	
Past History	
1. Previous problems with skin, hair, or nails (treatment and surgery)	
2. Allergic reactions	
Family History	
1. Family history of skin problems or skin cancer	
Lifestyle and Health Practices	
1. Exposure to sun or chemicals	
2. Daily care of skin, hair, and nails	
3. Usual diet and exercise patterns	

Activity E PERFORMING PHYSICAL ASSESSMENT OF THE SKIN, HAIR, AND NAILS

Use the following Physical Assessment Guide to examine the skin, hair, and nails of a lab partner, peer, or client. Column 1 will serve as a reminder as to what part of the exam you will do next. Column 2 will be used to record your findings. Your instructor may ask you to turn this in to be evaluated. Forms are also available on thePoint *website.*

Physical Assessment Guide to Collect Objective Client Data

Questions	Findings
1. Gather equipment (gloves, exam light, penlight, magnifying glass, centimeter ruler, Wood lamp if available).	
2. Explain procedure to client.	
3. Ask client to gown.	
Skin	
1. Note any distinctive odor.	
2. Inspect for generalized color variations (brownness, yellow, redness, pallor, cyanosis, jaundice, erythema, vitiligo).	
3. Inspect for skin breakdown (use staging criteria given in Chapter 13).	

Copyright © 2014. Wolters Kluwer Health | Lippincott Williams & Wilkins. Lab Manual for Health Assessment in Nursing, 5e.

Physical Assessment Guide to Collect Objective Client Data (continued)	
Questions	Findings
4. Inspect for primary, secondary, or vascular lesions. (Note size, shape, location, distribution, and configuration.) Use Wood lamp if fungus is suspected.	
5. Palpate lesions.	
6. Palpate texture (rough, smooth) of skin, using palmar surface of three middle fingers.	
7. Palpate temperature (cool, warm, hot) and moisture (dry, sweaty, oily) of skin, using dorsal side of hand.	
8. Palpate thickness of skin with fingerpads.	
9. Palpate mobility and turgor by pinching up skin over sternum.	
10. Palpate for edema, pressing thumbs over feet or ankles.	
Scalp and Hair	
1. Inspect color.	
2. Inspect amount and distribution.	
3. Inspect and palpate for thickness, texture, oiliness, lesions, and parasites.	
Nails	
1. Inspect for grooming and cleanliness.	
2. Inspect for color and markings.	
3. Inspect shape.	
4. Palpate texture and consistency.	
5. Test for capillary refill.	
Analysis of Data	
1. Formulate nursing diagnoses (wellness, risk, actual).	
2. Formulate collaborative problems.	
3. Make necessary referrals.	

CHAPTER POSTTEST

Activity F   MULTIPLE CHOICE QUESTIONS

Choose the one best answer for each of the following multiple choice questions.

_____   **1.** An adult female client visits the clinic for the first time. The client has many bruises around her neck and face, and she tells the nurse that the bruises are the "result of an accident." The nurse suspects that the client may be experiencing

    a. leukemia.

    b. diabetes mellitus.

    c. melanoma.

    d. domestic abuse.

Copyright © 2014. Wolters Kluwer Health | Lippincott Williams & Wilkins. Lab Manual for Health Assessment in Nursing, 5e.

____ 2. An adult male client visits the outpatient center and tells the nurse that he has been experiencing patchy hair loss. The nurse should further assess the client for

    a. symptoms of stress.

    b. recent radiation therapy.

    c. pigmentation irregularities.

    d. allergies to certain foods.

____ 3. The nurse is instructing a group of high school students about risk factors associated with various skin cancers. The nurse should instruct the group that

    a. melanoma skin cancers are the most common type of cancers.

    b. African Americans are the least susceptible to skin cancers.

    c. usually there are precursor lesions for basal cell carcinomas.

    d. squamous cell carcinomas are most common on body sites with heavy sun exposure.

____ 4. The nurse is assessing an African American client's skin. After the assessment, the nurse should instruct the client that African American persons are more susceptible to

    a. skin cancers than persons of European origin.

    b. melanomas if they reside in areas without ozone depletion.

    c. chronic discoid lupus erythematosus.

    d. genetic predisposition to melanomas.

____ 5. A 20-year-old client visits the outpatient center and tells the nurse that he has been experiencing sudden generalized hair loss. After determining that the client has not received radiation or chemotherapy, the nurse should further assess the client for signs and symptoms of

    a. hypothyroidism.

    b. hyperthyroidism.

    c. infectious conditions.

    d. hypoparathyroidism.

____ 6. A client visits the clinic for a routine physical examination. The nurse prepares to assess the client's skin. The nurse asks the client if there is a family history of skin cancer and should explain to the client that there is a genetic component with skin cancer, especially

    a. basal cell carcinoma.

    b. actinic keratoses.

    c. squamous cell carcinoma.

    d. malignant melanoma.

____ 7. A female client visits the clinic and complains to the nurse that her skin feels "dry." The nurse should instruct the client that skin elasticity is related to adequate

    a. calcium.

    b. vitamin D.

    c. carbohydrates.

    d. fluid intake.

____ 8. An adult white client visits the clinic for the first time. During assessment of the client's skin, the nurse should assess for central cyanosis by observing the client's

    a. nail beds.

    b. oral mucosa.

    c. sclera.

    d. palms.

Copyright © 2014. Wolters Kluwer Health | Lippincott Williams & Wilkins. Lab Manual for Health Assessment in Nursing, 5e.

____ **9.** To assess for anemia in a dark-skinned client, the nurse should observe the client's skin for a color that appears
- **a.** greenish.
- **b.** ashen.
- **c.** bluish.
- **d.** olive.

____ **10.** The nurse is assessing a dark-skinned client who has been transported to the emergency room by ambulance. When the nurse observes that the client's skin appears pale, with blue-tinged lips and oral mucosa, the nurse should document the presence of
- **a.** a great degree of cyanosis.
- **b.** a mild degree of cyanosis.
- **c.** lupus erythematosus.
- **d.** hyperthyroidism.

____ **11.** A dark-skinned client visits the clinic because he "hasn't been feeling well." To assess the client's skin for jaundice, the nurse should inspect the client's
- **a.** abdomen.
- **b.** arms.
- **c.** legs.
- **d.** sclera.

____ **12.** While assessing the skin of an older adult client, the nurse observes that the client has small yellowish brown patches on her hands. The nurse should instruct the client that these spots are
- **a.** signs of an infectious process.
- **b.** caused by aging of the skin in older adults.
- **c.** precancerous lesions.
- **d.** signs of dermatitis.

____ **13.** While assessing an adult client's feet for fungal disease using a Wood light, the nurse documents the presence of a fungus when the fluorescence is
- **a.** blue.
- **b.** red.
- **c.** yellow.
- **d.** purple.

____ **14.** The nurse assesses an older adult bedridden client in her home. While assessing the client's buttocks, the nurse observes that a small area of the skin is broken and resembles an erosion. The nurse should document the client's pressure ulcer as
- **a.** stage I.
- **b.** stage II.
- **c.** stage III.
- **d.** stage IV.

____ **15.** To assess an adult client's skin turgor, the nurse should
- **a.** press down on the skin of the feet.
- **b.** use the dorsal surfaces of the hands on the client's arms.
- **c.** use the fingerpads to palpate the skin at the sternum.
- **d.** use two fingers to pinch the skin under the clavicle.

____ **16.** While assessing the nails of an adult client, the nurse observes Beau lines. The nurse should ask the client if he has had
- **a.** chemotherapy.
- **b.** radiation.
- **c.** a recent illness.
- **d.** steroid therapy.

___ 17. While assessing the nails of an older adult, the nurse observes early clubbing. The nurse should further evaluate the client for signs and symptoms of

    a. hypoxia.

    b. trauma.

    c. anemia.

    d. infection.

___ 18. While assessing an adult client, the nurse observes freckles on the client's face. The nurse should document the presence of

    a. macules.

    b. papules.

    c. plaques.

    d. bulla.

___ 19. While assessing an adult client, the nurse observes an elevated, palpable, solid mass with a circumscribed border that measures 1 cm. The nurse documents this as a

    a. plaque.

    b. macule.

    c. papule.

    d. patch.

___ 20. The nurse is preparing to examine the skin of an adult client with a diagnosis of herpes simplex. The nurse plans to measure the client's symptomatic lesions and measure the size of the client's

    a. nodules.

    b. bullae.

    c. vesicles.

    d. wheals.

___ 21. An adult male client visits the clinic and tells the nurse that he believes he has athlete's foot. The nurse observes that the client has linear cracks in the skin on both feet. The nurse should document the presence of

    a. ulcers.

    b. erosion.

    c. scales.

    d. fissures.

___ 22. An African American female client visits the clinic. She tells the nurse that she had her ears pierced several weeks ago, and an elevated, irregular, reddened mass has now developed at the ear lobe. The nurse should document a

    a. cyst.

    b. lichenification.

    c. bulla.

    d. keloid.

___ 23. A client who is an active outdoor swimmer recently received a diagnosis of discoid systemic lupus erythematosus. The client visits the clinic for a routine examination and tells the nurse that she continues to swim in the sunlight three times per week. She has accepted her patchy hair loss and wears a wig on occasion. A priority nursing diagnosis for the client is

    a. ineffective individual coping related to changes in appearance.

    b. anxiety related to loss of outdoor activities and altered skin appearance.

    c. dry flaking skin and dull dry hair as a result of disease.

    d. risk for ineffective health maintenance related to deficient knowledge of effects of sunlight on skin lesions.

Copyright © 2014. Wolters Kluwer Health | Lippincott Williams & Wilkins. Lab Manual for Health Assessment in Nursing, 5e.

Activity G **MATCHING**

Match the terms in the left column with the correct description in the right column.

Term

_____ **1.** Lichenification

_____ **2.** Urticaria

_____ **3.** Papule

_____ **4.** Wheal

_____ **5.** Keloid

_____ **6.** Nevus

_____ **7.** Petechiae

_____ **8.** Annular

_____ **9.** Induration

_____ **10.** Bulla

Description

a. Hardening of the skin, usually caused by edema

b. Solid, elevated, circumscribed, superficial lesion; 1 cm or less in diameter

c. Elevated, solid, transient lesion; often irregularly shaped; an edematous

d. Thickening of the skin characterized by accentuated skin markings

e. An elevated, circumscribed, fluid-filled lesion; greater than 1 cm in diameter

f. Describes a lesion that forms a ring around a clear center of normal skin

g. Tiny, flat, purple, or red spots on the surface of the skin resulting from minute hemorrhage

h. Hypertrophic scar tissue; prevalent in nonwhite races

i. Congenital pigmented area on the skin, for example, mole, birthmark

j. Hives; pruritic wheals, often transient and allergic in origin

Activity H **CRITICAL THINKING ACTIVITY**

1. Discuss how you would assess for pallor, cyanosis, jaundice, and erythema in a dark-skinned client.

2. Read the following case study. Then analyze the client's risk for skin cancer.

Mike McDaniel is a 47-year-old construction worker, who has lived for 20 years in southern Florida. He has blond hair and tanned, leathery, freckled skin. He is 177.8 cm (5 ft 10 in) tall and weighs 90.7 kg (200 lb). He smokes two packs of cigarettes and drinks a six-pack of beer per day. He describes himself as a "meat and potatoes man." He has a history of mild hypertension, and several members of his family have heart disease.

Activity I **CASE STUDY**

Read the following case study. Then, work through the steps of analyzing the case study data. First identify abnormal data and strengths in **subjective and objective findings**, assemble **cue clusters**, draw **inferences**, make possible **nursing diagnoses**, identify **defining characteristics**, **confirm or rule out** the diagnoses, and **document** your conclusions. Use the blank diagnostic analysis charts provided at the end of this book (also available on thePoint website) to guide your thinking. Propose nursing diagnoses that are specific to the client in the case study. Identify collaborative problems, if any, for this client. Finally, identify data, if any, which point toward a medical problem requiring a referral.

Evelyn Vaughn is a 47-year-old white woman, who comes to the clinic for evaluation. She is a single mother and sells cosmetics in her home. She is lethargic and walks slowly into the room. She asks if she can have some "special lotion" for her dry skin.

When interviewed, Evelyn states that her skin has been dry and scaly for the past several months, unrelieved by numerous moisturizers. She expresses concern about "fly-away hair that I can't do anything with" and about brittle, easily broken fingernails. When asked about medications, she explains that she is supposed to take Synthroid daily for "my low thyroid" but cannot afford to get the prescription filled. She has a poor appetite, and with "not enough money to go around," she has been nibbling on crackers, lunch meat, and sodas daily. Exercise is out of the question because she lacks energy, and she is rarely able to get through a day without one or two 30-minute naps. Evelyn takes a shower and washes her hair using ivory soap and baby shampoo. She applies moisturizer to her skin and conditioner to her hair but states that neither helps for any length of time. She keeps her nails cut short because they break so easily. She states that she has cut down on her cosmetic sales appointments because "I look like I never use my own products."

Copyright © 2014. Wolters Kluwer Health | Lippincott Williams & Wilkins. Lab Manual for Health Assessment in Nursing, 5e.

Your physical assessment reveals dry flaking skin that is cool to the touch and yellow tinged. Facial and periorbital edema are present. The client's facial expression is blank. She has multiple bruises on both forearms and anterior lower legs, which are in various stages of healing and tender when touched. Her scalp hair is dry and dull and breaks easily. Her scalp is scaling. Sparse hair is noted in the axillae and the pubic area. Her fingernails are short and dry; her cuticles are dry and torn. Her toenails are thick and yellow.

How Well Did You Do?

After you have read the chapter and completed the exercises in this chapter, visit the Point to access the Self-Reflection Activity. This activity will help you identify to what degree you have met each of the chapter objectives. You can then review the chapter for objectives you have met partially or not at all.

Other tools to help you, like the Diagnostic Reasoning Guides, Nursing Interview Guides, Physical Assessment Guides, and NCLEX-Style Chapter Review Questions, are also available on the Point.

Copyright © 2014. Wolters Kluwer Health | Lippincott Williams & Wilkins. Lab Manual for Health Assessment in Nursing, 5e.

15

Assessing Head and Neck

Chapter Overview

Assessment of the head and neck focuses on the cranium, face, thyroid gland, and lymph node structures contained within the head and neck. Remember normal facial structures and features tend to vary widely among individuals and cultures. The client's health history is particularly important in this assessment because it provides clues to abnormalities that cannot be directly observed, for example, headaches and possible systemic problems. Some clients may be anxious as you palpate the neck for lymph nodes, especially if they have a history of cancer that caused lymph node enlargement. Use the following quizzes and activities to improve your head and neck assessment skills.

Chapter Learning Objectives

1. Describe the structures and functions of the head and neck.
2. Discuss the risk factors for head and neck disorders across cultures and ways to reduce one's risks.
3. Interview a client for an accurate nursing history of his/her head and neck.
4. Use the HEADACHE IMPACT TEST with a client to determine how his/her headaches affect his/her activities of daily living (see http://www.qualitymetric.com/demos/hit-6.aspx).
5. Perform a physical assessment of the heart and neck vessels using the correct techniques.
6. Differentiate between normal and abnormal findings of the head and neck.
7. Describe the findings frequently seen when assessing the older client's head and neck.
8. Analyze the data from the interview and physical assessment of the head and neck to formulate valid nursing diagnoses, collaborative problems, and/or referrals.

CHAPTER PRETEST

Activity A **MATCHING**

Match the terms in the left column with the correct descriptions in the right column.

Term

_____ **1.** Parotid gland

_____ **2.** Sublingual gland

_____ **3.** Trachea

_____ **4.** Hyoid bone

_____ **5.** Cricoid cartilage

_____ **6.** Thyroid gland

_____ **7.** Cranial nerve XI

_____ **8.** Trapezius and sternocleidomastoid

_____ **9.** Adam's apple

_____ **10.** Vertebra prominens

Description

a. The air passage extending from the throat and larynx to the main bronchi

b. Ring-like cartilage forming the lower and back part of the larynx

c. Spinal accessory nerve-contraction of trapezius and sternocleidomastoid muscles

d. The largest of the three main parts of salivary glands, located on either side of the face, just below and in front of the ears

e. Paired muscles that allow movement and provide support to the head and neck

f. The largest of the endocrine glands, situated in the front and sides of the neck just below the thyroid cartilage

g. Cervical vertebra (C7) that can be easily palpated when the neck is flexed

h. A salivary gland on either side of the tongue

i. A horseshoe-shaped bone at the base of the tongue; the only bone in the body not directly attached to another bone

j. The thyroid cartilage located just above the cricoid cartilage

Activity B **LABELING ACTIVITIES**

Label the structures of the neck in the following figure. Check your answer with Figure 15-2 in your textbook.

Label the neck muscles and landmarks in the following figure. Check your answers with Figure 15-3 in your textbook.

Label the lymph nodes in the neck in the following figure. Match your answers with Figure 15-5 in your textbook.

Activity C **LEARNER ACTIVITIES**

After reading Chapter 15, participate in the following learning activities.

1. Review Abnormal Findings 15-1 in the textbook pages 290–292, *Types and Characteristics of Headaches*. If you have a history of headaches, compare your symptoms to this table. Next, interview your lab partner to determine whether he or she has ever had a headache. Determine the type it might have been, based on the information in Abnormal Findings 15-1.

2. Practice the correct method for palpating the thyroid gland on your lab partner. Discuss your findings: size, texture, smoothness, presence of nodules or masses.

3. Auscultate your lab partner's thyroid gland and carotid arteries. Discuss the significance of this exam and what would indicate an abnormality.

4. Demonstrate on your lab partner how to inspect and palpate the C7 vertebra. Discuss the changes that may occur with aging, such as kyphosis of the spine or dowager hump.

5. Assess the lymph nodes of your lab partner. Discuss the normal and abnormal characteristics of the lymph nodes.

Activity D **INTERVIEWING AND RECORDING ASSESSMENT FINDINGS**

After reading Chapter 15, use the following Nursing Interview Guide to interview and record your subjective findings for an assessment of the head and neck of a lab partner, peer, or client. Your instructor may ask you to turn this in to be evaluated. Forms are also available on thePoint *website.*

Nursing Interview Guide to Collect Subjective Data From the Client	
Questions	**Findings**
Current Symptoms	
1. Lumps or lesions on head or neck that do not heal or disappear.	
2. Difficulty moving head or neck.	
3. Facial or neck pain or frequent headaches.	
4. Dizziness, lightheadedness, spinning sensation, or loss of consciousness.	
Past History	
Previous head or neck problems/trauma/injury (surgery, medication, physical or radiation therapy) results.	
Family History	
1. Family history of head and/or neck cancer.	
2. Family history of migraine headaches.	
Lifestyle and Health Practices	
1. Do you smoke or chew tobacco? Amount? Secondhand smoke?	
2. Do you wear a helmet or hard hat?	
3. Typical posture when relaxing, during sleep, and when working.	
4. Type of recreational activities.	
5. Satisfaction with appearance.	

Activity E **PERFORMING PHYSICAL ASSESSMENT OF THE HEAD AND NECK**

Use the following Physical Assessment Guide to examine the head and neck of a lab partner, peer, or client. Column 1 will serve as a reminder as to what part of the exam you will do next. Column 2 will be used to record your findings. Your instructor may ask you to turn this in to be evaluated. Forms are also available on thePoint *website.*

Physical Assessment Guide to Collect Objective Client Data

Questions	Findings
1. Gather equipment (gloves, penlight or flashlight, small glass of water, stethoscope).	
2. Explain procedure to client.	
Head and Face	
1. Inspect head for size, shape, and configuration.	
2. Palpate head for consistency while wearing gloves.	
3. Inspect face for symmetry, features, movement, expression, and skin condition.	
4. Palpate temporal artery for tenderness and elasticity.	
5. Palpate temporomandibular joint for range of motion, swelling, tenderness, or crepitation by placing index finger over the front of each and asking client to open mouth. Ask if client has history of frequent headaches.	
Neck	
1. Inspect neck while it is in a slightly extended position (and using a light) for position, symmetry, and presence of lumps and masses.	
2. Inspect movement of thyroid and cricoid cartilage and thyroid gland by having client swallow a small sip of water.	
3. Inspect cervical vertebrae by having client flex neck.	
4. Inspect neck range of motion by having client turn chin to right and left shoulder, touch each ear to the shoulder, touch chin to chest, and lift chin to ceiling.	
5. Palpate trachea by placing your finger in the sternal notch, feeling to each side, and palpating the tracheal rings.	
6. Palpate the thyroid gland.	
7. Auscultate thyroid gland for bruits if the gland is enlarged (use bell of stethoscope).	

Physical Assessment Guide to Collect Objective Client Data (continued)	
Questions	Findings
8. Palpate lymph nodes for size/shape, delimitation, mobility, consistency, and tenderness (refer to display on characteristics of lymph nodes). a. Preauricular nodes (front of ears) b. Postauricular nodes (behind the ears) c. Occipital nodes (posterior base of skull) d. Tonsillar nodes (angle of the mandible, on the anterior edge of the sternocleidomastoid muscle) e. Submandibular nodes (medial border of the mandible); do not confuse with the lobulated submandibular gland f. Submental nodes (a few centimeters behind the tip of the mandible); use one hand g. Superficial cervical nodes (superficial to the sternomastoid muscle) h. Posterior cervical nodes (posterior to the sternocleidomastoid and anterior to the trapezius in the posterior triangle) i. Deep cervical chain nodes (deep within and around the sternomastoid muscle) j. Supraclavicular nodes (hook fingers over clavicles and feel deeply between the clavicles and the sternomastoid muscles)	
Analysis of Data	
1. Formulate nursing diagnoses (wellness, risk, actual).	
2. Formulate collaborative problems.	
3. Make necessary referrals.	

CHAPTER POSTTEST

Activity F MULTIPLE CHOICE QUESTIONS

Choose the one best answer for each of the following multiple choice questions.

____ **1.** The nurse assesses an adult client's head and neck. While examining the carotid arteries, the nurse assesses each artery individually to prevent a

   a. reduction of the blood supply to the brain.

   b. rapid rise in the client's pulse rate.

   c. premature ventricular heart sound.

   d. decreased pulse pressure.

____ **2.** A client visits the outpatient center with a complaint of sudden head and neck pain and stiffness. The client's oral temperature is 37.7 °C (100 °F). The nurse suspects the client is experiencing symptoms of

   a. migraine headache.

   b. meningeal irritation.

   c. trigeminal neuralgia.

   d. otitis media.

Copyright © 2014. Wolters Kluwer Health | Lippincott Williams & Wilkins. Lab Manual for Health Assessment in Nursing, 5e.

_____ **3.** While assessing the head and neck of an adult client, the client tells the nurse that she has been experiencing sharp shooting facial pains that last from 10 to 20 seconds but are occurring more frequently. The nurse should refer the client for possible

    a. cancerous lesions.

    b. arterial occlusion.

    c. inner ear disease.

    d. trigeminal neuralgia.

_____ **4.** A female client visits the clinic and tells the nurse that she frequently experiences severe recurring headaches that sometimes last for several days and are accompanied by nausea and vomiting. The nurse determines that the type of headache the client is describing is a

    a. migraine headache.

    b. cluster headache.

    c. tension headache.

    d. tumor-related headache.

_____ **5.** An adult client visits the clinic and tells the nurse that she has had headaches recently that are intense and stabbing and often occur in the late evening. The nurse should suspect the presence of

    a. cluster headaches.

    b. migraine headaches.

    c. tension headaches.

    d. tumor-related headaches.

_____ **6.** A client visits the clinic and tells the nurse that he is depressed because of a recent job loss. He complains of dull, aching, tight, and diffuse headaches that have lasted for several days. The nurse should recognize that these are symptoms of

    a. cluster headaches.

    b. tumor-related headaches.

    c. migraine headaches.

    d. tension headaches.

_____ **7.** An older client visits the clinic accompanied by his daughter. The daughter tells the nurse that her father has been experiencing severe headaches that usually begin in the morning and become worse when he coughs. The client tells the nurse that he feels dizzy when he has the headaches. The nurse refers the client for further evaluation because these symptoms are characteristic of a

    a. migraine headache.

    b. cluster headache.

    c. tension headache.

    d. tumor-related headache.

_____ **8.** The nurse is preparing to perform a head and neck assessment of an adult client who has immigrated to the United States from Cambodia. The nurse should first

    a. explain to the client why the assessment is necessary.

    b. ask the client if touching the head is permissible.

    c. determine whether the client desires a family member present.

    d. examine the lymph nodes of the neck before examining the head.

_____ **9.** While assessing an adult client's skull, the nurse observes that the client's skull and facial bones are larger and thicker than usual. The nurse should assess the client for

    a. parotid gland enlargement.

    b. acromegaly.

    c. Paget disease.

    d. Cushing syndrome.

_____ 10. While assessing an adult client's head and neck, the nurse observes asymmetry in front of the client's ear lobes. The nurse refers the client to the physician because the nurse suspects the client is most likely experiencing a/an

   a. enlarged thyroid.

   b. lymph node abscess.

   c. neurologic disorder.

   d. parotid gland enlargement.

_____ 11. The nurse is preparing to assess the neck of an adult client. To inspect movement of the client's thyroid gland, the nurse should ask the client to

   a. inhale deeply.

   b. swallow a small sip of water.

   c. cough deeply.

   d. flex the neck to each side.

_____ 12. While assessing an older adult client's neck, the nurse observes that the client's trachea is pulled to the left side. The nurse should

   a. ask the client to flex his neck to the left side.

   b. observe whether the client has difficulty swallowing water.

   c. refer the client to a physician for further evaluation.

   d. palpate the cricoid cartilage for smoothness.

_____ 13. The nurse is planning to assess an adult client's thyroid gland. The nurse should plan to

   a. ask the client to raise the chin.

   b. approach the client posteriorly.

   c. turn the client's neck slightly backward.

   d. place the fingers above the cricoid cartilage.

_____ 14. The nurse is preparing to assess the lymph nodes of an adult client. The nurse should instruct the client to

   a. lie in a supine position.

   b. lie in a side-lying position.

   c. stand upright in front of the nurse.

   d. sit in an upright position.

_____ 15. A female client visits the clinic and tells the nurse that she wants to "stay healthy." The nurse observes that the client has diffuse neck enlargement, is perspiring, and is quite fidgety. The client tells the nurse that she is "hungry all the time, but I have lost weight." A priority nursing diagnosis for the client is

   a. imbalanced nutrition: less than body requirements related to excessive energy level and nervousness.

   b. ineffective health maintenance related to increased metabolism, diaphoresis, and hunger.

   c. health-seeking behaviors related to verbalization of wanting to stay healthy and concerns over weight loss.

   d. thyroid dysfunction related to neck swelling, perspiration, and fidgeting and concern over weight loss.

Activity G CRITICAL THINKING ACTIVITIES

1. Explain how head sizes and shapes vary among different cultures.

2. Discuss the significance of abnormal facial features described as asymmetric, moon-shaped, mask-like, tightened-hard, sunken, or pale and edematous. What underlying conditions may these represent?

3. Marie Lawsome is a 26-year-old woman, who is having frequent headaches in the frontal region of her head. She states that the headaches are dull and aching and have lasted days and occasionally weeks at a time. Ms. Lawsome reports using a warm cloth on her forehead and taking over-the-counter analgesics to help the pain, though the headaches are not always completely relieved.

   a. Describe the type of headache the client is most likely experiencing.

   b. Analyze what type of precipitating factors are likely to be revealed from your interview with Ms. Lawsome.

Copyright © 2014. Wolters Kluwer Health | Lippincott Williams & Wilkins. Lab Manual for Health Assessment in Nursing, 5e.

Activity H   CASE STUDY

Read the following case study. Then, work through the steps of analyzing the case study data. First identify abnormal data and strengths in **subjective and objective findings**, assemble **cue clusters**, draw **inferences**, make possible **nursing diagnoses**, identify **defining characteristics**, **confirm or rule out** the diagnoses, and **document** your conclusions. Use the blank diagnostic analysis charts provided at the end of this book (also available on thePoint website) to guide your thinking. Propose nursing diagnoses that are specific to the client in the case study. Identify collaborative problems, if any, for this client. Finally, identify data, if any, which point toward a medical problem requiring a referral.

Dorothy Grant is a married, 38-year-old, white woman who has come to the office of the school nurse with what she describes as a migraine headache. She is employed by the school system as a music teacher for grades K through 8. She has had a long history of migraine headaches and experienced her first episode at the age of 16. Her father also had migraine headaches until his mid-50s. She is employed full time and is the mother of two school-aged children. She states that she is 162.5 cm (5 ft 4 in) tall and weighs 63.5 kg (140 lb).

Dorothy relates that she has severe throbbing pain in the right temporal region. On a scale of 0 to 5 (with 5 being the worst), she rates her pain as a 4.5. She says she feels nauseated but denies vomiting. Although she is not currently experiencing visual disturbances, she did experience some about 2 hours ago. She describes them as beginning with loss of her central field of vision, followed by flashing lights and then "orange and blue triangles moving from left to right" across her visual field. About an hour later, she experienced the pain. She also reports feeling "a little lightheaded."

She took 600 mg of ibuprofen about 20 minutes ago. She states that sleeping for several hours is the best remedy. Although she usually sleeps well for 7 hours a night, lately she has not been getting adequate sleep and has been "eating cheeseburgers on the run." This is a departure from her usual habit of eating three healthy meals a day with a snack of fruit or popcorn. Dorothy routinely attends a step aerobics class four to five times a week, although she has not attended any classes for the past 2 weeks because of late practices for the annual Christmas program. There is no other history of head or neck problems.

Physical assessment reveals that her skin is warm, pale, and dry to touch. Her voice trembles slightly when she is speaking. Her pulse is 78 beats/minute, her respirations are 24 breaths/minute, her blood pressure is 128/74 mm Hg, and her temperature is 37.1 °C (98.8 °F). Her head and face are round and symmetric, with her head in a central position; no masses are noted. The client demonstrates normal range of motion of the head and neck, with no abnormal movements. The trachea is in the midline; the thyroid gland is nonpalpable. The cervical and supraclavicular lymph nodes are nonpalpable and nontender. The temporal area is tender to touch; the temporal artery is palpated. Test results of cranial nerves V, VII, and XI are normal. Her posture is erect, but she is holding her head with her hand.

How Well Did You Do?

After you have read the chapter and completed the exercises in this chapter, visit thePoint to access the Self-Reflection Activity. This activity will help you identify to what degree you have met each of the chapter objectives. You can then review the chapter for objectives you have met partially or not at all.

Other tools to help you, like the Diagnostic Reasoning Guides, Nursing Interview Guides, Physical Assessment Guides, and NCLEX-Style Chapter Review Questions, are also available on thePoint.

Copyright © 2014. Wolters Kluwer Health | Lippincott Williams & Wilkins. Lab Manual for Health Assessment in Nursing, 5e.

CHAPTER 16

Assessing Eyes

Chapter Overview

Assessment of vision provides important information about the client's ability to interact with the environment because healthy eyes are essential for vision and to perform activities of daily living. Vision informs our lives, permits mobility, and assists learning. People without vision are handicapped indeed. Changes in vision often occur gradually and go unrecognized by clients until a severe problem develops. Thus, an accurate history and exam are essential to detect any abnormalities. Clients may be anxious about their eyes being examined. Therefore it is imperative to explain in detail what you will be doing and answer any questions the client may have. This chapter reviews the structures and functions of the eye and the tests and techniques used by nurses to evaluate a client's visual acuity.

Chapter Learning Objectives

1. Describe the structures and function of the eyes.
2. Discuss the risk factors for cataracts and ways to reduce those risk factors.
3. Interview a client for an accurate nursing history of the eyes and vision.
4. Perform a physical assessment of the eyes and visual acuity correctly using inspection, visual testing, and the ophthalmoscope.
5. Differentiate between normal and abnormal findings of the eyes and visual acuity.
6. Describe the findings frequently seen when assessing the older client's eyes and visual acuity.
7. Analyze the data from the interview and physical assessment of the eyes and visual acuity to formulate valid nursing diagnoses, collaborative problems, and/or referrals.

CHAPTER PRETEST

Activity A MULTIPLE CHOICE QUESTIONS

Choose the one best answer for each of the following multiple choice questions.

_____ 1. The bony orbit and fat cushion of the eye serves as a
   a. caruncle.
   b. channel.
   c. protector.
   d. filter.

_____ 2. The tarsal plates of the upper eyelid contain
   a. meibomian glands.
   b. sebaceous glands.
   c. tear ducts.
   d. ocular muscles.

____ **3.** The conjunctiva of the eye is divided into the palpebral portion and the
   a. canthus portion.
   b. intraocular portion.
   c. nasolacrimal portion.
   d. bulbar portion.

____ **4.** Straight movements of the eye are controlled by the
   a. lacrimal muscles.
   b. oblique muscles.
   c. corneal muscles.
   d. rectus muscles.

____ **5.** The middle layer of the eye is known as the
   a. choroid layer.
   b. scleral layer.
   c. retinal layer.
   d. optic layer.

____ **6.** Photoreceptors of the eye are located in the eye's
   a. ciliary body.
   b. lens.
   c. retina.
   d. pupil.

____ **7.** The meibomian glands secrete
   a. an oily substance to lubricate the eyes.
   b. sweat.
   c. hormones.
   d. clear liquid tears.

____ **8.** The chambers of the eye contain aqueous humor, which helps to maintain intraocular pressure and
   a. transmit light rays.
   b. maintain the retinal vessels.
   c. change refractory of the lens.
   d. cleanse the cornea and the lens.

____ **9.** The optic nerves from each eyeball cross at the
   a. optic chiasma.
   b. vitreous humor.
   c. optic disc.
   d. visual cortex.

____ **10.** The functional reflex that allows the eyes to focus on near objects is termed
   a. pupillary reflex.
   b. accommodation.
   c. refraction.
   d. indirect reflex.

Copyright © 2014. Wolters Kluwer Health | Lippincott Williams & Wilkins. Lab Manual for Health Assessment in Nursing, 5e.

Activity B **LABELING ACTIVITIES**

Label the structures of the external eye in the following figure. Then check your answer with the matching figure, Figure 16-1, Chapter 16 of your textbook.

Label the structures of the lacrimal apparatus in the following figure. Then check your answers with the matching figure, Figure 16-2, in Chapter 16 of your textbook.

Label the structures of the anatomy of the eye in the following figure. Then check your answers with the matching figure, Figure 16-3, in Chapter 16 of your textbook.

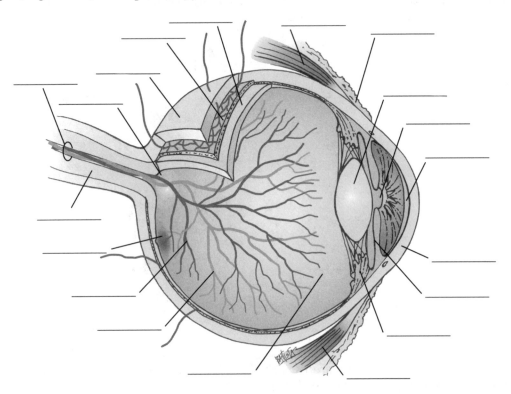

Label the structures of the fundus of the eye in the following figure. Then check your answers with the matching figure, Figure 16-4, in Chapter 16 of your textbook.

Copyright © 2014. Wolters Kluwer Health | Lippincott Williams & Wilkins. Lab Manual for Health Assessment in Nursing, 5e.

Activity C LEARNER ACTIVITIES

After reading Chapter 16, participate in the following learning activities.

1. Review the information in the "EVIDENCE-BASED HEALTH PROMOTION AND DISEASE PREVENTION" boxes on GLAUCOMA, MACULAR DEGENERATION, and CATARACTS on pages 303–306 in your textbook and determine your lab partner's risk for glaucoma, cataracts, or macular degeneration. Discuss ways to reduce these risks.

2. Inspect your lab partner's external eye structures. Describe the eyelids, lashes, position of eyeballs, bulbar conjunctiva and sclera, palpebral conjunctiva, and lacrimal apparatus.

3. Assess your lab partner's pupillary reaction to light and accommodation.

4. Assess your lab partner's vision, using the Snellen chart (see Assessment Guide 16-2, Ophthalmoscope, on page 308 in the textbook). Interpret the results.

5. Assess your lab partner's visual fields. Describe your findings.

6. Obtain an ophthalmoscope in your school lab. Follow the directions in Assessment Guide 16-2 on page 308 in the textbook to turn it on. Operate the apertures to learn how it works. Practice holding it to view your lab partner's red reflex and internal eye structures. Describe the red reflex, optic disc, retinal vessels, retinal background, fovea and macula, and anterior chamber.

Activity D INTERVIEWING AND RECORDING ASSESSMENT FINDINGS

After reading Chapter 16, use the following Nursing Interview Guide to interview and record your subjective findings for an assessment of the eyes and visual acuity of your lab partner, peer, or client. Your instructor may ask you to turn this in to be evaluated. Forms are also available on thePoint *website.*

Nursing Interview Guide to Collect Subjective Data From the Client

Questions	Findings
Current Symptoms	
1. Recent changes in vision?	
2. Spots or floaters in front of eyes?	
3. Blind spots, halos, or rings around lights?	
4. Trouble seeing at night?	
5. Double vision?	
6. Eye pain?	
7. Redness or swelling in eyes?	
8. Excessive watering or tearing or other discharge from eyes?	
Past History	
1. Previous eye or vision problems (medication, surgery, laser treatments, corrective lenses)?	
Family History	
1. Family history of eye problems or vision loss?	
Lifestyle and Health Practices	
1. Exposure to chemicals, fumes, smoke, dust, flying sparks, etc.?	
2. Use of safety glasses?	
3. Use of sunglasses?	

Copyright © 2014. Wolters Kluwer Health | Lippincott Williams & Wilkins. Lab Manual for Health Assessment in Nursing, 5e.

Nursing Interview Guide to Collect Subjective Data From the Client (continued)

Questions	Findings
4. Medications (corticosteroids, lovastatin, pyridostigmine, quinidine, risperdal, and rifampin) may have ocular side effects?	
5. Has vision loss affected ability to work or care for self or others?	
6. Date of last eye examination?	
7. Have glasses or contacts? Are they worn regularly?	
8. Live or work around frequent or continuous loud noise?	
9. Use of ear protection from noise or while in water?	

Activity E   PERFORMING PHYSICAL ASSESSMENT OF THE EYES AND VISUAL ACUITY

Use the following Physical Assessment Guide to examine the eyes and visual acuity of a lab partner, peer, or client. Column 1 will serve as a reminder as to what part of the exam you will do next. Column 2 will be used to record your findings. Your instructor may ask you to turn this in to be evaluated. Forms are also available on thePoint *website.*

Questions	Findings
1. Gather equipment (Snellen chart, handheld Snellen chart or near vision screener, penlight, opaque card, and ophthalmoscope).	
2. Explain procedures to client.	
Perform Vision Tests	
1. Distant visual acuity (with Snellen chart, normal acuity is 20/20 with or without corrective lenses).	
2. Near visual acuity (with a handheld vision chart, normal acuity is 14/14 with or without corrective lenses).	
3. Visual fields (use procedure discussed in textbook to test peripheral vision).	
Perform Extraocular Muscle Function Tests	
1. Corneal light reflex (using a penlight to observe parallel alignment of light reflection on corneas).	
2. Cover test (using an opaque card to cover an eye to observe for eye movement).	
3. Positions test (observing for eye movement).	
External Eye Structures	
1. Inspect eyelids and lashes (width and position of palpebral fissures, ability to close eyelids, direction of eyelids in comparison with eyeballs, color, swelling, lesions, or discharge).	

Copyright © 2014. Wolters Kluwer Health | Lippincott Williams & Wilkins. Lab Manual for Health Assessment in Nursing, 5e.

Questions	Findings
2. Inspect positioning of eyeballs (alignment in sockets, protruding or sunken).	
3. Inspect bulbar conjunctiva and sclera (clarity, color, and texture).	
4. Inspect the palpebral conjunctive (eversion of upper eyelid is usually performed only with complaints of eye pain or sensation of something in eye).	
5. Inspect the lacrimal apparatus over the lacrimal glands (lateral aspect of upper eyelid) and the puncta (medial aspect of lower eyelid). Observe for swelling, redness, or drainage.	
6. Palpate the lacrimal apparatus, noting drainage from the puncta when palpating the nasolacrimal duct.	
7. Inspect the cornea and lens by shining a light to determine transparency.	
8. Inspect the iris and pupil for shape and color of the iris and size and shape of the pupil.	
9. Test pupillary reaction to light (in a darkened room, have client focus on a distant object, shine a light obliquely into the pupil, and observe the pupil's reaction to light—normally, pupils constrict).	
10. Test accommodation of pupils by shifting gaze from far to near (normally, pupils constrict).	
Internal Eye Structure	
1. Inspect the red reflex by using an ophthalmoscope to shine the light beam toward the client's pupil (normally, a red reflex is easily seen and should appear round with regular borders).	
2. Inspect the optic disc by using the ophthalmoscope focused on the pupil and moving very close to the eye. Rotate the diopter setting until the retinal structures are in sharp focus (observe disc for shape, color, size, and physiologic cup).	
3. Inspect the retinal vessels using the above technique (observe vessels for numbers of sets, color, diameter, arteriovenous ratio, and arteriovenous crossings).	
4. Inspect retinal background for color and the presence of lesions.	
5. Inspect the fovea and macula for lesions.	
6. Inspect the anterior chamber for transparency.	
Analysis of Data	
1. Formulate nursing diagnoses (health promotion, risk, actual).	
2. Formulate collaborative problems.	
3. Make necessary referrals.	

Copyright © 2014. Wolters Kluwer Health | Lippincott Williams & Wilkins. Lab Manual for Health Assessment in Nursing, 5e.

CHAPTER POSTTEST

Activity F **MULTIPLE CHOICE QUESTIONS**

Choose the one best answer for each of the following multiple choice questions.

_____ 1. While assessing the eyes of an adult client, the nurse uses a wisp of cotton to stimulate the client's
a. eyelid reflexes.
b. refractory mechanism.
c. lacrimal reflexes.
d. corneal reflexes.

_____ 2. An adult client visits the clinic and tells the nurse that she has had a sudden change in her vision. The nurse should explain to the client that sudden changes in vision are often associated with
a. diabetes.
b. the aging process.
c. hypertension.
d. head trauma.

_____ 3. An adult client tells the nurse that he has been experiencing gradual vision loss. The nurse should
a. ask about the client's diet.
b. determine whether there is a history of glaucoma.
c. check the client's blood pressure.
d. ask the client if he has any known allergies.

_____ 4. A 45-year-old client tells the nurse that he occasionally sees spots in front of his eyes. The nurse should
a. tell the client that these often occur with aging.
b. refer the client to an ophthalmologist.
c. re-examine the client in 2 weeks.
d. assess the client for signs of diabetes.

_____ 5. An adult client tells the nurse that her peripheral vision is not what it used to be and she has a blind spot in her left eye. The nurse should refer the client for evaluation of possible
a. glaucoma.
b. increased intracranial pressure.
c. bacterial infection.
d. migraine headaches.

_____ 6. A client visits the local clinic after experiencing head trauma. The client tells the nurse that he has a consistent blind spot in his right eye. The nurse should
a. examine the area of head trauma.
b. refer the client to an ophthalmologist.
c. assess the client for double vision.
d. ask the client if he sees "halos."

_____ 7. A client tells the nurse that she has difficulty seeing while driving at night. The nurse should explain to the client that night blindness is often associated with
a. retinal deterioration.
b. head trauma.
c. migraine headaches.
d. vitamin A deficiency.

____ 8. An adult client visits the clinic and tells the nurse that he has been experiencing double vision for the past few days. The nurse refers the client to a physician for evaluation of possible
   a. glaucoma.
   b. increased intracranial pressure.
   c. hypertension.
   d. ophthalmic migraine.

____ 9. An adult client tells the nurse that she frequently experiences burning and itching of both eyes. The nurse should assess the client for
   a. a foreign body.
   b. recent trauma.
   c. blind spots.
   d. allergies.

____ 10. An adult client visits the outpatient clinic and tells the nurse that he has a throbbing aching pain in his right eye. The nurse should assess the client for
   a. recent exposure to irritants.
   b. increased intracranial pressure.
   c. excessive tearing.
   d. a foreign body in the eye.

____ 11. An adult client visits the clinic and tells the nurse that he has had excessive tearing in his left eye. The nurse should assess the client's eye for
   a. viral infection.
   b. double vision.
   c. allergic reactions.
   d. lacrimal obstruction.

____ 12. The nurse is caring for a healthy adult client with no history of vision problems. The nurse should tell the client that a thorough eye examination is recommended every
   a. year.
   b. 2 years.
   c. 3 years.
   d. 4 years.

____ 13. An adult client tells the nurse that his eyes are painful because he left his contact lenses in too long the day before yesterday. The nurse should instruct the client that prolonged wearing of contact lenses can lead to
   a. retinal damage.
   b. cataracts.
   c. myopia.
   d. corneal damage.

____ 14. An adult client tells the nurse that his father had cataracts. He asks the nurse about risk factors for cataracts. The nurse should instruct the client that a potential risk factor is
   a. lack of vitamin C in the diet.
   b. ultraviolet light exposure.
   c. obesity.
   d. use of antibiotics.

____ 15. The nurse is preparing to examine an adult client's eyes, using a Snellen chart. The nurse should
   a. position the client 609.6 cm (20 ft) away from the chart.
   b. ask the client to remove his glasses.
   c. ask the client to read each line with both eyes open.
   d. instruct the client to begin reading from the bottom of the chart.

Copyright © 2014. Wolters Kluwer Health | Lippincott Williams & Wilkins. Lab Manual for Health Assessment in Nursing, 5e.

___ **16.** A client has tested 20/40 on the distant visual acuity test using a Snellen chart. The nurse should

    a. document the results in the client's record.

    b. ask the client to read a handheld vision chart.

    c. ask the client to return in 2 weeks for another examination.

    d. refer the client to an optometrist.

___ **17.** The nurse has tested an adult client's visual fields and determined that the temporal field is 90 degrees in both eyes. The nurse should

    a. refer the client for further evaluation.

    b. examine the client for other signs of glaucoma.

    c. ask the client if there is a genetic history of blindness.

    d. document the findings in the client's records.

___ **18.** The nurse has tested the near visual acuity of a 45-year-old client. The nurse explains to the client that the client has impaired near vision and discusses a possible reason for the condition. The nurse determines that the client has understood the instructions when the client says that presbyopia is usually due to

    a. congenital cataracts.

    b. decreased accommodation.

    c. muscle weakness.

    d. constant misalignment of the eyes.

___ **19.** While assessing the eye of an adult client, the nurse observes an inward turning of the client's left eye. The nurse should document the client's

    a. esotropia.

    b. strabismus.

    c. phoria.

    d. exotropia.

___ **20.** The nurse is examining an adult client's eyes. The nurse has explained the positions test to the client. The nurse determines that the client needs further instructions when the client says that the positions test

    a. assesses the muscle strength of the eye.

    b. assesses the functioning of the cranial nerves innervating the eye muscles.

    c. requires the covering of each eye separately.

    d. requires the client to focus on an object.

Activity G CRITICAL THINKING ACTIVITY

A 62-year-old woman, arrives for an eye examination complaining of blurred vision. You find out from the nursing history that she has smoked a half pack of cigarettes a day for 30 years and spends a lot of time at the beach. She also tells you that she is taking medication for high blood pressure but often forgets to take it.

Describe what areas you will focus on during her eye examination, and analyze her possible risk factors for eye disorders.

Copyright © 2014. Wolters Kluwer Health | Lippincott Williams & Wilkins. Lab Manual for Health Assessment in Nursing, 5e.

Activity H CASE STUDY

Read the following case study. Then, work through the steps of analyzing the case study data. First identify abnormal data and strengths in **subjective and objective findings**, assemble **cue clusters**, draw **inferences**, make possible **nursing diagnoses**, identify **defining characteristics**, **confirm or rule out** the diagnoses, and **document** your conclusions. Use the blank diagnostic analysis charts provided at the end of this book (also available on thePoint website) to guide your thinking. Propose nursing diagnoses that are specific to the client in the case study. Identify collaborative problems, if any, for this client. Finally, identify data, if any, which point toward a medical problem requiring a referral.

Mrs. Hira is a 68-year-old woman, of Indian descent who comes to the community outpatient clinic for evaluation because she states that she "can't see as well as I used to." She has been retired from the telephone company for 3 years. Her 71-year-old husband had a major stroke 1 year ago, and she is solely responsible for his care. They live in a small one-story house and have a car, which Mrs. Hira uses for grocery shopping and to go to church. Their daughter and her family live 321.8 km (200 miles) away.

When interviewed, Mrs. Hira reports progressive changes in her vision over the past 5 months. She reports changes in her vision as "blurring that seems to be getting worse" and reports a halo effect at night when looking at lights. She said that she does not drive much at night anymore because of this. She has worn glasses for reading for the past 20 years. She denies eye pain, swelling, excessive tearing, or discharge. Mrs. Hira says that she had an eye examination 4 years ago. She states that she has never experienced any trauma to her eyes or head and has never had any serious eye problems or surgery. She does not know of any family history of eye problems.

Your physical assessment reveals distant visual acuity in the right eye (OD) 20/40, in the left eye (OS) 20/40. No lid lag is noted. The extraocular muscles are intact. The visual fields are equal to the examiner's. No excessive tearing or blinking is noted. The conjunctivae are smooth and without redness. The pupils are bilaterally round, equal in size, and reactive to light and accommodation. No nystagmus is noted. You are unable to assess the red reflex or perform an ophthalmic examination because of bilateral opacities of the lens.

How Well Did You Do?

After you have read the chapter and completed the exercises in this chapter, visit thePoint to access the Self-Reflection Activity. This activity will help you identify to what degree you have met each of the chapter objectives. You can then review the chapter for objectives you have met partially or not at all.

Other tools to help you, like the Diagnostic Reasoning Guides, Nursing Interview Guides, Physical Assessment Guides, and NCLEX-Style Chapter Review Questions, are also available on thePoint.

Copyright © 2014. Wolters Kluwer Health | Lippincott Williams & Wilkins. Lab Manual for Health Assessment in Nursing, 5e.

CHAPTER 17

Assessing Ears

Chapter Overview

The sense organ of hearing and equilibrium is the ear, which consists of the external ear, the middle ear, and the inner ear. Healthy ears are essential to effective communication and balance. When the nurse first meets the client, cues of hearing ability provide important information about the client's interaction with others and the environment. This assessment should be explained thoroughly to guarantee accurate results and to ease any client anxiety. This chapter reviews the structure and functions connected with hearing and balance as well as the techniques used in physical assessment of hearing acuity and sound conduction.

Chapter Learning Objectives

1. Describe the functions and the structures of the ear.
2. Discuss the risk factors for hearing loss across cultures and ways to reduce one's risks.
3. Interview a client for an accurate nursing history of the ears and hearing.
4. Perform a physical assessment of the ears and hearing ability using the correct techniques.
5. Correctly use the otoscope to inspect the auditory canal and the tympanic membrane.
6. Differentiate between normal and abnormal findings of the ear and hearing.
7. Describe the findings frequently seen when assessing the older client's ears and hearing.
8. Analyze the data from the interview and physical assessment of the ears and hearing to formulate valid nursing diagnoses, collaborative problems, and/or referrals.

CHAPTER PRETEST

Activity A MULTIPLE CHOICE QUESTIONS

Choose the one best answer for each of the following multiple choice questions.

_____ 1. The cone of light is located in the

   a. inner ear.

   b. middle ear.

   c. external ear.

   d. semicircular canal.

_____ 2. The ossicles contained in the middle ear include the malleus, the incus, and the

   a. pars tensa.

   b. pars flaccida.

   c. umbo.

   d. stapes.

_____ **3.** Sensory receptors in the ear that help to maintain both static and dynamic equilibrium are located in the semicircular canals and the

    a. vestibule.

    b. tympanic membrane.

    c. cone of light.

    d. eustachian tube.

_____ **4.** In the hearing pathway, hair cells of the spiral organ of Corti are stimulated by movement of

    a. fluid.

    b. sound.

    c. air.

    d. bone.

_____ **5.** Transmission of sound waves in the inner ear is known as

    a. conductive hearing.

    b. tympanic hearing.

    c. neuromotor hearing.

    d. perceptive hearing.

Activity B LABELING ACTIVITIES

Label the structures of the ear in the following figure that illustrates the external, middle, and inner ear. Match your answers with Figure 17-1 on page 329 of your textbook.

Label the structures of the tympanic membrane in the following figure. Then check your answer with Figure 17-2A on page 329 of your textbook.

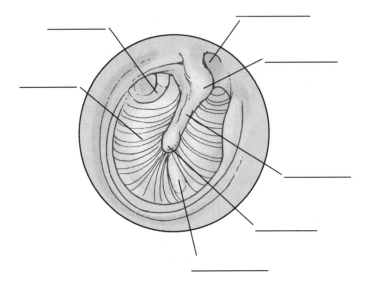

Label the pathways of hearing in the following figure. Then check your answer with Figure 17-3 on page 330 in your textbook.

Activity C LEARNER ACTIVITIES

After reading Chapter 17, participate in the following learning activities.

1. Use Box 17-1: TEN WAYS TO RECOGNIZE HEARING LOSS, on page 333 of your textbook to assess your own hearing ability.

2. Obtain a tuning fork. Practice using it after reading the instructions in your textbook (see pages 338–339). Explain how to perform both the Weber test and the Rinne test, and discuss the significance of each. Perform the Weber and Rinne tests on your lab partner and record your findings.

3. Obtain an otoscope. Read ASSESSMENT GUIDE 17-1: OTOSCOPE on page 335 of your textbook. Practice handling and operating the otoscope before using it to inspect the eardrum of your lab partner. Follow the instructions in your book taking caution to follow the safety measures. Record your findings.

4. Examine the ears of an elderly client, friend, or relative, and report your findings. Compare your findings with the variation of findings in the elderly discussed in the textbook.

Copyright © 2014. Wolters Kluwer Health | Lippincott Williams & Wilkins. Lab Manual for Health Assessment in Nursing, 5e.

Activity D INTERVIEWING AND RECORDING ASSESSMENT FINDINGS

After reading Chapter 17, use the following Nursing Interview Guide to interview and record your subjective findings for an assessment of the ears of a lab partner, peer, or client. Your instructor may ask you to turn this in to be evaluated. Forms are also available on thePoint *website.*

Nursing Interview Guide to Collect Subjective Data From the Client	
Questions	**Findings**
Current Symptoms	
1. Recent changes in hearing (if yes, were all or just some sounds affected)?	
2. Ear discharge (if yes, amount/odor)?	
3. Ear pain (if yes, is there accompanying sore throat, sinus infection, or problem with teeth or gums)?	
4. Ringing or crackling in ears?	
Past History	
1. Previous ear or hearing problems such as infections, trauma, or earaches (medications, surgery, hearing aids)?	
Family History	
1. Family history of ear problems or hearing loss?	
Lifestyle and Health Practices	
1. Live or work around frequent or continuous loud noise?	
2. Use of ear protection from noise or while in water?	
3. Has hearing loss affected ability to work or care for self or others?	

Activity E PERFORMING PHYSICAL ASSESSMENT OF THE EARS

Use the following Physical Assessment Guide to examine the ears of a lab partner, peer, or client. Column 1 will serve as a reminder as to what part of the exam you will do next. Column 2 will be used to record your findings. Your instructor may ask you to turn this in to be evaluated. Forms are also available on thePoint *website.*

Physical Assessment Guide to Collect Objective Client Data	
Questions	**Findings**
External Ear Structures	
1. Inspect the auricle, tragus, and lobule for size and shape, position, lesions/discoloration, and discharge.	
2. Palpate the auricle and mastoid process for tenderness.	
Otoscopic Examination	
1. Inspect the external auditory canal with the otoscope for discharge, color and consistency of cerumen, color and consistency of canal walls, and nodules.	
2. Inspect the tympanic membrane, using the otoscope, for color and shape, consistency, and landmarks.	

Copyright © 2014. Wolters Kluwer Health | Lippincott Williams & Wilkins. Lab Manual for Health Assessment in Nursing, 5e.

Physical Assessment Guide to Collect Objective Client Data (continued)

Questions	Findings
3. Have the client perform the Valsalva maneuver, and observe the center of the tympanic membrane for a flutter. (Do not do this procedure on an older client, as it may interfere with equilibrium and cause dizziness.)	
Hearing and Equilibrium Tests	
1. Perform the whisper test by having the client place a finger on the tragus of one ear. Whisper a two-syllable word 30.4–60.9 cm (1–2 ft) behind the client. Repeat on the other ear.	
2. Perform the Weber test by using a tuning fork placed on the center of the head or forehead and asking whether the client hears the sound better in one ear or the same in both ears.	
3. Perform the Rinne test by using a tuning fork and placing the base on the client's mastoid process. When the client no longer hears the sound, note the time interval, and move it in front of the external ear. When the client no longer hears a sound, note the time interval.	
4. Perform the Romberg test to evaluate equilibrium. With feet together and arms at the side, close eyes for 20 seconds. Observe for swaying. (Refer to textbook, Chapters 16 and 26.)	
Analysis of Data	
1. Formulate nursing diagnoses (wellness, risk, actual).	
2. Formulate collaborative problems.	
3. Make necessary referrals.	

CHAPTER POSTTEST

Activity F MULTIPLE CHOICE QUESTIONS

Choose the one best answer for each of the following multiple choice questions.

_____ 1. An adult client visits the clinic and complains of tinnitus. The nurse should ask the client if she has been
   a. dizzy.
   b. hypotensive.
   c. taking antibiotics.
   d. experiencing ear drainage.

_____ 2. An adult client tells the nurse that his 80-year-old father is almost completely deaf. After an explanation to the client about risk factors for hearing loss, the nurse determines that the client needs further instruction when the client says
   a. "There is a genetic predisposition to hearing loss."
   b. "Certain cultural groups have a higher rate of hearing loss."
   c. "It is difficult to prevent hearing loss or worsening of hearing."
   d. "Chronic otitis media has been associated with hearing loss."

Copyright © 2014. Wolters Kluwer Health | Lippincott Williams & Wilkins. Lab Manual for Health Assessment in Nursing, 5e.

_____ **3.** The nurse is planning to perform an ear examination on an adult client. After explaining the procedures to the client, the nurse should

    a. ask the client to remain standing.

    b. show the client the otoscope.

    c. ask the client to remove his contact lenses.

    d. observe the client's response to the explanations.

_____ **4.** The nurse is preparing to examine the ears of an adult client with an otoscope. The nurse should plan to

    a. ask the client to tilt the head slightly forward.

    b. release the auricle during the examination.

    c. use a speculum that measures 10 mm in diameter.

    d. firmly pull the auricle out, up, and back.

_____ **5.** While assessing the ears of an adult client, the nurse observes bloody drainage in the client's ear. The nurse should

    a. document the finding in the client's chart.

    b. determine whether a foreign body is present in the ear.

    c. assess the client for further signs of otitis media.

    d. refer the client to a physician.

_____ **6.** While assessing the ears of an adult client, the nurse observes that the tympanic membrane is completely immobile. The nurse should further assess the client for signs and symptoms of

    a. infection.

    b. skull injury.

    c. vestibular disorders.

    d. healed perforations.

_____ **7.** The nurse is planning to conduct the Weber test on an adult male client. To perform this test, the nurse should plan to

    a. strike a tuning fork and place it at the base of the client's mastoid process.

    b. whisper a word with two distinct syllables to the client.

    c. ask the client to close his eyes while standing with feet together.

    d. strike a tuning fork and place it on the center of the client's head or forehead.

_____ **8.** The nurse has performed the Rinne test on an older adult client. After the test, the client reports that her bone conduction sound was heard longer than the air conduction sound. The nurse determines that the client is most likely experiencing

    a. normal hearing.

    b. sensorineural hearing loss.

    c. conductive hearing loss.

    d. central hearing loss.

_____ **9.** The transmission of sound waves through the external ear and the middle ear is known as

    a. perceptive hearing.

    b. conductive hearing.

    c. external hearing.

    d. connective hearing.

_____ **10.** After examining the client's tympanic membranes, the nurse documents "Right tympanic membrane, red and bulging with no light reflex." The nurse recognizes that these are signs of

    a. acute otitis media.

    b. serous otitis media.

    c. skull trauma.

    d. trauma from infection.

Copyright © 2014. Wolters Kluwer Health | Lippincott Williams & Wilkins. Lab Manual for Health Assessment in Nursing, 5e.

Activity G **MATCHING**

Match the terms in the left column with the correct descriptions in the right column.

Term

____ **1.** Conductive hearing

____ **2.** Perceptive or sensorineural hearing

____ **3.** Presbycusis

____ **4.** Otorrhea

____ **5.** Otalgia

____ **6.** Tinnitus

____ **7.** Vertigo

____ **8.** Swimmer's ear

____ **9.** Cerumen

____ **10.** Umbo

Description

a. Gradual hearing loss

b. Infection of the ear canal

c. Drainage from the ear

d. Ringing in the ears

e. Earache

f. Ear wax

g. Transmission of sound waves through the external and middle ear

h. True spinning motion

i. Base of the malleus but also serves as a center point landmark

j. Transmission of sound waves in the inner ear

Activity H **CRITICAL THINKING ACTIVITIES**

1. Discuss what may be occurring if tenderness is noted when palpating the mastoid process during the ear exam.

2. Discuss ethnic variations that may be found during the ear exam.

3. Discuss the differences between conductive and sensorineural hearing.

4. Explain the meaning of the findings identified during a Weber test and a Rinne test.

Activity I **CASE STUDY**

Read the following case study. Then, work through the steps of analyzing the case study data. First identify abnormal data and strengths in **subjective and objective findings**, assemble **cue clusters**, draw **inferences**, make possible **nursing diagnoses**, identify **defining characteristics**, **confirm or rule out** the diagnoses, and **document** your conclusions. Use the blank diagnostic analysis charts provided at the end of this book (also available on thePoint website) to guide your thinking. Propose nursing diagnoses that are specific to the client in the case study. Identify collaborative problems, if any, for this client. Finally, identify data, if any, which point toward a medical problem requiring a referral.

Jack Jones, a 28-year-old man, currently works in an industrial plant as a supervisor. He has noticed lately that he is having trouble hearing conversations with his friends, but of even more concern is that he misunderstands his workers when they are giving him information about the projects they are working on. He denies any major current or past illnesses—"just the kid stuff, you know, colds and fevers. I do have trouble with ringing in my ears." He admits that when he was in his teens he frequently attended music concerts that were often loud, and he still goes occasionally. He tells you that he likes to listen to loud—"the louder the better"—rock music, using tight earphones. When he watches TV in the evening, he has to turn up the volume to hear clearly.

He denies any ear drainage or pain and has not experienced any spinning sensations. He states he had one ear infection several years ago and had several ear infections as a young child. Has had no surgeries and does not use a hearing aid device. He mows his lawn once a week on a riding mower and does wood working with loud saws in his home. He does not wear protective ear plugs during these activities. His last hearing examination was as a child in grade school.

Upon examination, the nurse observes the following.

Ears equal size bilaterally. Auricles line up within a 10-degree angle of vertical position. Auricles, tragus, and lobules smooth, no lumps, lesions, or nodules. No ear discharge. Mastoid process nontender on palpation. Small amount of moist, yellow cerumen in external canals, no nodules present. Tympanic membranes grey, transparent, no bulging or retraction, scarring noted on left tympanic membrane. Cone-shaped light reflex in 5-o'clock position in right ear and 7-o'clock position in left ear. Short process, handle of malleus, and umbo visible in both ears. Whisper test: Client unable to repeat two-syllable whispered word. Weber Test: sound lateralizes to right ear. Rinne Test: air conduction (AC) > bone conduction (BC) both ears. Romberg Test: Maintains position for 20 seconds without swaying.

Copyright © 2014. Wolters Kluwer Health | Lippincott Williams & Wilkins. Lab Manual for Health Assessment in Nursing, 5e.

How Well Did You Do?

After you have read the chapter and completed the exercises in this chapter, visit thePoint to access the Self-Reflection Activity. This activity will help you identify to what degree you have met each of the chapter objectives. You can then review the chapter for objectives you have met partially or not at all.

Other tools to help you, like the Diagnostic Reasoning Guides, Nursing Interview Guides, Physical Assessment Guides, and NCLEX-Style Chapter Review Questions, are also available on thePoint.

Copyright © 2014. Wolters Kluwer Health | Lippincott Williams & Wilkins. Lab Manual for Health Assessment in Nursing, 5e.

Assessing Mouth, Throat, Nose, and Sinuses

Chapter Overview

The mouth, throat, nose, and sinuses are the structures associated with eating, smell and taste, swallowing, speech, and purifying and warming the air that is transported to the lungs. Use the following activities and quizzes to review the structure and function of these very important tissues.

Chapter Learning Objectives

1. Describe the structure and functions of the mouth, throat, nose, and sinuses.
2. Discuss the risk factors for oral cancer across cultures and ways to reduce one's risks.
3. Interview a client for an accurate nursing history of the mouth, throat, nose, and sinuses.
4. Perform an accurate assessment of the mouth, throat, nose, and sinuses.
5. Differentiate between normal and abnormal findings of the mouth, throat, nose, and sinuses.
6. Describe the cultural variations seen with assessment findings of the mouth, throat, nose, and sinuses.
7. Describe the findings frequently seen when assessing the older client's mouth, throat, nose, and sinuses.
8. Analyze the data from the interview and physical assessment of the nose, mouth, throat, and sinuses to formulate valid nursing diagnoses, collaborative problems, and/or referrals.

CHAPTER PRETEST

Activity A MULTIPLE CHOICE QUESTIONS

Choose the one best answer for each of the following multiple choice questions.

_____ 1. The roof of the oral cavity of the mouth is formed by the anterior hard palate and the
   a. teeth.
   b. gums.
   c. muscles.
   d. soft palate.

_____ 2. An extension of the soft palate of the mouth, which hangs in the posterior midline of the oropharynx, is the
   a. uvula.
   b. frenulum.
   c. taste buds.
   d. sublingual fold.

____ **3.** The tongue is attached to the hyoid bone and styloid process of the temporal bone and is connected to the floor of the mouth by the

    a. mandible.

    b. frenulum.

    c. gums.

    d. soft palate.

____ **4.** The submandibular glands open under the tongue through openings called

    a. parasinal ducts.

    b. Stensen ducts.

    c. Wharton ducts.

    d. lacrimonasal ducts.

____ **5.** The rich blood supply of the nose serves to

    a. help propel moist air to the body.

    b. propel debris to the throat.

    c. filter large particles from the air.

    d. warm the inspired air.

Activity B MATCHING

Match the terms in the left column with the correct descriptions in the right column.

Term

____ **1.** Transillumination

____ **2.** Palpation and percussion

____ **3.** Kiesselbach area

____ **4.** Stensen ducts

____ **5.** Wharton ducts

____ **6.** Side of tongue

____ **7.** Torus palatinus

____ **8.** Bifid uvula

____ **9.** Grade 3 tonsils

____ **10.** Method for assessing the internal nose

____ **11.** Method used to palpate frontal sinuses

____ **12.** Method used to palpate maxillary sinuses

____ **13.** Significance of a red glow with transillumination

____ **14.** Absence of a red glow with transillumination

____ **15.** Cheilosis

____ **16.** Lip pits

Description

a. Press up with thumbs on sinuses

b. Touch the uvula

c. Most common site of tongue cancer

d. Cracking at the corner of the lips seen in riboflavin deficiency

e. Method used to test for fluid in the sinuses

f. Sinus filled with air

g. Inspection using otoscope with short wide tip attachment

h. Methods used to test for sinus tenderness

i. Press up on brow on each side of the nose

j. Openings found on buccal mucosa across from second upper molars

k. Bony protuberance in the midline of the hard palate

l. Sinus filled with fluid or pus

m. Common site of nasal bleeding

n. A variation that looks split or partially severed and may be associated with a submucous cleft palate

o. Normal variation that occurs in the crease between the upper and the lower lip

p. Openings found on either side of the frenulum of the floor of the mouth

Copyright © 2014. Wolters Kluwer Health | Lippincott Williams & Wilkins. Lab Manual for Health Assessment in Nursing, 5e.

Activity C **LABELING ACTIVITIES**

Label the structures of the mouth in the following figure. Check your answers with Figure 18-1 on page 347 in the textbook.

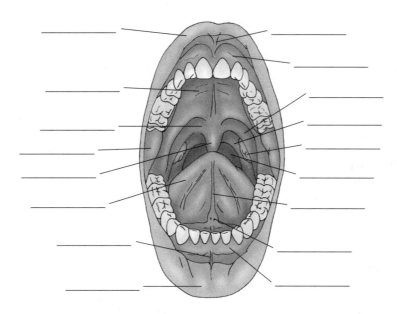

Label the teeth in the following figure. Check your answers with Figure 18-2 on page 347 in the textbook.

Label the structures of the salivary glands in the following figure. Check your answers with Figure 18-3 on page 347 in the textbook.

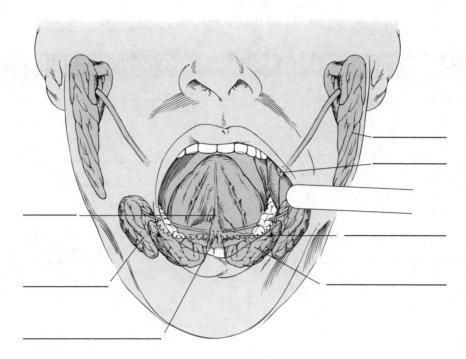

Label the structures of the nasal cavity and throat in the following figure. Check your answers with Figure 18-4 on page 347 in the textbook.

Activity D LEARNER ACTIVITIES

After reading Chapter 18 in the textbook, participate in the following learning activities.

1. Review the information in EVIDENCE-BASED HEALTH PROMOTION AND DISEASE PREVENTION: OROPHARYNGEAL CANCER (see pages 348–349 in your textbook). Determine your own risk for mouth cancer. Next, identify ethnic groups that are at highest risk for mouth cancer. Discuss what teaching could be implemented to reduce these risks.

2. Perform an assessment of the mouth, throat, nose, and sinuses on an elderly client, friend, or relative. Discuss with peers your findings as they compare with those of a younger person's mouth, throat, nose, and sinuses.

Copyright © 2014. Wolters Kluwer Health | Lippincott Williams & Wilkins. Lab Manual for Health Assessment in Nursing, 5e.

Activity E   **INTERVIEWING AND RECORDING ASSESSMENT FINDINGS**

After reading Chapter 18 in the textbook, use the following Nursing Interview Guide to interview and record your subjective findings for an assessment of the mouth, throat, nose, and sinuses of a lab partner, peer, or client. Your instructor may ask you to turn this in to be evaluated. Forms are also available on thePoint *website.*

Nursing Interview Guide to Collect Subjective Data From the Client	
Questions	Findings
Current Symptoms	
1. Mouth problems (tongue or mouth sores or lesions, gum or mouth redness, swelling, bleeding, or pain)?	
2. Sinus problems (pain over sinuses, postnasal drip)?	
3. Nose problems (nosebleeds, stuffy nose, cannot breath through one or both nostrils, change in ability to smell or taste)?	
Past History	
1. Previous problems with mouth, throat, nose, or sinuses (surgeries or treatment; how much and how often)?	
2. Use of nasal sprays?	
3. History of tooth grinding?	
4. Last dental exam? Fit of dentures?	
Family History	
1. Family history of oral, nasal, or sinus cancer or chronic problems?	
Lifestyle and Health Practices	
1. Daily practice of oral care, tooth care, or denture care?	
2. Usual diet?	
3. History of smoking, use of, how much, and how often?	
4. Use of alcohol (how much and how often)?	

Activity F   **PERFORMING PHYSICAL ASSESSMENT OF THE MOUTH, THROAT, NOSE, AND SINUSES**

Use the following Physical Assessment Guide to examine the mouth, throat, nose, and sinuses of a lab partner, peer, or client. Column 1 will serve as a reminder as to what part of the exam you will do next. Column 2 will be used to record your findings. Your instructor may ask you to turn this in to be evaluated. Forms are also available on thePoint *website.*

Physical Assessment Guide to Collect Objective Client Data	
Questions	Findings
Current Symptoms	
1. Gather equipment (gloves, cotton gauze pads, penlight, speculum attached to otoscope, tongue blade).	
2. Explain the procedure to client.	

Copyright © 2014. Wolters Kluwer Health | Lippincott Williams & Wilkins. Lab Manual for Health Assessment in Nursing, 5e.

Physical Assessment Guide to Collect Objective Client Data (continued)

Questions	Findings
Mouth	
1. Note any distinctive odors.	
2. Inspect and palpate lips, buccal mucosa, gums, and tongue for color variations (pallor, redness, white patches, bluish hue), moisture, tissue consistency, or lesions (induration, roughness, vesicles, crusts, plaques, nodules, ulcers, cracking, patches, bleeding, Koplik spots, cancer sores), Stensen and Wharton ducts.	
3. Inspect gums for hyperplasia, blue-black line.	
4. Inspect teeth for number and shape, color (white, brown, yellow, chalky white areas), occlusion.	
5. Inspect and palpate tongue for color, texture, and consistency (black, hairy, white patches, smooth, reddish, shiny without papillae), moisture, and size (enlarged or very small).	
Throat	
1. Inspect the throat for color, consistency, torus palatinus, uvula (singular).	
2. Inspect the tonsils for color and consistency; grading scale (1+, 2+, 3+, 4+).	
Nose	
1. Inspect and palpate the external nose for color, shape, consistency, tenderness, and patency of airflow.	
2. Inspect the internal nose for color, swelling, exudate, bleeding, ulcers, perforated septum, or polyps.	
Sinuses	
1. Palpate the sinuses for tenderness.	
2. Percuss and transilluminate the sinuses for air versus fluid or pus.	
Analysis of Data	
1. Formulate nursing diagnoses (wellness, risk, actual).	
2. Formulate collaborative problems.	
3. Make necessary referrals.	

Copyright © 2014. Wolters Kluwer Health | Lippincott Williams & Wilkins. Lab Manual for Health Assessment in Nursing, 5e.

CHAPTER POSTTEST

Activity G **MULTIPLE CHOICE QUESTIONS**

Choose the one best answer for each of the following multiple choice questions.

_____ 1. The nurse is preparing to examine the sinuses of an adult client. After examining the frontal sinuses, the nurse should proceed to examine the

    a. ethmoidal sinuses.

    b. laryngeal sinuses.

    c. maxillary sinuses.

    d. sphenoidal sinuses.

_____ 2. An adult client visits the clinic complaining of recurrent ulcers in the mouth. The nurse assesses the client's mouth and observes a painful ulcer. The nurse should document the presence of

    a. a cancerous lesion.

    b. *Candida albicans* infection.

    c. an oral ulceration.

    d. aphthous stomatitis.

_____ 3. A nurse assesses the mouth of an adult male client and observes a rough, crusty, eroded area. The nurse should

    a. refer the client for further evaluation.

    b. document the presence of herpes simplex.

    c. ask the client if his gums bleed.

    d. document the presence of a canker sore.

_____ 4. An adult client visits the clinic and tells the nurse that she has been experiencing frequent nosebleeds for the past month. The nurse should

    a. ask the client if she has had recent oral surgery.

    b. assess the client's nasal passages for blockage.

    c. ask the client if she is a smoker.

    d. refer the client for further evaluation.

_____ 5. The nurse is assessing the mouth of an older adult and observes that the client appears to have poorly fitting dentures. The nurse should instruct the client that she may be at greater risk for

    a. aspiration.

    b. malocclusion.

    c. gingivitis.

    d. throat soreness.

_____ 6. An adolescent client tells the nurse that her mother says she grinds her teeth when she sleeps. The nurse should explain to the client that grinding the teeth may be a sign of

    a. precancerous lesions.

    b. poor oral hygiene.

    c. malabsorption.

    d. stress and anxiety.

_____ 7. The nurse is planning a presentation to a group of high school students about the risk factors for oral cancer. Which of the following should be included in the nurse's plan?

    a. Diets low in fruits and vegetables are a possible risk factor for oral cancer.

    b. About 40% of all cancers occur in the lips, mouth, and tongue.

    c. The incidence of oral cancers is higher in women than in men.

    d. Most oral cancers are detected in people in their 70s.

Copyright © 2014. Wolters Kluwer Health | Lippincott Williams & Wilkins. Lab Manual for Health Assessment in Nursing, 5e.

____   **8.** Before examining the mouth of an adult client, the nurse should first

   a. ask the client to leave dentures in place.

   b. don sterile gloves for the procedure.

   c. offer the client mouthwash.

   d. don clean gloves for the procedure.

____   **9.** A client visits the clinic and tells the nurse that she has painful cracking in the corners of her lips. The nurse should assess the client's diet for a deficiency of

   a. vitamin C.

   b. fluoride.

   c. vitamin A.

   d. riboflavin.

____   **10.** The nurse is assessing a client who has been taking antibiotics for an infection for 10 days. The nurse observes whitish curd-like patches in the client's mouth. The nurse should explain to the client that these spots are most likely

   a. *Candida albicans* infection.

   b. Koplik spots.

   c. leukoplakia.

   d. Fordyce spots.

____   **11.** The nurse is assessing an adult client's oral cavity for possible oral cancer. The nurse should explain to the client that the most common site of oral cancer is the

   a. area on top of the tongue.

   b. area underneath the tongue.

   c. inside of the cheeks.

   d. area near the salivary glands.

____   **12.** The nurse is planning to inspect an adult client's mouth, using a tongue depressor. The nurse should plan to

   a. depress the tongue blade slightly off center.

   b. depress the tongue blade as close to the center as possible.

   c. ask the client to keep the mouth partially open.

   d. insert the tongue blade at the back of the client's tongue.

____   **13.** An adult client visits the clinic complaining of a sore throat. After assessing the throat, the nurse documents the client's tonsils as 4+. The nurse should explain to the client that 4+ tonsils are present when the nurse observes tonsils that are

   a. touching the uvula.

   b. visible upon inspection.

   c. touching each other.

   d. midway between the tonsillar pillars and uvula.

____   **14.** The nurse is preparing to inspect the nose of an adult client with an otoscope. The nurse plans to

   a. position the handle of the otoscope to one side.

   b. tip the client's head as far back as possible.

   c. direct the otoscope tip quickly back and down the nostril.

   d. position the handle of the otoscope straight and up.

____ **15.** The nurse has assessed the nose of an adult client and has explained to the client about her thick yellowish nasal discharge. The nurse determines that the client understands the instructions when the client says that the yellowish discharge is most likely due to

    a. too much smoking.

    b. chronic allergies.

    c. trauma to the nasal passages.

    d. an upper respiratory infection.

Activity H   CRITICAL THINKING ACTIVITIES

1. Discuss how you would distinguish between allergic conditions and infections.

2. Analyze the following client's risk factors for oral cancer.

Clara B. is a 25-year-old college student, with chronic rhinitis. She says that she has a history of sinus infections about twice a year. She smokes two packs of cigarettes a day, drinks beer every weekend and occasionally during the week, and eats a poorly balanced diet on the run. Her father smoked a pipe and had lip cancer.

Activity I   CASE STUDY

Read the following case study. Then, work through the steps of analyzing the case study data. First identify abnormal data and strengths in **subjective and objective findings**, assemble **cue clusters**, draw **inferences**, make possible **nursing diagnoses**, identify **defining characteristics**, **confirm or rule out** the diagnoses, and **document** your conclusions. Use the blank diagnostic analysis charts provided at the end of this book (also available on thePoint website) to guide your thinking. Propose nursing diagnoses that are specific to the client in the case study. Identify collaborative problems, if any, for this client. Finally, identify data, if any, that point toward a medical problem requiring a referral.

Alice K. is a 50-year-old divorced woman, with a medical diagnosis of carcinoma of the sphenoid sinus and nasal pharynx. She has been referred by the physician to the hospital's home health service for weekly skilled nursing visits by an RN. She lives in her own home and is currently being cared for by her younger sister. Alice has two grown sons. One son lives close by; the other lives in another state.

    Ms. K. is currently being treated with radiation therapy, which she receives three times weekly. She states that she is experiencing some pain across the bridge of her nose (2 on a scale of 0 to 5, with 5 being the worst). She uses cold compresses to help relieve the pain. Three small oral ulcers approximately 3 to 5 cm wide are noted on the left buccal mucosa. Ms. Kennedy reports that she has no difficulty swallowing, but the sores are painful when she eats, especially when she eats citrus fruits. She uses a soft-bristled toothbrush and brushes her teeth gently after eating, and she tries to avoid irritating food. The findings in the rest of the oral examination are within normal limits.

    The nasal examination reveals a slightly reddened color of the nose, with some tenderness noted across the bridge of the nose. There is no occlusion of either nostril. The nasal septum is intact, with no ulcers or perforations. The nasal mucosa is red and slightly swollen. Both frontal and maxillary sinuses transilluminate; the frontal sinus area is slightly tender to palpation.

    Ms. K's sister has taken over most of the housekeeping responsibilities. She says that she is currently able to keep up with everything but is concerned about whether she will be able to continue to care for her sister as her condition worsens.

How Well Did You Do?

After you have read the chapter and completed the exercises in this chapter, visit thePoint to access the Self-Reflection Activity. This activity will help you identify to what degree you have met each of the chapter objectives. You can then review the chapter for objectives you have met partially or not at all.

    Other tools to help you, like the Diagnostic Reasoning Guides, Nursing Interview Guides, Physical Assessment Guides, and NCLEX-Style Chapter Review Questions, are also available on thePoint.

Copyright © 2014. Wolters Kluwer Health | Lippincott Williams & Wilkins. Lab Manual for Health Assessment in Nursing, 5e.

Assessing Thorax and Lungs

Chapter Overview

Respiration is a life-sustaining function which makes precise assessment of the chest and breathing structures an essential nursing skill. This chapter reviews the structures and functions of the lungs and the assessment tests and techniques used by nurses to evaluate a client's thorax and lungs.

Chapter Learning Objectives

1. Describe the structures and functions of the thorax and lungs.
2. Identify the thoracic landmarks in relation to underlying structures of the thorax.
3. Discuss the risk factors for lung cancer across cultures and ways to reduce one's risks.
4. Describe the teaching opportunities to reduce risks and promote health of the thorax and lungs.
5. Interview a client for an accurate nursing history of the thorax and lungs.
6. Perform a physical assessment of the thorax and lungs using the correct techniques of inspection, auscultation, palpation, and percussion.
7. Differentiate between normal and abnormal findings of the thorax and lungs.
8. Describe the findings frequently seen when assessing the older client's thorax and lungs.
9. Analyze the data from the interview and physical assessment of the thorax and lungs to formulate valid nursing diagnoses, collaborative problems, and/or referrals.

CHAPTER PRETEST

Activity A   MULTIPLE CHOICE QUESTIONS

Choose the one best answer for each of the following multiple choice questions.

_____ **1.** The clavicles extend from the acromion of the scapula to the part of the sternum termed the

    a. body.

    b. xiphoid process.

    c. angle.

    d. manubrium.

_____ **2.** A bony ridge located at the point where the manubrium articulates with the body of the sternum is termed the sternal

   a. angle.

   b. notch.

   c. space.

   d. prominens.

_____ **3.** The spinous process termed the vertebra prominens is in which cervical vertebra?

   a. Fifth.

   b. Sixth.

   c. Seventh.

   d. Eighth.

_____ **4.** The apex of each lung is located at the

   a. level of the diaphragm.

   b. area slightly above the clavicle.

   c. level of the sixth rib.

   d. left oblique fissure.

_____ **5.** The thin double-layered serous membrane that lines the chest cavity is termed

   a. parietal pleura.

   b. pulmonary pleura.

   c. visceral pleura.

   d. thoracic pleura.

_____ **6.** The lining of the trachea and bronchi, which serves to remove dust, foreign bodies, and bacteria, is termed the

   a. bronchioles.

   b. alveolar sacs.

   c. alveolar ducts.

   d. cilia.

_____ **7.** Under normal circumstances, the strongest stimulus to breathe is

   a. hypoxemia.

   b. hypocapnia.

   c. pH changes.

   d. hypercapnia.

_____ **8.** The nurse assesses an adult client's thoracic area and observes a markedly sunken sternum and adjacent cartilages. The nurse should document the client's

   a. pectus thorax.

   b. pectus excavatum.

   c. pectus carinatum.

   d. pectus diaphragm.

_____ **9.** The nurse has assessed the respiratory pattern of an adult client. The nurse determines that the client is exhibiting Kussmaul respirations with hyperventilation. The nurse should contact the client's physician because this type of respiratory pattern usually indicates

   a. diabetic ketoacidosis.

   b. central nervous system injury.

   c. drug overdose.

   d. congestive heart failure.

Copyright © 2014. Wolters Kluwer Health | Lippincott Williams & Wilkins. Lab Manual for Health Assessment in Nursing, 5e.

____ **10.** The client has been admitted through the emergency department with chronic bronchitis, has elevated CO_2 levels, and has been placed on O_2. What priority assessment would the nurse include?

    a. Assess for signs of nonproductive cough.

    b. Review blood work including RBC and WBC.

    c. Assess the characteristics of sputum.

    d. Evaluate changes in respiratory pattern and rate.

Activity B MATCHING

Match the terms in the left column with the correct description in the right column.

Term

____ **1.** Promotes the strongest stimulus to breathe

____ **2.** Orthopnea

____ **3.** Crepitus

____ **4.** Pectus excavatum

____ **5.** Pectus carinatum

____ **6.** Pleural friction rub

____ **7.** Wheeze (sibilant)

____ **8.** Wheeze (sonorous)

____ **9.** Crackles (fine)

____ **10.** Crackles (coarse)

Description

a. High-pitched, short, popping sounds

b. Forward protrusion of the sternum

c. High-pitched musical sounds

d. An increase in carbon dioxide in the blood

e. Low-pitched, bubbling, moist sounds

f. Low-pitched snoring or moaning sounds

g. Difficulty breathing when lying supine

h. Markedly sunken sternum and adjacent cartilage

i. Low-pitched, dry, grating sounds

j. A "crackling" sensation

Activity C LABELING ACTIVITIES

Label the structures of the anterior thoracic cage in the following figure. Check your answers with Figure 19-1 on page 370 in the textbook.

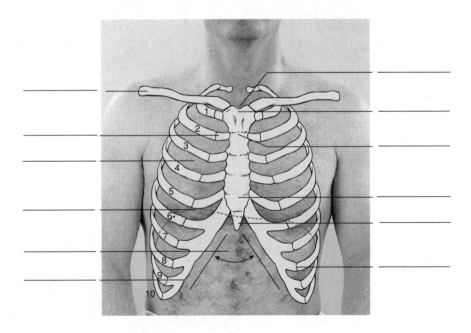

Label the structures of the posterior thoracic cage in the following figure. Check your answers with Figure 19-2 on page 370 in the textbook.

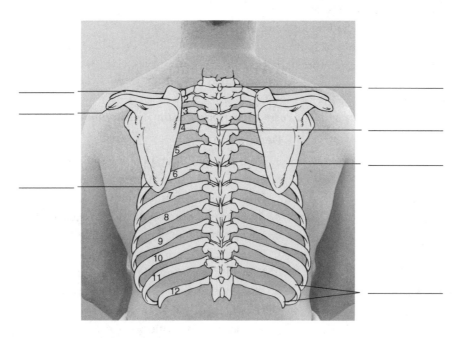

Label the structures of the anterior vertical lines of the chest in the following figure. Check your answers with Figure 19-3 on page 371 in the textbook.

Label the structures of the posterior vertical lines of the chest in the following figure. Check your answers with Figure 19-4 on page 371 in the textbook.

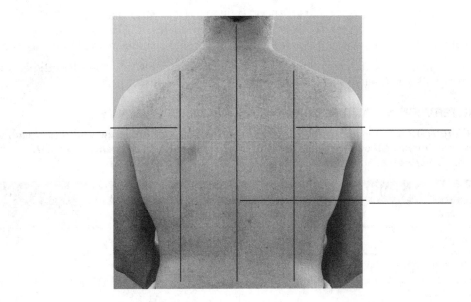

Label the structures of the lateral vertical lines of the chest in the following figure. Check your answers with Figure 19-5 on page 371 in the textbook.

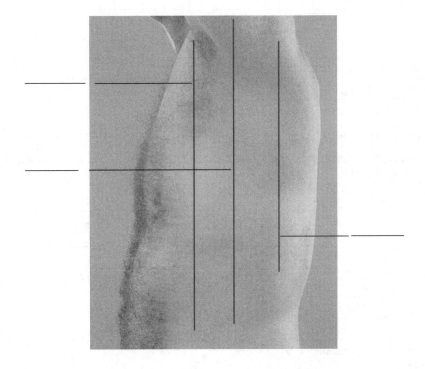

Copyright © 2014. Wolters Kluwer Health | Lippincott Williams & Wilkins. Lab Manual for Health Assessment in Nursing, 5e.

Activity D **LEARNER ACTIVITIES**

After reading Chapter 19 in the textbook, participate in the following learning activities.

1. Review the information in EVIDENCE-BASED HEALTH PROMOTION AND DISEASE PREVENTION: LUNG CANCER (see page 378 in your textbook). Determine your own risk for lung cancer. Next, identify ethnic groups that are at highest risk for lung cancer. Discuss what teaching could be implemented to reduce these risks.

2. Perform an assessment of the thorax and lungs on a client, friend, or relative. Discuss with peers your findings as they compare with the findings in a younger person's thorax and lungs.

Activity E **INTERVIEWING AND RECORDING ASSESSMENT FINDINGS**

After reading Chapter 19, use the following Nursing Interview Guide to interview and record your subjective findings for an assessment of the thorax and lungs of a lab partner, peer, or client. Your instructor may ask you to turn this in to be evaluated. Forms are also available on thePoint *website.*

Nursing Interview Guide to Collect Subjective Data From the Client

Questions	Findings
Current Symptoms	
1. Difficulty breathing (at rest, with specific activities, while sleeping, other symptoms when having trouble breathing)?	
2. Chest pain associated with a cold, fever, or deep breathing?	
3. Cough, with or without sputum?	
Past History	
1. Prior respiratory problems?	
2. Previous thoracic surgery, biopsy, or trauma?	
3. Allergies, symptoms/treatments?	
4. Pulmonary studies/tests: chest x-ray, TB skin test, or influenza immunization?	
Family History	
1. Family history of lung disease?	
Lifestyle and Health Practices	
1. Use of tobacco products, cigarettes or cigars (number of years, number per day)?	
2. Exposure to environmental conditions that affect breathing at work or at home, including secondhand smoke?	
3. Difficulty performing usual daily activities?	
4. Degree of stress, effect on breathing?	
5. Medications for breathing (prescribed or OTC), other breathing treatments?	

Copyright © 2014. Wolters Kluwer Health | Lippincott Williams & Wilkins. Lab Manual for Health Assessment in Nursing, 5e.

Activity F PERFORMING PHYSICAL ASSESSMENT OF THE THORAX AND LUNGS

Use the following Physical Assessment Guide to examine the thorax and lungs of a lab partner, peer, or client. Column 1 will serve as a reminder as to what part of the exam you will do next. Column 2 will be used to record your findings. Your instructor may ask you to turn this in to be evaluated. Forms are also available on thePoint *website.*

Physical Assessment Guide to Collect Objective Client Data

Questions	Findings
Current Symptoms	
1. Gather equipment (gown and drape, gloves, stethoscope, exam light, mask, skin marker, metric ruler).	
2. Explain the procedure to client.	
3. Ask the client to put on a gown.	
Posterior Thorax	
1. Inspect for shape and configuration of the chest wall and position of scapulae.	
2. Inspect for use of accessory muscles.	
3. Inspect the client's positioning noting posture and ability to support weight while breathing.	
4. Palpate for tenderness and sensation with gloved fingers.	
5. Palpate for surface characteristics such as lesions or masses with gloved fingers.	
6. Palpate for fremitus, using the ball or ulnar edge of one hand while the client says "ninety-nine." Assess for symmetry and intensity of vibration.	
7. Palpate for chest expansion. Place hands on the posterior chest wall with your thumbs at the level of T9 or T10, and observe the movement of your thumbs as the client takes a deep breath.	
8. Percuss for tone, starting at the apices above the scapulae and across the tops of both shoulders.	
9. Percuss intercostal spaces across and down, comparing sides.	
10. Percuss to the lateral aspects at the bases of the lungs, and compare sides.	
11. Percuss for diaphragmatic excursion, using the procedure in Chapter 18 of the textbook.	
12. Auscultate for breath sounds (normal: bronchial, bronchovesicular, and vesicular), noting location.	
13. Auscultate for adventitious sounds (crackles, fine or coarse, pleural friction rub, wheeze, sibilant, or sonorous).	
14. Auscultate for voice sounds over the chest wall: Bronchophony—ask the client to repeat the phrase "ninety-nine"; egophony—ask the client to repeat the letter "E"; whispered pectoriloquy—ask the client to whisper the phrase "one-two-three."	

Copyright © 2014. Wolters Kluwer Health | Lippincott Williams & Wilkins. Lab Manual for Health Assessment in Nursing, 5e.

Physical Assessment Guide to Collect Objective Client Data (continued)

Questions	Findings
Anterior Thorax	
1. Inspect for shape and configuration to determine the ratio of anteroposterior diameter to transverse diameter (normally 1:2).	
2. Inspect for position of sternum from anterior and lateral viewpoints.	
3. Inspect for slope of the ribs from anterior and lateral viewpoints.	
4. Inspect for quality and pattern of respiration, noting breathing characteristics, rate, rhythm, and depth.	
5. Inspect intercostal spaces while client breathes normally.	
6. Inspect for use of accessory muscles.	
7. Palpate for tenderness and sensation, using fingers.	
8. Palpate surface characteristics such as lesions or masses, using fingers of gloved hand.	
9. Palpate for fremitus while the client says "ninety-nine."	
10. Palpate for chest expansion by placing hands on anterolateral wall with the thumbs along the costal margins and pointing toward the xiphoid process. Observe the movement of the thumbs as the client takes a deep breath.	
11. Percuss for tone above the clavicles and then the intercostal spaces across and down, comparing sides.	
12. Auscultate for breath sounds, adventitious sounds, and voice sounds.	
Analysis of Data	
1. Formulate nursing diagnoses (wellness, risk, actual).	
2. Formulate collaborative problems.	
3. Make necessary referrals.	

CHAPTER POSTTEST

Activity G   MULTIPLE CHOICE QUESTIONS

Choose the one best answer for each of the following multiple choice questions.

_____ 1. While assessing an adult client, the client tells the nurse that she "has had difficulty catching her breath since yesterday." The nurse should assess the client further for signs and symptoms of

     a. emphysema.

     b. cardiac disease.

     c. trauma to the chest.

     d. infection.

Copyright © 2014. Wolters Kluwer Health | Lippincott Williams & Wilkins. Lab Manual for Health Assessment in Nursing, 5e.

_____ 2. An adult client visits the clinic and tells the nurse that he has been "spitting up rust-colored sputum." The nurse should refer the client to the physician for possible

    a. pulmonary edema.

    b. bronchitis.

    c. asthma.

    d. tuberculosis.

_____ 3. The nurse is planning a presentation to a group of high school students on the topic of lung cancer. Which of the following should the nurse plan to include in the presentation?

    a. Compared with whites in the United States, African Americans have a lower incidence of lung cancer.

    b. Lung cancer is the third leading cause of death in the United States.

    c. There is a higher incidence of lung cancer in women than men in the United States.

    d. Studies have indicated that there is a genetic component in the development of lung cancer.

_____ 4. While assessing an adult client, the nurse observes decreased chest expansion at the bases of the client's lungs. The nurse should refer the client to a physician for possible

    a. atelectasis.

    b. pneumonia.

    c. chest trauma.

    d. chronic obstructive pulmonary disease.

_____ 5. The nurse is planning to percuss the chest of an adult male client for diaphragmatic excursion. The nurse should begin the assessment by

    a. asking the client to take a deep breath and hold it.

    b. percussing upward from the base of the lungs.

    c. percussing downward until the tone changes to resonance.

    d. asking the client to exhale forcefully and hold his breath.

_____ 6. The nurse is preparing to auscultate the posterior thorax of an adult female client. The nurse should

    a. place the bell of the stethoscope firmly on the posterior chest wall.

    b. auscultate from the base of the lungs to the apices.

    c. ask the client to breathe deeply through her mouth.

    d. ask the client to breathe normally through her nose.

_____ 7. While assessing the thoracic area of an adult client, the nurse plans to auscultate for voice sounds. To assess bronchophony, the nurse should ask the client to

    a. repeat the phrase "ninety-nine."

    b. repeat the letter "E."

    c. whisper the phrase "one-two-three."

    d. repeat the letter "A."

_____ 8. The nurse assesses an adult client and observes that the client's breathing pattern is very labored and noisy, with occasional coughing. The nurse should refer the client to a physician for possible

    a. chronic bronchitis.

    b. atelectasis.

    c. renal failure.

    d. congestive heart failure.

_____ 9. While assessing an adult client's lungs during the postoperative period, the nurse detects coarse crackles. The nurse should refer the client to a physician for possible

    a. pneumonia.

    b. pleuritis.

    c. bronchitis.

    d. asthma.

Copyright © 2014. Wolters Kluwer Health | Lippincott Williams & Wilkins. Lab Manual for Health Assessment in Nursing, 5e.

____ **10.** The nurse assesses an adult client's breath sounds and hears sonorous wheezes, primarily during the client's expiration. The nurse should refer the client to a physician for possible

    a. asthma.

    b. chronic emphysema.

    c. pleuritis.

    d. bronchitis.

Activity H CRITICAL THINKING ACTIVITY

Bob T., age 61, arrives at the outpatient clinic complaining of shortness of breath. He tells you that he has been employed by an asbestos removal company for the past 15 years. He says he has followed safety precautions "most of the time." He also tells you that on weekends he always relaxes by drinking beer and smoking a little at his favorite bar. He is divorced and has two grown sons, who live about 32.1 km (20 miles) away. There is no history of lung cancer in his family that he can remember. He says, "I know I don't live a very healthy life, but I'm too old to change my ways now."

1. Develop appropriate nursing diagnoses for this client.

2. What teaching would be appropriate for this client?

Activity I CASE STUDY

Read the following case study. Then, work through the steps of analyzing the case study data. First identify abnormal data and strengths in **subjective and objective findings**, assemble **cue clusters**, draw **inferences**, make possible **nursing diagnoses**, identify **defining characteristics**, **confirm or rule out** the diagnoses, and **document** your conclusions. Use the blank diagnostic analysis charts provided at the end of this book (also available on thePoint website) to guide your thinking. Propose nursing diagnoses that are specific to the client in the case study. Identify collaborative problems, if any, for this client. Finally, identify data, if any, which point toward a medical problem requiring a referral.

Theresa J. is a 55-year-old white woman. She is a part-time secretary for a local businessman and is very active in her community. She is married and has two children. She presents at the nursing clinic this morning with a complaint of extreme shortness of breath. When entering the examination room, she appears very anxious and states that she has experienced this problem since yesterday afternoon.

    Theresa J. has no previous diagnosis of asthma, allergies, or respiratory problems, but her brother and father have cases of mild asthma. The client has smoked for 35 years but reports limiting her smoking to a pack every 2 to 3 days for the past 10 years. Before that, she reports having smoked a pack every day. She worked in her office yesterday and reports having felt fine. She met friends at a local park for lunch but denies anything unusual about her daily activity. She states she has experienced "tightness in my chest," increasing in severity since about 5 PM yesterday. She denies any other associated symptoms such as pain or cough. Her discomfort made sleeping difficult last night, and she states that she has not eaten today because of her shortness of breath.

    Theresa J. currently takes no medications. She reports having no regular exercise program but denies any intolerance to activity until the onset of dyspnea. She reports having tried only rest to alleviate the problem and knows "nothing else to do but go to the doctor."

    Theresa J.'s respiratory rate is 26 breaths/minute and appears somewhat labored. The client seems somewhat apprehensive and experiences obvious dyspnea on even mild exertion. Her anteroposterior diameter is within normal limits. The use of accessory muscles is noted, with respiration immediately after exertion. Expiration is somewhat labored and prolonged. Tactile fremitus is decreased, especially in lower lobes. Percussion tones are resonant over all lung fields. Breath sounds are decreased, with prolonged expiration. Voice sounds are also decreased. Expiratory wheeze is noted throughout the lung fields, especially bilaterally in the lower lobes.

How Well Did You Do?

After you have read the chapter and completed the exercises in this chapter, visit thePoint to access the Self-Reflection Activity. This activity will help you identify to what degree you have met each of the chapter objectives. You can then review the chapter for objectives you have met partially or not at all.

    Other tools to help you, like the Diagnostic Reasoning Guides, Nursing Interview Guides, Physical Assessment Guides, and NCLEX-Style Chapter Review Questions, are also available on thePoint.

Copyright © 2014. Wolters Kluwer Health | Lippincott Williams & Wilkins. Lab Manual for Health Assessment in Nursing, 5e.

CHAPTER 20

Assessing Breasts and Lymphatic System

Chapter Overview

Breast and lymphatic health is an important issue, not only for women during their childbearing years and throughout their lives, but also for men, whose breast development and health may be affected by various factors such as medications and hormonal problems. Use the following exercises and quizzes to guide your physical assessment of the breast and lymphatic structures.

Chapter Learning Objectives

1. Describe the structure and functions of the breast and major axillary lymph nodes.
2. Discuss the risk factors for breast cancer across cultures and ways to reduce one's risks.
3. Interview a client for an accurate nursing history of the breast and axillary lymph region.
4. Perform a physical assessment of the breast and lymphatic tissues using the correct techniques of inspection, auscultation, palpation, and percussion.
5. Differentiate between normal and abnormal findings of the breasts and lymphatic system.
6. Explain how to teach clients how to perform breast self-examinations.
7. Describe the findings frequently seen when assessing the older client's breasts and axillary lymph nodes.
8. Analyze the data from the interview and physical assessment of the breasts and axillary lymph nodes to formulate valid nursing diagnoses, collaborative problems, and/or referrals.

CHAPTER PRETEST

Activity A MULTIPLE CHOICE QUESTIONS

Choose the one best answer for each of the following multiple choice questions.

____ 1. At puberty, the female breasts enlarge in response to estrogen and

    a. progesterone.

    b. aldosterone.

    c. lactogen.

    d. prolactin.

____ **2.** Elevated sebaceous glands, known as Montgomery glands, are located in the breast's
 a. nipples.
 b. hair follicles.
 c. lactiferous ducts.
 d. areolas.

____ **3.** The functional part of the breast that allows for milk production consists of tissue termed
 a. fibrous.
 b. glandular.
 c. adipose.
 d. lactiferous.

____ **4.** Fibrous tissue that provides support for the glandular tissue of the breasts is termed
 a. lateral ligaments.
 b. Wharton ligaments.
 c. pectoral ligaments.
 d. Cooper ligaments.

____ **5.** The size and shape of the breasts in females are related to the amount of
 a. glandular tissue.
 b. fibrous tissue.
 c. lactiferous ducts.
 d. fatty tissue.

Activity B MATCHING

Match the terms in the left column with the correct descriptions in the right column.

Term

____ **1.** Axillary lymph nodes

____ **2.** Mammary gland

____ **3.** Mastectomy

____ **4.** Lactiferous duct

____ **5.** Lactiferous sinus

____ **6.** Cooper ligaments

____ **7.** Tail of spence

____ **8.** Areola

____ **9.** Nipple

____ **10.** Paget disease

____ **11.** Peau d'orange

____ **12.** Mastitis

____ **13.** Mammography

____ **14.** Gynecomastia

____ **15.** Lateral lymph nodes

Description

a. Lymphatic obstruction, causing edema, which thickens the skin, exaggerates the hair follicles, and gives the breast an orange peel or pigskin look

b. Darkly pigmented area surrounding the nipple of the mammary gland

c. Enlargement of one or both male breasts, seen more frequently in adolescent boys and elderly men

d. Reservoirs for storing milk, located behind the nipple

e. Pigmented projection at the tip of each breast, which allows passage of milk from the breast

f. Specialized gland of the skin of females, which secretes milk for nourishment of the young

g. Roentgenography of the breast to detect any underlying mass

h. Ducts conveying the milk secreted by the lobes of the breast to and through the nipples

i. Groups of lymph nodes located under the arm (the axilla)

j. Inflammation of the breast

k. Cone-shaped breast tissue that projects up into the axillae

l. Surgical removal of breast tissue

m. Fibrous glands extending vertically from the breast surface to attach on the chest wall muscles

n. Erythematous scaling lesion of the breast, involving the nipple and areola unilaterally, and associated with an underlying malignancy

o. Responsible for drainage from arms

Copyright © 2014. Wolters Kluwer Health | Lippincott Williams & Wilkins. Lab Manual for Health Assessment in Nursing, 5e.

Activity C **LABELING ACTIVITIES**

Label the structures of the anterior chest in the following figure. Check your answers with Figure 20-1 on page 397 in the textbook.

Label the breast quadrants in the following figure. Check your answers with Figure 20-2 on page 397 in the textbook.

Copyright © 2014. Wolters Kluwer Health | Lippincott Williams & Wilkins. Lab Manual for Health Assessment in Nursing, 5e.

Label the internal anatomic structures of the breast in the following figure. Check your answers with Figure 20-4 on page 398 in the textbook.

Label the major axillary lymph nodes in the following figure. Check your answers with Figure 20-5 on page 398 in the textbook.

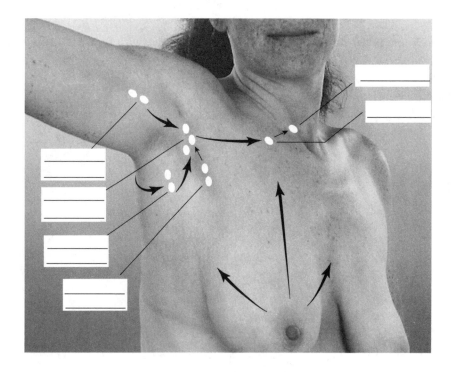

Activity D **LEARNER ACTIVITIES**

After reading Chapter 20 in the textbook, participate in the following learning activities.

1. Review the information in EVIDENCE-BASED HEALTH PROMOTION AND DISEASE PREVENTION: BREAST CANCER (see pages 402–403 in your textbook). Determine your own risk for breast cancer. Next, identify ethnic groups that are at highest risk for breast cancer. Discuss what teaching could be implemented to reduce these risks.

2. Use a breast model to review the anatomy and function of each anatomic structure. Discuss the changes of the breast and surrounding tissue that occur with aging.

3. Obtain an information packet from a local agency that performs mammograms. Review the material with a lab partner. Discuss when it is appropriate to teach a client the breast self-examination. Teach your lab partner how to do a breast self-examination.

Activity E **INTERVIEWING AND RECORDING ASSESSMENT FINDINGS**

After reading Chapter 20, use the following Nursing Interview Guide to interview and record your subjective findings for an assessment of the breasts and lymphatic tissue. Your instructor may ask you to turn this in to be evaluated. Forms are also available on thePoint *website.*

Nursing Interview Guide to Collect Subjective Data From the Client

Questions	Findings
Current Symptoms	
1. Changes in breasts (lumps, swelling, redness, warmth, dimpling, size, firmness, pain, discharge)?	
Past History	
1. Previous problems with breasts (treatment and surgery)?	
2. Age at menses?	
3. Age at menopause?	
4. Given birth?	
5. Age at first birth?	
6. First and last day of menstrual cycle?	
Family History	
1. Family history of breast cancer?	
Lifestyle and Health Practices	
1. Use of hormones, contraceptives, or antidepressants?	
2. Exposure to radiation, benzene, or asbestos?	
3. Usual diet, including intake of alcohol, coffee, tea, soft drinks, and chocolate?	
4. Usual exercise patterns?	
5. Type of bra worn during exercise?	
6. Examine own breasts/frequency?	
7. Last breast exam by physician?	
8. Last mammogram?	

Copyright © 2014. Wolters Kluwer Health | Lippincott Williams & Wilkins. Lab Manual for Health Assessment in Nursing, 5e.

Activity F   PERFORMING PHYSICAL ASSESSMENT OF THE BREAST AND LYMPHATIC TISSUE

Use the following Physical Assessment Guide to examine the breast model. Column 1 will serve as a reminder as to what part of the exam you will do next. Column 2 will be used to record your findings. Your instructor may ask you to turn this in to be evaluated. Forms are also available on thePoint *website.*

Physical Assessment Guide to Collect Objective Client Data	
Questions	**Findings**
Current Symptoms	
1. Gather equipment (centimeter ruler, small pillow, gloves, client handout on breast self-examination, slide for specimen).	
2. Explain the procedure to client.	
3. Ask the client to put on a gown.	
Female Breasts	

1. Inspect the breasts
   a. Size and symmetry
   b. Color and texture
   c. Superficial venous patterns
   d. Retraction and dimpling
   e. Bilaterally; note color, size, shape, and texture of areolas
   f. Bilaterally; note size and direction of nipples	

2. Palpate the breasts
   a. Texture and elasticity
   b. Tenderness and temperature
   c. Masses: noting location, size in centimeters, shape, mobility, consistency, and tenderness
   d. Palpate nipples by compressing nipple gently between thumb and index finger; observe for discharge
   e. Palpate mastectomy site, if applicable, observing the scar and any remaining breast or axillary tissue for redness, lesions, lumps, swelling, or tenderness	

Male Breasts	
1. Inspect and palpate the breasts, areolas, and nipples for swelling, nodules, or ulcerations.	
Axillae	
1. Inspect for rashes or infection.	
2. Hold the elbow with one hand and use the three fingerpads of your other hand to palpate firmly the axillary lymph nodes.	
3. Palpate high into the axillae, moving downward against the ribs to feel for the central nodes. Continue down the posterior axillae to feel for the posterior nodes.	
4. Use bimanual palpation to feel for the anterior axillary nodes.	
5. Palpate down the inner aspect of the upper arm.	
Analysis of Data	
1. Formulate nursing diagnoses (wellness, risk, actual).	
2. Formulate collaborative problems.	
3. Make necessary referrals.	

CHAPTER POSTTEST

Activity G **MULTIPLE CHOICE QUESTIONS**

Choose the one best answer for each of the following multiple choice questions.

_____   **1.** After assessing the breasts of a female client, the nurse should explain to the client that most breast tumors occur in the

    a. upper inner quadrant.

    b. lower inner quadrant.

    c. upper outer quadrant.

    d. lower outer quadrant.

_____   **2.** A female client tells the nurse that her breasts become lumpy and sore before menstruation but get better at the end of the menstrual cycle. The nurse should explain to the client that these symptoms are often associated with

    a. malignant tumors.

    b. fibroadenoma.

    c. fibrocystic breast disease.

    d. increased estrogen production.

_____   **3.** The nurse has discussed the risks for breast cancer with a group of high school seniors. The nurse determines that one of the students needs further instructions when the student says that one risk factor is

    a. having a baby before the age of 20 years.

    b. a family history of breast cancer.

    c. consumption of a high-fat diet.

    d. late menopause.

_____   **4.** Cultural beliefs about the causes of breast cancer do not always agree with medical findings. Hispanic Americans often associate breast cancer with

    a. improper diet.

    b. punishment from God.

    c. physical stress.

    d. evil thoughts.

_____   **5.** The nurse is working with a community group to set up teaching programs to increase awareness among African American women about preventive screening techniques for breast cancer. In the teaching program, the nurse should plan to include

    a. local female physicians who work with cancer clients.

    b. hospital clinic workers from various racial backgrounds.

    c. nurses who work in outpatient centers.

    d. breast cancer patients of the same race.

_____   **6.** The nurse is caring for an adult female client when the client tells the nurse that she has had a clear discharge from her nipples for the past month. The nurse should ask the client if she has been taking

    a. antidepressants.

    b. antibiotics.

    c. insulin.

    d. contraceptives.

_____   **7.** The nurse is assessing an adult male client when the nurse observes gynecomastia in the client. The nurse should ask the client if he is taking any medications for

    a. inflammation.

    b. depression.

    c. infection.

    d. ulcers.

____ **8.** The nurse is caring for a female client who has received a diagnosis of fibrocystic breast disease. The nurse has instructed the client about the disease. The nurse determines that the client needs further instructions when the client says she should avoid drinking

  a. regular coffee.

  b. regular tea.

  c. diet colas.

  d. grapefruit juice.

____ **9.** The nurse plans to instruct an adult female client with regular menstrual cycles, who is not taking oral contraceptives, about breast self-examination. The nurse should plan to instruct the client to perform breast self-examination

  a. during menstruation.

  b. on the same day every month.

  c. midway between the cycles.

  d. right after menstruation.

____ **10.** The nurse observes an orange peel appearance, or peau d'orange, of the areolae of a client's breasts. The nurse should explain to the client that this is most likely due to

  a. blocked lymphatic drainage.

  b. fibrocystic breast disease.

  c. fibroadenomas.

  d. radiation therapy.

____ **11.** The nurse is assessing a 50-year-old client's breasts and observes a spontaneous discharge of fluid from the left nipple. The nurse should

  a. document this as a normal finding.

  b. ask the client if she has had retracted nipples.

  c. refer the client for a cytology examination.

  d. determine whether the client wears a supportive bra.

____ **12.** The nurse observes dimpling in an adult female client's breasts. The nurse should explain to the client that dimpling of the breast may indicate a

  a. fibroadenoma.

  b. tumor.

  c. genetic deviation.

  d. fibrocystic breast.

____ **13.** The nurse is preparing to examine the breasts of a female client who had a left radical mastectomy 3 years ago. When examining the client, the nurse observes redness at the scar area. The nurse should explain to the client that this may be indicative of

  a. additional tumors.

  b. poor lymphatic drainage.

  c. an infectious process.

  d. metastasis to the right breast.

____ **14.** A client has had a recent mastectomy and visits the clinic for postoperative evaluation. The client tells the nurse that she has been depressed and feels as if she is less of a woman. The most appropriate nursing diagnosis for this client is

  a. ineffective individual coping related to mastectomy.

  b. fear of additional breast cancer related to the presence of risk factors.

  c. PC: hematoma after mastectomy.

  d. disturbed body image related to mastectomy.

Copyright © 2014. Wolters Kluwer Health | Lippincott Williams & Wilkins. Lab Manual for Health Assessment in Nursing, 5e.

_____ **15.** The lymph nodes that are responsible for drainage from the arms are the

    a. lateral lymph nodes.

    b. central lymph nodes.

    c. anterior lymph nodes.

    d. posterior lymph nodes.

Activity H CRITICAL THINKING ACTIVITY

1. Analyze the following client's risk factors for the development of breast cancer.

Julia H. is a 67-year-old retired secretary. Her mother and a sister have been treated for breast cancer, but Ms. H. has no personal history of cancer. She gave birth to her only child when she was 37 years of age. She states that her daughter was a "bottle baby" and that breastfeeding was not "proper" back when her daughter was a baby. Ms. H. states that she went through the "change" (menopause) in her late 40s. Although she understands how to perform breast self-examinations, Ms. H. states that she does not do them on a regular basis. Her chart indicates that her last mammogram was 6 years ago.

2. Explain how you would assess the male breast and the surrounding tissue. What would you explain to the male client about this part of the examination?

Activity I CASE STUDY

Read the following case study. Then, work through the steps of analyzing the case study data. First identify abnormal data and strengths in **subjective and objective findings**, assemble **cue clusters**, draw **inferences**, make possible **nursing diagnoses**, identify **defining characteristics**, **confirm or rule out** the diagnoses, and **document** your conclusions. Use the blank diagnostic analysis charts provided at the end of this book (also available on thePoint website) to guide your thinking. Propose nursing diagnoses that are specific to the client in the case study. Identify collaborative problems, if any, for this client. Finally, identify data, if any that point toward a medical problem requiring a referral.

Carol L., a teacher, is a 42-year-old white woman. She is married and has three children. She has a history of fibrocystic breast disease. She felt a distinct tender lump in her left breast while taking a shower 2 days ago. At age 56, the client's mother died of breast cancer. Carol had one breast biopsy years ago, and the results were negative for cancer. At that time her mammography revealed fibrocystic breast disease. Carol has one natural child, aged 4 years, and two adopted children, aged 10 and 12 years. She states, "I'm so afraid that this might be cancer."

Physical examination reveals symmetric, round, smooth, pink breasts. The areolae are dark brown, and the nipples are everted. No rashes, lesions, dimpling, or retraction of breast tissue are noted while the client is in various positions. The client has tears in her eyes and a quavering voice. Palpation reveals generalized bilateral breast tenderness. Clear discharge is excreted from the left nipple. Bilateral, multiple, scattered, small, rubbery nodules are palpated bilaterally. No enlarged lumps or masses are palpated in the right breast. A 3 cm × 2 cm × 1 cm firm, oval, nonmobile, tender lump is palpated in the left breast. No lymph nodes are palpable. Demonstrates appropriate technique for breast self-examination.

How Well Did You Do?

After you have read the chapter and completed the exercises in this chapter, visit thePoint to access the Self-Reflection Activity. This activity will help you identify to what degree you have met each of the chapter objectives. You can then review the chapter for objectives you have met partially or not at all.

Other tools to help you, like the Diagnostic Reasoning Guides, Nursing Interview Guides, Physical Assessment Guides, and NCLEX-Style Chapter Review Questions, are also available on thePoint.

Copyright © 2014. Wolters Kluwer Health | Lippincott Williams & Wilkins. Lab Manual for Health Assessment in Nursing, 5e.

Assessing Heart and Neck Vessels

Chapter Overview

One of the most complex and important aspects of the physical examination is the assessment of heart function and neck vessel patency. The heart needs to pump blood efficiently, and the neck vessels need to deliver the blood to and from the brain to ensure health, life, and mental and physical function. Use the following quizzes and exercises as a guide to your physical assessment activities.

Chapter Learning Objectives

1. Describe the structure and functions of the heart and neck vessels.
2. Discuss the risk factors for coronary artery disease (CAD) across cultures and ways to reduce one's risks.
3. Interview a client for an accurate nursing history of the heart and neck vessels.
4. Perform a physical assessment of the heart and neck vessels using the correct techniques of inspection, auscultation, palpation, and percussion.
5. Differentiate between normal and abnormal findings of the heart and neck vessels.
6. Describe the findings frequently seen when assessing the older client's heart and neck vessels.
7. Analyze the data from the interview and physical assessment of the heart and neck vessels to formulate valid nursing diagnoses, collaborative problems, and/or referrals.

CHAPTER PRETEST

Activity A MULTIPLE CHOICE QUESTIONS

Choose the one best answer for each of the following multiple choice questions.

_____ 1. The anterior chest area that overlies the heart and great vessels is called the

    a. endocardium.

    b. epicardium.

    c. myocardium.

    d. precordium.

____ **2.** The bicuspid, or mitral, valve is located
   a. between the left atrium and the left ventricle.
   b. between the right atrium and the right ventricle.
   c. at the beginning of the ascending aorta.
   d. at the exit of each ventricle near the great vessels.

____ **3.** The semilunar valves are located
   a. between the left atrium and the left ventricle.
   b. between the right atrium and the right ventricle.
   c. at the exit of each ventricle at the beginning of the great vessels.
   d. at the beginning of the ascending aorta.

____ **4.** The sinoatrial node of the heart is located on the
   a. anterior wall of the left atrium.
   b. anterior wall of the right atrium.
   c. upper intraventricular system.
   d. posterior wall of the right atrium.

____ **5.** The P-wave phase of an electrocardiogram (ECG) represents
   a. conduction of the impulse throughout the ventricles.
   b. conduction of the impulse throughout the atria.
   c. ventricular repolarization.
   d. ventricular polarization.

Activity B MATCHING

Match the terms in the left column with the correct description in the right column.

Term

____ **1.** Pulmonic
____ **2.** Diaphragm
____ **3.** Infarct
____ **4.** Auscultation
____ **5.** Bell
____ **6.** Mitral
____ **7.** Thrill
____ **8.** Systole
____ **9.** Splitting
____ **10.** Aortic

Description

a. Assessment technique most often associated with evaluation of the cardiovascular system
b. Event of the heart when contraction of the ventricles forces blood into major vessels
c. Palpable murmur described as feeling like the throat of a purring cat
d. Audible variation between closure of two valves
e. Area of auscultation located at second ICS and left sternal border
f. Localized area of tissue necrosis caused by prolonged anoxia
g. Area of auscultation located at the apex and assessing the left ventricle; fourth to fifth ICS at left midclavicular line (MCL)
h. Area of auscultation at second ICS and right sternal border
i. Part of stethoscope used to auscultate normal heart sounds
j. The portion of the stethoscope used to assess for murmurs

Copyright © 2014. Wolters Kluwer Health | Lippincott Williams & Wilkins. Lab Manual for Health Assessment in Nursing, 5e.

Activity C   LABELING ACTIVITIES

Label the areas of the heart that are used for auscultation in the following figure. Check your answers with Figure 21-1 on page 417 in the textbook.

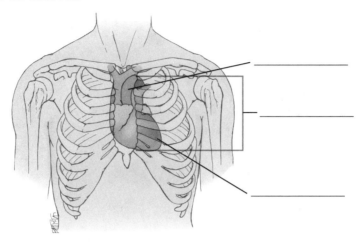

Label the heart chambers, valves, and direction of blood flow in the following figure. Check your answers with Figure 21-2 on page 417 in the textbook.

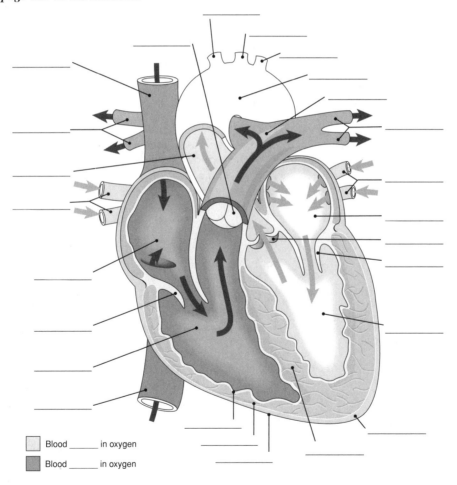

Blood _____ in oxygen

Blood _____ in oxygen

Label the major neck vessels in the following figure. Check your answers with Figure 21-5 on page 424 in the textbook.

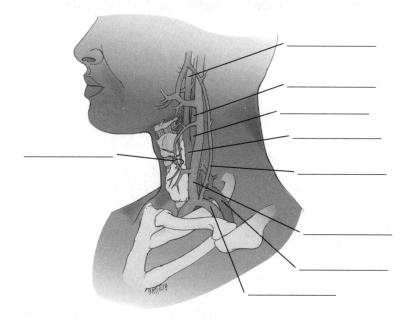

Activity D **LEARNER ACTIVITIES**

After reading Chapter 21 in the textbook, participate in the following learning activities.

1. Review the information in EVIDENCE-BASED HEALTH PROMOTION AND DISEASE PREVENTION: CORONARY HEART DISEASE (see pages 428–429 in your textbook). Determine your own risk for heart disease. Next, identify ethnic groups that are at highest risk for heart disease. Discuss what teaching could be implemented to reduce these risks.

2. Perform an assessment of the heart and neck vessels on an older client, friend, or relative. Discuss with peers your findings as they compare with the findings in a younger person's heart and neck vessels.

3. Discuss with your lab partner what teaching would be appropriate to reduce an individual's risk for heart disease.

Activity E **INTERVIEWING AND RECORDING ASSESSMENT FINDINGS**

After reading Chapter 21, use the following Nursing Interview Guide to interview and record your subjective findings for an assessment of the heart and neck vessels of a lab partner, peer, or client. Your instructor may ask you to turn this in to be evaluated. Forms are also available on thePoint *website.*

Nursing Interview Guide to Collect Subjective Data From the Client

Questions	Findings
Current Symptoms	
1. Chest pain (type, location, radiation, duration, frequency, intensity)?	
2. Palpitations?	
3. Dizziness?	
4. Swollen ankles?	
Past History	
1. Previous heart problems: heart defect, murmur, heart attack (MI)?	
2. Previous diagnosis of rheumatic fever, hypertension, elevated cholesterol, diabetes mellitus?	
3. Heart surgery or cardiac balloon intervention?	

Copyright © 2014. Wolters Kluwer Health | Lippincott Williams & Wilkins. Lab Manual for Health Assessment in Nursing, 5e.

Nursing Interview Guide to Collect Subjective Data From the Client (continued)

Questions	Findings
Family History	
1. Hypertension?	
2. Myocardial infarction?	
3. Coronary heart disease?	
4. Elevated cholesterol?	
5. Diabetes mellitus?	
Lifestyle and Health Practices	
1. Cigarette smoking pattern?	
2. Life stress—type and amount?	
3. Usual diet and exercise patterns?	
4. Use of alcohol?	
5. Sleep routine (use of extra pillows, up to urinate, feels rested)?	
6. Use of medications or treatments for heart disease?	
7. Self-monitoring of heart rate or blood pressure?	
8. Screenings for blood pressure, cholesterol, ECG?	
9. Impact of CHD on sexual activity?	

Activity F PERFORMING PHYSICAL ASSESSMENT OF THE HEART AND NECK VESSELS

Use the following Physical Assessment Guide to examine the heart and neck vessels of a lab partner, peer, or client. Column 1 will serve as a reminder as to what part of the exam you will do next. Column 2 will be used to record your findings. Your instructor may ask you to turn this in to be evaluated. Forms are also available on thePoint *website.*

Physical Assessment Guide to Collect Objective Client Data

Questions	Findings
Current Symptoms	
1. Gather equipment (stethoscope with bell diaphragm, small pillow, penlight or movable exam light, watch with second hand, two centimeter rulers).	
2. Explain the procedure to client.	
3. Ask the client to put on a gown.	
Neck Vessels	
1. Auscultate carotid arteries for bruits.	
2. Palpate each carotid artery for amplitude and contour of the pulse, elasticity of the vessel, and thrills.	
3. Inspect for jugular venous pulse.	
4. Measure jugular venous pressure.	

Copyright © 2014. Wolters Kluwer Health | Lippincott Williams & Wilkins. Lab Manual for Health Assessment in Nursing, 5e.

Physical Assessment Guide to Collect Objective Client Data (continued)	
Questions	Findings
Heart (Precordium)	
1. Inspect for visible pulsations (note if apical or other).	
2. Palpate apical pulse for location, size, strength, and duration of pulsation.	
3. Palpate for abnormal pulsations or vibrations at apex, left sternal border, and base.	
4. Auscultate heart sounds for rate and rhythm (apical and radial pulses, pulse rate deficit, S_1 and S_2).	
5. Auscultate S_1 and S_2 heart sounds for sound location and strength pattern (louder/softer at locations and with respiration, splitting of S_2).	
6. Auscultate for extra heart sounds (clicks, rubs) and murmurs (systolic or diastolic, intensity grade, pitch, quality, shape or pattern, location, transmission, effect of ventilation and position).	
7. Auscultate with the client in the left lateral position and with the client sitting up, leaning forward, and exhaling.	
Analysis of Data	
1. Formulate nursing diagnoses (wellness, risk, actual).	
2. Formulate collaborative problems.	
3. Make necessary referrals.	

CHAPTER POSTTEST

Activity G MULTIPLE CHOICE QUESTIONS

Choose the one best answer for each of the following multiple choice questions.

_____ 1. During a cardiac examination, the nurse can best hear the S_1 heart sound by placing the stethoscope at the client's
  a. base of the heart.
  b. pulmonic valve area.
  c. apex of the heart.
  d. second left interspace.

_____ 2. The S_4 heart sound
  a. can be heard during systole.
  b. is often termed *ventricular gallop*.
  c. is usually due to a heart murmur.
  d. can be heard during diastole.

_____ 3. An adult client visits the clinic and tells the nurse that she feels chest pain and pain down her left arm. The nurse should refer the client to a physician for possible
  a. congestive heart failure.
  b. angina.
  c. palpitations.
  d. acute anxiety reaction.

Copyright © 2014. Wolters Kluwer Health | Lippincott Williams & Wilkins. Lab Manual for Health Assessment in Nursing, 5e.

_____ **4.** An adult client tells the nurse that his father died of a massive coronary attack at the age of 65. The nurse should explain to the client that one of the risk factors for coronary heart disease is

     a. high serum level of low-density lipoproteins.

     b. low-carbohydrate diets.

     c. high serum level of high-density lipoproteins.

     d. diets that are high in antioxidant vitamins.

_____ **5.** The nurse is planning a presentation about coronary heart disease for a group of middle-aged adults. Which of the following should be included in the nurse's teaching plan?

     a. Hispanic clients have a higher incidence of CHD than black or white Americans.

     b. The incidence of hypertension in the white population of the United States is greater than in the black population.

     c. Women are more likely to have serious stenosis after a heart attack.

     d. Estrogen replacement therapy in postmenopausal women decreases the risk of heart attack.

_____ **6.** The nurse is preparing to assess the cardiovascular system of an adult client with emphysema. The nurse anticipates that there may be some difficulty palpating the client's

     a. apical pulse.

     b. breath sounds.

     c. jugular veins.

     d. carotid arteries.

_____ **7.** The nurse is planning to auscultate a female adult client's carotid arteries. The nurse should plan to

     a. ask the client to hold her breath.

     b. palpate the arteries before auscultation.

     c. place the diaphragm of the stethoscope over the artery.

     d. ask the client to breathe normally.

_____ **8.** While assessing an older adult client, the nurse detects a bruit over the carotid artery. The nurse should explain to the client that a bruit is

     a. a normal sound heard in adult clients.

     b. a wheezing sound.

     c. associated with occlusive arterial disease.

     d. heard when the artery is almost totally occluded.

_____ **9.** The nurse assesses a hospitalized adult client and observes that the client's jugular veins are fully extended. The nurse contacts the client's physician because the client's signs are indicative of

     a. pulmonary emphysema.

     b. diastolic murmurs.

     c. patent ductus arteriosus.

     d. increased central venous pressure.

_____ **10.** While palpating the apex, left sternal border, and base in an adult client, the nurse detects a thrill. The nurse should further assess the client for

     a. cardiac murmur.

     b. left-sided heart failure.

     c. constrictive pericarditis.

     d. congestive heart failure.

Copyright © 2014. Wolters Kluwer Health | Lippincott Williams & Wilkins. Lab Manual for Health Assessment in Nursing, 5e.

____ **11.** The nurse is auscultating the heart sounds of an adult client. To auscultate Erb point, the nurse should place the stethoscope at the

   a. second intercostal space at the right sternal border.

   b. third to fifth intercostal space at the left sternal border.

   c. apex of the heart near the midclavicular line (MCL).

   d. fourth or fifth intercostal space at the left lower sternal border.

____ **12.** While auscultating an adult client's heart rate and rhythm, the nurse detects an irregular pattern. The nurse should

   a. assess the client for signs and symptoms of pulmonary disease.

   b. document this as a normal finding.

   c. schedule the client for an ECG.

   d. refer the client to a physician.

____ **13.** The nurse has assessed the heart sounds of an adolescent client and detects the presence of an S_3 heart sound at the beginning of the diastolic pause. The nurse should instruct the client that she should

   a. be referred to a cardiologist for further evaluation.

   b. be examined again in 6 months.

   c. restrict exercise and strenuous activities.

   d. recognize that this finding is normal in adolescents.

____ **14.** While assessing an adult client, the nurse detects opening snaps early in diastole during auscultation of the heart. The nurse should refer the client to a physician because this is usually indicative of

   a. pulmonary hypertension.

   b. aortic stenosis.

   c. mitral valve stenosis.

   d. pulmonary hypotension.

____ **15.** The nurse detects paradoxical pulses in an adult client during an examination. The nurse should explain to the client that paradoxical pulses are usually indicative of

   a. obstructive lung disease.

   b. left-sided heart failure.

   c. premature ventricular contractions.

   d. aortic stenosis.

Activity H **CRITICAL THINKING ACTIVITY**

Your client states that his physician informed him that he has a new grade 3 heart murmur. He asks you to explain the following to him in layman's terms:

a. What is a heart murmur?

b. What does grade 3 mean?

c. What causes a heart murmur?

d. What does my murmur sound like?

Copyright © 2014. Wolters Kluwer Health | Lippincott Williams & Wilkins. Lab Manual for Health Assessment in Nursing, 5e.

Activity 1 **CASE STUDY**

Read the following case study. Then, work through the steps of analyzing the case study data. First identify abnormal data and strengths in **subjective and objective findings**, assemble **cue clusters**, draw **inferences**, make possible **nursing diagnoses**, identify **defining characteristics**, **confirm or rule out** the diagnoses, and **document** your conclusions. Use the blank diagnostic analysis charts provided at the end of this book (also available on thePoint website) to guide your thinking. Propose nursing diagnoses that are specific to the client in the case study. Identify collaborative problems, if any, for this client. Finally, identify data, if any, which point toward a medical problem requiring a referral.

Larry M. is a 37-year-old African American male client. He is a registered nurse and works 12-hour night shifts (7 PM to 7 AM) in an intensive care unit. He is married and has two daughters, aged 9 and 6. He has come to a local nurse practitioner for an annual physical examination. He is particularly worried about his risk for cardiac problems.

When interviewed, Mr. M. describes his general health as good. He denies any history of heart problems, surgery, or rheumatic fever and is not currently taking any medications. No previous lipid screening results are available. Mr. M. states that he believes his father has high blood pressure. He states that he drinks socially: one to two beers two to three times per week. He smokes about a half pack of cigarettes per day. He says, "I try to quit, but my job is so stressful, and smoking relaxes me." He states that he does not follow any specific diet, and he admits a weakness for sweets and chocolate. He denies any cough, dyspnea, chest pain, dizziness, palpitations, or swelling in his feet or legs. He states that he exercises sporadically, mainly playing tennis and basketball. He relates that he sometimes has difficulty sleeping during the day and then uses that time to get some chores done.

Physical examination reveals a blood pressure of 160/84 mm Hg. The carotid pulses are equal bilaterally, 2+, elastic; no bruits are auscultated. Jugular venous pulsation disappears when the client is upright. The precordium is intact with uniform color and no visible pulsations, heaves, or lifts. The apical impulse palpated in the fifth intercostal space (ICS) at the left MCL and is approximately the size of a nickel, with no thrill. The apical heart rate is auscultated at 88 beats/minute with regular rhythm; S₁ is heard best at the apex, S₂ is heard best at the base. No splitting, snaps, clicks, or murmurs are noted.

How Well Did You Do?

After you have read the chapter and completed the exercises in this chapter, visit thePoint to access the Self-Reflection Activity. This activity will help you identify to what degree you have met each of the chapter objectives. You can then review the chapter for objectives you have met partially or not at all.

Other tools to help you, like the Diagnostic Reasoning Guides, Nursing Interview Guides, Physical Assessment Guides, and NCLEX-Style Chapter Review Questions, are also available on thePoint.

22

Assessing Peripheral Vascular System

Chapter Overview

The arteries and veins of the arms and legs, the lymphatic system, and the capillaries are the vessels of peripheral vascular circulation. They deliver and exchange blood and fluids to and from the arms, legs, hands, and feet. As such, their function is a key factor in mobility and health. Use the following exercises and quizzes to help you review and master basic techniques and skills for peripheral vascular assessment.

Chapter Learning Objectives

1. Describe the structure and functions of blood vessels, including capillaries, and lymphatic circulation.
2. Discuss risk factors for peripheral vascular disease across cultures and ways to reduce one's risks.
3. Interview a client for an accurate nursing history of the peripheral vascular system.
4. Perform an accurate peripheral vascular assessment.
5. Differentiate between normal and abnormal findings of the peripheral vascular system.
6. Describe findings frequently seen when assessing the older client's peripheral vascular system.
7. Analyze data from the interview and physical assessment of the peripheral vascular system to formulate valid nursing diagnoses, collaborative problems, and/or referrals.

CHAPTER PRETEST

Activity A MULTIPLE CHOICE QUESTIONS

Choose the one best answer for each of the following multiple choice questions.

_____ 1. The major artery that supplies blood to the arm is the
   a. radial artery.
   b. ulnar artery.
   c. posterior artery.
   d. brachial artery.

_____ 2. The popliteal artery can be palpated at the
   a. knee.
   b. great toe.
   c. ankle.
   d. inguinal ligament.

____ **3.** The posterior tibial pulse can be palpated at the

    a. great toe.

    b. knee.

    c. top of the foot.

    d. ankle.

____ **4.** Blood from the lower trunk and legs drains upward into the inferior vena cava. The percentage of the body's blood volume that is contained in the veins is nearly

    a. 50%.

    b. 60%.

    c. 70%.

    d. 80%.

____ **5.** The nurse is planning to perform the Trendelenburg test on an adult client. The nurse should explain to the client that this test is used to determine the

    a. degree of arterial occlusion that exists.

    b. pulse of a client with poor elasticity.

    c. competence of the saphenous vein valves.

    d. severity of thrombophlebitis.

Activity B MATCHING

Match the terms in the left column with the correct descriptions in the right column.

Term

____ **1.** Doppler ultrasound probe

____ **2.** Edema

____ **3.** Clubbing

____ **4.** Raynaud disease

____ **5.** Capillary refill time

____ **6.** Allen test

____ **7.** Varicose veins

____ **8.** Thrombophlebitis

____ **9.** Arterial ulcer

____ **10.** Venous ulcer

____ **11.** Ischemia

____ **12.** Arteriosclerosis

Description

a. Deficient supply of oxygenated arterial blood to a tissue; caused by obstruction of a blood vessel

b. Swollen, distended, and knotted veins; occur most commonly in the legs

c. Usually occur on tips of toes, metatarsal heads, and lateral malleoli; ulcers have pale ischemic base, well-defined edges, and no bleeding

d. Swelling caused by excess fluid

e. Usually occur on medial malleoli; ulcers have bleeding uneven edges

f. The time it takes for color to return to the nail beds after they have been blanched by pressure; a good measure of peripheral perfusion and cardiac output

g. Rigid peripheral blood vessels; occurs more commonly in older adults

h. Used to detect a weak peripheral pulse to monitor blood pressure in infants or children and to measure blood pressure in a lower extremity; it magnifies pulse sounds from the heart and blood vessels

i. Inflammation of a vein associated with thrombus formation

j. Diffuse enlargement of terminal phalanges

k. Determines the patency of the radial and ulnar arteries

l. A vasospastic disorder, primarily affects the hands, characterized by color change from pallor, to cyanosis, to rubor; attacks precipitated by cold or emotional upset and relieved by warmth

Copyright © 2014. Wolters Kluwer Health | Lippincott Williams & Wilkins. Lab Manual for Health Assessment in Nursing, 5e.

Activity C LABELING ACTIVITIES

Label the major arteries of the arms and legs in the following figure. Check your answers with Figure 22-2 on page 449 in the textbook.

Label the major leg veins in the following figure. Check your answers with Figure 22-3 on page 450 in the textbook.

Copyright © 2014. Wolters Kluwer Health | Lippincott Williams & Wilkins. Lab Manual for Health Assessment in Nursing, 5e.

Label the superficial lymph nodes of the arms and legs in the following figure. Match your answers with Figure 22-6 on page 451 in the textbook.

Activity D **LEARNER ACTIVITIES**

After reading Chapter 22 in the textbook, participate in the following learning activities.

1. Review the information in EVIDENCE-BASED HEALTH PROMOTION AND DISEASE PREVENTION: PERIPHERAL ARTERY DISEASE (PAD) (see pages 454–455 in your textbook). Then interview your lab partner to determine their risk for peripheral artery disease (PAD). Discuss ways to reduce these risks with this person.

2. Perform a peripheral vascular assessment on an elderly client, friend, or relative. Discuss your assessment findings with your lab partner as they compare to those of a younger person.

3. Discuss with your lab partner what teaching would be appropriate to reduce an individual's risk for peripheral vascular disease.

Copyright © 2014. Wolters Kluwer Health | Lippincott Williams & Wilkins. Lab Manual for Health Assessment in Nursing, 5e.

Activity E **INTERVIEWING AND RECORDING ASSESSMENT FINDINGS**

After reading Chapter 22, use the following Nursing Interview Guide to interview and record your subjective findings for an assessment of peripheral vascular status of a lab partner, peer, or client. Your instructor may ask you to turn this in to be evaluated. Forms are also available on thePoint *website.*

Nursing Interview Guide to Collect Subjective Data From the Client

Questions	Findings
Current Symptoms	
1. Skin changes (color, temperature, or texture)?	
2. Leg pain, heaviness, or aching? Does it awaken you at night?	
3. Leg veins (rope-like, bulging, or contorted)?	
4. Leg sores or open wounds (location, pain)?	
5. Swelling in legs or feet?	
6. Men: sexual activity changes?	
7. Swollen glands or nodules (pain)?	
Past History	
1. Previous problems with circulation in arms or legs (blood clots, ulcers, coldness, hair loss, numbness, swelling, or poor healing)?	
2. Heart or blood vessel surgeries or treatments (coronary artery bypass, repair of an aneurysm, or vein stripping)?	
Family History	
1. Family history of varicose veins, diabetes, hypertension, coronary heart disease, or elevated cholesterol or triglyceride levels?	
Lifestyle and Health Practices	
1. Cigarettes or other forms of tobacco, past or present use (explain: amount and length of time used)?	
2. Regular exercise?	
3. Women: use of oral contraceptives?	
4. Degree of stress?	
5. Peripheral vascular problems that interfere with ADLs?	
6. Use of medications to improve circulation or control blood pressure?	
7. Use of support hose?	

Copyright © 2014. Wolters Kluwer Health | Lippincott Williams & Wilkins. Lab Manual for Health Assessment in Nursing, 5e.

Activity F **PERFORMING PHYSICAL ASSESSMENT OF THE PERIPHERAL VASCULAR SYSTEM**

Use the following Physical Assessment Guide to examine the peripheral vascular status of a lab partner, peer, or client. Column 1 will serve as a reminder as to what part of the exam you will do next. Column 2 will be used to record your findings. Your instructor may ask you to turn this in to be evaluated. Forms are also available on thePoint *website.*

Physical Assessment Guide to Collect Objective Client Data

Questions	Findings
Current Symptoms	
1. Gather equipment (gloves, centimeter tape, stethoscope, Doppler ultrasound probe, and tourniquet).	
2. Ask client to put on a gown.	
Assess Arms	
1. Inspect bilaterally for size, presence of edema, and venous patterning.	
2. Inspect bilaterally for skin color.	
3. Inspect fingertips for clubbing.	
4. Palpate fingers, hands, and arms for temperature, using dorsal surface of your fingers.	
5. Determine capillary refill time.	
6. Palpate radial, ulnar, and brachial pulses.	
7. Palpate epitrochlear lymph nodes behind the elbow in the groove between the biceps and triceps muscles.	
8. Perform Allen test by occluding the radial and ulnar arteries and observing for palm pallor. Then, release the ulnar artery and watch for color to return to hand.	
Assess Legs	
1. Inspect bilaterally for skin color (client in supine position).	
2. Inspect bilaterally for distribution of hair.	
3. Inspect for lesions or ulcers (note whether margins are smooth and even, location such as at pressure points, size, depth, drainage, odor).	
4. Inspect for edema, unilateral or bilateral (if calves are asymmetric, measure calf circumference).	
5. If client has edema, determine whether it is pitting or nonpitting. If client has pitting edema, rate on a 1+ to 4+ scale.	
6. Palpate skin temperature (cool, warm, hot). Use dorsal surface of hands.	
7. Palpate the superficial inguinal lymph nodes while keeping the genitals draped. If detected, note size, mobility, or tenderness.	
8. Palpate and auscultate femoral pulses over artery. Listen for bruits.	

Copyright © 2014. Wolters Kluwer Health | Lippincott Williams & Wilkins. Lab Manual for Health Assessment in Nursing, 5e.

Physical Assessment Guide to Collect Objective Client Data (continued)	
Questions	**Findings**
9. Palpate popliteal, dorsalis pedis, and posterior tibial pulses.	
10. Inspect for varicosities and thrombophlebitis by asking client to stand.	
11. Perform position change test for arterial insufficiency while client is in the supine position by placing hands under both of the client's ankles. Raise legs 30.48 cm (12 in) above heart level, and ask client to pump feet up and down for 1 minute. Have client sit up and dangle legs. Note color of feet. Time the interval for color to return.	
12. If varicosities are present, perform the manual compression test by having client stand. Firmly compress the lower portion of the varicose vein with one hand. Place other hand 15.2 to 20.3 cm (6 to 8 in) above hand. Feel for pulsation in the upper hand.	
13. If varicosities are present, perform the Trendelenburg test with client in supine position. Elevate leg 90 degrees for 15 seconds. With legs elevated, apply a tourniquet to the upper thigh. Assist client to a standing position, and observe for venous filling. Remove tourniquet after 30 seconds, and watch for sudden filling of the varicose veins from above.	
Analysis of Data	
1. Formulate nursing diagnoses (wellness, risk, actual).	
2. Formulate collaborative problems.	
3. Make necessary referrals.	

CHAPTER POSTTEST

Activity G MULTIPLE CHOICE QUESTIONS

Choose the one best answer for each of the following multiple choice questions.

_____ 1. While assessing the peripheral vascular system of an adult client, the nurse detects cold clammy skin and loss of hair on the client's legs. The nurse suspects that the client may be experiencing

    a. venous stasis.

    b. varicose veins.

    c. thrombophlebitis.

    d. arterial insufficiency.

_____ 2. During a physical examination, the nurse detects warm skin and brown pigmentation around an adult client's ankles. The nurse suspects that the client may be experiencing

    a. venous insufficiency.

    b. arterial occlusive disease.

    c. venous ulcers.

    d. ankle edema.

Copyright © 2014. Wolters Kluwer Health | Lippincott Williams & Wilkins. Lab Manual for Health Assessment in Nursing, 5e.

____ 3. The nurse is assessing the peripheral vascular system of an older adult client. The client tells the nurse that her legs "seem cold all the time and sometimes feel tingly." The nurse suspects that the client may be experiencing

    a. varicose veins.

    b. intermittent claudication.

    c. edema.

    d. thrombophlebitis.

____ 4. The nurse is caring for a client who is employed as a typist and has a family history of peripheral vascular disease. The nurse should instruct the client to reduce her risk factors by

    a. eating a high-protein diet.

    b. resting frequently.

    c. drinking large quantities of milk.

    d. getting regular exercise.

____ 5. The nurse is preparing to use a Doppler ultrasound probe to detect blood flow in the femoral artery of an adult client. The nurse should

    a. apply K-Y jelly to the client's skin.

    b. place the client in a supine position with the head flat.

    c. place the tip of the probe in a 30-degree angle to the artery.

    d. apply gel used for ECG to the client's skin.

____ 6. A client visits the clinic and tells the nurse that she had a mastectomy 2 years ago. The nurse should assess the client for

    a. lymphedema.

    b. Raynaud disease.

    c. poor peripheral pulses.

    d. bruits over the radial artery.

____ 7. After palpating the radial pulse of an adult client, the nurse suspects arterial insufficiency. The nurse should next assess the client's

    a. femoral pulse.

    b. popliteal pulse.

    c. brachial pulse.

    d. tibial pulse.

____ 8. The nurse is preparing to palpate the epitrochlear lymph nodes of an adult male client. The nurse should instruct the client to

    a. assume a supine position.

    b. rest his arm on the examination table.

    c. flex his elbow about 90 degrees.

    d. make a fist with his left hand.

____ 9. While inspecting the skin color of a male client's legs, the nurse observes that the client's legs are slightly cyanotic while he is sitting on the edge of the examination table. The nurse should refer the client to a physician for possible

    a. arterial insufficiency.

    b. congestive heart failure.

    c. Raynaud disease.

    d. venous insufficiency.

____ **10.** While assessing the inguinal lymph nodes in an older adult client, the nurse detects that the lymph nodes are approximately 3 cm in diameter, nontender, and fixed. The nurse should refer the client to a physician because these findings are generally associated with

    a. localized infection.

    b. systemic infection.

    c. arterial insufficiency.

    d. malignancy.

Activity H **CRITICAL THINKING ACTIVITY**

1. Explain how to distinguish between arterial and venous insufficiency.

2. Explain how to distinguish between edema associated with lymphedema versus edema associated with chronic venous insufficiency.

Activity I **CASE STUDY**

Read the following case study. Then, work through the steps of analyzing the case study data. First, identify the abnormal data and strengths in **subjective and objective findings**, assemble **cue clusters**, draw **inferences**, make possible **nursing diagnoses**, identify **defining characteristics**, **confirm or rule out** the diagnoses, and **document** your conclusions. Use the blank diagnostic analysis charts provided at the end of this book (also available on thePoint website) to guide your thinking. Propose nursing diagnoses that are specific to the client in the case study. Identify collaborative problems, if any, for this client. Finally, identify data, if any, that point toward a medical problem requiring a referral.

Fran H. is an 84-year-old white widow, with a medical diagnosis of venous (stasis) ulcers on the medial surface of her right lower leg. She is 149.8 cm (4 ft 11 in) tall and weighs 45.3 kg (100 lb). She has been referred by her physician to the Visiting Nurse Association (VNA) for skilled visits three times a week by an R.N. She lives in a small rural community in her own home. She lives alone, but her older sister, aged 87 years, lives across the street and looks after her. Fran has one adult daughter, who is married and lives out of state.

    When interviewed, Fran says she has had a history of venous ulcers for the past 10 years and has been seen in the past by the VNA for treatment of these ulcers. The last time she was seen for this was approximately 8 months ago, when she had venous ulcers on the medial aspects of both legs. Both areas were well healed at the time of discharge.

    Although communication with Fran is difficult because of a hearing loss, she denies any pain from the ulcers. However, she does cry out at times during the dressing changes. Her sister provides most of the information for the nurses and states that Fran has been up more than usual during the past few weeks and does not rest with her legs elevated as much as she should. Fran can ambulate with the aid of a walker. Her sister checks on Fran several times during the day and prepares meals for her.

    Physical assessment reveals the following findings on the upper extremities: no edema, pink, and no areas of discoloration observed bilaterally. The nail beds have no signs of clubbing. The upper and lower arms are warm to touch; however, the hands are slightly cool to touch. Capillary refill time is normal. The radial and brachial pulses are strong bilaterally. The epitrochlear lymph nodes are nonpalpable. The ulnar pulses are nonpalpable. Results of Allen test are normal.

    Physical assessment of lower extremities reveals areas of brownish pigmentation at the ankles. The legs are warm to the touch. An area of ulceration approximately 4 cm × 7 cm is present on the medial aspect of the left ankle. The medial aspect of the right lower leg has an area of scar tissue approximately 3 cm × 8 cm. Both lower legs are thin, but the left leg is slightly swollen, with 1+ pitting edema. No varicosities are noted. The inguinal lymph nodes are nonpalpable, and the femoral pulses are strong and equal bilaterally. The popliteal pulses are absent, and the dorsalis pedal pulses are weak in both feet. The posterior tibial pulses are present but weak. The client is unable to complete testing for arterial insufficiency.

How Well Did You Do?

After you have read the chapter and completed the exercises in this chapter, visit thePoint to access the Self-Reflection Activity. This activity will help you identify to what degree you have met each of the chapter objectives. You can then review the chapter for objectives you have met partially or not at all.

    Other tools to help you, like the Diagnostic Reasoning Guides, Nursing Interview Guides, Physical Assessment Guides, and NCLEX-Style Chapter Review Questions, are also available on thePoint.

Copyright © 2014. Wolters Kluwer Health | Lippincott Williams & Wilkins. Lab Manual for Health Assessment in Nursing, 5e.

Assessing Abdomen

Chapter Overview

The abdomen houses the structures of several different body systems—gastrointestinal, reproductive (female), lymphatic, and urinary. Known as the solid or hollow abdominal viscera, these structures include the liver, pancreas, spleen, adrenal glands, kidneys, ovaries, and uterus (solid viscera) and the stomach, gallbladder, small intestine, colon, and bladder (hollow viscera). Abdominal assessment is complex, largely because of the many vital organs and blood vessels within the abdominal cavity and the life-sustaining functions such as digestion and elimination that are performed there.

Chapter Learning Objectives

1. Describe the structures and functions of the abdomen.
2. Identify the organs located in each of the quadrants and the nine regions of the abdomen.
3. Discuss the incidence of peptic ulcer disease and ways to reduce one's risks.
4. Describe the teaching opportunities to reduce the risks of peptic ulcer disease and to promote health.
5. Obtain an accurate nursing history of the client's abdomen and related functions.
6. Perform a physical assessment of the abdomen using the correct techniques of inspection, auscultation, palpation, and percussion.
7. Differentiate between normal and abnormal findings of the abdomen.
8. Describe the findings frequently seen when assessing the older client's abdomen.
9. Analyze the data from the interview and physical assessment of the abdomen to formulate valid nursing diagnoses, collaborative problems, and/or referrals.

CHAPTER PRETEST

Activity A MULTIPLE CHOICE QUESTIONS

Choose the one best answer for each of the following multiple choice questions.

_____ 1. The abdominal contents are enclosed externally by the abdominal wall musculature—three layers of muscle extending from the back, around the flanks, to the front. The outer muscle layer is the external

   a. rectal abdominis.

   b. transverse abdominis.

   c. abdominal oblique.

   d. umbilical oblique.

_____ **2.** The sigmoid colon is located in this area of the abdomen: the

    a. left upper quadrant.

    b. left lower quadrant.

    c. right upper quadrant.

    d. right lower quadrant.

_____ **3.** The pancreas of an adult client is located

    a. below the diaphragm and extending below the right costal margin.

    b. posterior to the left midaxillary line and posterior to the stomach.

    c. high and deep under the diaphragm and can be palpated.

    d. deep in the upper abdomen and is not normally palpable.

_____ **4.** The primary function of the gallbladder is to

    a. store and excrete bile.

    b. aid in the digestion of protein.

    c. produce alkaline mucus.

    d. produce hormones.

_____ **5.** The colon originates in this abdominal area: the

    a. right lower quadrant.

    b. right upper quadrant.

    c. left lower quadrant.

    d. left upper quadrant.

Activity B MATCHING

Match the terms in the left column with the correct descriptions in the right column.

Term

_____ **1.** Murphy sign

_____ **2.** Cholecystitis

_____ **3.** Peptic ulcer disease

_____ **4.** Ascites

_____ **5.** Ballottement test

_____ **6.** Paralytic ileus

_____ **7.** Positive psoas sign

_____ **8.** Rebound tenderness

_____ **9.** Hernia

_____ **10.** Intestinal obstruction

Description

a. Absent or high-pitched bowel sounds

b. Can identify a mass or enlarged organ in an ascitic abdomen

c. Release of pressure quickly after deep palpation

d. Protrusion of the bowel through the abdominal wall

e. Inspiratory arrest or causes client to hold breath

f. Bacterium *Helicobacter pylori*

g. RUQ pain or tenderness

h. Increased peristaltic waves

i. Shifting dullness and fluid wave tests

j. Assessed by raising right leg from hip

Copyright © 2014. Wolters Kluwer Health | Lippincott Williams & Wilkins. Lab Manual for Health Assessment in Nursing, 5e.

Activity C LABELING ACTIVITIES

Label the four quadrants of the abdomen in the following figure. Check your answers with Figure 23-1 on page 474 in the textbook.

Label the nine regions of the abdomen in the following figures. Check your answers with Figure 23-2 on page 474 in the textbook.

Label the organs and associated structures of the abdomen in the following figure. Check your answers with Figure 23-4 on page 475 in the textbook.

Label the palpable structures in the abdomen in the following figure. Check your answers with Figure 23-20 on page 493 in the textbook.

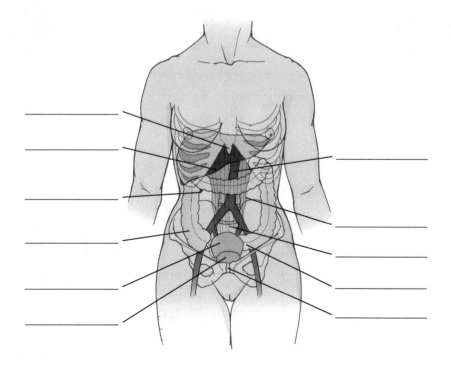

Copyright © 2014. Wolters Kluwer Health | Lippincott Williams & Wilkins. Lab Manual for Health Assessment in Nursing, 5e.

Activity D LEARNER ACTIVITIES

After reading Chapter 23 in the textbook, participate in the following learning activities.

1. Review the information in EVIDENCE-BASED HEALTH PROMOTION AND DISEASE PREVENTION: PEPTIC ULCER DISEASE (see pages 482–483 in your textbook). Determine your risk for peptic ulcer disease. Then, interview your lab partner to determine his/her risk for peptic ulcer disease. Discuss with your lab partner what teaching would be appropriate to reduce an individual's risk for peptic ulcer disease.

2. Perform an abdominal assessment on an elderly client, friend, or relative. Discuss your assessment findings with your lab partner as they compare to those of a younger person.

Activity E INTERVIEWING AND RECORDING ASSESSMENT FINDINGS

After reading Chapter 23, use the following Nursing Interview Guide to interview and record your subjective findings for an assessment of abdomen of a lab partner, peer, or client. Your instructor may ask you to turn this in to be evaluated. Forms are also available on thePoint *website.*

Nursing Interview Guide to Collect Subjective Data From the Client	
Questions	**Findings**
Current Symptoms	
1. Abdominal pain present?	
2. What factors precipitate the pain or make it worse?	
3. Description and location of the pain?	
4. Other symptoms present, such as nausea, vomiting, diarrhea, appetite changes, constipation?	
5. Recent weight gain or loss?	
Past History	
1. Previous abdominal surgery/trauma/injury/medications?	
2. Previous abdominal pain and treatment?	
3. Results of any lab work or gastrointestinal studies?	
Family History	
1. Stomach, colon, or liver cancer?	
2. Abdominal pain, appendicitis, colitis, bleeding, or hemorrhoids?	
3. Person responsible for nutrition in family?	
Lifestyle and Health Practices	
1. Smoking, amount?	
2. Alcohol use, amount?	
3. Diet (food and drink), past 24 hours?	
4. Antacid use, amount?	
5. Medication use?	
6. Fluid intake?	
7. Exercise, amount?	
8. Cause of stress in life; effect on eating and elimination patterns?	
9. Past actions with abdominal pain or problems?	

Activity F **PERFORMING PHYSICAL ASSESSMENT OF THE ABDOMEN**

Use the following Physical Assessment Guide to examine the abdomen of a lab partner, peer, or client. Column 1 will serve as a reminder as to what part of the exam you will do next. Column 2 will be used to record your findings. Your instructor may ask you to turn this in to be evaluated. Forms are also available on thePoint *website.*

Physical Assessment Guide to Collect Objective Client Data

Questions	Findings
Current Symptoms	
1. Gather equipment (pillow/towel, centimeter ruler, stethoscope, marking pen).	
2. Explain the procedure to client.	
3. Ask the client to put on a gown.	
Abdomen	
1. Inspect the skin, noting color, vascularity, striae, scars, and lesions (wear gloves to inspect lesions).	
2. Inspect the umbilicus, noting color, location, and contour.	
3. Inspect the contour of the abdomen.	
4. Inspect the symmetry of the abdomen.	
5. Inspect abdominal movement, noting respiratory movement, aortic pulsations, and/or peristaltic waves.	
6. Auscultate for bowel sounds, noting intensity, pitch, and frequency.	
7. Auscultate for vascular sounds and friction rubs.	
8. Percuss the abdomen for tone.	
9. Percuss the liver.	
10. Percuss the spleen.	
11. Perform blunt percussion on the liver and the kidneys.	
12. Perform light palpation, noting tenderness or guarding in all quadrants.	
13. Perform deep palpation, noting tenderness or masses in all quadrants.	
14. Palpate the umbilicus.	
15. Palpate the aorta.	
16. Palpate the liver, noting consistency and tenderness.	
17. Palpate the spleen, noting consistency and tenderness.	
18. Palpate the kidneys.	
19. Palpate the urinary bladder.	
20. Perform the test for shifting dullness.	
21. Perform the fluid wave test.	
22. Perform the ballottement test.	

Copyright © 2014. Wolters Kluwer Health | Lippincott Williams & Wilkins. Lab Manual for Health Assessment in Nursing, 5e.

Physical Assessment Guide to Collect Objective Client Data (continued)

Questions	Findings

23. Perform the tests for appendicitis.
     Rebound tenderness
     Rovsing sign
     Referred rebound tenderness
     Psoas sign
     Obturator sign
     Hypersensitivity test	

24. Perform the test for cholecystitis (Murphy sign).	
Analysis of Data	
1. Formulate nursing diagnoses (wellness, risk, actual).	
2. Formulate collaborative problems.	
3. Make necessary referrals.	

CHAPTER POSTTEST

Activity G   MULTIPLE CHOICE QUESTIONS

Choose the one best answer for each of the following multiple choice questions.

_____ 1. To percuss the liver of an adult client, the nurse should begin the abdominal assessment at the client's
   a. right upper quadrant.
   b. right lower quadrant.
   c. left upper quadrant.
   d. left lower quadrant.

_____ 2. To palpate for tenderness of an adult client's appendix, the nurse should begin the abdominal assessment at the client's
   a. left upper quadrant.
   b. left lower quadrant.
   c. right upper quadrant.
   d. right lower quadrant.

_____ 3. To palpate the spleen of an adult client, the nurse should begin the abdominal assessment of the client at the
   a. left lower quadrant.
   b. left upper quadrant.
   c. right upper quadrant.
   d. right lower quadrant.

_____ 4. The nurse plans to assess an adult client's kidneys for tenderness. The nurse should assess the area at the
   a. right upper quadrant.
   b. left upper quadrant.
   c. external oblique angle.
   d. costovertebral angle.

_____ **5.** A client visits the clinic because she experienced bright hematemesis yesterday. The nurse should refer the client to a physician because this symptom is indicative of

    a. stomach ulcers.

    b. pancreatic cancer.

    c. decreased gastric motility.

    d. abdominal tumors.

_____ **6.** The nurse is assessing an older adult client who has lost 2.27 kg (5 lb) since her last visit 1 year ago. The client tells the nurse that her husband died 2 months ago. The nurse should further assess the client for

    a. peptic ulcer.

    b. bulimia.

    c. appetite changes.

    d. pancreatic disorders.

_____ **7.** A client visits the clinic for a routine examination. The client tells the nurse that she has become constipated because she is taking iron tablets prescribed for anemia. The nurse has instructed the client about the use of iron preparations and possible constipation. The nurse determines that the client has understood the instructions when she says

    a. "I can decrease the constipation if I eat foods high in fiber and drink water."

    b. "I should cut down on the number of iron tablets I am taking each day."

    c. "Constipation should decrease if I take the iron tablets with milk."

    d. "I should discontinue the iron tablets and eat foods that are high in iron."

_____ **8.** The nurse is caring for a female client during her first postoperative day after a temporary colostomy. The client refuses to look at the colostomy bag or the area. A priority nursing diagnosis for this client is

    a. denial related to temporary colostomy.

    b. fear related to potential outcome of surgery.

    c. disturbed body image related to temporary colostomy.

    d. altered role functioning related to frequent colostomy bag changes.

_____ **9.** The nurse is preparing to assess the abdomen of a hospitalized client 2 days after abdominal surgery. The nurse should first

    a. palpate the incision site.

    b. auscultate for bowel sounds.

    c. percuss for tympany.

    d. inspect the abdominal area.

_____ **10.** The nurse is planning to assess the abdomen of an adult male client. Before the nurse begins the assessment, the nurse should

    a. ask the client to empty his bladder.

    b. place the client in a side-lying position.

    c. ask the client to hold his breath for a few seconds.

    d. tell the client to raise his arms above his head.

_____ **11.** The nurse is assessing the abdomen of an adult client and observes a purple discoloration at the flanks. The nurse should refer the client to a physician for possible

    a. liver disease.

    b. abdominal distention.

    c. Cushing syndrome.

    d. internal bleeding.

Copyright © 2014. Wolters Kluwer Health | Lippincott Williams & Wilkins. Lab Manual for Health Assessment in Nursing, 5e.

____ **12.** While assessing an adult client's abdomen, the nurse observes that the client's umbilicus is deviated to the left. The nurse should refer the client to a physician for possible

   a. gallbladder disease.

   b. cachexia.

   c. kidney trauma.

   d. masses.

____ **13.** While assessing an adult client's abdomen, the nurse observes that the client's umbilicus is enlarged and everted. The nurse should refer the client to a physician for possible

   a. umbilical hernia.

   b. ascites.

   c. intra-abdominal bleeding.

   d. pancreatitis.

____ **14.** The nurse assesses an adult male client's abdomen and observes diminished abdominal respiration. The nurse determines that the client should be further assessed for

   a. liver disease.

   b. umbilical hernia.

   c. intestinal obstruction.

   d. peritoneal irritation.

____ **15.** The nurse is assessing the bowel sounds of an adult client. After listening to each quadrant, the nurse determines that bowel sounds are not present. The nurse should refer the client to a physician for possible

   a. aortic aneurysm.

   b. paralytic ileus.

   c. gastroenteritis.

   d. fluid and electrolyte imbalances.

____ **16.** While assessing the abdominal sounds of an adult client, the nurse hears high-pitched tingling sounds throughout the distended abdomen. The nurse should refer the client to a physician for possible

   a. intestinal obstruction.

   b. gastroenteritis.

   c. inflamed appendix.

   d. cirrhosis of the liver.

____ **17.** During a physical examination of an adult client, the nurse is preparing to auscultate the client's abdomen. The nurse should

   a. palpate the abdomen before auscultation.

   b. listen in each quadrant for 15 seconds.

   c. use the diaphragm of the stethoscope.

   d. begin auscultation in the left upper quadrant.

____ **18.** To palpate the spleen of an adult client, the nurse should

   a. ask the client to exhale deeply.

   b. place the right hand below the left costal margin.

   c. point the fingers of the left hand downward.

   d. ask the client to remain in a supine position.

____ **19.** The nurse is planning to assess a client's abdomen for rebound tenderness. The nurse should

   a. perform this abdominal assessment first.

   b. ask the client to assume a side-lying position.

   c. palpate lightly while slowly releasing pressure.

   d. palpate deeply while quickly releasing pressure.

Copyright © 2014. Wolters Kluwer Health | Lippincott Williams & Wilkins. Lab Manual for Health Assessment in Nursing, 5e.

_____ **20.** To assess an adult client for possible appendicitis and a positive psoas sign, the nurse should

    a. rotate the client's knee internally.

    b. palpate at the lower right quadrant.

    c. raise the client's right leg from the hip.

    d. support the client's right knee and ankle.

Activity H CRITICAL THINKING ACTIVITIES

1. Imagine you find that your client's abdomen is distended, pale, and taut. Describe the tests you might perform, differentiating between the fluid wave test and the test for shifting dullness.

2. A client arrives in the emergency department with nausea, and localized, severe steady pain in the RLQ. You suspect that the client may have appendicitis. Describe the physical assessments that can be used to detect appendicitis.

3. A client presents with tenderness over the liver, right-sided guarding, and reports nausea and sharp pain in RUQ, particularly after eating fried foods. You suspect the client may have cholecystitis. Describe the physical assessment techniques used to detect cholecystitis.

4. Janet S. is 63 years old. She has a diagnosis of rheumatoid arthritis, for which she takes 8 to 10 aspirins daily to relieve pain. She states that for the past few days her stools have been dark and tarry-looking and her stomach has been upset and "queasy." Hoping to settle her stomach, she changed her diet in the past 2 days to include only soups and fluids. She tells you that the only other medication she takes is a calcium supplement.

    a. Describe the most likely cause for her upset stomach.

    b. Discuss the likely findings following an interview with her.

Activity I CASE STUDY

Read the following case study. Then, work through the steps of analyzing the case study data. First identify abnormal data and strengths in **subjective and objective findings**, assemble **cue clusters**, draw **inferences**, make possible **nursing diagnoses**, identify **defining characteristics**, **confirm or rule out** the diagnoses, and **document** your conclusions. Use the blank diagnostic analysis charts provided at the end of this book (also available on thePoint website) to guide your thinking. Propose nursing diagnoses that are specific to the client in the case study. Identify collaborative problems, if any, for this client. Finally, identify data, if any that point toward a medical problem requiring a referral.

Mrs. Vera W. is a 60-year-old white woman, who emigrated from Germany to the United States at the age of 18. She has come to her primary care physician's office with her daughter. She tells you, "My daughter made me come here because I have had bad stomach pains for about 6 weeks." After you ask about the character, onset, location, duration, severity, and pattern of the pain as well as associated symptoms (COLDSPA), such as what relieves the pain and what functions are affected by pain, you learn the following information. The pain is aching epigastric pain, fairly continuous, and worse at night. It radiates to her back when she lies down. The pain gets progressively worse, is not affected by eating, and interferes with her daily function (it prevented her from attending her grandson's birthday party and it also wakes her up at night). In addition, in the interview, Mrs. W. relates loss of appetite, mild nausea, heartburn, and fatigue. For the past several months she has felt full soon after beginning a meal. She tells you that she was afraid to tell her doctor this because "he always says I worry too much."

    A review of Mrs. W.'s chart discloses that she had four normal vaginal deliveries, several bladder and kidney infections, a total abdominal hysterectomy at age 50 for uterine fibroids, cholecystectomy at age 55, two episodes of deep vein thrombosis in the past few years, allergy to penicillin, and stomach sensitivity to medicines (e.g., aspirin). Four years ago she had gastric endoscopy and upper gastrointestinal (GI) barium swallow studies for complaints of heartburn and difficulty swallowing. The results revealed delayed esophageal peristalsis.

    Mrs. W. takes estrogen and calcium daily (in the form of Tums) as recommended by her physician as a source of hormone and calcium after surgical menopause. She tells you that she has recently started to take acetaminophen once—sometimes twice—daily in the hope that this will relieve her pain. She has had mild temporary relief as a result.

    Mrs. W.'s family history reveals that her mother died at age 58 from "liver problems after having half her stomach removed." She says she does not smoke, drink, or use illegal drugs. She says that she has eaten the same diet all her life. "I eat good German food, a lot of potatoes and meats. My children tell me I should eat more vegetables and drink more water, but I don't like fruits and vegetables and I'd rather drink coffee." In response to your question about exercise, you learn that Mrs. W. walks to the post office every day, and "I pick up after my

Copyright © 2014. Wolters Kluwer Health | Lippincott Williams & Wilkins. Lab Manual for Health Assessment in Nursing, 5e.

husband around the house—does that count?" You comment that Mrs. W. looks upset, and she tells you that she is very concerned about her pain. "I have always been strong and healthy, and now I am getting old and sick. It is depressing."

Your physical assessment reveals a firmly palpable left supraclavicular node, approximately 2 cm in diameter, nonmobile, and nontender, as well as the following abdominal findings: abdomen round and symmetric, hysterectomy scar, striae, umbilicus in the midline without inflammation or herniation, slight midline pulsation in the epigastrium. Soft bowel sounds are heard in all four quadrants; no audible bruits. Generalized tympany percussed throughout; span of liver dullness is 13 cm over the MCL, splenic dullness at the 10th intercostal space (ICS). The abdomen is soft and tender to palpation in the epigastrium; the liver edge descends 2 cm below the right costal margin (RCM) on deep inspiration; no splenomegaly is noted.

How Well Did You Do?

After you have read the chapter and completed the exercises in this chapter, visit thePoint to access the Self-Reflection Activity. This activity will help you identify to what degree you have met each of the chapter objectives. You can then review the chapter for objectives you have met partially or not at all.

Other tools to help you, like the Diagnostic Reasoning Guides, Nursing Interview Guides, Physical Assessment Guides, and NCLEX-Style Chapter Review Questions, are also available on thePoint.

Copyright © 2014. Wolters Kluwer Health | Lippincott Williams & Wilkins. Lab Manual for Health Assessment in Nursing, 5e.

CHAPTER 24

Assessing Musculoskeletal System

Chapter Overview

Muscles, bones, joints, ligaments, and tendons are the body's infrastructure—the elements that allow humans an upright posture and extensive mobility. Changes that occur in other body systems may have a profound effect on the musculoskeletal system, and changes that occur in the musculoskeletal system itself affect the activities of daily living and quality of life across the lifespan, making careful and accurate assessment extremely important. For example, musculoskeletal system problems may result in pain and reduced mobility leading to social isolation, limited ability to participate in family and recreational activities as well as lowered self-esteem. Use the following exercises and quizzes to guide your assessment of the musculoskeletal system.

Chapter Learning Objectives

1. Describe the structure and functions of the bones, skeletal muscles, and joints.
2. Discuss the incidence of osteoporosis across cultures and ways to reduce one's risks.
3. Describe the teaching opportunities to reduce risks for osteoporosis and promote joint health.
4. Obtain an accurate nursing history of the client's muscles, joints, and bones.
5. Perform a physical assessment of the musculoskeletal system using the correct techniques of inspection, auscultation, palpation, and percussion.
6. Differentiate between normal and abnormal findings of the musculoskeletal system.
7. Describe the expected aging changes of the bones, skeletal muscles, and joints.
8. Describe the findings frequently seen when assessing the older client's musculoskeletal system.
9. Analyze the data from the interview and physical assessment of the musculoskeletal system to formulate valid nursing diagnoses, collaborative problems, and/or referrals.

CHAPTER PRETEST

Activity A **MULTIPLE CHOICE QUESTIONS**

Choose the one best answer for each of the following multiple choice questions.

_____ **1.** One of the functions of a bone is to
   a. store fat.
   b. produce secretions.
   c. produce blood cells.
   d. store protein.

_____ **2.** Bones contain yellow marrow that is composed mainly of
   a. fat.
   b. protein.
   c. cartilage.
   d. carbohydrates.

_____ **3.** The external covering of the bone that contains osteoblasts and blood vessels is termed the
   a. cartilage.
   b. synovial membrane.
   c. connective tissue.
   d. periosteum.

_____ **4.** Skeletal muscles are attached to bones by
   a. tendons.
   b. cartilage.
   c. fibrous connective tissue.
   d. ligaments.

_____ **5.** Joints may be classified as cartilaginous, synovial, or
   a. articulate.
   b. flexible.
   c. immobile.
   d. fibrous.

_____ **6.** Bones in synovial joints are joined together by
   a. cartilage.
   b. ligaments.
   c. tendons.
   d. periosteal tissue.

_____ **7.** When the nurse moves the client's arm away from the midline of the body, the nurse is performing
   a. adduction.
   b. external rotation.
   c. retraction.
   d. abduction.

_____ **8.** When the nurse moves a client's leg upward, the nurse is performing
   a. supination.
   b. external rotation.
   c. eversion.
   d. internal rotation.

____ **9.** The subacromial bursae are contained in the

    a. temporomandibular joint.

    b. shoulder joint.

    c. elbow joint.

    d. wrist joint.

____ **10.** Articulation between the head of the femur and the acetabulum is in the

    a. knee joint.

    b. tibial joint.

    c. ankle joint.

    d. hip joint.

Activity B   MATCHING

Match the terms in the left column with the correct description in the right column.

Term

____ **1.** Adduction

____ **2.** Bursitis

____ **3.** Myalgia

____ **4.** Cogwheel

____ **5.** Dorsiflexion

____ **6.** Crepitus

____ **7.** Flexion

____ **8.** Plantar

____ **9.** Extension

____ **10.** Kyphosis

Description

a. Type of rigidity characterized by jerky movements with passive stretching

b. Crackling sound or sensation heard or felt with joint movement

c. Movement that brings a limb into or toward a bent condition

d. Inflammation of the bursa

e. Abnormal convexity of the posterior curve of spine

f. Movement bringing a limb into or toward a straight condition

g. Backward bending or flexion of a joint

h. Moving limbs toward median plane of body

i. Type of flexion associate with foot extension

j. Tenderness or pain in the muscle

Activity C   LABELING ACTIVITIES

Label the major structures of the shoulder in the following figure. Check your answers with the figure of the shoulder in Box 24-2 on page 511 in the textbook.

Copyright © 2014. Wolters Kluwer Health | Lippincott Williams & Wilkins. Lab Manual for Health Assessment in Nursing, 5e.

Label the major structures of the elbow in the following figure. Check your answers with the figure of the elbow in Box 24-2 on page 511 in the textbook.

Label the structures of the hip in the following figure. Check your answers with the figure of the hip in Box 24-2 on page 512 in the textbook.

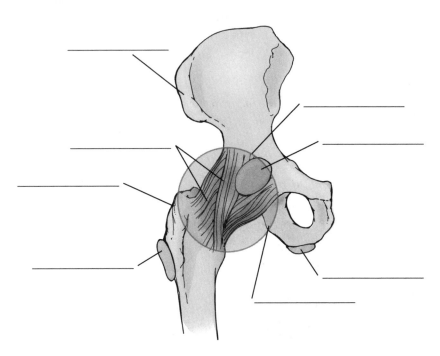

Copyright © 2014. Wolters Kluwer Health | Lippincott Williams & Wilkins. Lab Manual for Health Assessment in Nursing, 5e.

Label the structures of the knee in the following figure. Check your answers with figure of the knee in Box 24-2 on page 513 in the textbook.

Activity D LEARNER ACTIVITIES

After reading Chapter 24 in the textbook, participate in the following learning activities.

1. Review the information in EVIDENCE-BASED HEALTH PROMOTION AND DISEASE PREVENTION: OSTEOPOROSIS (see page 517 in your textbook). Determine your own risk of osteoporosis. Next, identify ethnic groups that are at highest risk for osteoporosis. Discuss what teaching could be implemented to reduce these risks.

2. Obtain brochures and literature on osteoporosis from the county health department or your local health care facility. Discuss with your lab partner how best to give a presentation on this topic to college-aged women and then to a group of middle-aged women.

3. Assess your lab partner's musculoskeletal system including gait and ROM of joints.

4. Perform an assessment of the musculoskeletal system on an older client, friend, or relative, including knees for the "bulge test," "ballottement test," and "McMurray test" as appropriate. Discuss with peers your findings as they compare with the findings in a younger person.

Copyright © 2014. Wolters Kluwer Health | Lippincott Williams & Wilkins. Lab Manual for Health Assessment in Nursing, 5e.

Activity E **INTERVIEWING AND RECORDING ASSESSMENT FINDINGS**

After reading Chapter 24, use the following Nursing Interview Guide to interview and record your subjective findings for an assessment of the musculoskeletal system of a lab partner, peer, or client. Your instructor may ask you to turn this in to be evaluated. Forms are also available on thePoint *website.*

Nursing Interview Guide to Collect Subjective Data From the Client	
Questions	**Findings**
Current Symptoms	
1. Recent weight gain?	
2. Difficulty chewing?	
3. Joint, muscle, or bone throbbing?	
Past History	
1. Past problems or injuries to joints, muscles, or bones?	
2. Past treatment: surgery, medications, physical therapy, exercise, rest?	
3. Tetanus and polio immunizations?	
4. Diagnosed with diabetes mellitus, lupus, or sickle cell anemia?	
5. How old at start of menstruation; started menopause; estrogen replacement therapy?	
Family History	
1. Family history of rheumatoid arthritis, gout, osteoporosis, psoriasis, infectious tuberculosis?	
Lifestyle and Health Practices	
1. Activities to promote musculoskeletal health?	
2. Home remedies to relieve musculoskeletal problems?	
3. Assistive devices to promote mobility?	
4. Smoking?	
5. Alcohol or caffeinated beverages?	
6. Typical diet, drink milk, take calcium supplements?	
7. Occupation?	
8. Time in sunlight?	
9. Routine exercise?	
10. Difficulty with ADL?	
11. Typical posture?	
12. Interference with sexual activities?	
13. Ability to interact/socialize?	
14. Body image?	
15. Stress?	

Activity F **PERFORMING PHYSICAL ASSESSMENT OF THE MUSCULOSKELETAL SYSTEM**

Use the following Physical Assessment Guide to examine the musculoskeletal system of a lab partner, peer, or client. Column 1 will serve as a reminder as to what part of the exam you will do next. Column 2 will be used to record your findings. Your instructor may ask you to turn this in to be evaluated. Forms are also available on thePoint *website.*

Physical Assessment Guide to Collect Objective Client Data

Questions	Findings
1. Gather equipment (tape measure, goniometer).	
2. Explain the procedure to client.	
3. Ask the client to put on a gown.	
Gait	
1. Observe gait for base, weight-bearing stability, feet position, stride, arm swing, and posture.	
Temporomandibular Joint	
1. Inspect, palpate, and test ROM.	
Sternoclavicular Joint	
1. Inspect and palpate for midline location, color, swelling, and masses.	
Spine	
1. Inspect and palpate cervical, thoracic, and lumbar spine for pain and tenderness.	
2. Test ROM of cervical spine.	
3. Test ROM of thoracic and lumbar spine.	
4. Test for leg and back pain.	
5. Measure leg length.	
Shoulders	
1. Inspect and palpate shoulders for symmetry, color, swelling, and masses.	
2. Test ROM of shoulders.	
Elbows	
1. Inspect and palpate elbows for size, shape, deformities, redness, or swelling.	
2. Test ROM of elbows.	
Wrists	
1. Inspect and palpate wrists for size, shape, symmetry, color, swelling, tenderness, and nodules.	
2. Test ROM of wrists.	
3. Test for carpal tunnel syndrome.	
Hands and Fingers	
1. Inspect and palpate hands and fingers for size, shape, symmetry, swelling, color, tenderness, and nodules.	
2. Test ROM of hands and fingers.	

Copyright © 2014. Wolters Kluwer Health | Lippincott Williams & Wilkins. Lab Manual for Health Assessment in Nursing, 5e.

Physical Assessment Guide to Collect Objective Client Data (continued)	
Questions	**Findings**
Hips	
1. Inspect and palpate hips for shape and symmetry.	
2. Test ROM of hips.	
Knees	
1. Inspect and palpate knees for size, shape, symmetry, deformities, pain, and alignment.	
2. Test knees for swelling. If small amount of fluid present, do "bulge test." If large amount of fluid present, do "ballottement test."	
3. Test ROM of knees.	
4. Perform McMurray test if client complains of "clicking" in knee.	
Ankles and Feet	
1. Inspect and palpate ankles and feet for position, alignment, shape, skin, tenderness, temperature, swelling, or nodules.	
2. Test ROM of ankles and toes.	
Analysis of Data	
1. Formulate nursing diagnoses (health promotion, risk, actual).	
2. Formulate collaborative problems.	
3. Make necessary referrals.	

CHAPTER POSTTEST

Activity G   MULTIPLE CHOICE QUESTIONS

Choose the one best answer for each of the following multiple choice questions.

_____   **1.** A client visits the clinic and tells the nurse that she has joint pain in her hands, especially in the morning. The nurse should assess the client further for signs and symptoms of

    a. arthritis.

    b. osteoporosis.

    c. carpal tunnel syndrome.

    d. a neurologic disorder.

_____   **2.** A client with insulin-dependent diabetes visits the clinic and complains of painful hip joints. The nurse should assess the client carefully for signs and symptoms of

    a. arthritis.

    b. gait difficulties.

    c. osteomyelitis.

    d. scoliosis.

Copyright © 2014. Wolters Kluwer Health | Lippincott Williams & Wilkins. Lab Manual for Health Assessment in Nursing, 5e.

____ **3.** A female client visits the clinic and tells the nurse that she began menarche at the age of 16 years. The nurse should instruct the client that she is at a higher risk for

  a. osteoporosis.

  b. osteomyelitis.

  c. rheumatoid arthritis.

  d. lordosis.

____ **4.** The nurse is planning a presentation on osteoporosis to a group of high school students. Which of the following should the nurse plan to include in the presentation?

  a. Bone density rises to a peak at age 50 for both sexes.

  b. Bone density in the Asian population is higher than in the white population.

  c. Moderate strenuous exercise tends to increase bone density.

  d. Approximately 5 million fractures in the United States are due to osteoporosis.

____ **5.** The nurse is caring for an adult client who is in a cast because of a fractured arm. To promote healing of the bone and tissue, the nurse should instruct the client to eat a diet that is high in

  a. whole grains.

  b. vitamin B.

  c. vitamin E.

  d. vitamin C.

____ **6.** An adult client tells the nurse that he eats sardines every day. The nurse should instruct the client that a diet high in purines can contribute to

  a. gouty arthritis.

  b. osteomalacia.

  c. bone fractures.

  d. osteomyelitis.

____ **7.** A client tells the nurse that his grandmother had a diagnosis of osteomalacia. The nurse should instruct the client that to decrease the risk factors for osteomalacia, the clients should have adequate amounts of

  a. vitamin E.

  b. riboflavin.

  c. β-carotene.

  d. vitamin D.

____ **8.** The nurse is preparing to perform a musculoskeletal examination on an adult client. The nurse has explained the examination procedure to the client. The nurse determines that the client needs further instructions when the client says

  a. "You will be asking me to change positions often."

  b. "You'll be comparing bilateral joints."

  c. "You'll be assessing the size and strength of my joints."

  d. "You'll continue with range of motion even if I have discomfort."

____ **9.** While assessing muscle strength in an older adult client, the nurse determines that the client's knee joint has a rating of 3 and exhibits active motion against gravity. The nurse should document the client's muscle strength as being/having

  a. normal.

  b. slight weakness.

  c. average weakness.

  d. poor range of motion.

Copyright © 2014. Wolters Kluwer Health | Lippincott Williams & Wilkins. Lab Manual for Health Assessment in Nursing, 5e.

____ **10.** While assessing an adult client's jaw, the nurse hears a clicking popping sound, and the client expresses pain in the joint. The nurse should further assess the client for

    a. arthritis.

    b. TMJ dysfunction.

    c. bruxism.

    d. previous fracture.

____ **11.** While examining the spine of an adult client, the nurse notes that the client has a flattened lumbar curvature. The nurse should refer the client to a physician for possible

    a. herniated disc.

    b. scoliosis.

    c. kyphosis.

    d. cervical disc degeneration.

____ **12.** The nurse is assessing the spine of an adult client and detects lateral curvature of the thoracic spine with an increase in convexity on the left curved side. The nurse suspects that the client is experiencing

    a. lordosis.

    b. arthritis.

    c. kyphosis.

    d. scoliosis.

____ **13.** A client visits the clinic and tells the nurse that he has had lower back pain for the past several days. To perform Lasègue test, the nurse should ask the client to

    a. bend backward toward the nurse.

    b. lean forward and touch his toes.

    c. twist the shoulders in both directions.

    d. lie flat and raise his leg to the point of pain.

____ **14.** An older adult client visits the clinic and tells the nurse that she has had shooting pain in both of her legs. The nurse should assess the client for signs and symptoms of

    a. herniated intervertebral disc.

    b. rheumatoid arthritis.

    c. osteoporosis.

    d. metastases.

____ **15.** While assessing the range of motion in an adult client's shoulders, the client expresses pain and exhibits limited abduction and muscle weakness. The nurse plans to refer the client to a physician for possible

    a. rotator cuff tear.

    b. nerve damage.

    c. cervical disc degeneration.

    d. tendonitis.

____ **16.** While assessing an older adult client, the client complains of chronic pain and severe limitation of all shoulder movements. The nurse should refer the client to a physician for possible

    a. rotator cuff tendonitis.

    b. rheumatoid arthritis.

    c. calcified tendinitis.

    d. chronic bursitis.

____ **17.** A client visits the clinic and tells the nurse that after playing softball yesterday, he thinks his knee is "locking up." The nurse should perform the McMurray test by asking the client to

    a. move from a standing to a squatting position.

    b. raise his leg while in a supine position.

    c. bend forward while trying to touch the toes.

    d. flex the knee and hip while in a supine position.

Copyright © 2014. Wolters Kluwer Health | Lippincott Williams & Wilkins. Lab Manual for Health Assessment in Nursing, 5e.

___ **18.** While assessing the elbow of an adult client, the client complains of pain and swelling. The nurse should further assess the client for

    a. arthritis.

    b. ganglion cyst.

    c. carpal tunnel syndrome.

    d. nerve damage.

___ **19.** While reviewing a client's chart before seeing the client for the first time, the nurse notes that the client has a diagnosis of Dupuytren contracture. The nurse anticipates that the client will exhibit

    a. inability to turn the wrists.

    b. ulnar deviation of the hands.

    c. flexion of the distal interphalangeal joints.

    d. inability to extend the ring and little finger.

___ **20.** While assessing the musculoskeletal system of an adult client, the nurse observes hard painless nodules over the distal interphalangeal joints. The nurse should document the presence of

    a. osteoarthritis.

    b. bursitis.

    c. tendonitis.

    d. rheumatoid arthritis.

Activity H CRITICAL THINKING ACTIVITIES

1. Compare and contrast how you would assess for muscle strength, gait, and stability in a 25-year-old client versus those in a 75-year-old client. Discuss your answers with your lab partner.

2. Describe what assessments you would make on a client who came into your clinic with the diagnosis of rheumatoid arthritis. Discuss with your lab partner how you would perform these assessments.

ACTIVITY I CASE STUDY

Read the following case study. Then, work through the steps of analyzing the case study data. First identify abnormal data and strengths in **subjective and objective findings**, assemble **cue clusters**, draw **inferences**, make possible **nursing diagnoses**, identify **defining characteristics, confirm or rule out** the diagnoses, and **document** your conclusions. Use the blank diagnostic analysis charts provided at the end of this book (also available on thePoint website) to guide your thinking. Propose nursing diagnoses that are specific to the client in the case study. Identify collaborative problems, if any, for this client. Finally, identify data, if any that point toward a medical problem requiring a referral.

Mrs. Marjorie C. is a 71-year-old woman, who has had diabetes mellitus for 15 years. Her diabetes is controlled by diet and insulin. A retired schoolteacher, she has lived alone for the past 7 years since her husband died of liver cancer. Living in the upper level of a two-story apartment, she socializes with her neighbor and regularly attends church. She has a grown son and a daughter, who both live out of state and call frequently but can visit only once a year. Because of her poor eyesight, her neighbor, a retired RN, helps her draw up her insulin. When visited by the home health care nurse, Mrs. C. states that she has had lower back and wrist pain for the past month.

    During the interview, Mrs. C. describes a sedentary lifestyle, spending much of her time watching TV, crocheting, or doing crossword puzzles. She uses a magnifying glass for close work. However, she has reduced her handwork because she has been having numbness and tingling in her right thumb and index finger. The pain is relieved by rest, but she often has sharp pain in the right wrist during the night. Mrs. C. has never smoked, does not drink alcohol, and has five cups of coffee a day. She does little cooking. Her diet primarily consists of TV dinners and canned soups, vegetables, and fruits, with very few dairy products. She reports that constipation has become a more frequent problem over the past month. She has maintained her weight of 63.5 kg (140 lb) for the past 10 years. She can do most activities of daily living unassisted, but her neighbor does the grocery shopping. She verbalizes embarrassment over the effects of the aging process and stooped posture, stating that she has noticed a decrease in her height over the past year. Mrs. C. reports frequent low back aches with occasional sharp pains. She tries to avoid bending to prevent pain, uses a heating pad, and takes Tylenol two or three times a day, which temporarily relieves the pain. She experienced menopause at the age of 50 years and has never used estrogen replacement therapy.

Copyright © 2014. Wolters Kluwer Health | Lippincott Williams & Wilkins. Lab Manual for Health Assessment in Nursing, 5e.

Physical examination reveals her to be 157.48 cm (5 ft 2 in) tall. Two years ago, her height was 161.29 cm (5 ft 3 1/2 in). Her gait is wide-based and slow. Her temporomandibular joint (TMJ) has full range of motion (ROM) against resistance. Mrs. C. has apparent kyphosis of the cervical spine. Her paravertebrals are tender to palpation. Lower back pain is aggravated by ROM, is limited to the lower lumbar area, and does not radiate down the leg. The result of Lasègue test is negative. No leg redness, nodules, tenderness, or swelling can be observed. The ROM of the cervical spine and upper extremities are within normal range against gravity but decreased against resistance. Lumbar flexion is 50 degrees; lateral bending is 25 degrees. The legs are equal in length. The shoulders, elbows, wrists, and fingers are symmetric, without redness, heat, swelling, or nodules. Some muscle atrophy is apparent in the upper extremities. The results of Phalen's test and Tinel's test are positive. The hips, knees, ankles, and toes are symmetric, without redness, swelling, heat, or nodules. The lower extremities have full ROM against gravity, but decreased ROM against resistance.

How Well Did You Do?

After you have read the chapter and completed the exercises in this chapter, visit thePoint to access the Self-Reflection Activity. This activity will help you identify to what degree you have met each of the chapter objectives. You can then review the chapter for objectives you have met partially or not at all.

Other tools to help you, like the Diagnostic Reasoning Guides, Nursing Interview Guides, Physical Assessment Guides, and NCLEX-Style Chapter Review Questions, are also available on thePoint.

Copyright © 2014. Wolters Kluwer Health | Lippincott Williams & Wilkins. Lab Manual for Health Assessment in Nursing, 5e.

Assessing Neurologic System

Chapter Overview

Just as the musculoskeletal system structures the body, so the nervous system structures thought, movement and balance, sensation, and communication, among other life functions. Quality of life is significantly affected by the health of the nervous system. This very complex system is responsible for coordinating and regulating all body functions. The neurologic system has two structural components: the central nervous system (CNS) and the peripheral nervous system. Assessment of this system includes mental status, cranial nerves, motor and cerebellar systems, sensory system, and reflexes. Determining mental status is discussed in the textbook in more detail in Chapter 6: *Assessing Mental Status* and motor assessment procedures are discussed in Chapter 24: *Assessing Musculoskeletal System*. Use the following exercises and quizzes to guide your assessment of the neurologic system.

Chapter Learning Objectives

1. Describe the structures and function of the central and peripheral nervous system.
2. Discuss the risk factors for stroke (also known as cerebral vascular accident [CVA]) across cultures and ways to reduce one's risks.
3. Describe the teaching opportunities to reduce a client's risk of stroke and to promote health.
4. Obtain an accurate nursing history of a client's neurologic system.
5. Perform a physical assessment of the nervous system using the correct techniques of inspection, auscultation, palpation, and percussion.
6. Differentiate between normal and abnormal findings of the nervous system.
7. Describe the findings frequently seen when assessing the older client's nervous system.
8. Analyze the data from the interview and physical assessment of the nervous system to formulate valid nursing diagnoses, collaborative problems, and/or referrals.

CHAPTER PRETEST

Activity A MULTIPLE CHOICE QUESTIONS

Choose the one best answer for each of the following multiple choice questions.

____ 1. The cerebrospinal fluid cushions the central nervous system (CNS), provides nourishment to the CNS, and

  a. transmits impulses.

  b. coats the brain.

  c. regulates heart rate.

  d. removes wastes.

____ **2.** The cerebrum is divided into right and left hemispheres, which are joined together by the
    a. corpus callosum.
    b. diencephalon.
    c. medulla oblongata.
    d. pons.

____ **3.** The portion of the brain that rims the surfaces of the cerebral hemispheres forming the cerebral cortex is the
    a. gray matter.
    b. cerebellum.
    c. diencephalon.
    d. brainstem.

____ **4.** The diencephalon of the brain consists of the
    a. pons and brainstem.
    b. medulla oblongata and cerebrum.
    c. cerebellum and midbrain.
    d. thalamus and hypothalamus.

____ **5.** The hypothalamus is responsible for regulating
    a. sleep cycles.
    b. nerve impulses.
    c. memory.
    d. eye reflexes.

Activity B   MATCHING

Match the terms in the left column with the correct descriptions in the right column.

Term

____ **1.** Spinal accessory

____ **2.** Glossopharyngeal

____ **3.** Olfactory

____ **4.** Facial

____ **5.** Hypoglossal

____ **6.** Acoustic

____ **7.** Optic

____ **8.** Vagus

____ **9.** Abducens

____ **10.** Oculomotor

____ **11.** Trigeminal

____ **12.** Trochlear

Description

a. Carries sensations from the throat, larynx, heart, lungs, bronchi, gastrointestinal tract, and abdominal viscera

b. Innervates neck muscles that promote movement of the shoulders and head rotation

c. Carries visual impulses from the eye to the brain

d. Contracts eye muscles to control eye movement, constricts pupils, and elevates eyelids

e. Contains sensory fibers for taste on posterior one third of the tongue; responsible for "gag reflex" when stimulated

f. Contracts one eye muscle to control inferomedial eye movement

g. Innervates tongue muscles that promote the movement of food and talking

h. Carries smell impulses from nasal mucous membrane to brain

i. Carries sensory impulses of pain, touch, and temperature from the face to the brain

j. Controls lateral eye movements

k. Contains sensory fibers for hearing and balance

l. Contains sensory fibers for taste on anterior two thirds of the tongue, and stimulates secretions from the salivary glands and tears from lacrimal glands

Activity C LABELING ACTIVITIES

Label the structures of the brain in the following figure. Check your answers with Figure 25-1A on page 546 in the textbook.

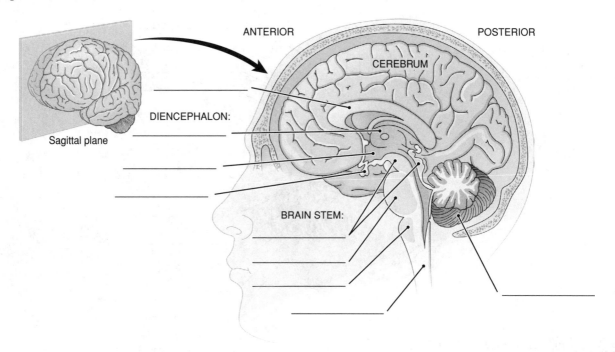

Label the cross-section of the spinal cord in the following figure. Check your answers with Figure 25-3 on page 547 in the textbook.

Copyright © 2014. Wolters Kluwer Health | Lippincott Williams & Wilkins. Lab Manual for Health Assessment in Nursing, 5e.

Label the cranial nerves in the following figure. Check your answers with Figure 25-6 on page 548 in the textbook.

Activity D LEARNER ACTIVITIES

After reading Chapter 25 in the textbook, participate in the following learning activities.

1. Review the information in EVIDENCE-BASED HEALTH PROMOTION AND DISEASE PREVENTION: CEREBROVASCULAR ACCIDENT (STROKE) (see pages 555–556 in your textbook). Use this information to determine your own risk for stroke (also known as cerebral vascular accident [CVA]). Next, identify ethnic groups that are at the highest risk for stroke. Discuss what teaching could be implemented to reduce these risks.

2. Assess your lab partner for functioning of his/her 12 cranial nerves that you labeled in the diagram above. (See Figure 25-6 on page 548 in the textbook).

3. Obtain the necessary equipment and assess your lab partner's sensory system for touch, vibrations, position, and tactile discrimination.

4. Use a reflex hammer to test your lab partner's deep tendon reflexes. Next, test for superficial plantar and abdominal reflexes.

5. Practice testing balance and coordination safely with a lab partner.

6. Perform an assessment of the nervous system on an older client, friend, or relative. Discuss with peers your neurologic findings as they compare with the findings in a younger person.

Activity E INTERVIEWING AND RECORDING ASSESSMENT FINDINGS

After reading Chapter 25, use the following Nursing Interview Guide to interview and record your subjective findings for an assessment of the nervous system of a lab partner, peer, or client. Your instructor may ask you to turn this in to be evaluated. Forms are also available on thePoint *website.*

Nursing Interview Guide to Collect Subjective Data From the Client

Questions	Findings
Current Symptoms	
1. Headaches, numbness, or tingling?	
2. Seizure activity?	
3. Dizziness, lightheadedness, or problems with balance or coordination?	
4. Decrease in ability to smell or taste?	
5. Ringing in ears?	
6. Change in vision?	
7. Difficulty understanding when people are talking to you or when you talk to others?	
8. Difficulty swallowing?	
9. Loss of bowel or bladder control?	
10. Memory loss?	
11. Tremors?	
Past History	
1. Head injury?	
2. Meningitis?	
3. Encephalitis?	
4. Spinal cord injury?	
5. Stroke?	
6. Treatment received?	
Family History	
1. High blood pressure?	
2. Stroke?	
3. Alzheimer disease?	
4. Epilepsy?	
5. Brain cancer?	
6. Huntington chorea?	
Lifestyle and Health Practices	
1. Any prescription or nonprescription medications?	
2. Smoking?	
3. Wearing of seat belts/protective headgear?	
4. Daily diet?	
5. Exposure to lead, insecticides, pollutants, chemicals?	
6. Lifting of heavy objects?	

Copyright © 2014. Wolters Kluwer Health | Lippincott Williams & Wilkins. Lab Manual for Health Assessment in Nursing, 5e.

Nursing Interview Guide to Collect Subjective Data From the Client (continued)

Questions	Findings
7. Frequent repetitive movements?	
8. Functioning/daily activities?	
Analysis of Data	
1. Formulate nursing diagnoses (wellness, risk, actual).	
2. Formulate collaborative problems.	
3. Make necessary referrals.	

Activity F   PERFORMING PHYSICAL ASSESSMENT OF THE NERVOUS SYSTEM

Use the following Physical Assessment Guide to examine the nervous system of a lab partner, peer, or client. Column 1 will serve as a reminder as to what part of the exam you will do next. Column 2 will be used to record your findings. Your instructor may ask you to turn this in to be evaluated. Forms are also available on thePoint *website.*

Physical Assessment Guide to Collect Objective Client Data

Questions	Findings
Current Symptoms	
1. Gather equipment, such as examination gloves, pencil and paper, cotton-tipped applicators, newsprint to read, ophthalmoscope, paper clip, penlight, Snellen chart, sterile cotton ball, substances to smell and taste, tongue blade, tuning fork, tape measure, cotton balls, objects to feel, test tubes with hot and cold water, tuning fork (low-pitched), and reflex hammer.	
2. Explain the procedure to client.	
3. Ask the client to put on a gown.	
Mental Status	
1. Assess level of consciousness.	
2. Observe appearance and behavior.	
3. Observe mood, feelings, and expressions.	
4. Observe thought processes and perceptions.	
5. Observe cognitive abilities.	
Cranial Nerves	
1. Test cranial nerve I—olfactory.	
2. Test cranial nerve II—optic.	
3. Test cranial nerve III—oculomotor.	
4. Test cranial nerve IV—trochlear.	
5. Test cranial nerve V—trigeminal.	
6. Test cranial nerve VI—abducens.	
7. Test cranial nerve VII—facial.	
8. Test cranial nerve VIII—acoustic (vestibulocochlear).	
9. Test cranial nerve IX—glossopharyngeal.	

Copyright © 2014. Wolters Kluwer Health | Lippincott Williams & Wilkins. Lab Manual for Health Assessment in Nursing, 5e.

Physical Assessment Guide to Collect Objective Client Data (continued)	
Questions	Findings
10. Test cranial nerve X—vagus.	
11. Test cranial nerve XI—spinal accessory.	
12. Test cranial nerve XII—hypoglossal.	
Motor and Cerebellar Systems	
1. Test condition and movement of muscles.	
2. Test balance.	
3. Test coordination.	
Sensory System	
1. Test light touch, pain, and temperature sensations.	
2. Test vibratory sensations.	
3. Test position sensations.	
4. Test tactile discrimination (fine touch).	
Reflexes	
1. Test deep tendon reflexes (biceps, brachioradialis, triceps, patellar, Achilles, and ankle clonus).	
2. Test superficial reflexes (plantar, abdominal, cremasteric).	
3. Test for meningeal irritation/inflammation (Brudzinski and Kernig signs if indicated).	
Analysis of Data	
1. Formulate nursing diagnoses (wellness, risk, actual).	
2. Formulate collaborative problems.	
3. Make necessary referrals.	

CHAPTER POSTTEST

Activity G **MULTIPLE CHOICE QUESTIONS**

Choose the one best answer for each of the following multiple choice questions.

_____ **1.** Sensations of temperature, pain, and crude and light touch are carried by way of the
   a. extrapyramidal tract.
   b. corticospinal tract.
   c. spinothalamic tract.
   d. posterior tract.

_____ **2.** The cranial nerve that has sensory fibers for taste and fibers that result in the "gag reflex" is the
   a. vagus.
   b. hypoglossal.
   c. trigeminal.
   d. glossopharyngeal.

Copyright © 2014. Wolters Kluwer Health | Lippincott Williams & Wilkins. Lab Manual for Health Assessment in Nursing, 5e.

____ 3. The nurse is assessing an older adult client when the client tells the nurse that she has experienced transient blind spots for the last few days. The nurse should refer the client to a physician for possible

a. vagus nerve damage.

b. stroke.

c. spinal cord compression.

d. Parkinson disease.

____ 4. The nurse is planning a presentation to a group of adults on the topic of strokes. Which of the following should the nurse plan to include in the teaching plan?

a. Strokes are the number one cause of death in the United States.

b. Smoking and high cholesterol levels are risk factors for STROKE.

c. Clients who smoke while taking oral contraceptives are not at higher risk.

d. Postmenopausal women taking estrogen are at greater risk for STROKE.

____ 5. The nurse is caring for a client during the immediate postoperative period after abdominal surgery. While performing a "neuro check" the nurse should assess the client's

a. sensation in the extremities.

b. deep tendon reflexes.

c. ability to speak.

d. recent memory.

____ 6. The nurse is preparing to percuss a client's reflexes in his arms. To use the reinforcement technique, the nurse should ask the client to

a. clench his jaw.

b. stretch the opposite arm.

c. hold his neck toward the floor.

d. straighten his legs forward.

____ 7. The Glasgow Coma Scale measures the level of consciousness in clients who are at high risk for rapid deterioration of the nervous system. A score of 13 indicates

a. deep coma.

b. severe impairment.

c. no verbal response.

d. some impairment.

____ 8. A client visits the clinic and tells the nurse that he has not been feeling very well. The nurse observes that the client's speech is slow, the client has a disheveled appearance, and he maintains poor eye contact with the nurse. The nurse should further assess the client for

a. depression.

b. delirium.

c. hallucinations.

d. schizophrenia.

____ 9. While assessing the neurologic system of a confused older adult, the nurse observes that the client is unable to recall past events. The nurse suspects that the client may be exhibiting signs of

a. depression.

b. anxiety.

c. attention deficit disorder.

d. cerebral cortex disorder.

Copyright © 2014. Wolters Kluwer Health | Lippincott Williams & Wilkins. Lab Manual for Health Assessment in Nursing, 5e.

_____ **10.** The nurse is assessing the neurologic system of an adult client. To test the client's use of memory to learn new information, the nurse should ask the client

    a. "What did you have for breakfast?"

    b. "How old were you when you began working?"

    c. "Can you repeat _rose, hose, nose, clothes?_"

    d. "Can you repeat _brown, chair, textbook, tomato?_"

_____ **11.** While assessing the pupils of a hospitalized adult client, the nurse observes that the client's pupils are dilated to 6 cm. The nurse suspects that the client is exhibiting signs of

    a. oculomotor nerve paralysis.

    b. damage to the pons.

    c. alcohol abuse.

    d. cocaine abuse.

_____ **12.** The nurse is assessing the neurologic system of an adult client. To test the client's motor function of the facial nerve, the nurse should

    a. ask the client to purse the lips.

    b. ask the client to open the mouth and say "ah."

    c. note the presence of a gag reflex.

    d. observe the client swallow a sip of water.

_____ **13.** The nurse is assessing the neurologic system of a client who has spastic muscle tone. The nurse should explain to the client that spastic muscle tone is associated with impairment to the

    a. extrapyramidal tract.

    b. spinothalamic tract.

    c. posterior columns.

    d. corticospinal tract.

_____ **14.** The nurse is preparing to perform the Romberg test on an adult male client. The nurse should instruct the client to

    a. squat down as far as he is able to do so.

    b. keep his eyes open while he bends at the knees.

    c. stand erect with arms at the sides and feet together.

    d. touch the tip of his nose with his finger.

_____ **15.** The nurse is planning to test position sensation in an adult female client. To perform this procedure, the nurse should ask the client to close her eyes while the nurse moves the client's

    a. arm away from the body.

    b. toes up or down.

    c. hand forward and then backward.

    d. leg away from the body.

Activity H CRITICAL THINKING ACTIVITY

George R., aged 74, has had Parkinson disease for more than 10 years. His primary caregiver is his wife of 52 years, who is in good health except for rheumatoid arthritis. The couple's grown sons live in another state but visit the family once a year during the Christmas holidays. Recently Mr. R. has experienced a greater degree of twitching in his arms. He slurs his speech and is difficult to understand at times. He and his wife had enjoyed a wide range of activities such as bowling, going to the movies, and trying new restaurants. However, since his condition has deteriorated they rarely leave the house. Mr. R. has also experienced difficulty walking and getting up from the bed or chair. His wife must assist him in all activities of daily living.

    Using the information above, formulate health promotion, risk, and actual nursing diagnoses and identify collaborative problems for the client and his wife.

Activity I **CASE STUDY**

Read the following case study. Then, work through the steps of analyzing the case study data. First identify abnormal data and strengths in **subjective and objective findings**, assemble **cue clusters**, draw **inferences**, make possible **nursing diagnoses**, identify **defining characteristics**, **confirm or rule out** the diagnoses, and **document** your conclusions. Use the blank diagnostic analysis charts provided at the end of this book (also available on thePoint website) to guide your thinking. Propose nursing diagnoses that are specific to the client in the case study. Identify collaborative problems, if any, for this client. Finally, identify data, if any, which point toward a medical problem requiring a referral.

Robert K. is a 72-year-old man who had a right hemisphere thrombotic stroke 14 days ago and was discharged to his home from the 51st State Stroke Rehabilitation Center. His primary caregiver is his 68-year-old wife, who is in good health. He has a daughter and a son, who live within an 80.47-km (50-mile) radius and visit frequently. Before the stroke, Mr. K. was very active and independent, a retired banker who loved to golf and travel. He was diagnosed with hypertension 15 years ago but has not been consistent in taking his prescribed medications. "When my blood pressure was checked, it was normal, so why take the medicine if I don't need it!" The stroke resulted in deficits in his visual, tactile, and kinesthetic senses. He denies his disabilities and frequently displays poor judgment and impulsive behavior. Mr. K. requires partial assistance with activities of daily living, feeding, and mobility. While in rehabilitation he seemed to learn best if given brief simple cues. Because of visual disturbance, he has difficulty with visual cues.

When interviewed, Mr. K. states he has weakness and numbness of his left arm and leg and that he often has to look at his left arm and leg to determine where they are. He also states that he frequently loses his balance and has occasional dizziness when getting up in the morning. He has difficulty with dressing and grooming and frequently confuses his comb with his toothbrush and puts his clothes on inside out. He is frustrated at not being able to care for himself. He has been prescribed a 2-g sodium diet; however, he has a poor appetite. He states that the "food doesn't taste or smell good." His wife states that it often takes him a long time to complete a meal, and he frequently leaves food on the left side of the plate. When asked about changes in memory or concentration, his wife states, "Now, it's difficult for him to remember dates and phone numbers, but he knows people's names."

Your physical assessment reveals the following.

- *Mental status:* Awake, alert, oriented to person, place, and usually time. Communicates verbally, although comprehension is questionable at times. Eye contact poor. Mood seems anxious. Dress clean, shirt is on inside out. Difficulty in recalling recent dates and events. Unable to interpret written instructions. Reads a few sentences at a time; loses place on page frequently. Unable to recognize familiar objects such as toothbrush and comb. Unable to draw left side of clock. Saint Louis University Mental Status (SLUMS) Examination Score: 23.

- *Cranial nerves:* Intact except for cranial nerve II; loses place on page after reading a few sentences. Unable to record visual stimuli from the left side because of homonymous hemianopia.

- *Motor and cerebellar systems:* Gait slow and unsteady with one person assisting; abnormal tandem walk. Muscle strength weak in left upper and lower extremities. Unable to assess finger coordination and fine motor function of left upper and lower extremities.

- *Sensory system:* Decreased light, sharp, dull touch; vibratory, two-point sensation in left upper and lower extremity; unable to identify safety pin and number traced on the palm of left hand.

- *Reflexes:* 1+ left upper and lower extremities; 2+ right upper and lower extremities; down-going toes with plantar stimulation.

How Well Did You Do?

After you have read the chapter and completed the exercises in this chapter, visit thePoint to access the Self-Reflection Activity. This activity will help you identify to what degree you have met each of the chapter objectives. You can then review the chapter for objectives you have met partially or not at all.

Other tools to help you, like the Diagnostic Reasoning Guides, Nursing Interview Guides, Physical Assessment Guides, and NCLEX-Style Chapter Review Questions, are also available on thePoint.

Copyright © 2014. Wolters Kluwer Health | Lippincott Williams & Wilkins. Lab Manual for Health Assessment in Nursing, 5e.

Assessing Male Genitalia and Rectum

Chapter Overview

An assessment of male genital structures requires an understanding of the external and the internal genitalia as well as the inguinal (or groin) structures, because hernias are common in this area. In addition, the anus and rectum complete the gastrointestinal tract. In men, the prostate gland is integrally entwined with these structures. In both men and women, the colon is also examined during assessment of the rectum and anus. The colon assessment is particularly important for detecting signs and symptoms of colon cancer; prostatic conditions, which affect older men; and other intestinal disorders.

Throughout the assessment, the nurse should keep in mind that Western culture emphasizes the importance of the male sex role and that self-esteem and body image are entwined with the male sex role. Therefore, the assessment may be uncomfortable or embarrassing for the client as well as for the nurse. The key goals of the assessment are screening and detection of serious or life-threatening problems, such as testicular cancer, and patient education and health promotion. Use the following exercises and quizzes to help you review the basic techniques and skills.

Chapter Learning Objectives

1. Describe the structure and functions of the male genitalia, anus, rectum, and prostate.
2. Discuss the incidence of HIV/AIDS across cultures and ways to reduce these risk factors.
3. Describe the teaching opportunities to reduce risks of HIV/AIDS and promote health.
4. Discuss the incidence of prostate cancer across cultures and ways to promote health.
5. Discuss the incidence of testicular cancer across cultures and ways to promote health.
6. Obtain an accurate nursing history of the male client's genitalia, anus, rectum, and prostate.
7. Perform a physical assessment of the male genitalia, anus, rectum, and prostate using the correct techniques of inspection, auscultation, and palpation.
8. Differentiate between normal and abnormal findings of the male genitalia, anus, rectum, and prostate.
9. Describe the findings frequently seen when assessing the older client's male genitalia, anus, rectum, and prostate.
10. Analyze the data from the interview and physical assessment of the abdomen to formulate valid nursing diagnoses, collaborative problems, and/or referrals.

CHAPTER PRETEST

Activity A **MULTIPLE CHOICE QUESTIONS**

Choose the one best answer for each of the following multiple choice questions.

____ **1.** The corpora spongiosum extends distally to form the acorn-shaped
   a. glans.
   b. frenulum.
   c. corona.
   d. scrotum.

____ **2.** If a male client is uncircumcised, the glans of the penis is covered by the
   a. epididymis.
   b. frenulum.
   c. corona.
   d. foreskin.

____ **3.** The testes in the male scrotum are
   a. joined with the ejaculatory duct.
   b. suspended by the spermatic cord.
   c. able to produce progesterone.
   d. the location of the vas deferens.

____ **4.** The inguinal canal in a male client is located
   a. just above and parallel to the inguinal ligament.
   b. anteriorly above the symphysis pubis.
   c. anterior to the external inguinal ring.
   d. posterior to the superior iliac ring.

____ **5.** The external sphincter of the anus is
   a. composed of smooth muscle.
   b. composed of skeletal muscle.
   c. composed of striated muscle.
   d. under involuntary control.

____ **6.** The Cowper glands
   a. are located inside the rectum.
   b. produce a substance to aid in sperm motility.
   c. empty into the urethra.
   d. can be palpated through the rectum.

____ **7.** The external sphincter and internal sphincter of the rectum are divided by the
   a. anorectal junction.
   b. rectovesical pouch.
   c. median sulcus.
   d. intersphincteric groove.

____ **8.** The rectum is lined with folds of mucosa, and each fold contains a network of arteries, veins, and visceral nerves. When these veins undergo chronic pressure, the result may be
   a. polyps.
   b. tumors.
   c. fissures.
   d. hemorrhoids.

Copyright © 2014. Wolters Kluwer Health | Lippincott Williams & Wilkins. Lab Manual for Health Assessment in Nursing, 5e.

____ **9.** The prostate gland consists of two lobes separated by the

    a. median sulcus.

    b. rectovesical pouch.

    c. anorectal junction.

    d. valves of Houston.

____ **10.** The prostate functions to

    a. store sperm until ejaculation occurs.

    b. secrete a milky substance that neutralizes female acidic secretions.

    c. produce the ejaculate that nourishes and protects sperm.

    d. produce mucus-like fluid to assist in lubrication.

Activity B MATCHING

Match the terms in the left column with the correct descriptions in the right column.

Term

____ **1.** Corona

____ **2.** Hernia

____ **3.** Chancres

____ **4.** Phimosis

____ **5.** Paraphimosis

____ **6.** Hypospadias

____ **7.** Epispadias

____ **8.** Cryptorchidism

____ **9.** Pilonidal cyst

____ **10.** Hemorrhoids

Description

a. Retracted foreskin that cannot be returned to cover the glans

b. Displacement of the urinary meatus to the dorsal surface of the penis

c. Base of the glans

d. Undescended testicle

e. Protrusion of bowel through weakened muscles

f. A tight foreskin that cannot be retracted

g. Red oval ulcerations caused by syphilis

h. Displacement of the urinary meatus to the ventral surface of the penis

i. Painless flabby papules due to varicose veins; two types, external or internal

j. A hair-containing cyst located in the midline over the coccyx or lower sacrum

Activity C LABELING ACTIVITIES

Label the structures of the external and internal genitalia in the following figure. Check your answers with Figure 26-1 on page 583 in the textbook.

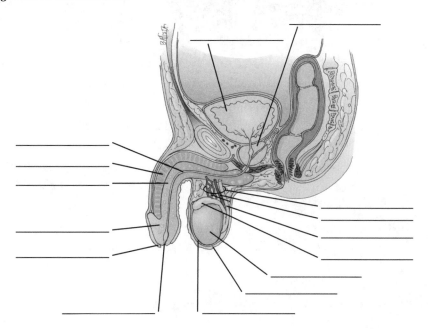

Copyright © 2014. Wolters Kluwer Health | Lippincott Williams & Wilkins. Lab Manual for Health Assessment in Nursing, 5e.

Label the structures of the inguinal area in the following figure. Check your answers with Figure 26-2 on page 583 in the textbook.

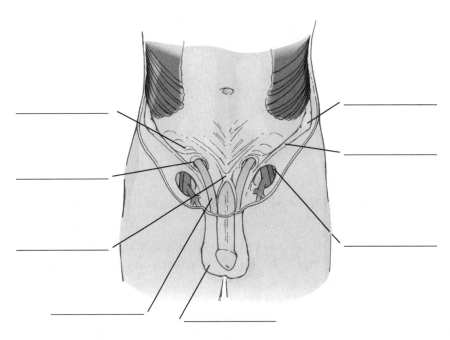

Label the anal and rectal structures in the following figure. Check your answers with Figure 26-3 on page 584 in the textbook.

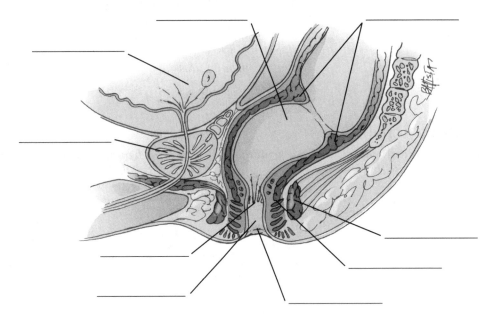

Copyright © 2014. Wolters Kluwer Health | Lippincott Williams & Wilkins. Lab Manual for Health Assessment in Nursing, 5e.

Label the prostate and nearby structures in the following figure. Check your answers with Figure 26-4 on page 585 in the textbook.

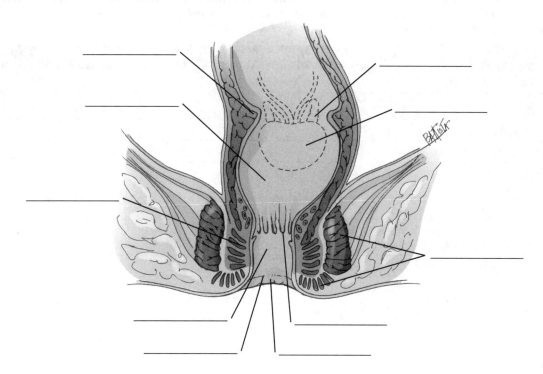

Activity D LEARNER ACTIVITIES

After reading Chapter 26 in the textbook, participate in the following learning activities.

1. Review the information in EVIDENCE-BASED HEALTH PROMOTION AND DISEASE PREVENTION: HIV/AIDS (see pages 590–591 in your textbook). Determine your own risk for HIV/AIDS. Identify ways to reduce your risk factors. Which groups are at higher risk for contracting HIV/AIDS?

2. Obtain brochures and literature on sexually transmitted infections (STIs) from the county health department or your campus student health center. Discuss with your lab partner the best way to give a presentation on this topic to teenagers and then to a college-aged group.

3. Review the information in EVIDENCE-BASED HEALTH PROMOTION AND DISEASE PREVENTION: PROSTATE CANCER (see page 591 in your textbook). Discuss with your lab partner the best way to give a presentation on early detection of prostate cancer and who would be your target audience.

4. Review the material from your textbook on testicular cancer and testicular self-examination with a lab partner, and discuss how you would teach a client how to examine himself.

5. Using a model of the male genitalia, anus, rectum, and prostate, review the anatomy and function of each anatomic structure. Discuss the assessment findings with your lab partner, and then compare those findings with what you would find in an elderly man.

Copyright © 2014. Wolters Kluwer Health | Lippincott Williams & Wilkins. Lab Manual for Health Assessment in Nursing, 5e.

Activity E INTERVIEWING AND RECORDING ASSESSMENT FINDINGS

After reading Chapter 26, use the following Nursing Interview Guide to interview and record your subjective findings for an assessment of male genitalia, anus, rectum, and prostate. Your instructor may ask you to turn this in to be evaluated. Forms are also available on thePoint *website.*

Nursing Interview Guide to Collect Subjective Data From the Client

Questions	Findings
Current Symptoms	
1. Pain in penis, scrotum, testes, or groin?	
2. Lesions on penis or genital area?	
3. Lumps, swelling, or masses in scrotum, genital, or groin area?	
4. Heaviness or dragging feeling in scrotum?	
5. Difficulty urinating (hesitancy, frequency, or difficulty starting or maintaining a stream)?	
6. Frequent nighttime urination?	
7. Changes in color, odor, or amount of urine?	
8. Pain or burning when urinating?	
9. Incontinence or dribbling of urine?	
10. Recent changes in sexual activity pattern or sexual desire?	
11. Difficulty attaining or maintaining an erection? Problems with ejaculation?	
12. Fertility problems?	
13. Problems with bowels (bowel pattern changes, constipation, diarrhea, bowel control, stool color, blood or mucus in stool, pain or itching in rectal area, hemorrhoids)?	
14. Anal and perianal problems (lumps, ulcers, lesions, rashes, redness)?	
Past History	
1. Previous problems related to your pelvic area (surgeries, treatments, and results)?	
2. Date of last testicular exam by physician or nurse practitioner? Results?	
3. Tested for HIV? Why tested? Results?	
4. Previous anal or rectal trauma or surgery, congenital deformities?	
5. History of blood in stool?	
6. History of prostate enlargement, treatment, or surgery on the prostate?	
7. Pattern of health screenings (occult blood, prostate-specific antigen, proctosigmoidoscopy, colonoscopy)?	

Copyright © 2014. Wolters Kluwer Health | Lippincott Williams & Wilkins. Lab Manual for Health Assessment in Nursing, 5e.

Nursing Interview Guide to Collect Subjective Data From the Client (continued)

Questions	Findings
Family History	
1. Family history of prostate or testicular cancer? What type and which family member?	
Lifestyle and Health Practices	
1. Number of sexual partners?	
2. Kind of birth control method?	
3. Current or past exposure to chemicals or radiation?	
4. Usual daily activity?	
5. Heavy lifting?	
6. Genital problems that affect daily activities?	
7. Fertility concerns? Effect on relationship?	
8. Sexual preference?	
9. Concerns related to sex?	
10. Stress related to sex?	
11. Knowledge of sexually transmitted diseases and prevention?	
12. Do you perform testicular self-examination? Date last performed?	
13. Use of laxatives, stool softeners, enemas, or other bowel medications?	
14. Practice anal sex?	
15. Daily water/fluid intake?	
16. Usual diet (high fiber and roughage, saturated fat content)?	
17. Usual exercise pattern?	
18. Any effect on daily life from anal, rectal, or bowel problems or from prostate problems?	

Activity F PERFORMING PHYSICAL ASSESSMENT OF THE MALE GENITALIA, ANUS, RECTUM, AND PROSTATE

Use the following Physical Assessment Guide to examine the male genitalia, anus, rectum, and prostate model. Column 1 will serve as a reminder as to what part of the exam you will do next. Column 2 will be used to record your findings. Your instructor may ask you to turn this in to be evaluated. Forms are also available on thePoint *website.*

Physical Assessment Guide to Collect Objective Client Data	
Questions	**Findings**
Current Symptoms	
1. Gather equipment (gloves, stool, gown, penlight).	
2. Explain the procedure to client.	
3. Ask the client to put on gown.	
Penis	
1. Inspect the base of penis and pubic hair for growth pattern and excoriation, erythema, or infestation (client is standing while you sit).	
2. Inspect the skin of the shaft for rashes, lesions, or lumps.	
3. Palpate the shaft for hardened areas or areas of tenderness.	
4. Inspect the foreskin (if present) for color, location, and integrity.	
5. Inspect the glans for size, shape, lesions or redness, and location of the urinary meatus on the glans (if uncircumcised, ask him to retract his foreskin to allow for observation).	
6. Palpate for urethral discharge by gently squeezing the glans between the index finger and the thumb.	
Scrotum	
1. Inspect the size, shape, and position (penis is held out of the way).	
2. Observe for swelling, lumps, or bulges.	
3. Inspect the skin for color, integrity, and the presence of lesions or rashes. (Spread out the scrotal folds of skin to perform an accurate inspection. Lift the sac to inspect the posterior skin.)	
4. Palpate the scrotal contents (testes and epididymis) between your thumb and first two fingers. Note size, shape, consistency, and presence of tenderness or nodules. Palpate each spermatic cord and vas deferens, noting nodules, swelling, or tenderness.	
5. Transilluminate the scrotal contents (if a mass or swelling was noted). Look for a red glow.	

Physical Assessment Guide to Collect Objective Client Data (continued)

Questions	Findings
Inguinal Area	
1. Inspect for inguinal and femoral hernia, watching for bulges while the client bears down.	
2. Palpate for inguinal hernia, observing for bulges or masses. Have the client shift weight to the left to palpate the right inguinal canal. Place index finger into the right scrotum and press upward to the slit-like opening of the external inguinal ring. With finger in canal or external inguinal ring, ask him to bear down or cough. Repeat for left side.	
3. Palpate for femoral hernia on the front of the thigh in the femoral canal area. Ask him to bear down or cough while feeling for bulges. Repeat on the other side.	
4. Inspect and palpate for scrotal hernia (if a mass was detected during inspection or palpation of the scrotum). Ask the client to lie down, and note whether the bulge disappears. If it remains, auscultate it for bowel sounds. Then gently palpate the mass and try to push it up into the abdomen unless it is too tender.	
Anus and Perianal Area	
1. Inspect for lumps, ulcers, lesions, rashes, redness (note size, shape, location, distribution, and configuration).	
2. Inspect sacrococcygeal area for swelling, redness, dimpling, or presence of hair in pilonidal area.	
3. Inspect for rectal prolapse with Valsalva maneuver.	
4. Palpate for anal sphincter tone, tenderness, nodules, or hardness.	
Rectum and Prostate	
1. Palpate rectal mucosa for tenderness, irregularities, nodules, and hardness.	
2. Palpate peritoneal cavity for tenderness or nodules, or "rectal shelf."	
3. Palpate the prostate gland for tenderness, size, shape, texture, or irregularities.	
4. Inspect the feces for blood and perform occult blood test.	
Analysis of Data	
1. Formulate nursing diagnoses (health promotion, risk, actual).	
2. Formulate collaborative problems.	
3. Make necessary referrals.	

Copyright © 2014. Wolters Kluwer Health | Lippincott Williams & Wilkins. Lab Manual for Health Assessment in Nursing, 5e.

CHAPTER POSTTEST

Activity G   MULTIPLE CHOICE QUESTIONS

Choose the one best answer for each of the following multiple choice questions.

_____ 1. During assessment of an elderly male client, the client tells the nurse that he has had difficulty urinating for the past few weeks. The nurse should refer the client to the physician for possible
   a. inguinal hernia.
   b. sexually transmitted disease.
   c. impotence.
   d. prostate enlargement.

_____ 2. A 25-year-old client asks the nurse how often he should have a testicular examination. After instructing the client about the American Cancer Society's guidelines, the nurse determines that the client has understood the instructions when he says he should have a testicular examination every
   a. year.
   b. 2 years.
   c. 3 years.
   d. 4 years.

_____ 3. A 45-year-old male client tells the nurse that he has had problems in having an erection for the last couple of weeks but is "doing better now." The nurse should explain to the client that
   a. transient periods of erectile dysfunction are common.
   b. impotence in males should be investigated.
   c. transient impotence may be indicative of prostate enlargement.
   d. inguinal hernias have been associated with transient impotence.

_____ 4. A male client tells the nurse that his occupation requires heavy lifting and a great deal of strenuous activity. The nurse should assess the client for
   a. signs and symptoms of prostate enlargement.
   b. erectile dysfunction.
   c. inguinal hernia.
   d. urinary tract infection.

_____ 5. During assessment of an adult client, which of the following lifestyle practices would indicate to the nurse that the client may be at high risk for HIV/AIDS? A client who
   a. uses a condom on a regular basis.
   b. has multiple female partners.
   c. smokes marijuana occasionally.
   d. has anal intercourse with other males.

_____ 6. During assessment of the genitalia of an adult male, the client has an erection. The nurse should
   a. explain to the client that this often happens during an examination.
   b. cover the client's genitals and discontinue the examination.
   c. allow the client time to rest before proceeding with the examination.
   d. continue the examination in an unhurried manner.

_____ 7. Before beginning the examination of the genitalia of an adult male client, the nurse should
   a. ask the client to empty his bladder.
   b. tell the client that he will remain in a supine position.
   c. ask the client to leave his shirt in place.
   d. tell the client that he may leave his underwear in place.

Copyright © 2014. Wolters Kluwer Health | Lippincott Williams & Wilkins. Lab Manual for Health Assessment in Nursing, 5e.

____ **8.** While assessing an adult male client, the nurse detects pimple-like lesions on the client's glans. The nurse explains the need for a referral to the client. The nurse determines that the client has understood the instructions when the client says he may have

    a. venereal warts.

    b. herpes infection.

    c. syphilis.

    d. gonorrhea.

____ **9.** While inspecting the genitalia of a male client, the nurse observes a chancre lesion under the foreskin. The nurse has explained this observation to the client. The nurse determines that the client understands the need for a referral when the client says that chancre lesions are associated with

    a. herpes virus.

    b. syphilis.

    c. papilloma virus.

    d. gonorrhea.

____ **10.** A male client visits the clinic and tells the nurse that he has had a white discharge from his penis for the past few days. The nurse should refer the client to a physician for possible

    a. urethritis.

    b. gonorrhea.

    c. herpes infection.

    d. syphilis.

____ **11.** The nurse has assessed a male client and determines that one of the testes is absent. The nurse should explain to the client that this condition is termed

    a. hypospadias.

    b. hematocele.

    c. cryptorchidism.

    d. orchitis.

____ **12.** The nurse is assessing the genitalia of an adult male client when he tells the nurse that his testes are swollen and painful. The nurse should refer the client to a physician for possible

    a. cancer.

    b. hydrocele.

    c. epididymitis.

    d. hematocele.

____ **13.** While transilluminating the scrotal contents in a male adult client, the nurse does not detect a red glow. The nurse should refer the client to a physician for possible

    a. spermatocele.

    b. orchitis.

    c. hydrocele.

    d. varicocele.

____ **14.** The nurse suspects that a male client may have a hernia. The nurse should further assess the client for

    a. bruising at the site.

    b. urinary tract infection.

    c. cysts at the spermatic cord.

    d. bowel sounds at the bulge.

Copyright © 2014. Wolters Kluwer Health | Lippincott Williams & Wilkins. Lab Manual for Health Assessment in Nursing, 5e.

____ **15.** A male client tells the nurse that he has received a diagnosis of hernia. He visits the clinic because he is nauseated and has extreme tenderness on the left side. The nurse should

    a. refer the client to an emergency room.

    b. try to push the mass into the abdomen.

    c. assess for a mass on the right side.

    d. assess the client's vital signs.

Activity H CRITICAL THINKING ACTIVITIES

1. Why would it be necessary to transilluminate the scrotal contents, and what are the possible findings and their significance?

2. During assessment for a hernia, what is the rationale for asking the client to cough or bear down?

3. Compare and contrast how you would focus the nursing history of the male genitalia for an 18-year-old versus that for an 80-year-old.

4. Describe your communication techniques, how you would word nursing history questions, and how you would conduct a physical examination of the anus, rectum, and prostate for a 26-year-old man who engages in anal sex. Include what and how you would teach about the risk factors for various diseases or conditions.

Activity I CASE STUDY

Read the following case study. Then, work through the steps of analyzing the case study data. First identify abnormal data and strengths in **subjective and objective findings**, assemble **cue clusters**, draw **inferences**, make possible **nursing diagnoses**, identify **defining characteristics**, **confirm or rule out** the diagnoses, and **document** your conclusions. Use the blank diagnostic analysis charts provided at the end of this book (also available on thePoint website) to guide your thinking. Propose nursing diagnoses that are specific to the client in the case study. Identify collaborative problems, if any, for this client. Finally, identify data, if any, which point toward a medical problem requiring a referral.

Don C. is a 32-year-old African American man who arrives at the clinic for an evaluation by a nurse practitioner. He complains that his right testicle feels heavy or weighted down. He appears very nervous and explains that he has been experiencing this feeling for about 3 months. He explains that he came in today because "my wife is very upset about it and pleaded with me to go to a doctor." When interviewed, the client reports that he does not have trouble becoming erect, but he states, "I feel like it takes longer to ejaculate." He denies past medical problems or a family history of cancer.

He explains that he has not had a genital examination in years—"I really don't like to go to the doctor unless I have a problem." He says he has never done, and does not really know how to do, a testicular self-examination. He tells you that he is afraid he might have cancer.

Your physical examination reveals a normal adult pubic hair pattern and no excoriation or infestation in the pubic hair or at the base of the penis. The penis is circumcised and free of rashes, lesions, and discoloration. No tenderness or nodules are noted on palpation. The urinary meatus is located in the mid-glans and no discharge is revealed on palpation. Inspection of the scrotum reveals an enlarged right scrotum and redness on the scrotal sac, but no lesions. Palpation of the left testicle, epididymis, and spermatic cord reveal no tenderness, nodules, or swelling. Palpation of the right testicle reveals a 2-cm, nonmobile, nontender nodule on the anterior portion of the testicle. The left epididymis and spermatic cord are free of tenderness, nodules, and swelling. No red glow is seen on transillumination of the scrotal contents on either side. No bulges are noted in the inguinal or femoral canal.

How Well Did You Do?

After you have read the chapter and completed the exercises in this chapter, visit thePoint to access the Self-Reflection Activity. This activity will help you identify to what degree you have met each of the chapter objectives. You can then review the chapter for objectives you have met partially or not at all.

    Other tools to help you, like the Diagnostic Reasoning Guides, Nursing Interview Guides, Physical Assessment Guides, and NCLEX-Style Chapter Review Questions, are also available on thePoint.

Copyright © 2014. Wolters Kluwer Health | Lippincott Williams & Wilkins. Lab Manual for Health Assessment in Nursing, 5e.

CHAPTER 27

Assessing Female Genitalia and Rectum

Chapter Overview

The female genitalia consist of internal and external structures, and assessment requires the nurse's tact and sensitivity. The key goals of the assessment are screening and detection of serious or life-threatening problems such as cervical cancer, and patient education and health promotion. Because the pelvic region is linked to a woman's sexuality, much care and sensitivity must be exercised by the nurse to promote the client's comfort, self-esteem, and body image. Use the following exercises and quizzes to help you review basic techniques and skills.

Chapter Learning Objectives

1. Describe the structure and functions of the female genitalia, anus, and rectum.
2. Discuss the incidence across cultures and risk factors for cervical cancer and ways to reduce these risks.
3. Describe the teaching opportunities to reduce risks of cervical cancer and ways to promote health.
4. Discuss the incidence across cultures and risk factors for colorectal cancer and ways to reduce these risks.
5. Obtain an accurate nursing history of the female client's genitalia, anus, and rectum and related functions.
6. Perform a physical assessment of the female client's genitalia, anus, and rectum using the correct techniques of inspection and palpation.
7. Differentiate between normal and abnormal findings of the female client's genitalia, anus, and rectum.
8. Describe the findings frequently seen when assessing the older female client's genitalia, anus, and rectum.
9. Analyze data from the interview and physical assessment of the client's genitalia, anus, and rectum to formulate valid nursing diagnoses, collaborative problems, and/or referrals.

CHAPTER PRETEST

Activity A MULTIPLE CHOICE QUESTIONS

Choose the one best answer for each of the following multiple choice questions.

_____ 1. The skin folds of the labia majora are composed of adipose tissue, sebaceous glands, and

    a. Skene ducts.

    b. vestibular glands.

    c. sweat glands.

    d. Bartholin glands.

____ **2.** The visible portion of the clitoris is termed the

    a. corpus.

    b. crura.

    c. vestibule.

    d. glans.

____ **3.** The skin folds of the labia majora and the labia minora form a boat-shaped area termed the

    a. vestibule.

    b. corpus.

    c. Skene glands.

    d. urethral meatus.

____ **4.** The outermost layer of the vaginal wall is composed of

    a. pink squamous epithelium and connective tissue.

    b. the vascular supply, nerves, and lymphatic channels.

    c. smooth muscle and connective tissue.

    d. connective tissue and the vascular network.

____ **5.** The outer layer of the vaginal wall is under the direct influence of

    a. androgen.

    b. progesterone.

    c. aldosterone.

    d. estrogen.

Activity B MATCHING

Match the terms in the left column with the correct description in the right column.

Term

____ **1.** Skene glands

____ **2.** Bartholin glands

____ **3.** Os

____ **4.** Libido

____ **5.** Pediculosis pubis

____ **6.** Chadwick sign

____ **7.** Mons pubis

____ **8.** Menopause

____ **9.** Amenorrhea

____ **10.** Menorrhagia

____ **11.** Dysmenorrhea

____ **12.** Dysuria

____ **13.** Valves of Houston

____ **14.** Valsalva maneuver

____ **15.** Proctosigmoidoscopy

Description

a. Painful menstruation

b. Cessation of menstruation

c. "Crabs"

d. Heavy menstruation

e. Secrete mucus to aid in lubrication during intercourse

f. Desire for sexual activity

g. Secrete mucus to lubricate and maintain moist vaginal environment

h. Cervix appears blue rather than pink

i. Painful urination

j. Absence of menstruation

k. Opening in center of cervix

l. Round firm pad of adipose tissue that covers the symphysis pubis

m. Client holds breath and bears down

n. Examination of the rectum and sigmoid colon using a sigmoidoscope

o. Three semilunar transverse folds within the rectal interior

Copyright © 2014. Wolters Kluwer Health | Lippincott Williams & Wilkins. Lab Manual for Health Assessment in Nursing, 5e.

Activity C LABELING ACTIVITIES

Label the external female genitalia in the following figure. Check your answers with Figure 27-1 on page 613 in the textbook.

Label the internal female genitalia in the following figure. Check your answers with Figure 27-2 on page 613 in the textbook.

Copyright © 2014. Wolters Kluwer Health | Lippincott Williams & Wilkins. Lab Manual for Health Assessment in Nursing, 5e.

Activity D LEARNER ACTIVITIES

After reading Chapter 27 in the textbook, participate in the following learning activities.

1. Review the information in EVIDENCE-BASED HEALTH PROMOTION AND DISEASE PREVENTION: CERVICAL CANCER (see page 621–622 in your textbook). Discuss ways to reduce a woman's risk factors for cervical cancer. Next, identify and discuss ethnic groups that are at high risk for cervical cancer.

2. Obtain brochures and literature on cervical cancer and Pap smear testing from the county health department, your campus student health center, or the American Cancer Society. Discuss with your lab partner how to best give a presentation on this topic to teenagers and then to a college-aged group.

3. Using a model of the female genitalia, review the anatomy and function of each anatomic structure. Discuss the assessment findings with your lab partner as they compare with those of an elderly woman.

4. Review the information in EVIDENCE-BASED HEALTH PROMOTION AND DISEASE PREVENTION: COLORECTAL CANCER (see pages 622–623 in the textbook). Discuss ways to reduce a woman's risk factors for colorectal cancer. Next, identify and discuss ethnic groups that are at high risk for colorectal cancer.

Activity E INTERVIEWING AND RECORDING ASSESSMENT FINDINGS

After reading Chapter 27, use the following Nursing Interview Guide to interview and record your subjective findings for an assessment of a female genitalia, anus, and rectum. Your instructor may ask you to turn this in to be evaluated. Forms are also available on thePoint *website.*

Nursing Interview Guide to Collect Subjective Data From the Client	
Questions	**Findings**
Current Symptoms	
1. Menstrual cycles (date of last period, regular cycles, length, describe typical amount of blood flow, symptoms experienced before or during period)?	
2. Age at the time of first menstrual period?	
3. Menopause: Stopped menstruating (if yes, at what age?) or having irregular periods? What symptoms experienced?	
4. Vaginal discharge (unusual in color, amount, or odor)?	
5. Pain or itching in genitalia or groin?	
6. Lumps, swelling, or masses in genital area?	
7. Urinating difficulty, change in urine color, or developed an odor? Difficulty controlling urine?	
8. Problems with sexual performance?	
9. Recent change in sexual activity pattern or libido?	
10. Fertility problems now or in the past?	
Past History	
1. Previous gynecologic problems and results of any treatment?	
2. Date of last pelvic exam by a physician? Date of last Pap smear? Results?	
3. Ever diagnosed with a sexually transmitted disease (STD)? How treated?	

Nursing Interview Guide to Collect Subjective Data From the Client (continued)	
Questions	**Findings**
4. Past pregnancies? Number of pregnancies? Number of children? Possibility of being pregnant now?	
5. Previous anal or rectal trauma or surgery, congenital deformities?	
6. History of blood in stool?	
7. Pattern of health screenings (occult blood, proctosigmoidoscopy, colonoscopy)?	
Family History	
1. Family history of reproductive or genital cancer? Type? How is the family member related to you?	
Lifestyle and Health Practices	
1. Do you smoke or have you smoked in the past? Amount and length of time?	
2. Number of sexual partners?	
3. Use of contraceptives? Type? Frequency?	
4. Problems with your genitalia that affect your functioning?	
5. What is your sexual preference?	
6. Comfort level communicating with your partner your sexual likes and dislikes?	
7. Fears related to sex? Do you have stress related to sex?	
8. Fertility concerns? If so, has this affected your relationship with partner or family?	
9. Feelings about going through menopause?	
10. Do you perform monthly genital self-exams?	
11. Tested for HIV? Results? Why tested?	
12. Taking estrogen replacement? Length of treatment? Dosage?	
13. Knowledge of toxic shock syndrome?	
14. Knowledge of sexually transmitted diseases and their prevention?	
15. Use of laxatives, stool softeners, enemas, or other bowel medications?	
16. Practice anal sex?	
17. Daily water/fluid intake?	
18. Usual diet (high fiber and roughage, saturated fat content)?	
19. Usual exercise pattern?	
20. Any effect on daily life from anal, rectal, or bowel problems?	

Copyright © 2014. Wolters Kluwer Health | Lippincott Williams & Wilkins. Lab Manual for Health Assessment in Nursing, 5e.

Activity F PERFORMING PHYSICAL ASSESSMENT OF THE FEMALE GENITALIA, ANUS, AND RECTUM

Use the following Physical Assessment Guide to examine the female genitalia, anus, and rectum model. Column 1 will serve as a reminder as to what part of the exam you will do next. Column 2 will be used to record your findings. Your instructor may ask you to turn this in to be evaluated. Forms are also available on thePoint *website.*

Physical Assessment Guide to Collect Objective Client Data	
Questions	**Findings**
Current Symptoms	
1. Gather equipment (stool, light, speculum, emesis basin filled with warm tap water, Surgilube, cotton-tipped applicators, *Chlamydia* culture tube, culturette, test tube with water, sterile gloves, Ayre spatula [wood stick], and feminine napkins).	
2. Explain the procedure to client.	
3. Ask client to put on a gown.	
External Genitalia	
1. Inspect the mons pubis. Note pubic hair distribution, signs of infestation.	
2. Inspect the labia majora and perineum. Note lesions, swelling, excoriation.	
3. Inspect the labia minora, clitoris, urethral meatus, and vaginal opening. Note lesions, excoriation, swelling, discharge.	
4. Palpate the Bartholin glands (if history of swelling or current swelling noted). Note swelling, tenderness, discharge.	
5. Palpate the urethra (if client complains of urethral symptoms or urethritis, or inflammation of Skene glands is suspected) by inserting gloved index finger into the superior portion of the vagina and milking the urethra from the inside, pushing up and out. Observe for drainage.	
Internal Genitalia	
1. Inspect the size of the vaginal opening and the angle of the vagina by moistening gloved index finger with warm water and gently inserting the finger into the vagina.	
2. Assess the vaginal musculature by keeping index finger inserted in the vaginal opening and asking the client to squeeze around your finger. Using middle and index fingers to separate the labia minora, ask client to bear down. Observe for bulging or discharge of urine.	
3. Perform the speculum examination.	
a. Inspect the cervix for color, size, position, surface, os, discharge, or lesions.	
b. Obtain specimens for the Pap smear and, if indicated, cultures to test for STDs.	
c. Inspect the vagina, unlocking the speculum and inspecting the vagina as the partially open speculum is slowly rotated and removed. Note color, surface, consistency, and discharge.	

Copyright © 2014. Wolters Kluwer Health | Lippincott Williams & Wilkins. Lab Manual for Health Assessment in Nursing, 5e.

Physical Assessment Guide to Collect Objective Client Data (continued)

Questions	Findings
4. Perform the bimanual examination by placing nondominant hand on lower abdomen and inserting gloved lubricated index and middle fingers into the vaginal opening, applying pressure to the posterior wall, and waiting for the opening to relax. Palpate the ovaries by sliding your intravaginal fingers to the right lateral fornix and attempting to palpate the left and then the right ovaries. Note size, shape, consistency, mobility, and tenderness. Observe for secretions as fingers are withdrawn.	
5. Perform the rectovaginal examination by changing gloves on dominant hand and lubricating index and middle fingers. Ask client to bear down. Insert index finger into the vagina and middle finger into the rectum. While pushing down on the abdominal wall with the other hand, palpate the internal reproductive structures through the anterior rectal wall, with attention to the area behind the cervix, the rectovaginal septum, the cul-de-sac, and the posterior uterine wall.	
Anus and Perianal Area	
1. Inspect for lumps, ulcers, lesions, rashes, redness (note size, shape, location, distribution, and configuration).	
2. Inspect the sacrococcygeal area for swelling, redness, dimpling, or presence of hair in pilonidal area.	
3. Inspect for rectal prolapse with Valsalva maneuver.	
4. Palpate for anal sphincter tone, tenderness, nodules, or hardness.	
Rectum	
1. Palpate rectal mucosa for tenderness, irregularities, nodules, and hardness.	
2. Palpate peritoneal cavity for tenderness or nodules, or "rectal shelf."	
3. Inspect the feces for blood and perform occult blood test.	
Analysis of Data	
1. Formulate nursing diagnoses (health promotion, risk, actual).	
2. Formulate collaborative problems.	
3. Make necessary referrals.	

Copyright © 2014. Wolters Kluwer Health | Lippincott Williams & Wilkins. Lab Manual for Health Assessment in Nursing, 5e.

CHAPTER POSTTEST

Activity G   MULTIPLE CHOICE QUESTIONS

Choose the one best answer for each of the following multiple choice questions.

____ 1. A female client tells the nurse that she may be experiencing premenstrual syndrome. An appropriate question for the nurse to ask the client is
   a. "How often are your menstrual periods?"
   b. "Do you experience mood swings or bloating?"
   c. "Are you experiencing regular menstrual cycles?"
   d. "How old were you when you began to menstruate?"

____ 2. A 53-year-old client tells the nurse that she thinks she is starting the menopausal phase of her life. The nurse should instruct the client that she may experience
   a. hot flashes.
   b. increased appetite.
   c. vaginal discharge.
   d. urinary frequency.

____ 3. During assessment of the vaginal area of an adult client, the client tells the nurse that she has had pain in her vaginal area. The nurse should further assess the client for
   a. trauma.
   b. cancer.
   c. pregnancy.
   d. infection.

____ 4. A female client tells the nurse that she has pain while urinating. Besides obtaining a urinalysis, the nurse should assess the client for
   a. kidney trauma.
   b. sexually transmitted disease.
   c. tumors.
   d. infestation.

____ 5. An older adult client visits the clinic complaining of urinary incontinence. The nurse should explain to the client that this is often due to
   a. decreased urethral elasticity.
   b. atrophy of the vaginal mucosa.
   c. change in the vaginal pH.
   d. decreased estrogen production.

____ 6. A female client has scheduled a physical examination, including a Pap smear. The nurse should instruct the client to
   a. refrain from douching 48 hours before the examination.
   b. bring in a urine sample for testing.
   c. drink a large volume of fluid before the examination.
   d. refrain from using talcum powder after her shower.

____ 7. The nurse is preparing to perform a speculum examination on an adult woman. To lubricate the speculum before insertion, the nurse should use
   a. sterile water.
   b. K-Y jelly.
   c. warm tap water.
   d. petroleum jelly.

Copyright © 2014. Wolters Kluwer Health | Lippincott Williams & Wilkins. Lab Manual for Health Assessment in Nursing, 5e.

____ **8.** The nurse is performing a speculum examination on an adult woman. The nurse is having difficulty inserting the speculum because the client is unable to relax. The nurse should ask the client to

 a. bear down.

 b. hold her breath.

 c. use imagery to relax.

 d. take a deep breath.

____ **9.** The nurse is assessing the genitalia of a female client and detects a bulging anterior wall in the vagina. The nurse should plan to refer the client to a physician for

 a. stress incontinence.

 b. rectocele.

 c. tumor of the vagina.

 d. cystocele.

____ **10.** An older adult client visits the clinic for a gynecologic examination. The client tells the nurse that she has been told that she has uterine prolapse. The nurse should further assess the client for

 a. stress incontinence.

 b. cystocele.

 c. a retroverted uterus.

 d. diastasis recti.

____ **11.** While assessing the cervix of an adult client, the nurse observes a yellowish discharge from the cervix. The nurse should further assess the client for a/an

 a. infection.

 b. abnormal lesion.

 c. positive pregnancy test result.

 d. polyp.

____ **12.** While performing a gynecologic examination, the nurse observes small, painful, ulcer-like lesions with red bases on the client's labia. The nurse should refer the client to a physician for possible

 a. herpes simplex virus infection.

 b. syphilis.

 c. lice.

 d. herpes zoster virus infection.

____ **13.** While assessing the genitalia of a female client, the nurse observes moist fleshy lesions on the client's labia. The nurse should refer the client to a physician for possible

 a. gonorrhea.

 b. herpes simplex virus infection.

 c. nabothian cysts.

 d. genital warts.

____ **14.** During a gynecologic examination, the nurse observes that the client has a yellow-green frothy vaginal discharge. The nurse should plan to test the client for possible

 a. *Trichomonas vaginalis* infection.

 b. bacterial vaginosis.

 c. atrophic vaginitis.

 d. *Chlamydia trachomatis* infection.

Copyright © 2014. Wolters Kluwer Health | Lippincott Williams & Wilkins. Lab Manual for Health Assessment in Nursing, 5e.

_____ **15.** A client visits the clinic because she has missed one period and suspects she is pregnant. While assessing the client, the nurse detects a solid, mobile, tender, unilateral adnexal mass. The client's cervix is soft. The nurse suspects that the client may be experiencing

    a. normal pregnancy.

    b. endometriosis.

    c. pelvic inflammatory disease.

    d. ectopic pregnancy.

_____ **16.** A client visits the clinic and tells the nurse that her stools have been black for the past 3 days. The nurse should assess the client for

    a. gallbladder disease.

    b. colitis.

    c. polyps.

    d. gastrointestinal bleeding.

_____ **17.** A client visits the clinic and tells the nurse that her stools have been pale for the past 2 days and her skin has been itching. The nurse should refer the client to a physician for possible

    a. biliary disease.

    b. cancer.

    c. gastrointestinal infection.

    d. hemorrhoids.

_____ **18.** The nurse is planning to inspect the anal area of an adult female client. To assess for any bulges or lesions, the nurse should ask the client to

    a. hold her breath.

    b. breathe deeply through her mouth.

    c. breathe normally.

    d. bear down.

_____ **19.** While assessing the anal area of an adult client, the nurse detects redness and excoriation. The nurse determines that this sign is most likely due to

    a. internal hemorrhoids.

    b. an anorectal fistula.

    c. a fungal infection.

    d. previous surgery.

_____ **20.** While assessing the anus of an adult client, the nurse detects the presence of small nodules. The nurse should refer the client to a physician for possible

    a. polyps.

    b. anorectal fistula.

    c. hemorrhoids.

    d. rectocele.

Activity H   CRITICAL THINKING ACTIVITIES

1. Develop a seminar on prevention of sexually transmitted infections (STIs) for a group of college freshmen. Include what and how you would teach risks factors for various diseases.

2. You are to do a presentation on the topic of constipation in a series of talks at the Senior Center. You have decided to present your material by developing a questionnaire. What questions will you include? Why?

3. What variations of the cervix are considered normal?

4. Compare and contrast how you would focus the nursing history of the female genitalia for an 18-year-old versus that for an 80-year-old.

Copyright © 2014. Wolters Kluwer Health | Lippincott Williams & Wilkins. Lab Manual for Health Assessment in Nursing, 5e.

5. Andrea S., 37 years old, has made an appointment with the OB/GYN nurse practitioner. You are asked to compile the nursing history. When you ask Mrs. S. why she is here today, she looks somewhat embarrassed and answers quietly, "I am having trouble with sexual intercourse." She goes on to explain that she has had decreased interest in sex, and her vagina seems drier than usual. When asked whether she has been able to discuss this problem with her husband, she says, "No … it is embarrassing … we have always enjoyed sex, and I feel I am not meeting his needs any more. I can tell he is getting very frustrated. My husband asks me why we never have sex any more, and I just give excuses of having headaches, being tired, or being too busy."

In your interview, you ask her what is going on in her life right now, and Mrs. S. tells you that she is under a lot of stress at her marketing job and that lately she has had to help her two children, aged 10 and 8, with numerous school projects. She is also worried about her mother, who is undergoing tests to determine whether she has cancer.

Develop possible nursing diagnoses that are appropriate for this client.

6. Mrs. Norman C. is 85 years old and has a long history of chronic constipation, internal and external hemorrhoids, and heavy use of laxatives. She describes another bout of constipation with no bowel movement for 5 days, but with a feeling of fullness in her rectum. She says that she eats many vegetables when she feels better but gets too weak to cook or exercise, or even to get dressed, when she has these bouts of constipation. On examination, you note internal and external hemorrhoids, a moderate amount of hard-formed stool in the rectum, and an area of hardness and irregularity about 2 cm in size in the distal portion of the rectum. The results of her stool test are positive for occult blood.

Develop possible appropriate nursing diagnoses and collaborative problems for this client.

Activity I CASE STUDY

Read the following case study. Then, work through the steps of analyzing the case study data. First identify abnormal data and strengths in **subjective and objective findings**, assemble **cue clusters**, draw **inferences**, make possible **nursing diagnoses**, identify **defining characteristics**, **confirm or rule out** the diagnoses, and **document** your conclusions. Use the blank diagnostic analysis charts provided at the end of this book (also available on thePoint website) to guide your thinking. Propose nursing diagnoses that are specific to the client in the case study. Identify collaborative problems, if any, for this client. Finally, identify data, if any, that point toward a medical problem requiring a referral.

Tina K. is a 26-year-old white woman. She is a single mother of two and is employed as a paralegal in a law firm. She comes to the clinic appearing anxious. She states she is experiencing a brown vaginal discharge that started 2 days ago. When interviewed, she states that her last pelvic examination was 6 months ago. She denies any history of cancer or abnormal Pap smear results. Her last menstrual period was normal and ended 1 week ago today. She has never been tested for HIV. She admits to unprotected sex 3 weeks ago with her boyfriend. A Norplant birth control device was placed in her left arm 1 year ago. Ms. K. denies smoking, states that she does not follow any special diet, and does not exercise on a regular basis. She explains that she is not comfortable discussing this problem with her new boyfriend—"I am afraid he might leave me."

Your physical assessment reveals normal hair distribution and no lesions, masses, or swelling. The labia majora and labia minora are pink, moist, and free of lesions, excoriation, and swelling. A small amount of malodorous brown discharge is noted at the vaginal orifice. There is no bulging at the vaginal orifice. The perineum is intact with a healed episiotomy scar. No discharge is observed on urethral palpation. Internal examination reveals cervix to be slightly anterior and pink, with a slit-like os, and free of lesions. A brown discharge is noted on the cervix. The vaginal walls are pink and moist with streaks of brown discharge. Bimanual examination reveals a mobile, firm, but tender cervix. The fundus is palpated at the level of the symphysis pubis. The ovaries are palpated bilaterally without lesions and are approximately 3 cm. The right ovary is very tender on palpation. A routine Pap smear is performed and culture specimens are taken. A smooth, firm, mobile, nontender posterior uterine wall and a smooth, firm, thin, movable rectovaginal septum are palpated during rectovaginal palpation.

How Well Did You Do?

After you have read the chapter and completed the exercises in this chapter, visit thePoint to access the Self-Reflection Activity. This activity will help you identify to what degree you have met each of the chapter objectives. You can then review the chapter for objectives you have met partially or not at all.

Other tools to help you, like the Diagnostic Reasoning Guides, Nursing Interview Guides, Physical Assessment Guides, and NCLEX-Style Chapter Review Questions, are also available on thePoint.

Copyright © 2014. Wolters Kluwer Health | Lippincott Williams & Wilkins. Lab Manual for Health Assessment in Nursing, 5e.

CHAPTER 28

Pulling It All Together: Integrated Head-to-Toe Assessment

Chapter Overview

Let the pages of this chapter help you pull all your assessment skills together to integrate the examination of all the body systems into an organized process that flows comfortably for you and the client. A head-to-toe approach to perform a comprehensive assessment saves time and energy for both the client and the nurse. It is important to be familiar with your state's Nurse Practice Act to find out what you can legally assess and diagnose.

Chapter Learning Objectives

1. Explain how to prepare yourself and the client for a holistic nursing interview and head-to-toe integrated physical examination.
2. List all the equipment needed for a total physical examination.
3. Describe the parts of the physical examination that can be integrated within assessment of each of the body systems.
4. Correctly interview a client for an accurate holistic nursing history.
5. Correctly perform a total head-to-toe integrated physical examination, identifying normal and abnormal findings.
6. Analyze data from a holistic nursing interview and head-to-toe integrated physical assessment to formulate valid nursing diagnoses, collaborative problems, and/or referrals.

CHAPTER PRETEST

Activity A MULTIPLE CHOICE QUESTIONS

Choose the one best answer for each of the following multiple choice questions.

_____ 1. The best approach to use when performing a total physical examination on a client is

    a. a toe-to-head integrated assessment of body systems.

    b. a head-to-toe integrated assessment of body systems.

    c. a total body system approach examining each body system individually.

    d. any approach that is convenient for you and the client.

____ **2.** Before beginning a physical assessment it is important for the nurse to
  a. explain to the client in detail how each body system will be assessed.
  b. explain to the client the purpose of every physical assessment technique you will be using.
  c. acquire your client's verbal permission to perform the physical examination.
  d. acquire your client's written permission to perform the physical examination.

____ **3.** Two body systems that may be logically integrated and assessed at the same time are the
  a. eye and ear exams.
  b. eye exam and cranial nerves II, III, IV, and VI.
  c. ear exam and cranial nerves IV, VI, and VIII.
  d. ear and nose exams.

____ **4.** Examination of the skin should be
  a. integrated throughout the head-to-toe examination.
  b. completed at the beginning of the physical assessment before proceeding to other parts of the exam.
  c. performed at the very end of the physical assessment.
  d. integrated and completed only with the musculoskeletal examination.

____ **5.** When integrating the total physical examination the nurse should
  a. perform the Mental Status Exam after examining all other body systems.
  b. assess cranial nerve I (olfactory) with the other 11 cranial nerves at the same time.
  c. assess peripheral vascular status when examining the lower extremities.
  d. integrate the rectal examination with the abdominal examination.

Activity B LEARNER ACTIVITY

After reading Chapter 28 in the textbook, participate in the following learning activity.

Practice performing an integrated head-to-toe examination on your lab partner without referring to the chapter. When you are finished, have your lab partner identify anything he or she feels you may have omitted during the examination. Check his or her report against the Physical Assessment Guide provided in this workbook chapter. Discuss which parts might have been better integrated for a smoother transition process for both the examiner and the client. Then repeat the process with you being the client and your lab partner being the examiner.

Activity C INTERVIEWING AND RECORDING ASSESSMENT FINDINGS

After reading Chapter 28, use the following Nursing Interview Guide to interview and record your subjective findings for a holistic assessment of a lab partner, peer, or client. Your instructor may ask you to turn this in to be evaluated. Forms are also available on thePoint *website.*

Nursing Interview Guide to Collect Subjective Data From the Client	
Questions	**Findings**
Biographic Data	
1. Name?	
2. Address?	
3. Phone?	
4. Birthdate?	
5. Provider history?	
6. Ethnicity?	
7. Educational level?	
8. Occupation?	

Nursing Interview Guide to Collect Subjective Data From the Client (continued)

Questions	Findings
Current Symptoms	
1. History of present concern (COLDSPA)?	
Past History	
1. Birth problems?	
2. Childhood illnesses?	
3. Immunizations?	
4. Illnesses?	
5. Surgeries?	
6. Accidents?	
7. Pain?	
8. Allergies?	
Family History	
1. Family genogram?	
Review of Body Systems	
1. Skin, hair, nails?	
2. Ears?	
3. Mouth, throat, nose, sinuses?	
4. Thorax and lungs?	
5. Breasts and regional lymph nodes?	
6. Heart and neck vessels?	
7. Peripheral vascular?	
8. Abdomen?	
9. Male/female genitalia?	
10. Anus, rectum, and prostate?	
11. Musculoskeletal?	
12. Neurologic?	
Lifestyle and Health Practices	
1. ADLs in a typical day?	
2. Diet for past 24 hours?	
3. Exercise regimen?	
4. Sleep patterns?	
5. Medications?	
6. Use of recreation drugs, alcohol, nicotine, or caffeine?	
7. Self-concept?	
8. Life stressors and coping strategies?	
9. Responsibilities and role at home and at work?	
10. Type of work and level of satisfaction?	

Nursing Interview Guide to Collect Subjective Data From the Client (continued)

Questions	Findings
11. Finances?	
12. Educational plans?	
13. Social activities?	
14. Relationships with others?	
15. Values?	
16. Spirituality?	
17. Religious affiliations?	
18. Environment, residency, and neighborhood?	

Activity D PERFORMING A HOLISTIC PHYSICAL ASSESSMENT

Use the following Physical Assessment Guide for a holistic assessment of a lab partner, peer, or client. Column 1 will serve as a reminder as to what part of the exam you will do next. Column 2 will be used to record your findings. Your instructor may ask you to turn this in to be evaluated. Forms are also available on thePoint *website.*

Physical Assessment Guide to Collect Objective Client Data

Questions	Findings
1. Gather all equipment needed for a head-to-toe exam.	
2. Prepare client by explaining what you will be doing.	
General Survey	
1. Observe appearance.	
2. Assess vital signs.	
3. Take body measurements.	
4. Calculate ideal body weight, body mass index, waist-to-hip ratio, mid-arm muscle area and circumference.	
5. Test vision.	
Mental Status Examination	
1. Observe LOC.	
2. Observe posture and body movements.	
3. Observe facial expressions.	
4. Observe speech.	
5. Observe mood, feelings, and expressions.	
6. Observe thought processes and perceptions.	
7. Assess cognitive abilities.	
8. Give client a specimen cup if sample is needed, and ask client to empty bladder and change into gown. Ask client to sit on examination table.	
Skin	
1. Throughout examination, assess skin for color variations, texture, temperature, turgor, edema, and lesions.	
2. Teach skin self-examination.	

Copyright © 2014. Wolters Kluwer Health | Lippincott Williams & Wilkins. Lab Manual for Health Assessment in Nursing, 5e.

Physical Assessment Guide to Collect Objective Client Data (continued)

Questions	Findings
Head and Face	
1. Inspect and palpate head.	
2. Note consistency, distribution, color of hair.	
3. Observe face for symmetry, features, expressions, condition of skin.	
4. Have client smile, frown, show teeth, blow out cheeks, raise eyebrows, and tightly close eyes (CN VII).	
5. Test sensations of forehead, cheeks, and chin (CN V).	
6. Palpate temporal arteries for elasticity and tenderness.	
7. Palpate temporomandibular joint.	
Eyes	
1. Assess visual function.	
2. Inspect external eye.	
3. Test papillary reaction to light.	
4. Test accommodation of pupils.	
5. Assess corneal reflex (CN VII facial).	
6. Use ophthalmoscope to inspect interior of eye.	
Ears	
1. Inspect auricle, tragus, and lobule.	
2. Palpate auricle and mastoid process.	
3. Use otoscope to inspect auditory canal.	
4. Use otoscope to inspect tympanic membrane.	
5. Test hearing.	
Nose and Sinuses	
1. Inspect external nose.	
2. Palpate external nose for tenderness.	
3. Check patency of airflow through nostrils.	
4. Occlude each nostril and ask client to smell for soap, coffee, or vanilla (CN I).	
5. Use otoscope to inspect internal nose.	
6. Transilluminate maxillary sinuses.	
Mouth and Throat	
1. Put on gloves.	
2. Inspect lips.	
3. Inspect teeth.	
4. Check gums and buccal mucosa.	
5. Inspect hard and soft palates.	
6. Observe uvula.	

Copyright © 2014. Wolters Kluwer Health | Lippincott Williams & Wilkins. Lab Manual for Health Assessment in Nursing, 5e.

Physical Assessment Guide to Collect Objective Client Data (continued)

Questions	Findings
7. Assess for gag reflex (CN X).	
8. Inspect tonsils.	
9. Inspect and palpate tongue.	
10. Assess tongue strength (CN IX and X).	
11. Check taste sensation (CN VII and IX).	
Neck	
1. Inspect appearance of neck.	
2. Test ROM of neck.	
3. Palpate preauricular, postauricular, occipital, tonsillar, submandibular, and submental nodes.	
4. Palpate trachea.	
5. Palpate thyroid gland.	
6. If enlarged, auscultate thyroid gland for bruits.	
7. Palpate and auscultate carotid arteries.	
Arms, Hands, and Fingers	
1. Inspect upper extremities.	
2. Test shoulder shrug and ability to turn head against resistance (CN XI spinal).	
3. Palpate arms.	
4. Assess epitrochlear lymph nodes.	
5. Test ROM of elbows.	
6. Palpate brachial pulse.	
7. Palpate ulnar and radial pulses.	
8. Test ROM of wrist.	
9. Inspect and palpate palms of hands.	
10. Test ROM of fingers.	
11. Use reflex hammer to test biceps, triceps, and brachioradialis reflexes.	
12. Test rapid alternating movements of hands.	
13. Test sensation in arms, hands, and fingers.	
Posterior and Lateral Chest	
1. Ask the client to continue sitting with arms at sides and stand behind the client. Untie gown to expose posterior chest.	
2. Inspect scapulae and chest wall.	
3. Note the use of accessory muscles when breathing.	
4. Palpate chest.	
5. Evaluate chest expansion at T9 or T10.	
6. Percuss at posterior intercostal spaces.	

Copyright © 2014. Wolters Kluwer Health | Lippincott Williams & Wilkins. Lab Manual for Health Assessment in Nursing, 5e.

Physical Assessment Guide to Collect Objective Client Data (continued)

Questions	Findings
7. Determine diaphragmatic excursion.	
8. Auscultate posterior chest.	
9. Test for two-point discrimination on back.	
10. Auscultate apex and left sternal border of heart during exhalation.	
Anterior Chest	
1. Inspect chest.	
2. Note quality and pattern of respirations.	
3. Observe intercostal spaces.	
4. Palpate anterior chest.	
5. Percuss anterior chest.	
6. Auscultate anterior chest.	
7. Test skin mobility and turgor.	
8. Ask client to fold gown to waist and sit with arms hanging freely.	
Female Breasts	
1. Inspect both breasts, areolas, and nipples.	
2. Inspect for retractions and dimpling of nipples.	
3. Palpate axillae.	
Male Breasts	
1. Inspect breast tissue.	
2. Palpate breast tissue and axillae.	
3. Assist client to supine position with the head elevated to 30 to 45 degrees. Stand on client's right side.	
Neck	
1. Evaluate jugular venous pressure.	
2. Assist client to supine position (lower examination table).	
Breasts (Female)	
1. Palpate breasts for masses and nipples for discharge.	
2. Teach breast self-examination.	
Heart	
1. Inspect and palpate for apical impulse.	
2. Palpate the apex, left sternal border, and base of the heart.	
3. Auscultate over aortic area, pulmonic area, Erb point, tricuspid area, and apex.	
4. Auscultate apex of heart as client lays on left side.	

Copyright © 2014. Wolters Kluwer Health | Lippincott Williams & Wilkins. Lab Manual for Health Assessment in Nursing, 5e.

Physical Assessment Guide to Collect Objective Client Data (continued)	
Questions	**Findings**
Abdomen	
1. Cover chest with gown and arrange draping to expose abdomen.	
2. Inspect abdomen.	
3. Auscultate abdomen.	
4. Percuss abdomen.	
5. Palpate abdomen.	
Legs, Feet, and Toes	
1. Observe muscles.	
2. Note hair distribution.	
3. Palpate joints of hips and test ROM.	
4. Palpate legs and feet.	
5. Palpate knees.	
6. Palpate ankles.	
7. Assess capillary refill.	
8. Test sensations (dull and sharp), two-point discrimination, reflexes, position sense, and vibratory sensation.	
9. Perform heel-to-shin test.	
10. Perform any special tests as warranted.	
11. Secure gown and assist client to standing position.	
Musculoskeletal and Neurologic Systems	
1. Observe for spinal curvatures and check for scoliosis.	
2. Observe gait.	
3. Observe tandem walk.	
4. Observe hopping on each leg.	
5. Perform Romberg test.	
6. Perform finger-to-nose test.	
Female Genitalia	
1. Have the female client assume the lithotomy position. Apply gloves. Apply lubricant as appropriate.	
2. Inspect pubic hair.	
3. Inspect mons pubis, labia majora, and perineum.	
4. Inspect labia minora, clitoris, urethral meatus, and vaginal opening.	
5. Palpate Bartholin glands, urethra, and Skene glands.	
6. Inspect cervix.	
7. Inspect vagina.	
8. Obtain cytologic smears and culture.	

Copyright © 2014. Wolters Kluwer Health | Lippincott Williams & Wilkins. Lab Manual for Health Assessment in Nursing, 5e.

Physical Assessment Guide to Collect Objective Client Data (continued)

Questions	Findings
9. Palpate cervix.	
10. Palpate uterus.	
11. Palpate ovaries.	
12. Discard gloves and apply clean gloves and lubricant.	
13. Palpate rectovaginal septum.	
Male Genitalia	
1. Sit on a stool and have the client stand and face you with gown raised. Apply gloves.	
2. Inspect penis.	
3. Palpate for urethral discharge.	
4. Inspect scrotum.	
5. Palpate both testis and epididymis.	
6. Transilluminate scrotal contents.	
7. Inspect for bulges in inguinal and femoral areas.	
8. Palpate for scrotal hernia.	
9. Palpate for inguinal hernia.	
10. Teach testicular self-examination.	
11. Inspect perineal area.	
12. Inspect sacrococcygeal area.	
13. Inspect for bulges or lesions as Valsalva maneuver is performed.	
Rectal	
1. Ask the client to remain standing and to bend over the exam table. Change gloves.	
2. Palpate anus.	
3. Palpate external sphincter.	
4. Palpate rectum.	
5. Palpate peritoneal cavity.	
6. Palpate prostate.	
7. Inspect stool.	

Copyright © 2014. Wolters Kluwer Health | Lippincott Williams & Wilkins. Lab Manual for Health Assessment in Nursing, 5e.

CHAPTER POSTTEST

Activity E MATCHING

Match the section of the head-to-toe examination on the left with the assessment on the right that would best be integrated there.

Section

_____ **1.** General survey

_____ **2.** Mental Status Exam

_____ **3.** Head and face

_____ **4.** Eye

_____ **5.** Ear

_____ **6.** Mouth and throat

_____ **7.** Neck

_____ **8.** Arms, hands, and fingers

_____ **9.** Male examination

Assessment

a. Biceps, triceps, and brachioradialis reflexes

b. Vital signs and anthropometric measurements

c. Mood, feelings, and perceptions

d. Cervical lymph nodes

e. Cranial nerve VII (facial)

f. Cranial nerve VIII

g. Cremasteric reflex

h. Cranial nerves IX and X

i. Cranial nerves II, III, IV, and VI

Activity F CRITICAL THINKING ACTIVITY

Take turns with your partner stating one way to integrate different parts of a head-to-toe physical examination. Try to generate as many ways as possible without looking at your textbook. Then review your textbook to see which areas you may have missed.

How Well Did You Do?

After you have read the chapter and completed the exercises in this chapter, visit thePoint to access the Self-Reflection Activity. This activity will help you identify to what degree you have met each of the chapter objectives. You can then review the chapter for objectives you have met partially or not at all.

Other tools to help you, like the Diagnostic Reasoning Guides, Nursing Interview Guides, Physical Assessment Guides, and NCLEX-Style Chapter Review Questions, are also available on thePoint.

Copyright © 2014. Wolters Kluwer Health | Lippincott Williams & Wilkins. Lab Manual for Health Assessment in Nursing, 5e.

CHAPTER 29

Assessing Childbearing Women

Chapter Overview

Women in the childbearing years have unique health care needs, particularly during pregnancy. The nursing assessment focuses generally on the various needs and changes specific to women and particularly on the related issues of hormones and hormonal balance.

Chapter Learning Objectives

1. Explain the dynamic cardiovascular changes that occur during pregnancy.
2. Describe the skin changes that occur during pregnancy.
3. Measure the progressional growth of the uterus during pregnancy.
4. Discuss common concerns and complaints experienced by the pregnant client.
5. Obtain an accurate nursing history by conducting a prenatal interview.
6. Demonstrate how to correctly perform Leopold maneuvers.
7. Analyze data from the client interview and physical assessment of a childbearing woman to formulate valid nursing diagnoses, collaborative problems, and/or referrals.

CHAPTER PRETEST

Activity A MULTIPLE CHOICE QUESTIONS

Choose the one best answer for each of the following multiple choice questions.

_____ **1.** While assessing the abdomen of a pregnant client, the nurse observes striae gravidarum. The nurse should instruct the client that after delivery, the striae gravidarum will

   a. completely disappear.

   b. remain the same.

   c. disappear if a special ointment is used.

   d. fade to a white or silvery color.

_____ **2.** While assessing the abdomen of a pregnant woman, the nurse observes a dark line from the client's umbilicus to the mons pubis. The nurse should explain to the client that this is called

   a. linea nigra.

   b. chloasma.

   c. melanin.

   d. epulis.

_____ **3.** During pregnancy, a relaxation of the ligaments and joints is caused by the increase in

   a. estrogen.

   b. chorionic gonadotropin.

   c. lactation hormone.

   d. progesterone.

_____ **4.** The nurse is caring for a client who is 24 weeks pregnant. The client tells the nurse that she has been secreting colostrum for the past few days. The nurse should instruct the client that colostrum secretion

   a. does not normally occur until delivery of the baby.

   b. may be indicative of a problem with the breasts.

   c. is normal for some women in the second and third trimesters.

   d. may be indicative of preterm labor ensuing.

_____ **5.** One cardiac change that commonly occurs in a pregnant client is

   a. an increase in maternal blood volume by 40% to 50%.

   b. a decrease in plasma volume by 20%.

   c. physiologic hypertension that stabilizes by 24 weeks' gestation.

   d. a decrease in the heart rate of the client.

_____ **6.** As pregnancy progresses, the abdominal muscles may stretch to the point of separation. This condition is termed

   a. herniation.

   b. McDonald sign.

   c. Goodell sign.

   d. diastasis recti abdominis.

_____ **7.** The nurse has instructed a pregnant client about changes that may occur to the client's gastrointestinal system during pregnancy. The nurse determines that the client needs further instructions when the client says

   a. "As a result of pregnancy, diarrhea may occur more often."

   b. "Gastric motility is decreased from the pressure of the fetus."

   c. "Constipation may occur because gastric tone is decreased."

   d. "Gallstone formation may occur because of prolonged emptying time of the gallbladder."

_____ **8.** While interviewing a pregnant client, the nurse determines that the client has pica. The nurse should assess the client's

   a. blood sugar.

   b. teeth and gums.

   c. nutritional status.

   d. emotional status.

_____ **9.** During pregnancy, the uterus enlarges as a result of hypertrophy of existing myometrial cells and hyperplasia of new cells. This growth is due to

   a. estrogen.

   b. progesterone.

   c. growth hormone.

   d. lactation hormone.

_____ **10.** The nurse is caring for a pregnant client who is at approximately 20 weeks' gestation. The nurse is planning to measure the client's fundal height. At 20 weeks' gestation, the nurse should locate the top of the fundus

   a. at the top of the symphysis pubis.

   b. midway between the symphysis pubis and the umbilicus.

   c. at the level of the umbilicus.

   d. above the level of the umbilicus.

Copyright © 2014. Wolters Kluwer Health | Lippincott Williams & Wilkins. Lab Manual for Health Assessment in Nursing, 5e.

Activity B LEARNER ACTIVITIES

After reading Chapter 29 in the textbook, participate in the following learning activity.

1. With a lab partner, role-play nurse and childbearing client. Have the client present with common complaints of pregnancy. Have the nurse reassure the client, explain in layperson's terms the reasons for these symptoms, and offer recommendations for relief. (Also have the nurse refer any problems that are not normal to an appropriate health care provider, such as midwife or a physician.)

Activity C INTERVIEWING AND RECORDING ASSESSMENT FINDINGS

After reading Chapter 29, use the following Nursing Interview Guide to interview and record your subjective findings for an assessment of the childbearing woman. Your instructor may ask you to turn this in to be evaluated. Forms are also available on thePoint *website.*

Nursing Interview Guide to Collect Subjective Data From the Client	
Questions	**Findings**
Current Symptoms	
1. Weight changes?	
2. Upper respiratory symptoms?	
3. Stomach or bowel problems?	
4. Urinary tract symptoms?	
5. Vaginal discharge, bleeding, or leaking fluid?	
6. Psychological problems?	
7. Breast changes?	
Past History	
1. Past pregnancy history (include all previous deliveries and miscarriages)?	
2. Neonatal problems at delivery or within the first 2 weeks of life?	
3. Complicated pregnancies requiring termination, molar pregnancy, ectopic pregnancy, etc.?	
4. Last menstrual period (LMP) and duration, bleeding since that time?	
5. Type of birth control used, if any?	
6. Infertility problems?	
7. Reproductive surgeries, abnormal Pap smears, etc.?	
8. History of sexually transmitted diseases, treatment, vaginal infections, etc.?	
9. Blood type?	
10. Medical history?	
11. Hospitalizations?	
12. Surgeries?	
Family History	
1. History of birth defects in the family?	
2. Ethnic background?	
3. Heart disease, lung disease, diabetes, asthma, cancer, birth defects, blood disorders, mental retardation, sickle cell disease?	

Nursing Interview Guide to Collect Subjective Data From the Client (continued)

Questions	Findings
Lifestyle and Health Practices	
1. Age at delivery?	
2. Current medications?	
3. Alcohol/cigarette use?	
4. Street drug use?	
5. Family members who consider social habits to be a problem?	
6. Diet evaluation?	
7. Weight/baseline?	
8. Exercise routine?	
9. Client's occupation/highest degree?	
10. Work routine?	
11. Chemical/radiation exposure?	
12. Risk for toxoplasmosis?	
13. Partner profile?	
14. Social support systems?	
15. Siblings?	

Activity D PERFORMING PHYSICAL ASSESSMENT

Use the following Physical Assessment Guide to examine the childbearing woman. Column 1 will serve as a reminder as to what part of the examination you will do next. Column 2 will be used to record your findings. Your instructor may ask you to turn this in to be evaluated. Forms are also available on thePoint *website.*

Physical Assessment Guide to Collect Objective Client Data

Questions	Findings
1. Gather equipment (ophthalmoscope, otoscope, stethoscope, speculum, sphygmomanometer, light, tape measure, fetal Doppler, gloves, lubricant, slides).	
2. Explain procedure to client.	
3. Ask client to put on a gown.	
4. Assess vital signs.	
5. Measure weight/height.	
6. Observe behavior.	
7. Inspect skin.	
8. Inspect hair/nails.	
9. Inspect neck.	
10. Inspect mouth/nose/throat.	
11. Inspect, palpate, percuss, and auscultate chest.	

Copyright © 2014. Wolters Kluwer Health | Lippincott Williams & Wilkins. Lab Manual for Health Assessment in Nursing, 5e.

Physical Assessment Guide to Collect Objective Client Data (continued)

Questions	Findings
12. Inspect and palpate breasts.	
13. Auscultate heart.	
14. Inspect and palpate abdomen.	
15. Measure fundal height.	
16. Assess fetal position.	
17. Auscultate fetal heart tones.	
18. Inspect external genitalia.	
19. Palpate Bartholin and Skene glands.	
20. Inspect vaginal opening.	
21. Perform speculum examination.	
22. Obtain specimens.	
23. Perform pelvic examination.	
24. Inspect anus/rectum.	
25. Auscultate blood pressure.	
26. Inspect face and extremities.	
27. Percuss deep tendon reflexes.	
28. Determine pelvic adequacy.	
29. Determine height/inclination of symphysis pubis.	
30. Palpate lateral walls of pelvis.	
31. Palpate ischial spines.	
32. Palpate sacrum/coccyx.	
33. Measure diagonal conjugate.	
34. Calculate obstetric conjugate.	
35. Measure transverse diameter of the pelvic outlet.	
36. Assess for complaints of common neurologic discomforts during pregnancy.	
37. Formulate nursing diagnoses (wellness, risk, actual).	
38. Formulate collaborative problems.	
39. Make necessary referrals.	
Analysis of Data	
1. Formulate nursing diagnoses (wellness, risk, actual).	
2. Formulate collaborative problems.	
3. Make necessary referrals.	

Copyright © 2014. Wolters Kluwer Health | Lippincott Williams & Wilkins. Lab Manual for Health Assessment in Nursing, 5e.

CHAPTER POSTEST

Activity E MULTIPLE CHOICE QUESTIONS

Choose the one best answer for each of the following multiple choice questions.

____ 1. A pregnant client who is at approximately 36 weeks' gestation tells the nurse that she experiences dizziness while in bed. The nurse should instruct the client to avoid which position?

   a. side-lying.
   b. left lateral.
   c. prone.
   d. supine.

____ 2. A client who is of normal weight just learned that she is 10 weeks pregnant. The client asks the nurse about weight gain during pregnancy. The nurse should instruct the client that the recommended weight gain is

   a. 15 to 20 pounds.
   b. 20 to 25 pounds.
   c. 25 to 35 pounds.
   d. 35 to 45 pounds.

____ 3. A pregnant client at 12 weeks' gestation visits the clinic and tells the nurse that she has been vomiting severely for the past 5 days. The nurse should refer the client to a physician for possible

   a. hyperemesis gravidarum.
   b. viral infection.
   c. fetal anomalies.
   d. peptic ulcer.

____ 4. A pregnant client visits the clinic for the first time. She tells the nurse that she has had two spontaneous abortions before this pregnancy. The nurse should refer the client to a physician for possible

   a. incompetent cervix.
   b. substance abuse.
   c. Rh incompatibility.
   d. hyperthyroidism.

____ 5. A pregnant client visits the clinic for the first time. The client tells the nurse that this is her first pregnancy and that she and her husband are Ashkenazi Jews and immigrated to the United States from Israel. The nurse should encourage the client to be tested for

   a. sickle cell anemia.
   b. cystic fibrosis.
   c. cerebral palsy.
   d. Tay-Sachs disease.

____ 6. A pregnant client near term is admitted to the hospital with scant vaginal bleeding, mild contractions, very firm uterus, and pain on palpation of uterus. The client tells the nurse that she uses cocaine occasionally. The nurse should assess the client for signs and symptoms of

   a. oligohydramnios.
   b. polyhydramnios.
   c. placenta previa.
   d. abruptio placentae.

____ 7. A pregnant client visits the clinic for the first time. The nurse should explain to the client that she will have initial routine blood tests, which include testing for

   a. α-fetoprotein levels.
   b. chromosomal anomalies.
   c. cystic fibrosis.
   d. Rh status.

____ 8. A pregnant client visits the clinic at 36 weeks' gestation. The nurse weighs the client and determines that the client has gained 5 pounds in 1 week. The nurse should assess the client's

    a. dietary patterns.

    b. edema of the lower extremities.

    c. urinary patterns.

    d. blood pressure.

____ 9. The nurse is planning to perform Leopold maneuvers on a pregnant client. To perform the first maneuver, the nurse should place his or her hands on the

    a. upper quadrant of the maternal abdomen.

    b. lateral sides of the maternal abdomen.

    c. presenting part.

    d. top of the symphysis pubis.

____ 10. While caring for a pregnant client at 8 weeks' gestation, the client asks the nurse, "When can you hear the baby's heartbeat?" The nurse should instruct the client that when a Doppler device is used, the earliest time when the fetal heart rate can be heard is the gestational age of

    a. 10 weeks.

    b. 14 weeks.

    c. 18 weeks.

    d. 22 weeks.

____ 11. While assessing a pregnant client, the nurse detects fetal heart rate decelerations that occur after a contraction. The nurse should notify the client's physician because this may be indicative of

    a. fetal demise.

    b. cardiac disease.

    c. head compression.

    d. poor placental perfusion.

____ 12. The nurse is preparing to assess the fetal heart rate of a pregnant client near term. When the nurse hears the fetal heart rate above the maternal umbilicus, the fetus is most likely in which position?

    a. transverse.

    b. breech.

    c. vertex.

    d. face.

____ 13. A pregnant client visits the clinic and complains of a thick purulent vaginal discharge. The nurse should obtain a specimen of the vaginal discharge because this type of discharge is usually indicative of

    a. gonorrhea.

    b. bacterial vaginosis.

    c. *Candida albicans* infection.

    d. chlamydial infection.

____ 14. While assessing a pregnant client at 36 weeks' gestation, the nurse observes that the client's face is edematous and she has 3+ reflexes with mild clonus. The nurse should refer the client to a physician for possible

    a. hydatidiform mole.

    b. multiple gestation.

    c. pregnancy-induced hypertension.

    d. hyperthyroidism.

Copyright © 2014. Wolters Kluwer Health | Lippincott Williams & Wilkins. Lab Manual for Health Assessment in Nursing, 5e.

___ **15.** The nurse is caring for a pregnant client at 14 weeks' gestation and determines that the measurement between the client's ischial tuberosities is 10.5 cm. The nurse should

   a. instruct the client that a vaginal delivery is likely.

   b. refer the client to a physician for small pelvic size.

   c. measure the pubic arch to validate the measurement.

   d. estimate the size of the fetus.

Activity F CASE STUDY

1. Read the following case study. Then, work through the steps of analyzing the case study data. First, identify abnormal data and strengths in **subjective and objective findings**, assemble **cue clusters**, draw **inferences**, make possible **nursing diagnoses**, identify **defining characteristics**, **confirm or rule out** the diagnoses, and **document** your conclusions. Use the blank diagnostic analysis charts provided at the end of this book (also available on thePoint website) to guide your thinking. Propose nursing diagnoses that are specific to the client in the case study. Identify collaborative problems, if any, for this client. Finally, identify data, if any, that point toward a medical problem requiring a referral.

Kaitlin presents to your office today, thinking that she may be pregnant. Kaitlin is a 20-year-old primigravida, who remembers her LMP as having been November 13, 2013, which would make her at approximately 20 weeks' gestation. She states that she did have some irregular spotting in December for approximately 2 days.

Kaitlin's medical and surgical history is unremarkable. Her family history is also noncontributory. Her social history is negative for alcohol and drugs. She is single and lives at home with her parents while attending college. The father of the baby is involved but is unsure about his feelings regarding the pregnancy. This pregnancy was not planned, and he wants to finish college and develop his career. Marriage plans are not in the father's schedule at this time.

How Well Did You Do?

After you have read the chapter and completed the exercises in this chapter, visit thePoint to access the Self-Reflection Activity. This activity will help you identify to what degree you have met each of the chapter objectives. You can then review the chapter for objectives you have met partially or not at all.

Other tools to help you, like the Diagnostic Reasoning Guides, Nursing Interview Guides, Physical Assessment Guides, and NCLEX-Style Chapter Review Questions, are also available on thePoint.

Copyright © 2014. Wolters Kluwer Health | Lippincott Williams & Wilkins. Lab Manual for Health Assessment in Nursing, 5e.

Assessing Newborns and Infants

Chapter Overview

During the first year of life, the newborn undergoes rapid physical and mental growth and development. Routine preventive health care is important for the early detection of medical disorders/abnormalities and intervention that may grossly affect proper growth and development of the newborn.

Chapter Learning Objectives

1. Evaluate the growth and development patterns of infants.
2. Describe the components needed to assess general appearance, and differentiate between norms and variations of normal and abnormal general appearances.
3. Demonstrate proper method for assessing vital signs and temperature in newborns and infants. Discuss the normal ranges for each measurement.
4. Explain the technique used to measure head circumference and why it is measured.
5. Explain how skin, hair, and nails are assessed in newborns and infants, and discuss possible norms, variations, and abnormalities that may be noted.
6. Explain how head, neck, and cervical lymph nodes are assessed in newborns and infants, and discuss possible norms, variations, and abnormalities that may be noted.
7. Explain how eyes are assessed in newborns and infants, and discuss possible norms, variations, and abnormalities that may be noted.
8. Explain how ears are assessed in newborns and infants, and discuss possible norms, variations, and abnormalities that may be noted.
9. Explain how mouth, throat, nose, and sinuses are assessed in newborns and infants, and discuss possible norms, variations, and abnormalities that may be noted.
10. Explain how thorax is assessed in newborns and infants, and discuss possible norms, variations, and abnormalities that may be noted.
11. Explain how breasts are assessed in newborns and infants, and discuss possible norms, variations, and abnormalities that may be noted.
12. Explain how heart is assessed in newborns and infants, and discuss possible norms, variations, and abnormalities that may be noted.
13. Explain how abdomen is assessed in newborns and infants, and discuss possible norms, variations, and abnormalities that may be noted.
14. Explain how male and female genitalia are assessed in newborns and infants, and discuss possible norms, variations, and abnormalities that may be noted.
15. Explain how the anus and rectum are assessed in newborns and infants, and discuss possible norms, variations, and abnormalities that may be noted.
16. Explain how to assess the musculoskeletal system in newborns and infants, and discuss possible variations.

17. Explain how to assess the neurologic system in newborns and infants, and discuss possible variations.
18. Explain the common infantile reflexes.
19. Explain how to document and interpret assessment findings.
20. Discuss various nursing diagnoses and collaborative problems commonly seen with assessment of infants and children.
21. Analyze data from the client interview and physical assessment of a newborn to formulate valid nursing diagnoses, collaborative problems, and/or referrals.

CHAPTER PRETEST

Activity A MULTIPLE CHOICE QUESTIONS

Choose the one best answer for each of the following multiple choice questions.

____ 1. The anterior fontanelle of a neonate closes between
    a. 2 and 3 months.
    b. 4 and 6 months.
    c. 7 and 11 months.
    d. 12 and 18 months.

____ 2. The nurse is planning to instruct a first time mother about her newborn. The nurse should plan to instruct the mother that the newborn
    a. is an obligatory nose breather.
    b. will have deciduous teeth by 3 months.
    c. who drools is preparing for tooth eruption.
    d. will develop permanent teeth in the jaw by 6 years of age.

____ 3. Normal breathing pattern for a full-term infant may include
    a. abdominal breathing with a rate of 80 to 100 breaths/minute.
    b. chest breathing with nasal flaring of 20 to 40 breaths/minute.
    c. shallow and irregular breathing with a rate of 80 to 100 breaths/minute.
    d. abdominal/chest breathing movements at a rate of 30 to 60 breaths/minute.

____ 4. The Moro reflex is
    a. a response to sudden stimulation or an abrupt change in position.
    b. fanning of the toes.
    c. stepping of the feet.
    d. extension of one arm and leg when turning the head.

Activity B LEARNER ACTIVITIES

Working with peers in the learning lab, discuss the following scenario:

A 4-month-old is brought in for well-child care. The mother asks, "What is my baby going to have done today?" What would you include in your reply.

Copyright © 2014. Wolters Kluwer Health | Lippincott Williams & Wilkins. Lab Manual for Health Assessment in Nursing, 5e.

Activity C INTERVIEWING AND RECORDING ASSESSMENT FINDINGS

After reading Chapter 30 in the textbook, use the following Nursing Interview Guide to interview and record your subjective findings for a pediatric assessment. Your instructor may ask you to turn this in to be evaluated. Forms are also available on thePoint *website.*

Nursing Interview Guide to Collect Subjective Data From the Client

Questions	Findings
Current Symptoms	
1. Parent's (informant's) reason for seeking health care for the newborn or infant?	
Current Health/Illness Status	
1. Symptom analysis of chief complaint?	
2. Other current or recurrent illnesses or problems?	
3. Any other health concerns?	
4. Current medication used?	
Past History	
1. Birth history (pregnancy, labor and delivery, perinatal history)?	
2. Previous illnesses, injuries, or surgeries?	
3. Allergies (and reactions to same)?	
4. Immunization status?	
5. Growth and developmental milestones?	
6. Habits?	
Review of Systems	
1. General: overall health status?	
2. Integument: lesions, bruising, care habits?	
3. Head: trauma?	
4. Eyes: visual acuity, last eye exam, drainage, infections?	
5. Ears: hearing acuity, last hearing exam, drainage, infections?	
6. Nose: bleeding, congestion, discharge?	
7. Mouth: lesions, tooth eruption, last dental exam?	
8. Throat: hoarseness, difficulty swallowing?	
9. Neck: limited range of motion?	
10. Chest: cough, wheezing, shortness of breath, asthma, infections?	
11. Breasts: lesions, discharge, swelling?	
12. Cardiovascular: history of murmurs, congenital defects?	
13. Gastrointestinal: change in appetite, bowel habits, food intolerances, nausea, vomiting, history of parasites?	
14. Genitourinary: discharge, urinary tract infections?	

Nursing Interview Guide to Collect Subjective Data From the Client (continued)

Questions	Findings
15. Musculoskeletal: pain, swelling, fractures, mobility problems, scoliosis?	
16. Neurologic: ataxia, tremors, unusual movements, seizures?	
17. Lymphatic: pain, swelling or tenderness, enlargement of spleen or liver?	
18. Endocrine/metabolic: growth patterns, polyuria, polydipsia, polyphagia?	
19. Psychiatric history: any psychiatric, developmental, substance abuse, or eating disorder?	
Family History	
1. Family genetic traits or diseases with familial tendencies?	
2. Communicable diseases?	
3. Psychiatric disorders?	
4. Substance abuse?	
Nutritional History	
1. Quantity and the types of food or formula ingested daily (use 24-hour recall, food diary for 3 days [2 weekdays and 1 weekend day], or food frequency record)?	
2. Newborn or infant has any problem with feeding?	
Sleep History	
1. Sleep patterns of newborn or infant?	
Developmental Assessment	
1. Reflexes?	
2. Denver Developmental Screening Test results?	

Activity D   PERFORMING PHYSICAL ASSESSMENT OF NEWBORNS AND INFANTS

Use the following Physical Assessment Guide to perform a pediatric assessment examination. Column 1 will serve as a reminder as to what part of the exam you will do next. Column 2 will be used to record your findings. Your instructor may ask you to turn this in to be evaluated. Forms are also available on thePoint *website.*

Physical Assessment Guide to Collect Objective Client Data

Questions	Findings
1. In most cases, physical assessment involves a head-to-toe examination that covers each body system.	
General Appearance	
1. Inspect physical appearance.	
2. Assess nutritional state.	
3. Assess behavior.	
4. Assess overall development.	

Copyright © 2014. Wolters Kluwer Health | Lippincott Williams & Wilkins. Lab Manual for Health Assessment in Nursing, 5e.

Physical Assessment Guide to Collect Objective Client Data (continued)

Questions	Findings
Vital Signs	
1. Measure blood pressure.	
2. Measure pulse rate.	
3. Measure respirations.	
4. Measure temperature.	
5. Measure height and weight.	
6. Measure head circumference.	
Skin, Hair, and Nails	
1. Inspect and palpate skin.	
2. Inspect and palpate hair (distribution, characteristics).	
3. Inspect and palpate nails (texture, shape, color, condition).	
Head, Neck, and Cervical Lymph Nodes	
1. Inspect and palpate the head (symmetry, condition of fontanelles).	
2. Inspect and palpate the face.	
3. Inspect and palpate the neck (suppleness, lymph nodes for swelling, mobility, temperature, and tenderness).	
Mouth, Throat, Nose, and Sinuses	
1. Inspect mouth and throat (tooth eruption, condition of gums, lips, teeth, palpates, tonsils, tongue, buccal mucosa).	
2. Inspect nose and sinuses (discharge, tenderness, turbinates [color, swelling]).	
Eyes	
1. Inspect external eye.	
2. Perform visual acuity tests.	
3. Perform extraocular muscle tests.	
4. Perform internal (ophthalmoscopic) examination.	
Ears	
1. Inspect external ears.	
2. Perform otoscopic examination.	
3. Assess hearing acuity.	
Thorax and Lungs	
1. Inspect shape of thorax and respiratory effort.	
2. Percuss the lungs.	
3. Auscultate for breath sounds and adventitious sounds.	

Copyright © 2014. Wolters Kluwer Health | Lippincott Williams & Wilkins. Lab Manual for Health Assessment in Nursing, 5e.

Physical Assessment Guide to Collect Objective Client Data (continued)

Questions	Findings
Breasts	
1. Inspect and palpate breasts (shape, discharge, lesions).	
Heart	
1. Inspect and palpate the precordium.	
2. Auscultate heart sounds.	
Abdomen	
1. Inspect shape.	
2. Inspect umbilicus.	
3. Auscultate bowel sounds.	
4. Palpate softness.	
5. Palpate for masses and tenderness.	
6. Palpate liver.	
7. Palpate spleen.	
8. Palpate kidneys.	
9. Palpate bladder.	
Male Genitalia	
1. Inspect penis and urinary meatus.	
2. Inspect and palpate scrotum and testes.	
3. Inspect and palpate inguinal area for hernias.	
Female Genitalia	
1. Inspect external genitalia.	
2. Inspect internal genitalia.	
Anus and Rectum	
1. Inspect anus.	
2. Palpate rectum.	
Musculoskeletal	
1. Assess feet and legs.	
2. Assess for congenital hip dysplasia.	
3. Assess spine and posture.	
4. Assess gait.	
5. Assess joints.	
6. Assess muscles.	
Neurologic	
1. Perform newborn assessment.	
2. Test cranial nerve function.	
3. Test deep tendon and superficial reflexes.	
4. Test sensory function.	

Copyright © 2014. Wolters Kluwer Health | Lippincott Williams & Wilkins. Lab Manual for Health Assessment in Nursing, 5e.

Physical Assessment Guide to Collect Objective Client Data (continued)	
Questions	**Findings**
5. Test motor function and infantile reflexes.	
6. Observe for "soft" signs.	
Analysis of Data	
1. Formulate nursing diagnoses (wellness, risk, actual).	
2. Formulate collaborative problems.	
3. Make necessary referrals.	

CHAPTER POSTTEST

Activity E   MULTIPLE CHOICE QUESTIONS

Choose the one best answer for each of the following multiple choice questions.

_____ 1. While assessing a young infant's musculoskeletal system, the nurse anticipates that the anterior curve in the cervical region will be developed by

     a. 1 to 2 months.

     b. 3 to 4 months.

     c. 6 to 8 months.

     d. 9 to 12 months.

_____ 2. The nurse is assessing a 1-year-old infant who weighed 3.6 kg (8 lb) at birth. When the nurse prepares to weigh the infant, the nurse anticipates that this infant should weigh approximately

     a. 7.2 kg (16 lb).

     b. 9.07 kg (20 lb).

     c. 10.8 kg (24 lb).

     d. 12.7 kg (28 lb).

_____ 3. A mother visits the clinic with her 2-month-old son for a routine visit. The mother has been bottle feeding the infant and asks the nurse, "When can I start giving him solid foods?" The nurse should instruct the mother that solid foods can be introduced when the infant is

     a. 2 to 4 months old.

     b. 4 to 6 months old.

     c. 6 to 8 months old.

     d. 8 to 10 months old.

_____ 4. The nurse is assessing a newborn with the mother present. When the nurse observes an irregularly shaped red patch on the back of the newborn's neck, the nurse should explain to the mother that this is termed

     a. port wine stain.

     b. hemangioma.

     c. cafe au lait spot.

     d. stork bite.

_____ 5. While assessing a newborn infant, the nurse observes yellow–white retention cysts in the newborn's mouth. The nurse should explain to the infant's parents that these spots are usually indicative of

     a. Epstein pearls.

     b. thrush.

     c. allergic reactions.

     d. dehydration.

___ **6.** The nurse is preparing to inspect a newborn's inner ear with an otoscope. The nurse should pull the pinna

   a. down and back.

   b. up and back.

   c. down and forward.

   d. sideways and forward.

Activity F CRITICAL THINKING ACTIVITY

Carsen is a 2-week-old infant brought into the clinic today for a weight check and his regular 2-week visit. His mother, a 22-year-old gravida 1, is concerned that he is not eating well. She started out breastfeeding him but had difficulty and stopped breastfeeding 2 days ago. She is not sure how much formula he should be taking now. She is here for his physical exam and to learn how to determine if he is getting the proper nutrition he needs.

   What questions would you ask Carsen's mother about her experience with breastfeeding? Based on the data provided and the further data from your questions, what cue clusters would you identify? What nursing diagnoses would you formulate for this mother and baby?

Activity G CASE STUDY

Read the following case study. Then, work through the steps of analyzing the case study data. First identify the abnormal data and strengths in **subjective and objective findings**, assemble **cue clusters**, draw **inferences**, make possible **nursing diagnoses**, identify **defining characteristics, confirm or rule out** the diagnoses, and **document** your conclusions. Use the blank diagnostic analysis charts provided at the end of this book (also available on thePoint website) to guide your thinking. Propose nursing diagnoses that are specific to the client in the case study. Identify collaborative problems, if any, for this client. Finally, identify data, if any, that point toward a medical problem requiring a referral.

Kaylee, an 18-month-old, returns to the operating room 4 days post-op for cauterization of posttonsillectomy bleed. Vital signs upon returning to the pediatric floor after surgery are weight 11.83 kg, BP 109/71 mm Hg, apical heart rate 144 beats/minute, respiratory rate 28 breaths/minute, temperature 37.4 °C (99.4 °F) axillary, and pulse ox 96% room air. An IV is in place with an initial D5LR 200 cc bolus followed by D5.225% NS at 60 cc/hour. Initial lab results indicate moderate dehydration and moderate anemia. Physical exam reveals pale skin tones, tacky mucous membranes, with no active tonsillectomy bleeding. Tylenol with Codeine 3/4 teaspoon is ordered q4h prn pain. Kaylee remains on the floor for 4 subsequent days—continuing to refuse PO fluids even with regular administration of analgesic. Two days after admission, a trial of locking IV fluids is initiated with plan to discharge if Kaylee tolerates PO fluids through supper. If unable to tolerate PO, restart IV fluids at 50 cc/hour. This trial fails this day and the following day has a total PO intake of sips and urine output of 141 cc for the 24-hour period. A repeat IV bolus is given and the same course of action is taken the next day. Again, this trial fails and IV fluids are re-initiated. Several days after returning to the OR for cauterization, Kaylee still refused to drink anything at all. Kaylee's behavior consisted of continually holding a blue blanket and watching the door, crying "Bubby … Bubby" repeatedly. After having much interaction with Kaylee and her family, and assessing the situation, the nurse realized that Kaylee was missing her twin brother so much that it was affecting everything she could see or do. Apparently, these siblings had never been separated. The brother's visitation had been restricted by the other shifts—because of his age—he was well below the required 6 years of age to visit on the pediatric floor. Two evenings in a row, the nurse allowed the parents to bring him into the room to visit with the understanding that he was not allowed in the hallway, but would always remain in the room. During both of these visits, Kaylee began to drink normally during a "pretend picnic" on the floor with her brother. She was discharged home on the fourth post-op day of hospitalization with optimal PO intake.

How Well Did You Do?

After you have read the chapter and completed the exercises in this chapter, visit thePoint to access the Self-Reflection Activity. This activity will help you identify to what degree you have met each of the chapter objectives. You can then review the chapter for objectives you have met partially or not at all.

   Other tools to help you, like the Diagnostic Reasoning Guides, Nursing Interview Guides, Physical Assessment Guides, and NCLEX-Style Chapter Review Questions, are also available on thePoint.

Copyright © 2014. Wolters Kluwer Health | Lippincott Williams & Wilkins. Lab Manual for Health Assessment in Nursing, 5e.

Assessing Children and Adolescents

Chapter Overview

The special data collected during the nursing assessment of children and adolescents play a key role in supporting the health of these growing young people. The nurse should be aware of the differences between a child/adolescent and an adult and incorporate the special needs of both the pediatric client and his or her parent into the assessment.

Chapter Learning Objectives

1. Briefly describe how children differ in structure and function from adults, and discuss how these differences affect physical assessment.
2. Differentiate the interviewing techniques used for parents, toddlers, preschoolers, school-agers, and adolescents.
3. Explain how play techniques can be used for distraction purposes during assessment.
4. Explain the components of the pediatric history.
5. Evaluate the growth and development patterns of toddlers.
6. Evaluate the growth and development patterns of preschoolers.
7. Evaluate the growth and development patterns of school-aged children.
8. Evaluate the growth and development patterns of adolescents.
9. Describe the components needed in the assessment of the general appearance, and differentiate between norms and variations of normal and abnormal general appearances.
10. Demonstrate the proper method for assessing vital signs and temperature in children and adolescents. Discuss the normal ranges for each measurement for children and adolescents.
11. Explain the technique used to measure head circumference in toddlers younger than 2 years.
12. Explain how skin, hair, and nails are assessed in children and adolescents, and discuss the possible norms, variations, and abnormalities that may be noted.
13. Explain how head, neck, and cervical lymph nodes are assessed in children and adolescents, and discuss the possible norms, variations, and abnormalities that may be noted.
14. Explain how eyes are assessed in children and adolescents, and discuss the possible norms, variations, and abnormalities that may be noted.
15. Explain how ears are assessed in children and adolescents, and discuss the possible norms, variations, and abnormalities that may be noted.
16. Explain how thorax and lungs are assessed in children and adolescents, and discuss the possible norms, variations, and abnormalities that may be noted.
17. Explain how heart is assessed in children and adolescents, and discuss the possible norms, variations, and abnormalities that may be noted.

18. Explain how breasts are assessed in children and adolescents, and discuss the possible norms, variations, and abnormalities that may be noted. Explain the Tanner stages of female breast development and the method of teaching breast self-examination to adolescents.

19. Explain how the abdomen is assessed in children and adolescents, and discuss the possible norms, variations, and abnormalities that may be noted.

20. Explain how male genitalia are assessed in children and adolescents, and discuss the possible norms, variations, and abnormalities that may be noted. Explain the Tanner stages of male pubic hair and genital development and the method of teaching testicular self-examination to male adolescents.

21. Explain how female genitalia are assessed in children and adolescents, and discuss the possible norms, variations, and abnormalities that may be noted. Explain the Tanner stages of female pubic hair development.

22. Explain how the anus and rectum are assessed in children and adolescents, and discuss the possible norms, variations, and abnormalities that may be noted.

23. Explain how to assess the musculoskeletal system in children and adolescents, and discuss the possible norms, variations, and abnormalities that may be noted.

24. Explain how to assess the neurologic system in children and adolescents, and discuss the possible norms, variations, and abnormalities that may be noted.

25. Explain how to document and interpret assessment findings.

26. Discuss the various nursing diagnoses and collaborative problems commonly seen with assessment of children and adolescents.

27. Analyze data from the client interview and physical assessment of a child or adolescent to formulate valid nursing diagnoses, collaborative problems, and/or referrals.

CHAPTER PRETEST

Activity A MULTIPLE CHOICE QUESTIONS

Choose the one best answer for each of the following multiple choice questions.

_____ 1. While assessing the skin, hair, and nails of a 4-year-old boy, the nurse can anticipate that the child will have

   a. functioning apocrine glands.

   b. a thin layer of subcutaneous fat.

   c. fine, downy hairs on his body.

   d. smooth-textured skin.

_____ 2. The nurse is planning a presentation on childhood growth and development to a group of new parents. Which of the following should the nurse include in the teaching plan?

   a. A child's head reaches 90% of its full growth by 6 years of age.

   b. Half of a child's postnatal brain growth is achieved by 3 years of age.

   c. During the school-aged years, the cranium grows faster than the face.

   d. Lymphoid tissue reaches adult size by 4 years of age.

_____ 3. The nurse is preparing to assess the heart sounds in a 3-year-old child. To locate the apical impulse, the nurse should plan to place the stethoscope at the child's

   a. second intercostal space.

   b. third intercostal space.

   c. fourth intercostal space.

   d. fifth intercostal space.

Copyright © 2014. Wolters Kluwer Health | Lippincott Williams & Wilkins. Lab Manual for Health Assessment in Nursing, 5e.

Activity B　MATCHING

Match the following descriptions with the appropriate age group.

Description	Age Group
____　1. Engages in parallel play	**a.** Toddlers
____　2. Likes explanations and demonstrations in health teaching	**b.** Preschoolers
____　3. Peak age group for separation anxiety	**c.** School-agers
____　4. Confidentiality a must	**d.** Adolescents
____　5. Gains 6.8 to 29.4 kg (15 to 65 lb) during this stage	
____　6. Girls surpass boys in growth during this period	
____　7. Visual capacity reaches adult level of 20/20	
____　8. Sensorimotor stage is completed in this period	
____　9. Ability to listen and comprehend starts during this stage	
____　10. Vocabulary ranges from 900 to 2,100 words	
____　11. Develops ability to think beyond the present	
____　12. Has ability to decide between two socially accepted standards	
____　13. The age of "magical thinking"	
____　14. Learns rules and competition	
____　15. Develops lifelong eating patterns	

Activity C　LEARNER ACTIVITIES

After reading Chapter 31 in the textbook, participate in the following learning activities.

1. Describe how you would perform the following.
   a. An otoscopic examination on a feisty 2-year-old
   b. The patellar reflex on a 4-year-old who kicks before you strike
   c. Abdominal palpation on a ticklish 9-year-old
   d. The psychosocial history of a 16-year-old

2. Discuss with a lab partner how you would handle the following situations.
   a. While performing an assessment of a 15-year-old girl, you note that she is quiet and withdrawn. She complains of multiple vague physical complaints and gives you her favorite watch, stating, "I know you'll take real good care of this." Discuss what you would do next.
   b. You are going to give a 30-minute talk to a PTA group on the health needs of school-aged children. Considering that you are addressing a group whose children's ages range from 6 to 12 years, discuss what you would include in your talk.

Copyright © 2014. Wolters Kluwer Health | Lippincott Williams & Wilkins. Lab Manual for Health Assessment in Nursing, 5e.

Activity D INTERVIEWING AND RECORDING ASSESSMENT FINDINGS

After reading Chapter 31, use the following Nursing Interview Guide to interview and record your subjective findings for the assessment of a child or adolescent. Your instructor may ask you to turn this in to be evaluated. Forms are also available on thePoint website.

Nursing Interview Guide to Collect Subjective Data From the Client

Questions	Findings
Current Symptoms	
1. Child's reason for seeking health care or the parent's (informant's) reason for seeking health care for the child?	
Current Health/Illness Status	
1. Symptom analysis of chief complaint?	
2. Other current or recurrent illnesses or problems?	
3. Any other health concerns?	
4. Current medication used?	
Past History	
1. Birth history (pregnancy, labor and delivery, perinatal history)?	
2. Previous illnesses, injuries, or surgeries?	
3. Allergies (and reactions to same)?	
4. Immunization status?	
5. Growth and developmental milestones?	
6. Habits?	
Review of Systems	
1. General: overall health status?	
2. Integument: lesions, bruising, care habits?	
3. Head: trauma, headaches?	
4. Eyes: visual acuity, last eye exam, drainage, infections?	
5. Ears: hearing acuity, last hearing exam, drainage, infections?	
6. Nose: bleeding, congestion, discharge?	
7. Mouth: lesions, soreness, tooth eruption, patterns of dental care, last dental exam?	
8. Throat: sore throat frequency, hoarseness, difficulty swallowing?	
9. Neck: stiffness, tenderness?	
10. Chest: pain, cough, wheezing, shortness of breath, asthma, infections?	
11. Breasts: thelarche, lesions, discharge, performance of breast self-examination (BSE)?	
12. Cardiovascular: history of murmurs, exercise tolerance, dizziness, palpitations, congenital defects?	

Nursing Interview Guide to Collect Subjective Data From the Client (continued)

Questions	Findings
13. Gastrointestinal: appetite, bowel habits, food intolerances, nausea, vomiting, pain, history of parasites?	
14. Genitourinary: urgency, frequency, discharge, urinary tract infections, sexually transmitted diseases, enuresis, sexual problems or dysfunctions (male), performance of testicular self-examination?	
15. Gynecologic: menarche, menstrual history, sexual problems or dysfunctions?	
16. Musculoskeletal: pain, swelling, fractures, mobility problems, scoliosis?	
17. Neurologic: ataxia, tremors, unusual movements, seizures?	
18. Lymphatic: pain, swelling or tenderness, enlargement of spleen or liver?	
19. Endocrine/metabolic: growth patterns, polyuria, polydypsia, polyphagia?	
20. Psychiatric history: any psychiatric, developmental, substance abuse, or eating disorder?	
Family History	
1. Family genetic traits or diseases with familial tendencies?	
2. Communicable diseases?	
3. Psychiatric disorders?	
4. Substance abuse?	
Nutritional History	
1. Determine the quantity and the types of food or formula ingested daily: use 24-hour recall, food diary for 3 days (2 weekdays and 1 weekend day), or food frequency record.	
2. Ask if child has any problem with feeding.	
3. Ask if child uses any vitamin supplements.	
4. Ask if child is on special diet.	
5. Ask if there are any cultural or religious preferences.	
6. Assess dieting behaviors: include body image, types of diets, frequency of weighing, and use of self-induced vomiting, laxatives, and diuretics.	
Sleep History	
1. Time child goes to bed and awakens?	
2. Quality of sleep?	
3. Nap history?	
4. Sleep aids (blanket, toy)?	

Copyright © 2014. Wolters Kluwer Health | Lippincott Williams & Wilkins. Lab Manual for Health Assessment in Nursing, 5e.

Nursing Interview Guide to Collect Subjective Data From the Client (continued)

Questions	Findings
Psychosocial History	
1. Home: composition of family members, occupation/ education of members, culture and religion, communication patterns, family roles and relationships, financial status?	
2. School: grades, behavior, relationship with teachers and peers?	
3. Activities: types of play, number of hours of TV viewing per day, amount of nonschool-related reading, hobbies?	
4. Discipline: type and frequency used at home?	
5. Sex: child's/adolescent's concerns, abuse history, sexual activity patterns, number of partners, use of condoms and contraceptives, AIDS awareness?	
6. Substance use: amount, frequency, and circumstances of use for tobacco, alcohol, licit and illicit drugs, steroids, and substances such as inhalants?	
7. Violence: domestic violence, self-abusive behaviors, suicide ideation and attempts, violence perpetrated on others by child/adolescent being interviewed?	
Developmental Assessment	
1. Assess developmental milestones in a. gross motor skills. b. fine motor skills. c. language development. d. cognitive development. e. social and affective development.	
2. Observe the child's behavior before structured interaction for spontaneous activity; observe the child's responses to the environment.	
3. Administer developmental tests as appropriate for age (Denver Developmental Screening Test, Brazelton Neonatal Behavior Assessment Scale, Goodenough-Harris Draw-A-Person Test, temperament questionnaires).	

Activity E PERFORMING PHYSICAL ASSESSMENT OF A CHILD OR ADOLESCENT

Use the following Physical Assessment Guide for the assessment of a child or adolescent. Column 1 will serve as a reminder as to what part of the exam you will do next. Column 2 will be used to record your findings. Your instructor may ask you to turn this in to be evaluated. Forms are also available on thePoint website.

Physical Assessment Guide to Collect Objective Client Data

Questions	Findings

1. Uses general principles:
  a. In most cases, physical assessment involves a head-to-toe examination that covers each body system.
  b. Complete less threatening and least intrusive procedures first, to secure child's trust.
  c. Explain what you will be doing and what the child can expect to feel; allow the child to manipulate equipment before it is used.	

2. Uses developmental approaches:
  a. Toddlers: Allow to sit on parent's lap, enlist parent's aid, use play, praise cooperation.
  b. Preschoolers: Use story telling, use doll and puppet play, give choices when able.
  c. School-age: Maintain privacy, use gown, explain procedures and equipment, teach about their bodies.
  d. Adolescents: Provide privacy and confidentiality, provide option of having parent present or not, emphasize normality, provide health teaching.	

General Appearance	
1. Inspect physical appearance.	
2. Assess nutritional state.	
3. Assess hygiene.	
4. Assess behavior.	
5. Assess interactions with parents and nurse.	
6. Assess overall development and speech.	
Vital Signs	
1. Measure blood pressure.	
2. Measure pulse rate.	
3. Measure respirations.	
4. Measure temperature.	
5. Measure height and weight.	
Skin, Hair, and Nails	
1. Inspect and palpate skin.	
2. Inspect and palpate hair (distribution, characteristics).	
3. Inspect and palpate nails (texture, shape, color, condition).	

Copyright © 2014. Wolters Kluwer Health | Lippincott Williams & Wilkins. Lab Manual for Health Assessment in Nursing, 5e.

Physical Assessment Guide to Collect Objective Client Data (continued)

Questions	Findings
Head, Neck, and Cervical Lymph Nodes	
1. Inspect and palpate the head (symmetry, condition of fontanelles).	
2. Inspect and palpate the face.	
3. Inspect and palpate the neck (suppleness, lymph nodes for swelling, mobility, temperature, and tenderness).	
Mouth, Throat, Nose, and Sinuses	
1. Inspect mouth and throat (tooth eruption, condition of gums, lips, teeth, palpates, tonsils, tongue, buccal mucosa).	
2. Inspect nose and sinuses (discharge, tenderness, turbinates [color, swelling]).	
Eyes	
1. Inspect external eye.	
2. Perform visual acuity tests.	
3. Perform extraocular muscle tests.	
4. Perform internal (ophthalmoscopic) examination.	
Ears	
1. Inspect external ears.	
2. Perform internal (otoscopic) examination.	
3. Assess hearing acuity.	
Thorax and Lungs	
1. Inspect shape of thorax and respiratory effort.	
2. Percuss the lungs.	
3. Auscultate for breath sounds and adventitious sounds.	
Breasts	
1. Inspect and palpate breasts (shape, discharge, lesions).	
2. Assess stage of sexual development (for girls).	
Heart	
1. Inspect and palpate the precordium.	
2. Auscultate heart sounds.	
Abdomen	
1. Inspect shape.	
2. Inspect umbilicus.	
3. Auscultate bowel sounds.	
4. Palpate softness.	
5. Palpate for masses and tenderness.	
6. Palpate liver.	

Copyright © 2014. Wolters Kluwer Health | Lippincott Williams & Wilkins. Lab Manual for Health Assessment in Nursing, 5e.

Physical Assessment Guide to Collect Objective Client Data (continued)

Questions	Findings
7. Palpate spleen.	
8. Palpate kidneys.	
9. Palpate bladder.	
Male Genitalia	
1. Inspect penis and urinary meatus.	
2. Inspect and palpate scrotum and testes.	
3. Inspect and palpate inguinal area for hernias.	
4. Assess sexual development.	
Female Genitalia	
1. Inspect external genitalia.	
2. Inspect internal genitalia.	
3. Assess sexual development.	
Anus and Rectum	
1. Inspect anus.	
2. Palpate rectum.	
Musculoskeletal	
1. Assess feet and legs.	
2. Assess for congenital hip dysplasia.	
3. Assess spine and posture.	
4. Assess gait.	
5. Assess joints.	
6. Assess muscles.	
Neurologic	
1. Test cerebral function (language, memory, cognition).	
2. Test cranial nerve function.	
3. Test deep tendon and superficial reflexes.	
4. Test balance and coordination.	
5. Test sensory function.	
6. Test motor function and infantile reflexes.	
7. Observe for "soft" signs.	
Analysis of Data	
1. Formulate nursing diagnoses (wellness, risk, actual).	
2. Formulate collaborative problems.	
3. Make necessary referrals.	

Copyright © 2014. Wolters Kluwer Health | Lippincott Williams & Wilkins. Lab Manual for Health Assessment in Nursing, 5e.

CHAPTER POSTTEST

Activity F MULTIPLE CHOICE QUESTIONS

Choose the one best answer for each of the following multiple choice questions.

____ 1. The nurse is assessing a young adolescent female client using Tanner Sexual Maturity Rating for Breast Development. The nurse determines that the client has enlargement of the breasts and areolae, with no separation of contours. The client is in Tanner Stage

    a. two.

    b. three.

    c. four.

    d. five.

____ 2. A mother brings her 12-year-old son to the clinic for a routine physical. The mother tells the nurse that her son seems to be growing taller recently. The nurse should instruct the mother that the peak growth spurt in boys usually occurs by age

    a. 12 years.

    b. 13 years.

    c. 14 years.

    d. 15 years.

____ 3. A parent visits the clinic with her 4-year-old child. While communicating with the child, the nurse should

    a. touch the child gently but frequently during the interview.

    b. stand in front of the child so the child can see the nurse.

    c. use standard medical terminology so the child is not confused.

    d. talk to the child in simple terms at the child's eye level.

____ 4. While communicating with an ill 5-year-old child, one of the most valuable communication techniques that the nurse can use is

    a. play.

    b. direct communication.

    c. indirect communication.

    d. closed-ended questions.

____ 5. A mother visits the clinic with her toddler, who has injured himself in a fall. The nurse caring for the toddler should

    a. tell the child it is okay to cry in the clinic.

    b. play a game with the child.

    c. allow the child to identify the nurse with the parent.

    d. use demonstrations when providing health teaching to the child.

____ 6. The nurse is caring for an 11-year-old child who was hospitalized after an auto accident. While communicating with this child, the nurse should

    a. use simple questions.

    b. provide simple explanations.

    c. use peers as examples.

    d. allow the child to engage in the discussions.

____ 7. The nurse is caring for a hospitalized adolescent with sickle cell crisis. While communicating with the client, the nurse should

    a. give the client control whenever possible.

    b. provide simple explanations.

    c. use concrete terminology.

    d. provide concrete answers to questions.

____ **8.** A mother visits the clinic for a routine visit with her 5-year-old son. The mother asks the nurse when the child's permanent teeth will erupt. The nurse should explain to the mother that permanent teeth usually begin to erupt by age

    a. 5½ years.

    b. 6 years.

    c. 6½ years.

    d. 7 years.

____ **9.** A mother visits the clinic for a routine visit with her 11-year-old daughter. The mother tells the nurse that her daughter has just started puberty. The mother asks the nurse when she can expect the daughter to begin menstruation. The nurse should explain to the mother that menstruation usually begins about

    a. 1 year after the onset of puberty.

    b. 18 months after the onset of puberty.

    c. 24 months after the onset of puberty.

    d. 30 months after the onset of puberty.

____ **10.** The nurse is preparing to assess the gross motor development of a 4-year-old child. The nurse should ask the child to

    a. hop on one foot.

    b. skip a rope.

    c. throw a ball.

    d. balance on alternate feet with eyes closed.

____ **11.** The nurse is planning to assess the cognitive development of a 3-year-old child. The nurse plans to assess whether or not the child can

    a. classify complex objects.

    b. quantify objects.

    c. sort objects.

    d. make simple classifications.

____ **12.** A young mother visits the clinic with her 18-month-old child. The mother asks the nurse when she should begin toilet training with the child. The nurse should explain to the mother that

    a. she can begin bowel training as soon as the child appears ready.

    b. bladder training usually begins at 18 months of age.

    c. nighttime bladder control is usually achieved by 3 years of age.

    d. bowel training is usually started when the child is 3 years of age.

____ **13.** While assessing a 4-year-old child, the nurse observes that the child's nails are concave in shape. The nurse should assess the child for a deficiency of

    a. magnesium.

    b. vitamin C.

    c. zinc.

    d. iron.

____ **14.** The nurse is assessing a 4-year-old child with a temperature of 37.7 °C (100 °F). The nurse observes that the client has Koplik spots on his buccal mucosa. The nurse should explain to the client's parents that the child is most likely exhibiting signs of

    a. measles.

    b. mumps.

    c. chickenpox.

    d. tonsillitis.

Copyright © 2014. Wolters Kluwer Health | Lippincott Williams & Wilkins. Lab Manual for Health Assessment in Nursing, 5e.

_____ **15.** The nurse is preparing to assess a 5-year-old child. To perform the Hirschberg test, the nurse should

    a. ask the child to cover one eye.

    b. shine a light directly into the pupils.

    c. use an ophthalmoscope to check the eyes.

    d. ask the child to name various colors.

Activity G CASE STUDY

Read the following case study. Then, work through the steps of analyzing the case study data. First identify abnormal data and strengths in **subjective and objective findings**, assemble **cue clusters**, draw **inferences**, make possible **nursing diagnoses**, identify **defining characteristics**, **confirm or rule out** the diagnoses, and **document** your conclusions. Use the blank diagnostic analysis charts provided at the end of this book (also available on thePoint website) to guide your thinking. Propose nursing diagnoses that are specific to the client in the case study. Identify collaborative problems, if any, for this client. Finally, identify data, if any, that point toward a medical problem requiring a referral.

Sara Smith is a 12-year-old girl who has mild cerebral palsy and a seizure disorder. Sara has difficulty with gross and fine motor movement and must wear leg braces. However, she is a very intelligent child, who makes up for her disability with her gift for creativity. Recently she has experienced an increase in seizure activity. Her physician has related this to the changes of puberty and has altered her medications. You are making a home visit to see how she is adjusting to her new medications.

    During your interview, you find that Sara has just moved to this town. She states that she hates her new house and her new school. She tells you that everyone teases her because of the way she speaks and moves and because of her braces. She also states that she has not told her mother about this because she does not want to upset her. Sara has no siblings. Her mother is a single parent, who works full time and who still expresses some guilt over Sara's "condition," which has existed from birth.

How Well Did You Do?

After you have read the chapter and completed the exercises in this chapter, visit thePoint to access the Self-Reflection Activity. This activity will help you identify to what degree you have met each of the chapter objectives. You can then review the chapter for objectives you have met partially or not at all.

    Other tools to help you, like the Diagnostic Reasoning Guides, Nursing Interview Guides, Physical Assessment Guides, and NCLEX-Style Chapter Review Questions, are also available on thePoint.

Copyright © 2014. Wolters Kluwer Health | Lippincott Williams & Wilkins. Lab Manual for Health Assessment in Nursing, 5e.

Assessing Older Adults

Chapter Overview

What distinguishes a frail elderly adult from an elderly adult is his or her delicate balance of health and independence, which can easily be compromised by an acute illness, accidents such as a fall, or adverse medication reactions.

Chapter Learning Objectives

1. Describe the common structural changes brought on by aging in the various body systems.
2. Recognize the unique presentation of disease and illness in the very old (often referred to as the geriatric syndromes).
3. Effectively interview the frail elderly client by modifying interview techniques used for the adult client.
4. Effectively examine the frail elderly client by modifying the physical examination techniques used for the adult client.
5. Describe assessment abnormalities in the frail elderly client that may be the result of adverse drug effects.
6. Explain how to incorporate assessment of functional status when collecting subjective and objective data on the frail elderly client to accurately evaluate findings.
7. Analyze the data from the client interview and physical assessment of an elderly client to formulate valid nursing diagnoses, collaborative problems, and/or referrals.

CHAPTER PRETEST

Activity A MULTIPLE CHOICE QUESTIONS

Choose the one best answer for each of the following multiple choice questions.

_____ 1. The physical declines of aging often first become noticeable when
   a. approximately 50% of function is lost.
   b. the person is at least 75 years old.
   c. acute or chronic illness places excessive demands on the body.
   d. cognitive declines become significant.

_____ 2. A benign skin lesion commonly seen in the aged is
   a. squamous cell carcinoma.
   b. shingles.
   c. actinic keratosis.
   d. lentigines.

____ **3.** Diminished vibratory sensations and slowed motor responses in advanced age result in

    a. stiffness and rigidity.

    b. paresthesia.

    c. postural instability.

    d. tremors.

____ **4.** A sign of infection in the elder that is more common than fever is

    a. pain.

    b. confusion.

    c. diarrhea.

    d. cough.

____ **5.** By age 90, renal blood flow has usually decreased by approximately

    a. 5%.

    b. 10%.

    c. 25%.

    d. 50%.

____ **6.** A neurologic change associated with normal aging is

    a. loss of long-term memory.

    b. a decrease in reaction time.

    c. swaying or shuffling gait.

    d. a significant decline in judgment and cognition.

Activity B MATCHING

Match the terms in the left column with the correct descriptions in the right column.

Term

____ **1.** Calcification, stiffening, and dilation of the aortic valve

____ **2.** Decreased ventricular compliance

____ **3.** Loss of elasticity in aorta and arteries

____ **4.** Decreased baroreceptor sensitivity

Description

a. Rise in systolic blood pressure

b. Soft systolic murmur at base of heart

c. S_4

d. Orthostatic hypotension

Activity C MATCHING

Match the sign or symptom with the corresponding eye disorder (only one response per question and some disorders may not be used).

Symptoms

____ **1.** Noticeable loss of vision and distortion of familiar objects and occasional floaters

____ **2.** Floaters associated with flashes of light

____ **3.** Blurriness of words in center of the page

____ **4.** Significant decrease in central vision

Disorders

a. Macular degeneration

b. Retinal detachment

c. Cataract

d. Diabetic retinopathy

e. Oral corticosteroid

f. Steroidal inhalant

Copyright © 2014. Wolters Kluwer Health | Lippincott Williams & Wilkins. Lab Manual for Health Assessment in Nursing, 5e.

Activity D MATCHING

Match adverse side effect with the medication that may cause it (possibly more than one answer per question; some responses may not be used at all).

Adverse Effects

____ **1.** Whitish or yellow-tinged patches in mouth

____ **2.** Orthostatic hypotension

____ **3.** Erectile dysfunction

____ **4.** GI bleeding

____ **5.** Constipation

Medications

a. Antidepressants

b. Anticoagulants

c. Anticholinergics

d. Antihypertensives

Activity E LEARNER ACTIVITIES

After reading Chapter 32 in the textbook, participate in the following learning activities.

1. Practice the timed Get Up and Go test on your lab partner (see Fig. 32-13 on page 818 in the textbook). Then do the test again with your lab partner, using crutches to walk. Do it one more time with your partner's arm in a sling. How do these disabilities affect gait stability and timing?

2. Identify and discuss with your lab partner two risk factors for each problem included in the acronym SPICES (see Box 32-1 on page 788 in the textbook).

3. Find a frail elder 80 years or older who is not completely independent in some aspect of everyday life. Assess the degree to which he or she is dependent in activities of daily living (ADLs) and instrumental activities of daily living (IADLs). Also address this person's physical and social environment for barriers and for resources related to independent function.

4. Visit a retail supplier of rehabilitative aids or home medical equipment. Locate items that assist persons with various degrees of immobility. Itemize at least ten of them from least to most expensive.

5. Visit an intensive care unit. Identify as many factors as you can in the physical environment or the nursing practices that may contribute to delirium in a frail elder.

6. Review the medication profile of five hospitalized elders greater than the age of 80. Identify all the medications they are taking that have anticholinergic side effects. Describe the assessment parameters that are indicated.

Activity F INTERVIEWING AND RECORDING ASSESSMENT FINDINGS

Working with peers in the learning lab after reading Chapter 32, use the following Functional Status Guide to interview and record your findings for an assessment of an elder client. Your instructor may ask you to turn this in to be evaluated. Forms are also available on thePoint *website.*

Function Status Checklist	
Function	**Findings**
Activities of Daily Living (ADLs)	
1. Bathing	
2. Dressing	
3. Toileting	
4. Transferring	
5. Continence	
6. Feeding	

Copyright © 2014. Wolters Kluwer Health | Lippincott Williams & Wilkins. Lab Manual for Health Assessment in Nursing, 5e.

Function Status Checklist (continued)

Instrumental Activities of Daily Living (IADLs)	
1. Ability to use the telephone	
2. Shopping	
3. Food preparation	
4. Housekeeping	
5. Laundry	
6. Transportation	
7. Medication management	
8. Ability to handle finances	
Geriatric Syndromes	
1. Skin impairment	
2. Poor nutrition	
3. Incontinence	
4. Cognitive impairment	
5. Evidence of falls or functional decline	
6. Sleep disturbances	
Special Tests Indicated by History or Physical Examination	
1. Assessment of swallowing	
2. Voice-whisper examination	
3. Get Up and Go test	
4. 24-hour food and fluid diary	
5. Mini-nutritional assessment	
6. Short Blessed Test for memory and concentration	
7. Geriatric depression scale	
8. Assessment of urinary continence	

CHAPTER POSTTEST

Activity G MULTIPLE CHOICE QUESTIONS

Choose the one best answer for each of the following multiple choice questions.

_____ **1.** A risk factor for sinusitis in the frail elderly is

  a. a nasogastric feeding tube.

  b. an accumulation of ear wax.

  c. decreased ability to detect odors.

  d. conductive hearing loss.

_____ **2.** Some symptoms are common in elderly clients. Which of the following is less likely to be a common problem in old age?

  a. Weakness.

  b. Confusion.

  c. Falls.

  d. Fever.

Copyright © 2014. Wolters Kluwer Health | Lippincott Williams & Wilkins. Lab Manual for Health Assessment in Nursing, 5e.

____ 3. Any new onset of incontinence in the frail elder should be investigated for
   a. prostatitis.
   b. stroke.
   c. fecal impaction.
   d. urinary tract infection.

____ 4. An objective assessment that is frequently indicated when the subjective assessment reveals a history of falling is
   a. a 24-hour food diary.
   b. a Get Up and Go test.
   c. a tonometry exam.
   d. palpation of the joints for crepitus.

____ 5. A gastrointestinal problem that often requires emergency treatment in the frail elder is
   a. lactose intolerance.
   b. hiatal hernia.
   c. diverticulitis.
   d. Crohn disease.

____ 6. To compensate for a stooped posture and less flexible knee, hip, and shoulder joints, the elderly person often walks
   a. with a waddling type of gait.
   b. with one leg slightly dragging behind the other.
   c. with the feet farther apart and the knees slightly bent.
   d. with a slight swaying side-to-side motion.

____ 7. A common sign or symptom of depression in the elderly is
   a. rambling or incoherent speech.
   b. illusion or hallucinations.
   c. insomnia.
   d. cognitive impairment or pseudodementia.

____ 8. A key area to assess in older adults with chronic respiratory or cardiac problems and some constant degree of dyspnea is
   a. nutritional deficiency.
   b. dysphagia.
   c. the degree to which dyspnea affects daily function.
   d. a possible history of immunosuppression.

____ 9. A characteristic sign of delirium is
   a. a significant decline in memory.
   b. a chronic low mood.
   c. a rapid decline in level of alertness.
   d. disorientation to self.

____ 10. Some symptoms of dehydration are common to younger and older adults. Which one of the following cannot be used to determine dehydration in older adults?
   a. A furrowed tongue.
   b. Tenting of the skin when pinched.
   c. Dry warm skin.
   d. Sunken eyes.

Copyright © 2014. Wolters Kluwer Health | Lippincott Williams & Wilkins. Lab Manual for Health Assessment in Nursing, 5e.

Activity H CRITICAL THINKING ACTIVITIES

1. Explain the various ways in which falls or a history of falls should be assessed in the frail elder.

2. Identify an acute pathologic condition that may manifest as a decline in functional ability. Explain how you might identify the condition.

3. Compare and contrast the steps of a musculoskeletal and neurologic examination of a young adult with those for an adult greater than the age of 85. Pay close attention to the significance of those steps that assess functional status.

4. An 88-year-old woman is brought to the ER by her daughter-in-law who states that her mother fell in the bathtub and she is worried that she may have broken a bone. Upon initial examination, you notice that this thin, frail, elderly woman has bruises on her back, buttocks, and upper chest. She follows your actions with her eyes but mainly groans or cries out, "Oh take it away...take it away."

   How would you adjust the interview to adapt to the needs of this elderly woman? What key features of the musculoskeletal and neurologic examinations need to be undertaken? What aspects of a functional and psychosocial assessment should you perform?

How Well Did You Do?

After you have read the chapter and completed the exercises in this chapter, visit thePoint to access the Self-Reflection Activity. This activity will help you identify to what degree you have met each of the chapter objectives. You can then review the chapter for objectives you have met partially or not at all.

Other tools to help you, like the Diagnostic Reasoning Guides, Nursing Interview Guides, Physical Assessment Guides, and NCLEX-Style Chapter Review Questions, are also available on thePoint.

Copyright © 2014. Wolters Kluwer Health | Lippincott Williams & Wilkins. Lab Manual for Health Assessment in Nursing, 5e.

Assessing Families

Chapter Overview

In assessing the family, many nurses focus on the individual as client and the family as context for the client's health and care. This requires assessing family strengths and problem areas as they affect the family support system. If the whole family is viewed as the client, then nursing assessment is directed toward the family unit as a dynamic system.

Chapter Learning Objectives

1. Define family.
2. List three essential components of a family assessment (structure, development, and function) and the major elements of each component.
3. Determine a family's life cycle stage and the related tasks.
4. Construct a genogram for a three-generational family.
5. Construct a family attachment diagram.
6. Construct a family ecomap.
7. Discuss theoretic concepts of family function, including systems theory, Bowen's family system theory, and communication theory.
8. Use Bowen's theory to determine the level of self-differentiation of a family and its members and to detect triangles within a family.
9. Describe the importance of communication to family function.
10. Discuss various nursing diagnoses and collaborative problems commonly seen with assessment of the family.
11. Analyze the data from the client interview and physical assessment of a family to formulate valid nursing diagnoses, collaborative problems, and/or referrals.

CHAPTER PRETEST

Activity A MULTIPLE CHOICE QUESTIONS

Choose the one best answer for each of the following multiple choice questions.

_____ 1. A broad definition of the family includes two or more persons who
  a. are related by blood.
  b. live in the same household.
  c. are married.
  d. have mutual decision making.

____ 2. The internal structure of a family includes
   a. the gender of the members.
   b. ethnic identity.
   c. religious practices.
   d. social class.

____ 3. An example of a subsystem of a family is
   a. father–renter.
   b. mother–chairperson.
   c. father–leader.
   d. mother–son.

____ 4. According to the theory by Minuchin, disengaged families have boundaries that are
   a. open.
   b. diffuse.
   c. permeable.
   d. rigid.

____ 5. In the most functional families, parents have power that
   a. rests with the father.
   b. rests with the mother.
   c. is shared by both parents.
   d. is shared by all of the family members.

Activity B MATCHING

Match the terms in the left column with the correct descriptions in the right column.

Term	Description
____ 1. Ecomap	a. Feedback system of reciprocal communication between people
____ 2. Self-differentiation	b. Similarity of illness or behaviors that run through the family from one generation to the next
____ 3. Circular communication	c. Diagram of the family's contact with larger systems
____ 4. Gender role	d. Behaviors expected of family members based on their sex and family beliefs about masculinity and femininity
____ 5. Multigenerational patterns	e. Young adult's shift toward separation from the family of origin

Activity C MATCHING

Match the terms in the left column with the correct descriptions in the right column.

Term	Description
____ 1. Genogram	a. Messages sent through body position, eye contact, touch, gestures, tone of voice, crying, stammering, etc.
____ 2. Nuclear family	b. The position of the children within a family based on age and gender
____ 3. Rank order	c. The range and types of feelings that are openly expressed or acceptable to be communicated within a family
____ 4. Emotional communication	d. A diagram of the family tree showing genetics, generational information, and relationships of family members
____ 5. Nonverbal communication	e. Usually considered to include father, mother, and children

Copyright © 2014. Wolters Kluwer Health | Lippincott Williams & Wilkins. Lab Manual for Health Assessment in Nursing, 5e.

Activity D **LEARNER ACTIVITIES**

After reading Chapter 33 in the textbook, participate in the following learning activities.

1. Have a group of lab partners and make lists of words that each associates with family. Discuss the patterns and definitions of family revealed by the words.

2. Make a genogram of your family over three or four generations. Add causes and dates of illness or death for each family member. Note any repeating patterns.

Activity E **INTERVIEWING AND RECORDING ASSESSMENT FINDINGS**

After reading Chapter 33, use the following Nursing Interview Guide to interview and record your subjective findings for a family assessment. Your instructor may ask you to turn this in to be evaluated. Forms are also available on thePoint *website.*

Nursing Interview Guide to Collect Subjective Data From the Client

Questions	Findings
Internal Family Structure	
1. Construct genogram of family composition.	
2. Family type and who is considered to be family?	
3. Recent movement in or out?	
4. Gender role?	
5. Rank order?	
6. Family subsystems?	
7. Family boundaries (permeable, rigid, or diffuse)?	
8. Family power structure?	
External Family Structure	
1. Construct an ecomap.	
2. Extended family?	
3. External systems?	
4. Context?	
Family Development	
1. Life cycle stages and tasks?	
Instrumental Function	
1. Ability to carry out activities of daily living?	
Affecting and Socialization Function	
1. Support and nurturance of family members?	
2. Parenting practices for socialization of children?	
3. Subgroups for triangles and boundaries (permeable, rigid, diffuse boundaries; level of self-differentiation of family members)?	
Expressive Function	
1. Construct a family attachment diagram.	
2. Emotional communication?	
3. Verbal communication?	

Nursing Interview Guide to Collect Subjective Data From the Client (continued)	
Questions	**Findings**
4. Nonverbal communication?	
5. Circular communication?	
Health Care Function	
1. Family's health care function (beliefs and practices)?	
Multigenerational Patterns	
1. Data for multigenerational patterns of positive and negative behaviors?	
Analysis of Data	
1. Formulate nursing diagnoses (wellness, risk, actual).	
2. Formulate collaborative problems (if present).	
3. Make necessary referrals.	

CHAPTER POSTTEST

Activity F **MULTIPLE CHOICE QUESTIONS**

Choose the one best answer for each of the following multiple choice questions.

_____ **1.** The nurse is preparing to draw a genogram of a client's family. The symbol for male members of the family is a
   a. triangle.
   b. circle.
   c. oval.
   d. square.

_____ **2.** One element of the context of a family's structure is
   a. ethnicity.
   b. extended family members.
   c. gender.
   d. power.

_____ **3.** The ability of a family to carry out activities of daily living is a family function termed
   a. employment.
   b. exchanging.
   c. differentiation.
   d. instrumental.

_____ **4.** According to Bowen's family theory, differentiation of self is assessed by
   a. determining the number of members in the family.
   b. looking at the communication patterns of the family.
   c. documenting the roles of each family member.
   d. determining the boundaries of the subsystems in the family structure.

_____ **5.** Families with poorly differentiated members will exhibit

    a. rigid patterns of interactions.

    b. difficulties in delaying gratification.

    c. difficulties in maintaining intimate personal relations.

    d. family roles that are based on skills and interests.

_____ **6.** Cybernetics, as applied to families, combines communication with

    a. Minuchin's theory.

    b. general systems theory.

    c. Friedman's theory.

    d. Bowen's theory.

_____ **7.** One example of a complementary birth order of spouses is

    a. youngest son marries youngest daughter.

    b. middle son marries middle daughter.

    c. oldest son marries youngest daughter.

    d. oldest son marries oldest daughter.

_____ **8.** In the assessment of the family's home environment, an important characteristic for the nurse to assess is the

    a. neighborhood's safety.

    b. school system.

    c. public transportation.

    d. availability of churches.

_____ **9.** While assessing a family, the nurse determines that the family's parental practices are based on control, coercion, and punishment. These parenting practices discourage

    a. self-fulfillment.

    b. self-differentiation.

    c. circular communication.

    d. socialization.

_____ **10.** The nurse visits a family at home after the 16-year-old only son was injured severely in an automobile accident. The client is in a wheelchair and requires 24-hour care. The client's mother is the sole caregiver, and she tells the nurse that she is saddened because "my son was such a wonderful basketball player." A priority family nursing diagnosis is

    a. depression related to youthful family member's health status.

    b. ineffective community coping related to mother being sole caregiver.

    c. immobility related to severe injuries from automobile accident.

    d. risk for dysfunctional grieving related to loss of health status of youthful family member.

Activity G   CASE STUDY

Read the following case study. Then, work through the steps of analyzing the case study data. First, identify the abnormal data and strengths in **subjective and objective findings**, assemble **cue clusters**, draw **inferences**, make possible **nursing diagnoses**, identify **defining characteristics**, **confirm or rule out** the diagnoses, and **document** your conclusions. Use the blank diagnostic analysis charts provided at the end of this book (also available on thePoint website) to guide your thinking. Propose nursing diagnoses that are specific to the client in the case study. Identify collaborative problems, if any, for this client. Finally, identify data, if any, that point toward a medical problem requiring a referral.

The Harrison family has come to the clinic for a renewal of prescriptions. Mary Harrison begins to talk to the nurse about the increasing stress that she is under because of her parents' illnesses. In the course of the conversation, the nurse asks whether Mary believes that she and the family need help with deciding how to handle the many problems associated with caring for her mother with Alzheimer disease and her father with congestive heart failure. The Harrison family decides to arrange a meeting with the nurse to discuss these problems.

Copyright © 2014. Wolters Kluwer Health | Lippincott Williams & Wilkins. Lab Manual for Health Assessment in Nursing, 5e.

The Harrison family is composed of a couple (Mary and Richard), Mary's mother and father (Nan and Ned), and two grown children (Maria and Stan), who live and work in other cities. Mary is a 52-year-old schoolteacher who has had to take a leave of absence to care for her mother, Nan. Nan is 78 years old and has advancing Alzheimer disease. Richard, 53 years old, works in construction and on occasion is out of work. Ned is 80 years old and has congestive heart failure, which makes it difficult for him to care for his wife. Nan and Ned moved in with Mary and Richard when Maria and Stan moved away 2 years ago. Financial pressures are increasing because of Mary's 3-month leave of absence and Richard's variable annual income. Nan and Ned have no income other than Ned's social security.

Mary describes herself as less and less able to keep up with the house, the meals, and her mother's personal care needs. Richard says that Mary is becoming very grouchy and unpleasant and that she rarely wants to have sex. Mary accuses Richard of not doing anything to help her around the house. Richard says that housework and caring for people is women's work. No one in the family wants to put Nan in a nursing home.

How Well Did You Do?

After you have read the chapter and completed the exercises in this chapter, visit thePoint to access the Self-Reflection Activity. This activity will help you identify to what degree you have met each of the chapter objectives. You can then review the chapter for objectives you have met partially or not at all.

Other tools to help you, like the Diagnostic Reasoning Guides, Nursing Interview Guides, Physical Assessment Guides, and NCLEX-Style Chapter Review Questions, are also available on thePoint.

Copyright © 2014. Wolters Kluwer Health | Lippincott Williams & Wilkins. Lab Manual for Health Assessment in Nursing, 5e.

Assessing Communities

Community may be defined and classified in various ways depending on one's perspective. A nursing assessment of a community, however, aims to determine the health-related concerns of its members, regardless of the type of the community.

Chapter Learning Objectives

1. Discuss how the history of a community may affect its current health status.
2. Describe the types of demographic information necessary to complete a community assessment and the sources of this information.
3. Discuss ways in which cultural and religious values affect health behaviors and attitudes.
4. Describe factors that make up the physical environment of the community.
5. Describe types of primary care facilities and providers that should be available in a community.
6. Discuss types of programs/services that public health/home agencies can provide.
7. Describe types of agencies needed to provide necessary services within a community.
8. Describe types of long-term care options that may be available in a community.
9. Discuss how economic factors can affect the health of a community.
10. Describe services and programs essential to provide for the safety needs of a community.
11. Discuss the forms of transportation that may be available in a community and how lack of adequate transportation may impact health.
12. Assess education-related factors in a community, and discuss the relationship between education and health.
13. Describe the relationship of government officials and leaders to the overall welfare of the community.
14. Identify formal and informal means of communication that may exist within a community.
15. Describe ways in which recreation affects the health of individuals in a community.
16. Complete a community assessment.
17. Analyze the data from the client interview and physical assessment of a community to formulate valid nursing diagnoses, collaborative problems, and/or referrals.

CHAPTER PRETEST

Activity A **MULTIPLE CHOICE QUESTIONS**

Choose the one best answer for each of the following multiple choice questions.

_____ 1. The number one cause of childhood mortality in the United States for children between the ages of 5 and 14 years is
  a. malignant neoplasms.
  b. congenital anomalies.
  c. motor vehicle accidents.
  d. burns.

_____ 2. The number one cause of mortality in the United States for people between the ages of 45 and 64 years is
  a. cerebrovascular diseases.
  b. diseases of the heart.
  c. accidents.
  d. malignant neoplasms.

_____ 3. The number one cause of mortality in the United States for people of 65 years and older is
  a. diseases of the heart.
  b. malignant neoplasms.
  c. cerebrovascular diseases.
  d. accidents.

_____ 4. Since 1970, the number of divorces in the United States has
  a. declined.
  b. doubled.
  c. tripled.
  d. quadrupled.

_____ 5. In the United States, single parents are at a greater risk for health problems, especially those related to
  a. finances.
  b. housing.
  c. role overload.
  d. basic needs.

_____ 6. In the United States, the growing number of homeless individuals and families is related to the community's
  a. disregard for these individuals.
  b. lack of resources for assistance.
  c. high unemployment rates.
  d. lack of affordable housing.

_____ 7. Many communities, especially those in rural areas, cannot provide needed health care services, particularly those related to
  a. cardiac care.
  b. orthopedic care.
  c. dental care.
  d. obstetric care.

____ **8.** The primary purpose of a community assessment is to

    a. determine the tax base.

    b. determine health-related concerns.

    c. obtain federal funding for new programs.

    d. collect census data.

____ **9.** In many rural areas of the United States, one major problem that makes many social service programs inaccessible is

    a. a lack of community awareness.

    b. reliance on federal support monies.

    c. a lack of transportation.

    d. a limited number of welfare programs.

____ **10.** One major concern associated with higher morbidity and mortality rates in a community is

    a. limited athletic programs in schools.

    b. the number of long-term care facilities.

    c. the religious beliefs of the population.

    d. poverty.

Activity B LEARNER ACTIVITIES

After reading Chapter 34 in the textbook, participate in the following learning activities.

1. With a group of lab partners, assess the health and social services of a selected part of your community. Include items one through five on the Community Assessment Guide below. Discuss your findings regarding whether the resources are adequate for that community.

2. With a group of lab partners, have each group member take a specific age group and list the forms of recreation that might be of interest to that age group and how they might contribute to health.

3. Go to an inner city health clinic or a rural health clinic. Interview clients about their means of transportation to health and social service agencies. Note the difficulties and identify the resources that would be needed to improve access to these agencies.

Activity C INTERVIEWING AND RECORDING ASSESSMENT FINDINGS

Complete the following Community Assessment Guide for a selected community. Choose a small community or a section of a larger community, for example, an institution such as a university, a suburb, or an inner city residential section. Analyze the data as indicated.

Community Assessment Guide

Questions	Findings
Community of People	
1. Assess history.	
2. Assess age/gender distribution of community members.	
3. Assess racial/ethnic groups.	
4. Assess vital statistics (birth and death records).	
5. Assess household size/marital status/mobility.	
6. Assess values/religious beliefs.	
7. Assess geographic boundaries.	
8. Assess neighborhoods.	
9. Assess housing.	
10. Assess climate and terrain.	

Community Assessment Guide (continued)

Questions	Findings
Health and Social Services	
1. Assess hospitals/clinics/emergency care/private practitioners.	
2. Assess public health and home services.	
3. Assess social service agencies.	
4. Assess long-term care.	
5. Assess economics.	
6. Assess safety.	
7. Assess transportation.	
8. Assess education.	
9. Assess government and politics.	
10. Assess communication.	
11. Assess recreation.	
Analysis of Data	
1. Formulate nursing diagnoses (wellness, risk, and actual).	
2. Formulate collaborative problems.	
3. Make necessary referrals.	

CHAPTER POSTTEST

Activity D MULTIPLE CHOICE QUESTIONS

Choose the one best answer for each of the following multiple choice questions.

_____ 1. From a sociologic perspective, a community is defined as a group, population, or cluster of people with
  a. common geographic boundaries.
  b. a time–space relationship.
  c. similar religious practices.
  d. at least one common characteristic.

_____ 2. The definition of a community as defined by the World Health Organization includes
  a. a community functioning within a particular social structure.
  b. an open social system that is characterized by people in a place.
  c. a cluster of people with similar political preferences.
  d. a group of people with at least one common characteristic.

_____ 3. One example of a boundary for a geopolitical community is a
  a. religious organization.
  b. special-interest group.
  c. subway system.
  d. river.

Copyright © 2014. Wolters Kluwer Health | Lippincott Williams & Wilkins. Lab Manual for Health Assessment in Nursing, 5e.

____ **4.** The "Community as Partner" model is based on the work by the nursing theorist
- **a.** Madeleine Leininger.
- **b.** Sister Callista Roy.
- **c.** Imogene King.
- **d.** Betty Neuman.

____ **5.** The nurse is assessing demographic information about a particular community. To assess the risk factors for health-related problems, the nurse should assess the community members'
- **a.** ethnicity.
- **b.** age.
- **c.** housing density.
- **d.** growth within the population.

____ **6.** A nurse is assessing a community of Native Americans. One important piece of health-related information that the nurse should obtain is the incidence of
- **a.** tuberculosis.
- **b.** congenital anomalies.
- **c.** pregnancy-induced hypertension.
- **d.** diabetes mellitus.

____ **7.** The number one cause of infant mortality in the United States is
- **a.** sudden infant death syndrome.
- **b.** low birth weight/prematurity.
- **c.** respiratory distress syndrome.
- **d.** congenital anomalies.

____ **8.** The number one cause of childhood mortality in the United States for children between the ages of 1 and 4 years is
- **a.** unintentional injuries.
- **b.** malignant neoplasms.
- **c.** homicide.
- **d.** congenital anomalies.

____ **9.** Occupational-related deaths and injuries in the United States are usually due to
- **a.** musculoskeletal injuries.
- **b.** burns.
- **c.** chemical injuries.
- **d.** poisonings.

____ **10.** In the assessment of a community, it is important for the nurse to assess the educational institutions. One indicator that there are problems in the high school system is the
- **a.** low absenteeism of the teachers.
- **b.** number of GED programs available.
- **c.** special education programs available.
- **d.** low graduation rate.

____ **11.** After assessing a local community, the nurse determines that there is a lack of community areas for exercise and socialization, particularly for the elderly members of the population. A priority nursing diagnosis for this community is
- **a.** potential for enhanced community coping.
- **b.** ineffective community coping related to lack of funding.
- **c.** ineffective management of therapeutic regimen related to elderly population.
- **d.** risk for social isolation related to a lack of recreational activities and facilities.

Copyright © 2014. Wolters Kluwer Health | Lippincott Williams & Wilkins. Lab Manual for Health Assessment in Nursing, 5e.

Activity E CASE STUDY

Read the following assessment information about a community. Then, work through the steps of analyzing the data. First, identify the abnormal data and strengths in **subjective and objective findings**, assemble **cue clusters**, draw **inferences**, make possible **nursing diagnoses**, identify **defining characteristics**, **confirm or rule out** the diagnoses, and **document** your conclusions. Use the blank diagnostic analysis charts provided at the end of this book (also available on thePoint website) to guide your thinking. Propose nursing diagnoses that are specific to the community in the case study. Identify collaborative problems, if any, for this community. Finally, identify data, if any, that point toward a community problem requiring a referral to an appropriate agency.

History

The area known as Evansboro was first settled by French explorers and established as a military outpost. Soon afterward, the area was settled by other French immigrants because of its rich farmland. It was a busy trading post in the 1800s because of its location on the St. Croix River.

Demographics

The total population of Evansboro, as of the 2000 census, was 9,156. Of the total residents, the female-to-male ratio is 1.1:1. There are 1,767 persons who are 65 years of age or older and 2,287 who are 18 years or younger. Racial distribution data reveal that 64.2% of the residents are African American, 34.5% are white, 0.8% are Native American, and 0.5% belong to other racial groups. Most of Evansboro's residents are married (71.6%), 23.1% are single, and the remainder are either separated, divorced, or widowed. The leading causes of death are cardiovascular disease and lung cancer. Several religious denominations are represented in Evansboro; those with the greatest percentage of members include Southern Baptist, African Methodist Episcopal, and United Methodist.

Physical Characteristics

Evansboro is bordered on the west by the St. Croix River and is otherwise surrounded by farmland. It lies within the flood plain of the river and as a result is periodically threatened by flooding. The last time that homes were affected by flood waters was 3 years ago. Evansboro is located in Washington County. State Highway 25 borders the eastern limits of the town and intersects with U.S. Highway 62 along the northern border of Evansboro. The average temperature during the month of January is 15.7 °C (60.3 °F); during the month of July it is 35.05 °C (95.1 °F).

Health and Social Services

Evansboro has a small 50-bed general hospital with a 5-bed special care unit, an emergency room, and limited surgical services. No obstetric services are available. The hospital also provides hospice and home health services. Additional home health services are provided to the area through Housecalls, Inc. Twelve physicians provide services in Evansboro; seven are family practice specialists and the others include an internist, two pediatricians, and two general surgeons. There are also four dentists and three optometrists. The main office of the Washington County Health Department is in Evansboro and offers several services, including Women, Infants, and Children (WIC), immunizations, surveillance for sexually transmitted diseases (STDs), screening for chronic diseases, and a smoking cessation program. The health department does not provide family planning services and does not currently employ an environmental sanitarian. There is a small community counseling center that employs three full-time counselors, one full-time psychologist, and one part-time psychiatrist. Evansboro is the county seat and offers limited social welfare programs through government agencies such as Family and Children's Services. There are two long-term care facilities (with 100 beds and 65 beds), and both provide skilled nursing care. The county provides ambulance/EMT service but does not have a 911 system in place. The community has a Meals on Wheels program for the homebound. Civic and fraternal organizations, such as the Lions Club and the Business and Professional Women's Club, provide many services as well.

Economics

The median household income for Evansboro is $28,586; the median individual income is $15,356. Of the total population of Evansboro, 5.6% fall below the federal poverty guidelines. The major occupations in Evansboro are manufacturing, farming, and business, including agribusiness. The major crops include peanuts and tobacco. The manufacturers include Johnson's Peanut Processing Plant, Jordan Tobacco, Inc., and Pinewood Paper Mill. None of these companies employs a health nurse. The unemployment rate is 6.9%, which is near the state average.

Safety and Transportation

Evansboro employs seven full-time and four part-time policemen. The most frequently reported crimes are domestic assault, traffic violations, and vandalism. The crime rate is slightly lower than that for the state. The police department provides the DARE program to the local middle school. The local fire department includes six full-time and six part-time employees and has recently purchased a new fire truck. There are also several volunteers trained by the fire department who offer their services when needed. The primary means of transportation is the private automobile. There is a taxi service in Evansboro, and the local senior citizens' center

Copyright © 2014. Wolters Kluwer Health | Lippincott Williams & Wilkins. Lab Manual for Health Assessment in Nursing, 5e.

provides transportation to seniors within the city. There is a small county airport about 24.1 km (15 miles) away, which provides commuter service to larger airports in the region.

Education

There are three elementary schools (grades K through 3), one middle school (grades 4 through 6), one junior high school (grades 7 and 8), and one senior high school (grades 9 through 12). Together the schools have an enrollment of approximately 1,900 students. One school nurse provides services for the three elementary schools, one nurse provides services between the middle school and the junior high school, and one school nurse is employed at the high school. The elementary and middle schools have an after-school program, and all schools have a school lunch program. The schools require physical education for all grades. The junior high offers programs in softball, baseball, basketball, and track. The high school also offers these same athletic programs as well as golf, wrestling, football, and volleyball. There is a variety of other extracurricular school-sponsored activities as well. The nurses employed at the high school and the junior high expressed some concern about what they believe is a growing problem with illicit drug and alcohol use among students. The high school offers GED classes, and the district's junior college, which is 48.2 km (30 miles) away, offers some night classes in Evansboro. There is a community library, which is open 6 days a week. School officials and others in Evansboro are concerned about the condition of the junior high, which was built 70 years ago; the building is in need of many repairs and cannot adequately accommodate the number of students enrolled. The school board is considering a school bond referendum, but is not optimistic because of the reluctance of voters to pass any tax increase.

Recreation

Evansboro has a city park with ball fields, tennis courts, soccer fields, picnic facilities, hiking trails, and a municipal pool. The park district provides several programs, including Red Cross swimming instruction, water aerobics for seniors, a swim team, Little League baseball and softball, soccer teams, and a tag football program for children aged 8 to 14 years. Evansboro has a movie theater, a bowling alley, a senior citizens' center, and several Boy Scout and Girl Scout troops. There are several other activities, such as the county fair and "Christmas in the Park," when businesses in town provide a light display in the city park. Other special-interest groups include a fishing club, a 4-H club, and a club for those interested in collecting. Church groups also offer a variety of recreational opportunities.

Politics and Government

Evansboro has an aldermanic type of local government. The city council is composed of eight elected members, two from each ward. The chair of the council is the mayor, who is also elected. There is a city attorney, a city treasurer, and a city clerk. The mayor is quite positive about the ability of the city council members to work together as well as about the response of the community to the city government. Both major political parties are represented in the city.

Communication

Evansboro has one local AM radio station, which primarily broadcasts local news and country music, and various other AM and FM stations broadcast in the area. There is a weekly newspaper, the *Evansboro Chronicle*. The city has cable television access, and internet services are provided through Apex Internet, Inc. Evansboro has a post office and telephone services.

How Well Did You Do?

After you have read the chapter and completed the exercises in this chapter, visit thePoint to access the Self-Reflection Activity. This activity will help you identify to what degree you have met each of the chapter objectives. You can then review the chapter for objectives you have met partially or not at all.

Other tools to help you, like the Diagnostic Reasoning Guides, Nursing Interview Guides, Physical Assessment Guides, and NCLEX-Style Chapter Review Questions, are also available on thePoint.

Copyright © 2014. Wolters Kluwer Health | Lippincott Williams & Wilkins. Lab Manual for Health Assessment in Nursing, 5e.

Answers

CHAPTER 1

CHAPTER PRETEST

Activity A MATCHING

1. f
2. i
3. a
4. b
10. e

6. g
7. c
8. j
9. h
10. d

CHAPTER POSTTEST

Activity C MULTIPLE CHOICE QUESTIONS

1. **a.** physiologic status.
2. **d.** formulation of nursing diagnoses.
3. **a.** continuous.
4. **d.** comprehensive.
5. **b.** focused or problem-oriented assessment.
6. **c.** review the client's health care record.
7. **c.** avoid premature judgments about the client.
8. **a.** arrive at conclusions about the client's health.
9. **d.** check for the presence of defining characteristics.
10. **b.** rapid advances in biomedical knowledge and technology.

CHAPTER 2

CHAPTER PRETEST

Activity A MULTIPLE CHOICE QUESTIONS

1. **a.** perception of pain.
2. **d.** using closed-ended questions.
3. **a.** indicate acceptance of the client's cultural differences.
4. **c.** knowledge of his or her own thoughts and feelings about these issues.
5. **a.** use very basic lay terminology.
6. **d.** encourage the client to quit smoking.
7. **a.** avoids excessive eye contact with the client.
8. **b.** provide the client with information as questions arise.
9. **a.** maintain eye contact while asking the questions from the form.
10. **a.** assess the client's hearing acuity.

CHAPTER POSTTEST

Activity D MULTIPLE CHOICE QUESTIONS

1. **b.** rephrasing the client's statements.
2. **c.** working.
3. **d.** explain the role and purpose of the nurse.
4. **a.** allow the client to ventilate his or her feelings.
5. **d.** expressing interest in a neutral manner.
6. **b.** provide structure and set limits with the client.
7. **d.** identify risk factors to the client and his or her significant others.
8. **b.** review the ChooseMyPlate information with the client.
9. **d.** "How do you manage your stress?"

CHAPTER 3

CHAPTER PRETEST

Activity A MATCHING

1. b
2. c
3. d
4. f
5. h
6. k

7. g
8. i
9. a
10. j
11. e

CHAPTER POSTTEST

Activity C MULTIPLE CHOICE QUESTIONS

1. **a.** wash both hands with soap and water.
2. **b.** explain each procedure being performed and the reason for the procedure.
3. **d.** use minimal position changes.
4. **d.** inspection.
5. **c.** dorsal surface of the hand.
6. **c.** deep palpation.
7. **d.** percussion.
8. **d.** blunt percussion.
9. **d.** blunt percussion.
10. **c.** indirect percussion.
11. **a.** hyperresonance.
12. **b.** bone.
13. **b.** 1½-inch diaphragm.

CHAPTER 4

CHAPTER PRETEST

Activity A MULTIPLE CHOICE QUESTIONS

1. **d.** draw a line through the error, writing "error" and initialing.
2. **b.** avoid slang terms or labels unless they are direct quotes.
3. **a.** "bilateral lung sounds clear."
4. **d.** vital signs.
5. **d.** pain relief measures.
6. **c.** requires a lot of time to complete.
7. **a.** prevents missed questions during data collection.
8. **b.** may be easily used by different levels of caregivers, which enhances communication.
9. **a.** establishes comparability of nursing data across clinical populations.
10. **d.** focused.
11. **a.** validate all data before documentation of the data.

CHAPTER POSTTEST

Activity C MATCHING

1. S		6. S	
2. O		7. O	
3. S		8. O	
4. O		9. S	
5. O		10. O	

CHAPTER 5

CHAPTER PRETEST

Activity A MATCHING

1. f		7. k	
2. e		8. c	
3. a		9. d	
4. b		10. g	
5. h		11. j	
6. i			

CHAPTER POSTTEST

Activity C MULTIPLE CHOICE QUESTIONS

1. **d.** validate information and judgments.
2. **d.** perform the steps of the assessment process accurately.
3. **a.** fatigue related to excessive noise levels as manifested by the client's statements of chronic fatigue.
4. **d.** quickly make a diagnosis without hypothesizing several diagnoses.
5. **a.** NANDA label (for problem) + related to + etiology + AMB (as manifested by) + defining characteristics.

6. **c.** Risk for Impaired Skin Integrity related to immobility secondary to right-sided paralysis, dehydration, and reluctance to participate in physical therapy as manifested by reddened coccyx and very dry skin.
7. **a.** Identify abnormal data and strengths, cluster data, draw inferences, propose possible nursing diagnoses, check for the presence of defining characteristics, confirm or rule out nursing diagnoses, document conclusions.
8. **b.** Risk for osteoporosis.

CHAPTER 6

CHAPTER PRETEST

Activity A MATCHING

1. e		6. c	
2. d		7. h	
3. f		8. i	
4. a		9. g	
5. b			

CHAPTER POSTTEST

Activity E MULTIPLE CHOICE QUESTIONS

1. **a.** Eye opening, and appropriateness of verbal and motor responses.
2. **c.** depression often mimics signs and symptoms of dementia.
3. **b.** Orientation, memory, speech, and cognitive function.
4. **b.** Orientation to time is usually lost first and orientation to person is usually lost last.
5. **d.** Abstract reasoning.
6. **c.** a referral to the primary health care provided for further evaluation.
7. **b.** answered "yes" to three of the four CAGE questions.
8. **a.** has a hazardous alcohol consumption.

CHAPTER 7

CHAPTER PRETEST

Activity A MATCHING

1. e		6. c	
2. h		7. i	
3. a		8. f	
4. j		9. d	
5. b		10. g	

Copyright © 2014. Wolters Kluwer Health | Lippincott Williams & Wilkins. Lab Manual for Health Assessment in Nursing, 5e.

CHAPTER POSTTEST

Activity E MULTIPLE CHOICE QUESTIONS

1. **c.** Generativity.
2. **b.** Developmental theory often reflects the culture/life experiences of the theorist.
3. **b.** A person is generally not aware of the underlying reasons for his behavior.
4. **c.** puberty allows sexual impulses to reappear.
5. **c.** The *id* is controlling this patient's behavior.
6. **c.** the person must accomplish a healthy balance between these opposing viewpoints in order to progress to the next psychosocial stage 30 to 50 mm Hg.
7. **d.** positively resolving a sense of generativity versus stagnation.
8. **d.** "You are feeling like you have had a wasted life...?"
9. **a.** Cognitive development occurs as the result of the person's organization and adaptation to the perceived environment; **e.** Piaget did not believe absolute ages should be ascribed to each of his stages of cognitive development.
10. **c.** Formal operational.
11. **c.** Transductive thinking can be used by formal operational thinkers.
12. **c.** moral development is determined, in part, by decisions that challenge the person.
13. **b.** desiring to avoid disapproval from others and be considered a respectful, helpful person.

CHAPTER 8

CHAPTER PRETEST

Activity A MULTIPLE CHOICE QUESTIONS

1. **a.** The client has just run 4.82 km (3 miles) outside before coming to the interview.
2. **d.** Rectum.
3. **a.** Rate, rhythm, amplitude and contour, and elasticity.
4. **d.** cardiac output, distensibility of the arteries, blood volume, blood velocity and viscosity.
5. **d.** kyphosis.

Activity B MATCHING

1. c
2. f
3. e
4. g
5. b
6. j
7. i
8. h
9. d
10. a
11. k

CHAPTER POSTTEST

Activity F MULTIPLE CHOICE QUESTIONS

1. **c.** vital signs.
2. **a.** normal changes that occur with the aging process.
3. **b.** observe for equal bilateral chest expansion of 2.54 to 5.08 cm (1 to 2 in).
4. **a.** shorter inspiratory phase.
5. **c.** "Are you having pain from your surgery?"
6. **b.** 30 to 50 mm Hg.
7. **c.** lacking adequate finances.
8. **a.** decreased body metabolism.
9. **a.** Oral temperature of 37.7 °C (100 °F).
10. **b.** record the vital signs.

CHAPTER 9

CHAPTER PRETEST

Activity A MULTIPLE CHOICE QUESTIONS

1. **c.** believe the client when he or she claims to be in pain.
2. **b.** acute pain is associated with a recent onset of illness or injury with a duration of less than 6 months, whereas chronic pain persists longer than 6 months.
3. **c.** diaphoresis.
4. **a.** documents the exact description given by the client.

CHAPTER POSTTEST

Activity F MULTIPLE CHOICE QUESTIONS

1. c
2. b
3. a
4. a
5. a
6. d

CHAPTER 10

CHAPTER PRETEST

Activity A MULTIPLE CHOICE QUESTIONS

1. **b.** remain calm and accepting in response to any information the client discloses.
2. **b.** make sure that the assessment includes questions to ensure that Mr. Jenkins has access to food and needed medication.
3. **c.** Period of reconciliation.
4. **b.** Wife abuse is an accepted behavior in some societies.
5. **c.** Irregular pattern of small, circular reddened areas with healing blisters on various parts of his body.
6. **b.** economic exploitation.

Copyright © 2014. Wolters Kluwer Health | Lippincott Williams & Wilkins. Lab Manual for Health Assessment in Nursing, 5e.

CHAPTER POSTTEST

Activity E MULTIPLE CHOICE QUESTIONS

1. **a.** Assure confidentiality of all information revealed.
2. **c.** Hand or finger-patterned bruising around upper arm and leg.
3. **d.** Intimate partner violence is caused by the "victim" refusing her husband's desire for sex.
4. **b.** An abuser may use psychological behaviors such as belittling, exploiting, denigrating, or remaining emotionally unresponsive.
5. **a.** Universal screening for family and intimate partner violence is recommended.

CHAPTER 11

CHAPTER PRETEST

Activity A MATCHING

1. b	**4.** a
2. c	**5.** d
3. e	

Activity B MULTIPLE CHOICE QUESTIONS

1. **d.** expecting all members of a cultural group to hold the same beliefs and behave in the same way.
2. **c.** The family values taking sick roles and caregiver roles.
3. **a.** Both genetics and environment produce biologic variation.
4. **b.** Sickle cell disease
5. **b.** a genetic variation associated with distance from the equator.

Activity C CHOOSING

a. Do
b. Don't
c. Don't
d. Do
e. Do
f. Do
g. Do

CHAPTER POSTTEST

Activity F MULTIPLE CHOICE QUESTIONS

1. **b.** nutritional information specifically for a Hispanic client.
2. **a.** may be specific to an ethnic group.
3. **d.** spend time with a variety of individuals of that ethnic group.
4. **d.** the client may be well acculturated to your dominant culture, so don't assume.
5. **d.** No culture is without an element of the magicoreligious beliefs.
6. **c.** Mediterranean.
7. **a.** Diseases associated with black Africans.
8. **d.** Muslims eat pork and do not fast for religious festivals.

CHAPTER 12

CHAPTER PRETEST

Activity A MULTIPLE CHOICE QUESTIONS

1. **a.** religion.
2. **b.** Spirituality.
3. **c.** attempting to convert clients to your own beliefs.
4. **d.** All of the above.

CHAPTER POSTTEST

Activity D MULTIPLE CHOICE QUESTIONS

1. **d.** reveal beliefs that might affect client care.
2. **b.** spiritual distress.
3. **c.** promote harmony between health and spirituality.
4. **a.** individualizing interventions to meet specific needs.
5. **b.** share the same religious beliefs as the client to provide effective spiritual care.

CHAPTER 13

CHAPTER PRETEST

Activity A MATCHING

1. e	**4.** b
2. d	**5.** c
3. a	

CHAPTER POSTTEST

Activity E MULTIPLE CHOICE QUESTIONS

1. **a.** heart attack.
2. **c.** Body mass index (BMI).
3. **b.** Females with 88.9 cm (35 in) or greater waist circumference.
4. **a.** Waist circumference.
5. **d.** who is a bodybuilder.
6. **b.** altered nutrition, more than body requirements related to intake greater than calories expended.
7. **c.** repeat the procedure three times and average the measurements.
8. **c.** Body mass index.
9. **b.** To provide percentage of body fat and muscle tissue.
10. **d.** A nutritional screening tool.

Copyright © 2014. Wolters Kluwer Health | Lippincott Williams & Wilkins. Lab Manual for Health Assessment in Nursing, 5e.

CHAPTER 14

CHAPTER PRETEST

Activity A MULTIPLE CHOICE QUESTIONS

1. **d.** subcutaneous tissue.
2. **d.** D.
3. **a.** innermost layer of the epidermis.
4. **b.** volume of blood circulating in the dermis.
5. **d.** dermis.
6. **a.** areola of the breast.
7. **a.** vellus.
8. **b.** filter for dust.
9. **c.** keratinized epidermal cells.
10. **a.** overall amount of sun exposure.

CHAPTER POSTTEST

Activity F MULTIPLE CHOICE QUESTIONS

1. **d.** domestic abuse.
2. **a.** symptoms of stress.
3. **d.** squamous cell carcinomas are most common on body sites with heavy sun exposure.
4. **c.** chronic discoid lupus erythematosus.
5. **a.** hypothyroidism.
6. **d.** malignant melanoma.
7. **d.** fluid intake.
8. **b.** oral mucosa.
9. **b.** ashen.
10. **a.** a great degree of cyanosis.
11. **d.** sclera.
12. **b.** caused by aging of the skin in older adults.
13. **a.** blue.
14. **b.** stage II.
15. **d.** use two fingers to pinch the skin under the clavicle.
16. **c.** a recent illness.
17. **a.** hypoxia.
18. **a.** macules.
19. **a.** plaque.
20. **c.** vesicles.
21. **d.** fissures.
22. **d.** keloid.
23. **d.** risk for ineffective health maintenance related to deficient knowledge of effects of sunlight on skin lesions.

Activity G MATCHING

1. d
2. j
3. b
4. c
5. h
6. i
7. g
8. f
9. a
10. e

CHAPTER 15

CHAPTER PRETEST

Activity A MATCHING

1. d
2. h
3. a
4. i
5. b
6. f
7. c
8. e
9. j
10. g

CHAPTER POSTTEST

Activity F MULTIPLE CHOICE QUESTIONS

1. **d.** reduction of the blood supply to the brain.
2. **a.** meningeal irritation.
3. **d.** trigeminal neuralgia.
4. **c.** migraine headache.
5. **a.** cluster headaches.
6. **d.** tension headaches.
7. **d.** tumor-related headache.
8. **b.** ask the client if touching the head is permissible.
9. **b.** acromegaly.
10. **d.** parotid gland enlargement.
11. **b.** swallow a small sip of water.
12. **c.** refer the client to a physician for further evaluation.
13. **b.** approach the client posteriorly.
14. **d.** sit in an upright position.
15. **c.** health-seeking behaviors related to verbalization of wanting to stay healthy and concerns over weight loss.

CHAPTER 16

CHAPTER PRETEST

Activity A MULTIPLE CHOICE QUESTIONS

1. **c.** protector.
2. **a.** meibomian glands.
3. **d.** bulbar portion.
4. **d.** rectus muscles.
5. **a.** choroid layer.
6. **c.** retina.
7. **a.** an oily substance to lubricate the eyes.
8. **d.** cleanse the cornea and the lens.
9. **a.** optic chiasma.
10. **b.** accommodation.

CHAPTER POSTTEST

Activity F MULTIPLE CHOICE QUESTIONS

1. **d.** corneal reflexes.
2. **d.** head trauma.
3. **c.** check the client's blood pressure.
4. **a.** tell the client that these often occur with aging.
5. **a.** glaucoma.
6. **b.** refer the client to an ophthalmologist.
7. **d.** vitamin A deficiency.
8. **b.** increased intracranial pressure.
9. **d.** allergies.
10. **d.** a foreign body in the eye.
11. **d.** lacrimal obstruction.
12. **b.** 2 years.
13. **d.** corneal damage.
14. **b.** ultraviolet light exposure.
15. **a.** position the client 609.6 cm (20 ft) away from the chart.
16. **d.** refer the client to an optometrist.
17. **d.** document the findings in the client's records.
18. **b.** decreased accommodation.
19. **a.** esotropia.
20. **c.** requires the covering of each eye separately.

CHAPTER 17

CHAPTER PRETEST

Activity A MULTIPLE CHOICE QUESTIONS

1. **c.** external ear.
2. **d.** stapes.
3. **a.** vestibule.
4. **a.** fluid.
5. **d.** perceptive hearing.

CHAPTER POSTTEST

Activity F MULTIPLE CHOICE QUESTIONS

1. **c.** taking antibiotics.
2. **c.** "It is difficult to prevent hearing loss or worsening of hearing."
3. **d.** observe the client's response to the explanations.
4. **d.** firmly pull the auricle out, up, and back.
5. **d.** refer the client to a physician.
6. **a.** infection.
7. **d.** strike a tuning fork and place it on the center of the client's head or forehead.
8. **c.** conductive hearing loss.
9. **b.** conductive hearing.
10. **a.** acute otitis media.

Activity G MATCHING

1. g	6. d
2. j	7. h
3. a	8. b
4. c	9. f
5. e	10. i

CHAPTER 18

CHAPTER PRETEST

Activity A MULTIPLE CHOICE QUESTIONS

1. **d.** soft palate.
2. **a.** uvula.
3. **b.** frenulum.
4. **c.** Wharton ducts.
5. **d.** warm the inspired air.

Activity B MATCHING

1. e	9. b
2. h	10. g
3. m	11. i
4. j	12. a
5. p	13. f
6. c	14. l
7. k	15. d
8. n	16. o

CHAPTER POSTTEST

Activity G MULTIPLE CHOICE QUESTIONS

1. **c.** maxillary sinuses.
2. **d.** aphthous stomatitis.
3. **a.** refer the client for further evaluation.
4. **d.** refer the client for further evaluation.
5. **a.** aspiration.
6. **d.** stress and anxiety.
7. **a.** Diets low in fruits and vegetables are a possible risk factor for oral cancer.
8. **d.** don clean gloves for the procedure.
9. **d.** riboflavin.
10. **a.** *Candida albicans* infection.
11. **b.** area underneath the tongue.
12. **a.** depress the tongue blade slightly off center.
13. **c.** touching each other.
14. **a.** position the handle of the otoscope to one side.
15. **d.** an upper respiratory infection.

CHAPTER 19

CHAPTER PRETEST

Activity A MULTIPLE CHOICE QUESTIONS

1. **d.** manubrium.
2. **a.** angle.
3. **c.** Seventh.
4. **b.** area slightly above the clavicle.
5. **a.** parietal pleura.
6. **d.** cilia.
7. **d.** hypercapnia.
8. **b.** pectus excavatum.
9. **a.** diabetic ketoacidosis.
10. **d.** Evaluate changes in respiratory pattern and rate.

Activity B MATCHING

1. d	**6.** i
2. g	**7.** c
3. j	**8.** f
4. h	**9.** a
5. b	**10.** e

CHAPTER POSTTEST

Activity G MULTIPLE CHOICE QUESTIONS

1. **d.** infection.
2. **d.** tuberculosis.
3. **d.** Studies have indicated that there is a genetic component in the development of lung cancer.
4. **d.** chronic obstructive pulmonary disease.
5. **d.** asking the client to exhale forcefully and hold his breath.
6. **c.** ask the client to breathe deeply through her mouth.
7. **a.** repeat the phrase "ninety-nine."
8. **a.** chronic bronchitis.
9. **a.** pneumonia.
10. **d.** bronchitis.

CHAPTER 20

CHAPTER PRETEST

Activity A MULTIPLE CHOICE QUESTIONS

1. **a.** progesterone.
2. **d.** areolas.
3. **b.** glandular.
4. **d.** Cooper ligaments.
5. **d.** fatty tissue.

Activity B MATCHING

1. i	**9.** e
2. f	**10.** n
3. l	**11.** a
4. h	**12.** j
5. d	**13.** g
6. m	**14.** c
7. k	**15.** o
8. b	

CHAPTER POSTTEST

Activity G MULTIPLE CHOICE QUESTIONS

1. **c.** upper outer quadrant.
2. **c.** fibrocystic breast disease.
3. **a.** having a baby before the age of 20 years.
4. **c.** physical stress.
5. **d.** breast cancer patients of the same race.
6. **d.** contraceptives.
7. **b.** depression.
8. **d.** grapefruit juice.
9. **d.** right after menstruation.
10. **a.** blocked lymphatic drainage.

11. **c.** refer the client for a cytology examination.
12. **b.** tumor.
13. **c.** an infectious process.
14. **d.** disturbed body image related to mastectomy.
15. **a.** lateral lymph nodes.

CHAPTER 21

CHAPTER PRETEST

Activity A MULTIPLE CHOICE QUESTIONS

1. **d.** precordium.
2. **a.** between the left atrium and the left ventricle.
3. **c.** at the exit of each ventricle at the beginning of the great vessels.
4. **d.** posterior wall of the right atrium.
5. **b.** conduction of the impulse throughout the atria.

Activity B MATCHING

1. e	**6.** g
2. i	**7.** c
3. f	**8.** b
4. a	**9.** d
5. j	**10.** h

CHAPTER POSTTEST

Activity G MULTIPLE CHOICE QUESTIONS

1. **c.** apex of the heart.
2. **d.** can be heard during diastole.
3. **b.** angina.
4. **a.** high serum level of low-density lipoproteins.
5. **d.** Estrogen replacement therapy in postmenopausal women decreases the risk of heart attack.
6. **a.** apical pulse.
7. **a.** ask the client to hold her breath.
8. **c.** associated with occlusive arterial disease.
9. **d.** increased central venous pressure.
10. **a.** cardiac murmur.
11. **b.** third to fifth intercostal space at the left sternal border.
12. **d.** refer the client to a physician.
13. **d.** recognize that this finding is normal in adolescents.
14. **c.** mitral valve stenosis.
15. **a.** obstructive lung disease.

CHAPTER 22

CHAPTER PRETEST

Activity A MULTIPLE CHOICE QUESTIONS

1. **d.** brachial artery.
2. **a.** knee.
3. **d.** ankle.
4. **c.** 70%.
5. **c.** competence of the saphenous vein valves.

Copyright © 2014. Wolters Kluwer Health | Lippincott Williams & Wilkins. Lab Manual for Health Assessment in Nursing, 5e.

Activity B MATCHING

1. h
2. d
3. j
4. l
5. f
6. k

7. b
8. i
9. c
10. e
11. a
12. g

CHAPTER POSTTEST

Activity G MULTIPLE CHOICE QUESTIONS

1. **d.** arterial insufficiency.
2. **a.** venous insufficiency.
3. **b.** intermittent claudication.
4. **d.** getting regular exercise.
5. **a.** apply K-Y jelly to the client's skin.
6. **a.** lymphedema.
7. **c.** brachial pulse.
8. **c.** flex his elbow about 90 degrees.
9. **d.** venous insufficiency.
10. **d.** malignancy.

CHAPTER 23

CHAPTER PRETEST

Activity A MULTIPLE CHOICE QUESTIONS

1. **c.** abdominal oblique.
2. **b.** left lower quadrant.
3. **d.** deep in the upper abdomen and is not normally palpable.
4. **a.** store and excrete bile.
5. **a.** right lower quadrant.

Activity B MATCHING

1. e
2. g
3. f
4. i
5. b

6. a
7. j
8. c
9. d
10. h

CHAPTER POSTTEST

Activity G MULTIPLE CHOICE QUESTIONS

1. **a.** right upper quadrant.
2. **d.** right lower quadrant.
3. **b.** left upper quadrant.
4. **d.** costovertebral angle.
5. **a.** stomach ulcers.
6. **c.** appetite changes.
7. **a.** "I can decrease the constipation if I eat foods high in fiber and drink water."
8. **c.** disturbed body image related to temporary colostomy.
9. **d.** inspect the abdominal area.
10. **a.** ask the client to empty his bladder.
11. **d.** internal bleeding.
12. **d.** masses.
13. **a.** umbilical hernia.

14. **d.** peritoneal irritation.
15. **b.** paralytic ileus.
16. **a.** intestinal obstruction.
17. **c.** use the diaphragm of the stethoscope.
18. **b.** place the right hand below the left costal margin.
19. **d.** palpate deeply while quickly releasing pressure.
20. **c.** raise the client's right leg from the hip.

CHAPTER 24

CHAPTER PRETEST

Activity A MULTIPLE CHOICE QUESTIONS

1. **c.** produce blood cells.
2. **a.** fat.
3. **d.** periosteum.
4. **a.** tendons.
5. **d.** fibrous.
6. **b.** ligaments.
7. **d.** abduction.
8. **a.** supination.
9. **b.** shoulder joint.
10. **d.** hip joint.

Activity B MATCHING

1. h
2. d
3. j
4. a
5. g

6. b
7. c
8. i
9. f
10. e

CHAPTER POSTTEST

Activity G MULTIPLE CHOICE QUESTIONS

1. **a.** arthritis.
2. **c.** osteomyelitis.
3. **a.** osteoporosis.
4. **c.** Moderate strenuous exercise tends to increase bone density.
5. **d.** vitamin C.
6. **a.** gouty arthritis.
7. **d.** vitamin D.
8. **d.** "You'll continue with range of motion even if I have discomfort."
9. **c.** average weakness.
10. **b.** TMJ dysfunction.
11. **a.** herniated disc.
12. **d.** scoliosis.
13. **d.** lie flat and raise his leg to the point of pain.
14. **a.** herniated intervertebral disc.
15. **a.** rotator cuff tear.
16. **c.** calcified tendinitis.
17. **d.** flex the knee and hip while in a supine position.
18. **a.** arthritis.
19. **d.** inability to extend the ring and little finger.
20. **a.** osteoarthritis.

Copyright © 2014. Wolters Kluwer Health | Lippincott Williams & Wilkins. Lab Manual for Health Assessment in Nursing, 5e.

CHAPTER 25

CHAPTER PRETEST

Activity A MULTIPLE CHOICE QUESTIONS

1. **d.** removes wastes.
2. **a.** corpus callosum.
3. **a.** gray matter.
4. **d.** thalamus and hypothalamus.
5. **a.** sleep cycles.

Activity B MATCHING

1. b
2. e
3. h
4. l
5. g
6. k
7. c
8. a
9. j
10. d
11. i
12. f

CHAPTER POSTTEST

Activity G MULTIPLE CHOICE QUESTIONS

1. **c.** spinothalamic tract.
2. **d.** glossopharyngeal.
3. **b.** stroke.
4. **b.** Smoking and high cholesterol levels are risk factors for STROKE.
5. **a.** sensation in the extremities.
6. **a.** clench his jaw.
7. **d.** some impairment.
8. **a.** depression.
9. **d.** cerebral cortex disorder.
10. **d.** "Can you repeat *brown, chair, textbook, tomato*?"
11. **a.** oculomotor nerve paralysis.
12. **a.** ask the client to purse the lips.
13. **d.** corticospinal tract.
14. **c.** stand erect with arms at the sides and feet together.
15. **b.** toes up or down.

CHAPTER 26

CHAPTER PRETEST

Activity A MULTIPLE CHOICE QUESTIONS

1. **a.** glans.
2. **d.** foreskin.
3. **b.** suspended by the spermatic cord.
4. **a.** just above and parallel to the inguinal ligament.
5. **b.** composed of skeletal muscle.
6. **c.** empty into the urethra.
7. **d.** intersphincteric groove.
8. **d.** hemorrhoids.
9. **a.** median sulcus.
10. **b.** secrete a milky substance that neutralizes female acidic secretions.

Activity B MATCHING

1. c
2. e
3. g
4. f
5. a
6. h
7. b
8. d
9. j
10. i

CHAPTER POSTTEST

Activity G MULTIPLE CHOICE QUESTIONS

1. **d.** prostate enlargement.
2. **c.** 3 years.
3. **a.** transient periods of erectile dysfunction are common.
4. **c.** inguinal hernia.
5. **d.** has anal intercourse with other males.
6. **d.** continue the examination in an unhurried manner.
7. **a.** ask the client to empty his bladder.
8. **b.** herpes infection.
9. **b.** syphilis.
10. **a.** urethritis.
11. **c.** cryptorchidism.
12. **c.** epididymitis.
13. **d.** varicocele.
14. **d.** bowel sounds at the bulge.
15. **a.** refer the client to an emergency room.

CHAPTER 27

CHAPTER PRETEST

Activity A MULTIPLE CHOICE QUESTIONS

1. **c.** sweat glands.
2. **d.** glans.
3. **a.** vestibule.
4. **a.** pink squamous epithelium and connective tissue.
5. **d.** estrogen.

Activity B MATCHING

1. g
2. e
3. k
4. f
5. c
6. h
7. l
8. b
9. j
10. d
11. a
12. i
13. o
14. m
15. n

CHAPTER POSTTEST

Activity G MULTIPLE CHOICE QUESTIONS

1. **b.** "Do you experience mood swings or bloating?"
2. **a.** hot flashes.
3. **d.** infection.
4. **b.** sexually transmitted disease.
5. **a.** decreased urethral elasticity.
6. **a.** refrain from douching 48 hours before the examination.
7. **c.** warm tap water.
8. **a.** bear down.
9. **d.** cystocele.
10. **a.** stress incontinence.
11. **a.** infection.
12. **a.** herpes simplex virus infection.
13. **d.** genital warts.
14. **a.** *Trichomonas vaginalis* infection.
15. **d.** ectopic pregnancy.
16. **d.** gastrointestinal bleeding.
17. **a.** biliary disease.
18. **d.** bear down.
19. **c.** a fungal infection.
20. **a.** polyps.

CHAPTER 28

CHAPTER PRETEST

Activity A MULTIPLE CHOICE QUESTIONS

1. **b.** a head-to-toe integrated assessment of body systems.
2. **c.** acquire your client's verbal permission to perform the physical examination.
3. **b.** eye exam and cranial nerves II, III, IV, and VI.
4. **a.** integrated throughout the head-to-toe examination.
5. **c.** assess peripheral vascular status when examining the lower extremities.

CHAPTER POSTTEST

Activity E MATCHING

1. b
2. c
3. e
4. i
5. f
6. h
7. d
8. a
9. g

CHAPTER 29

CHAPTER PRETEST

Activity A MULTIPLE CHOICE QUESTIONS

1. **d.** fade to a white or silvery color.
2. **a.** linea nigra.
3. **d.** progesterone.
4. **c.** is normal for some women in the second and third trimesters.
5. **a.** an increase in maternal blood volume by 40% to 50%.
6. **d.** diastasis recti abdominis.
7. **a.** "As a result of pregnancy, diarrhea may occur more often."
8. **c.** nutritional status.
9. **a.** estrogen.
10. **c.** at the level of the umbilicus.

CHAPTER POSTTEST

Activity E MULTIPLE CHOICE QUESTIONS

1. **d.** Supine.
2. **c.** 11.3 to 15.8 kg (25 to 35 lb).
3. **a.** hyperemesis gravidarum.
4. **a.** incompetent cervix.
5. **d.** Tay–Sachs disease.
6. **d.** abruptio placentae.
7. **d.** Rh status.
8. **d.** blood pressure.
9. **a.** upper quadrant of the maternal abdomen.
10. **a.** 10 weeks.
11. **d.** poor placental perfusion.
12. **b.** Breech.
13. **a.** gonorrhea.
14. **c.** pregnancy-induced hypertension.
15. **a.** instruct the client that a vaginal delivery is likely.

CHAPTER 30

CHAPTER PRETEST

Activity A MULTIPLE CHOICE QUESTIONS

1. **d.** 12 and 18 months.
2. **a.** is an obligatory nose breather.
3. **d.** abdominal/chest breathing movements at a rate of 30 to 60 breaths/minute.
4. **a.** a response to sudden stimulation or an abrupt change in position.

CHAPTER POSTTEST

Activity E MULTIPLE CHOICE QUESTIONS

1. **b.** 3 to 4 months.
2. **c.** 10.8 kg (24 lb).
3. **b.** 4 to 6 months old.
4. **d.** stork bite.
5. **a.** Epstein pearls.
6. **a.** down and back.

CHAPTER 31

CHAPTER PRETEST

Activity A MULTIPLE CHOICE QUESTIONS

1. **d.** smooth-textured skin.
2. **a.** A child's head reaches 90% of its full growth by 6 years of age.
3. **c.** fourth intercostal space.

Activity B MATCHING

1. a	**9.** a
2. c	**10.** b
3. a	**11.** d
4. d	**12.** d
5. d	**13.** b
6. c	**14.** c
7. c	**15.** c
8. a	

CHAPTER POSTTEST

Activity F MULTIPLE CHOICE QUESTIONS

1. **b.** three.
2. **c.** 14 years.
3. **d.** talk to the child in simple terms at the child's eye level.
4. **a.** play.
5. **a.** tell the child it is okay to cry in the clinic.
6. **d.** allow the child to engage in the discussions.
7. **a.** give the client control whenever possible.
8. **b.** 6 years.
9. **d.** 30 months after the onset of puberty.
10. **a.** hop on one foot.
11. **d.** make simple classifications.
12. **a.** she can begin bowel training as soon as the child appears ready.
13. **d.** iron.
14. **a.** measles.
15. **b.** shine a light directly into the pupils.

CHAPTER 32

CHAPTER PRETEST

Activity A MULTIPLE CHOICE QUESTIONS

1. **c.** acute or chronic illness places excessive demands on the body.
2. **d.** lentigines.
3. **c.** postural instability.
4. **b.** confusion.
5. **d.** 50%.
6. **b.** a decrease in reaction time.

Activity B MATCHING

1. b	**3.** a
2. c	**4.** d

Activity C MATCHING

1. d	**3.** a
2. b	**4.** c

Activity D MATCHING

1. a, b	**4.** d
2. c, e, f	**5.** c, e
3. c, f	

CHAPTER POSTTEST

Activity G MULTIPLE CHOICE QUESTIONS

1. **a.** a nasogastric feeding tube.
2. **d.** Fever.
3. **d.** urinary tract infection.
4. **b.** a Get Up and Go test.
5. **c.** diverticulitis.
6. **c.** with the feet farther apart and the knees slightly bent.
7. **d.** cognitive impairment or pseudodementia.
8. **c.** the degree to which dyspnea affects daily function.
9. **c.** a rapid decline in level of alertness.
10. **b.** Tenting of the skin when pinched.

CHAPTER 33

CHAPTER PRETEST

Activity A MULTIPLE CHOICE QUESTIONS

1. **d.** have mutual decision making.
2. **a.** the gender of the members.
3. **d.** mother–son.
4. **d.** rigid.
5. **c.** is shared by both parents.

Activity B MATCHING

1. c	**4.** d
2. e	**5.** b
3. a	

Activity C MATCHING

1. d	**4.** c
2. e	**5.** a
3. b	

CHAPTER POSTTEST

Activity F MULTIPLE CHOICE QUESTIONS

1. **d.** square.
2. **a.** ethnicity.
3. **d.** instrumental.
4. **d.** determining the boundaries of the subsystems in the family structure.
5. **a.** rigid patterns of interactions.
6. **b.** general systems theory.
7. **c.** oldest son marries youngest daughter.
8. **a.** neighborhood's safety.
9. **d.** socialization.
10. **d.** risk for dysfunctional grieving related to loss of health status of youthful family member.

Copyright © 2014. Wolters Kluwer Health | Lippincott Williams & Wilkins. Lab Manual for Health Assessment in Nursing, 5e.

CHAPTER 34

CHAPTER PRETEST

Activity A MULTIPLE CHOICE QUESTIONS

1. **c.** motor vehicle accidents.
2. **d.** malignant neoplasms.
3. **a.** diseases of the heart.
4. **d.** quadrupled.
5. **c.** role overload.
6. **d.** lack of affordable housing.
7. **d.** obstetric care.
8. **b.** determine health-related concerns.
9. **c.** a lack of transportation.
10. **d.** poverty.

CHAPTER POSTTEST

Activity D MULTIPLE CHOICE QUESTIONS

1. **d.** at least one common characteristic.
2. **a.** a community functioning within a particular social structure.
3. **d.** river.
4. **d.** Betty Neuman.
5. **b.** age.
6. **d.** diabetes mellitus.
7. **d.** congenital anomalies.
8. **a.** unintentional injuries.
9. **a.** musculoskeletal injuries.
10. **d.** low graduation rate.
11. **d.** risk for social isolation related to a lack of recreational activities and facilities.

Copyright © 2014. Wolters Kluwer Health | Lippincott Williams & Wilkins. Lab Manual for Health Assessment in Nursing, 5e.

Diagnostic Reasoning Guides

The following pages are included for use with the case studies in this book. They are designed to help guide your thinking and assist you in arriving at appropriate conclusions. Use them to work through the steps of data analysis. You may also want to refer to the concept maps in your textbook algorithms on thePoint for examples of how these will look after you fill them out. In addition, you will find a Diagnostic Reasoning Guide form on thePoint that you can download and print if you would like to have additional copies of the form.

1) Identify abnormal findings and client strengths

Subjective Data

Objective Data

2) Identify cue clusters

3) Draw Inferences

4) List possible nursing diagnoses

5) Check for defining characteristics

6) Confirm or rule out diagnoses

7) Document conclusions

Nursing diagnoses that are appropriate for this client include: Potential collaborative problems include the following:

Copyright © 2014. Wolters Kluwer Health | Lippincott Williams & Wilkins. Lab Manual for Health Assessment in Nursing, 5e.

1) Identify abnormal findings and client strengths

Subjective Data

Objective Data

2) Identify cue clusters

3) Draw Inferences

4) List possible nursing diagnoses

5) Check for defining characteristics

6) Confirm or rule out diagnoses

7) Document conclusions

Nursing diagnoses that are appropriate for this client include:

Potential collaborative problems include the following:

Copyright © 2014. Wolters Kluwer Health | Lippincott Williams & Wilkins. Lab Manual for Health Assessment in Nursing, 5e.

1) Identify abnormal findings and client strengths

Subjective Data

Objective Data

2) Identify cue clusters

3) Draw Inferences

4) List possible nursing diagnoses

5) Check for defining characteristics

6) Confirm or rule out diagnoses

7) Document conclusions

Nursing diagnoses that are appropriate for this client include:

Potential collaborative problems include the following:

Copyright © 2014. Wolters Kluwer Health | Lippincott Williams & Wilkins. Lab Manual for Health Assessment in Nursing, 5e.

1) Identify abnormal findings and client strengths

Subjective Data

Objective Data

2) Identify cue clusters

3) Draw Inferences

4) List possible nursing diagnoses

5) Check for defining characteristics

6) Confirm or rule out diagnoses

7) Document conclusions

Nursing diagnoses that are appropriate for this client include:

Potential collaborative problems include the following:

Copyright © 2014. Wolters Kluwer Health | Lippincott Williams & Wilkins. Lab Manual for Health Assessment in Nursing, 5e.

1) Identify abnormal findings and client strengths

Subjective Data   Objective Data

2) Identify cue clusters

3) Draw Inferences

4) List possible nursing diagnoses

5) Check for defining characteristics

6) Confirm or rule out diagnoses

7) Document conclusions

Nursing diagnoses that are appropriate for this client include: **Potential collaborative problems include the following:**

Copyright © 2014. Wolters Kluwer Health | Lippincott Williams & Wilkins. Lab Manual for Health Assessment in Nursing, 5e.

1) Identify abnormal findings and client strengths

Subjective Data

Objective Data

2) Identify cue clusters

3) Draw Inferences

4) List possible nursing diagnoses

5) Check for defining characteristics

6) Confirm or rule out diagnoses

7) Document conclusions

Nursing diagnoses that are appropriate for this client include:

Potential collaborative problems include the following:

Copyright © 2014. Wolters Kluwer Health | Lippincott Williams & Wilkins. Lab Manual for Health Assessment in Nursing, 5e.

1) Identify abnormal findings and client strengths

Subjective Data

Objective Data

2) Identify cue clusters

3) Draw Inferences

4) List possible nursing diagnoses

5) Check for defining characteristics

6) Confirm or rule out diagnoses

7) Document conclusions

Nursing diagnoses that are appropriate for this client include: Potential collaborative problems include the following:

Copyright © 2014. Wolters Kluwer Health | Lippincott Williams & Wilkins. Lab Manual for Health Assessment in Nursing, 5e.

1) Identify abnormal findings and client strengths

Subjective Data

Objective Data

2) Identify cue clusters

3) Draw Inferences

4) List possible nursing diagnoses

5) Check for defining characteristics

6) Confirm or rule out diagnoses

7) Document conclusions

Nursing diagnoses that are appropriate for this client include:

Potential collaborative problems include the following:

Copyright © 2014. Wolters Kluwer Health | Lippincott Williams & Wilkins. Lab Manual for Health Assessment in Nursing, 5e.

1) Identify abnormal findings and client strengths

Subjective Data

Objective Data

2) Identify cue clusters

3) Draw Inferences

4) List possible nursing diagnoses

5) Check for defining characteristics

6) Confirm or rule out diagnoses

7) Document conclusions

Nursing diagnoses that are appropriate for this client include:

Potential collaborative problems include the following:

Copyright © 2014. Wolters Kluwer Health | Lippincott Williams & Wilkins. Lab Manual for Health Assessment in Nursing, 5e.

1) Identify abnormal findings and client strengths

Subjective Data

Objective Data

2) Identify cue clusters

3) Draw Inferences

4) List possible nursing diagnoses

5) Check for defining characteristics

6) Confirm or rule out diagnoses

7) Document conclusions

Nursing diagnoses that are appropriate for this client include:

Potential collaborative problems include the following:

Copyright © 2014. Wolters Kluwer Health | Lippincott Williams & Wilkins. Lab Manual for Health Assessment in Nursing, 5e.

I) Identify abnormal findings and client strengths

Subjective Data   Objective Data

2) Identify cue clusters

3) Draw Inferences

4) List possible nursing diagnoses

5) Check for defining characteristics

6) Confirm or rule out diagnoses

7) Document conclusions

Nursing diagnoses that are appropriate for this client include: **Potential collaborative problems include the following:**

Copyright © 2014. Wolters Kluwer Health | Lippincott Williams & Wilkins. Lab Manual for Health Assessment in Nursing, 5e.

DRC0913